MANAGEMENT OF LABOR
Second Edition

Edited by

Wayne R. Cohen, MD
Associate Professor of Obstetrics and Gynecology
Albert Einstein College of Medicine
Director of Obstetrics and Gynecology
Bronx Municipal Hospital Center
Bronx, New York

David B. Acker, MD
Assistant Professor of Obstetrics and Gynecology
Harvard Medical School
Associate Chief of Obstetrics and Gynecology
Beth Israel Hospital
Boston, Massachusetts

Emanuel A. Friedman, MD, Med ScD
Professor of Obstetrics, Gynecology, and Reproductive Biology
Harvard Medical School
Professor of Health Science and Technology
Massachusetts Institute of Technology
Obstetrician-Gynecologist-in-Chief
Beth Israel Hospital
Boston, Massachusetts

AN ASPEN PUBLICATION®
Aspen Publishers, Inc.
Rockville, Maryland
Royal Tunbridge Wells
1989

Library of Congress Cataloging-in-Publication Data

Management of labor/edited by Wayne R. Cohen, David B. Acker,
Emanuel A. Friedman.--2nd. ed.
p. cm.
"An Aspen publication."
Bibliography: p.
Includes index.
ISBN: 0-87189-791-1
I. Labor (Obstetrics) I. Cohen, Wayne R. II. Acker, David B. III. Friedman, Emanuel A.
RG651.M3   1988   618.4--dc19
88-16783
CIP

The authors have made every effort to ensure the accuracy of the information herein.
However, appropriate information sources should be consulted, especially for new or
unfamiliar procedures. It is the responsibility of every practitioner to evaluate the
appropriateness of a particular opinion in the context of actual clinical situations and with
due consideration to new developments. Authors, editors, and the publisher cannot be
held responsible for any typographical or other errors found in this book.

Editorial Services: Ruth Bloom

Library of Congress Catalog Card Number: 88-16783
ISBN: 0-87189-791-1

Printed in the United States of America

1 2 3 4 5

To our most important teachers:
The women in whose labors we have
been privileged to participate

Table of Contents

Contributors

David B. Acker, MD
Assistant Professor of Obstetrics and
  Gynecology
Harvard Medical School
Associate Chief of Obstetrics and
  Gynecology
Beth Israel Hospital
Boston, Massachusetts

Max Borten, MD, JD
Associate Professor of Obstetrics and
  Gynecology
Harvard Medical School
Director of Medical Gynecology
Beth Israel Hospital
Boston, Massachusetts

Wayne R. Cohen, MD
Associate Professor of Obstetrics and
  Gynecology
Albert Einstein College of Medicine
Director, Obstetrics & Gynecology
Bronx Municipal Hospital Center
Bronx, New York

Michael F. Epstein, MD
Associate Professor of Medicine
Harvard Medical School
Chief, Division of Newborn Medicine
Children's Hospital Medical Center
Boston, Massachusetts

Scott Fisher, MD
Director of Anesthesiology
St. Margaret's Hospital
Boston, Massachusetts

Alan R. Fleischman, MD
Professor of Pediatrics
Director, Division of Neonatology
Albert Einstein College of Medicine
Bronx, New York

**Emanuel A. Friedman, MD,
  Med ScD**
Professor of Obstetrics, Gynecology, and
  Reproductive Biology
Harvard Medical School
Professor of Health Science and
  Technology
Massachusetts Institute of Technology
Obstetrician-Gynecologist-in-Chief
Beth Israel Hospital
Boston, Massachusetts

Ellen Harrison, MD
Assistant Professor of Medicine and
  Obstetrics and Gynecology
Albert Einstein College of Medicine
Associate Director of Medicine and
  Director, Medical Intensive Care Unit
North Central Bronx Hospital
Bronx, New York

Cassandra E. Henderson, MD
Assistant Professor of Obstetrics and
  Gynecology
Albert Einstein College of Medicine
Perinatologist
Bronx Municipal Hospital Center
Bronx, New York

Benjamin T. Jackson, MD
Professor of Surgery
Program in Medicine
Brown University
Chief, Surgical Service
Providence Veterans Administration
  Medical Center
Providence, Rhode Island

Eric D. Lichter, MD
Instructor of Obstetrics and Gynecology
Harvard Medical School
Director of Emergency Gynecology
Beth Israel Hospital
Boston, Massachusetts

Gertie F. Marx, MD
Professor of Anesthesia
Albert Einstein College of Medicine
Director of Obstetric Anesthesia
Bronx Municipal Hospital Center
Bronx, New York

**Maureen Guarino McRae, RN,
  MS**
Head Nurse, Labor and Delivery Unit
Beth Israel Hospital
Boston, Massachusetts

Frances V. Mervyn, PhD
Clinical Psychologist
Wellesley Hills, Massachusetts

Gerard W. Ostheimer, MD
Associate Professor of Anesthesia
Harvard Medical School
Director of Obstetric Anesthesia
Brigham and Women's Hospital
Boston, Massachusetts

Nigel Paneth, MD
Associate Professor of Public Health
  (Epidemiology) and Pediatrics
Columbia University
New York, New York
Research Scientist, Epidemiology of
  Developmental Brain Disorders,
  Research Department
New York State Department of Mental
  Hygiene
New York, New York

George J. Piasecki, MS
Associate in Research
Program in Medicine
Brown University
Providence, Rhode Island

Nancy K. Rhoden, JD
Professor of Law
University of North Carolina School of
  Law
Chapel Hill, North Carolina

Benjamin P. Sachs, MD, MPH
Assistant Professor of Obstetrics and
  Gynecology
Harvard Medical School
Director, Maternal-Fetal Medicine
Beth Israel Hospital
Boston, Massachusetts

Barry S. Schifrin, MD
Director, Maternal-Fetal Medicine
Tarzana Medical Center
Tarzana, California

Steven S. Schwalbe, MD
Clinical Assistant Professor of
  Anesthesiology
State University of New York Health
  Science Center
Brooklyn, New York

Jeffrey A. Shane, MD, JD
Attorney
Shulman, Rogers, Gandal, Pordy and
  Ecker
Rockville, Maryland

Raymond Stark, MD
Associate Professor of Pediatrics
Columbia University
New York, New York

Robert C. Vannucci, MD
Associate Professor of Pediatrics
Chief, Division of Pediatric Neurology
Milton S. Hershey Medical Center
Hershey, Pennsylvania

Thomas M. Warren, MD
Associate Professor of Anesthesia
Indiana University School of Medicine
Indianapolis, Indiana

Preface to the First Edition

The physician's ability to control or to intervene appropriately in the progress of labor has evolved in parallel with advances in our comprehension of the physiology of parturition and the widespread application of high-technology instrumentation and techniques. Recent improvements in the United States' perinatal mortality rate, which have reflected these changes, are the consequence of a panoply of innovations in obstetric and pediatric practice. Important among these advances have been improved means for objective evaluation of labor, early diagnosis and rational management of disordered labor, a trend away from potentially traumatic operative delivery, a refined ability to diagnose and manage fetal and neonatal hypoxemia, and new attitudes toward drug therapy and modes of anesthesia during labor and delivery.

These new clinical concepts have developed rapidly for helping obstetric attendants make critical decisions about obstetric intervention. There is, however, an ever-present risk that the information will be misused, and that intervention will be excessive or inappropriate. Thus, the clinician has the rather formidable responsibility of learning about modern trends in obstetric thought, interpreting them with sagacity and the perspective of experience, and deciding how (or indeed whether) to integrate them into practice.

This book is designed for the obstetric practitioner, whether generalist, specialist, or midwife. It reviews many of our current concepts regarding the management of labor. Our focus and direction derive from material that we have presented for several years in a popular postgraduate course at Harvard Medical School. We have not attempted to provide a text that exhaustively reviews all aspects of labor. We have chosen instead to focus on areas of special clinical interest and practical importance: the use of objective criteria for measuring the progress of cervical dilatation and fetal descent, and the use of bioelectronic techniques for the evaluation of intrapartum fetal oxygenation. In addition, we have dealt with some common specific problems to provide a summary of contemporary views and to illustrate more general means of interpreting and synthesizing available data to establish management programs.

Contemporary issues relating to the potential conflict between burgeoning technology and mounting pressures for more family oriented and emotionally fulfilling birth experiences are confronted, with the view toward reconciling both attitudes. Certainly the notion of delivering the highest quality of available medical and technical care and of providing a psychologically rewarding family experience are not mutually exclusive ideologies.

Finally, we have dealt with issues of communication. This is necessary because the consequences of medical judgments are influenced by the patient's comprehension of her problem and by the confidence and trust she places in her medical care providers. In fact, perceptions by the general public of obstetric care rest on a foundation of the quality of interactions between individual patients and doctors.

Although the wisdom of individual experience will result in some modifications of obstetric care, the practitioner cannot reasonably expect to accumulate enough data to appreciate the sundry subtle effects of obstetric procedures. Thus, the clinician must learn to interpret the collective experience of the specialty through the intermedium of relevant publications. We feel strongly that changes in clinical practice should be based only on substantive conclusions from well-designed research, and we have tried to present information with that perspective in mind. Thus, for example, one cannot have a clear comprehension of our suggested approach to fetal distress without first understanding the nature of the fetal adaptive cardiovascular responses to hypoxemia and the morphologic and epidemiologic evidence for the adverse consequences of fetal asphyxia. Similarly, the ability to resuscitate a depressed newborn infant successfully depends not only on technical facility, but also on a thorough understanding of the pathophysiology of neonatal asphyxia.

For obstetrics, a new era has dawned. Previously a specialty that depended largely on clinical experience and dexterity, obstetrics has become a complex discipline that requires its practitioners to be knowledgeable in several rapidly expanding areas of medical science, to be adroit and skillful surgeons, and to provide personalized and compassionate care. To meet such demands requires intense dedication.

The privilege of assisting women with the delivery of babies provides great joys and gratification; but it also implies enormous responsibilities. We have tried to provide information that the clinician will find useful in meeting the challenge of those responsibilities. Mother and fetus can thereby be provided with the best we can now offer in attainable safety, and be treated with the sensitivity and dignity that the process of childbirth demands.

Wayne R. Cohen
Emanuel A. Friedman

Preface to the Second Edition

The enthusiastic response to the first edition was gratifying, and the opportunity to prepare a second was met with an admixture of pride and eagerness. Despite some trepidation regarding the daunting task of assembling a multiauthor text, we welcomed the chance to add relevant material, to make amends for inaccuracies, and to clarify some of the concepts expressed in the first edition.

The basic format of the book is unchanged. Its major mission remains the presentation of our collective ideas concerning certain aspects of the clinical management of human labor and birth. We have emphasized the importance of fundamental aspects of obstetric medicine (thorough physical examination, graphic labor assessment, fetal monitoring), and have summarized contemporary approaches to several important obstetric problems encountered commonly during parturition. We have tried where possible to present a thorough analysis of available information pertaining to the range of options available for labor management. The conclusions about obstetric practice, some of which we acknowledge to be parochial, have been applied in our own institutions with gratifying improvements in perinatal outcome. Therefore, we feel justified in sharing our particular orientation to care with the reader.

During the past decade, interest has focused increasingly on the relation between events that occur during parturition and infant outcome. This emphasis has resulted from the confluence of several developments: the evolution of advanced imaging techniques to evaluate the neonatal brain; recent epidemiologic studies that addressed the etiology of perinatal injury; and a sense of urgency engendered by a crescendo of medical negligence lawsuits, the outcome of which often hinges on understanding the contribution of perinatal events to permanent neurologic handicap. Because of the importance of these issues to obstetric practice, we have dwelt at length upon them in chapters reviewing current knowledge about neurologic injury that can result from perinatal asphyxia and trauma. Although the clinician might feel some of this material is excessively detailed and of limited applicability, we hope this book will serve as a resource for those who require a timely summary of knowledge in this area. Much of this information is not available elsewhere in the obstetric literature.

Although most complications encountered in the labor and delivery suite can be managed readily, the rarity of some events may find even the competent obstetrician unprepared. This has become especially so as medical care has required use of increasingly complex and sophisticated technology. We have therefore included chapters intended to serve as a resource for the obstetric attendant to review principles of cardiopulmonary resuscitation and of the use of critical care techniques in obstetric patients. This should benefit both the generalist and perinatologist.

As the requirement for complex technical knowledge burgeons in obstetrics, new related issues reach the forefront. Ethical quandaries challenge the obstetrician almost daily, as does the shadow of possible litigation. We have confronted some of these complexities of contemporary practice as well, in a manner that we hope will be thought provoking.

The assistance of many individuals in the production of this text should be acknowledged. A debt of gratitude is owed to the contributors, who superimposed the labor of writing onto already sated schedules, and to their secretaries, who typed the original chapter drafts. Special approbation is due Ms. Linda Thompson-Biggs, who worked deftly and uncomplainingly on many drafts of the manuscript, all the while coping with the physiologic adventure of her own pregnancy. Finally, we are very grateful to Ms. Anne S. Patterson and to Ms. Ruth Bloom of Aspen Publishers for their patience, professionalism, and good advice. We hope that the aggregate of efforts has resulted in a volume that will find a useful niche in the obstetric literature, and that will contribute to the gentle and competent care of women in labor.

Wayne R. Cohen
David B. Acker
Emanuel A. Friedman

1

Normal and Dysfunctional Labor

Emanuel A. Friedman

Normal labor is traditionally defined as the physiologic process by which the gravid uterus evacuates its contents at or near term by a mechanism involving a coordinated sequence of periodic contractions of the myometrium effecting progressive cervical dilatation and fetal descent through the birth canal. Teleologic implications aside (to the effect that the uterus is willfully implementing its own purposeful objective), this definition does indeed describe the goal, conditions, methods, and results that are expected of normal parturition. Since it is all in qualitative terms, however, it cannot serve the pragmatic needs of the obstetric attendant who is called upon to recognize when the course of a given labor is becoming or has become abnormal. Thus, more specific and objective characteristics of the component events that make up this process are needed.

At the outset, it is important to appreciate that there is as yet no known laboratory test or physiologic measuring device capable of differentiating normal labor from abnormal or even true labor from false. This is so despite the large body of knowledge derived from the scientific study of how the human uterus functions in both the pregnant and nonpregnant states. In the absence of such a test or tool, clinical assessment of labor must be based on observation of those features of the phenomenon that are identifiable and quantifiable at the bedside. These include intensity, duration, and frequency of contractions; dilatation and effacement of the cervix; and descent of the fetus. Each of these six parameters can be readily studied by periodic examinations in the course of any given labor with reproducible accuracy. They serve as the primary clinical characteristics for evaluating labors in progress, providing the only really usable data for determining if a given patient may be developing a labor disorder.

1

UTERINE CONTRACTILITY

Measuring and recording devices, such as external (abdominal wall) tokodynamometer or internal (intrauterine) catheter with strain gauge attached, are widely available for purposes of registering the contractility pattern. They provide much more information on the wave configuration of the intermittent myometrial contractions over time than palpation, even by well-trained and dedicated personnel. Nonetheless, interpretation of that information is elusive insofar as it offers means for determining normalcy of the labor progress it is assessing. A number of interesting adaptations have been explored to correct this deficiency. As long ago as 1929, the practice of counting the number of contractions necessary to accomplish delivery was developed and reported by Frey.[14] This was a decidedly better conceptual approach than use of total duration of labor as a measure of abnormality then in wide use (and regrettably still used as a criterion by some). He determined that most nulliparas delivered with fewer than 300 contractions after membranes ruptured (200 for multiparas). In the 1940s, Calkins[7,8] affirmed this and further determined that the expectations of a given labor could be predicted on the basis of the number and intensity of contractions as modified by the consistency and effacement of the cervix and the station of the fetal presenting part. The less favorable the cervix and the station, the more contractions needed to achieve birth. However, Calkins showed a wide range for normal labor, reducing the value of these observations for diagnostic purposes.

With the introduction of objective pressure measurement techniques at midcentury, greater objectivity was attained. The classic observations of Caldeyro-Barcia and his colleagues[6] showed the intrinsic value of simple summation of the peak amplitude of all contractions occurring during a specific time unit, conventionally chosen as 10 min, to yield a uterine work unit called the Montevideo unit. Their foundational work demonstrated the feasibility of obtaining such information in clinically utilitarian form, although its applicability to resolving clinical problems of diagnosis and management of labor disorders proved disappointingly limited.[36,49] As to false labor, although there have been no comparable published reports of measurements of uterine activity, Schauberger[48] found essentially the same wide range of clinical patterns based on bedside recordings for both women in false labor and matched case controls, except for a somewhat diminished average frequency of contractions.

Several potentially important modifications of uterine pressure assessment have been forthcoming in recent years to help correct this apparent shortcoming. Principal among them was assessment of the shape of the contraction waveform by Seitchik and co-workers [51,52] and summary integration of the area under the curve as an index of the total force generated by contractions by Huey et al.[30] and Miller et al.,[38] among others. It was found, for example, that the uterus appeared to become more efficient as labor progressed so that the amount of uterine activity required to dilate the cervix 1 cm early in labor was two to three times that required to achieve the same change late in the first stage.[31] Thus, the rate of dilatation accelerated faster than could be accounted for by the increase in uterine activity alone.[38] This suggested that there were inherent changes occurring in the cervix as labor advanced and that the cervix was just not passively responding to the contractions by dilating in a constant manner. To support this, total uterine activity to achieve late labor dilatation[47] or vaginal delivery,[1] based on the summation of contractile energy, was shown to reflect cervical resistance. Moreover, patients with poor contractile activity levels were required to compensate for the reduced forces by experiencing longer labors to effect delivery.

The sophistication afforded by these indices of contractility has also proved useful for monitoring the impact and guiding the administration of oxytocin for use in induction or augmentation of labor. Steer and co-workers[55] determined that progress in dilatation could not be realized without a certain minimum uterine activity (nearly 440 kPas [kilopascal units]/15 min on average above the basal uterine tonus) and that a critical incremental level above this (to 700 kPas/15 min) was needed to produce a minimally acceptable dilatation rate of 1 cm/hr. The amount of oxytocin needed to accomplish this was relatively small, but more important, the rate of dilatation resulting from oxytocin enhancement of the uterine activity could not be predicted by the level of or the degree of increase in uterine activity.[56] This confirmed the work of Seitchik and Castillo,[50] who showed that it was not possible to identify the level of contractility necessary to promote cervical dilatation in cases with dysfunctional labor. They also verified that such patients do not require more uterine activity to progress to delivery than gravidas in otherwise normal labor.

These observations illustrate that while uterine contractions are an obvious *sine qua non* of labor, there are as yet neither qualitative nor quantitative characteristics of myometrial activity to help distinguish normal from abnormal labor. This limitation applies especially to the ability to evaluate an ongoing labor while it is in progress so as to detect abnormalities as they arise. In addition, investigations have shown that uterine contractility is not directly related to the effect it is expected to achieve, namely, timely cervical dilatation and fetal descent. This dissociation between the forces generated by the myometrium and its work output is well recognized by all who care for obstetric patients. Experience in bedside observations illustrates examples of gravidas with negligible contractions (characterized as infrequent, of short duration, and weak) whose cervix dilates and fetus descends rapidly and, about just as often, others with intensive contractions (frequent, long, and strong) whose labor progress is desultory. While one can generally expect faster progress with better contractions as a rough rule, this relationship is clearly neither universal nor sufficiently reliable to serve as a clinical index for flagging potentially aberrant labors. For clinical purposes, therefore, other means must be sought to identify disorders of labor progress.

CERVICAL DILATATION

In simplistic terms, the essential components of the phenomenon of labor are dilatation of the cervix and fetal descent. Cervical effacement, the only remaining clinical parameter available for determining labor progress, has proved to be almost of no value. Effacement is usually complete or nearly complete in nulliparas well before labor begins; and in multiparas, nearly all effacement takes place in the last few minutes of the first stage. Some degree of progressive effacement is known to occur during the weeks prior to onset of labor,[29] but the nonprogressive nature of effacement in labor makes it unacceptable as a marker for normal labor progress. Dilatation and descent, by contrast, serve this function well. Dilatation removes the barrier that acts so effectively in the course of pregnancy to prevent spontaneous uterine evacuation (except in the case of cervical incompetence). Once the cervical barrier is breached, fetal descent can follow in an unimpeded manner and lead to the birth of the baby. The mechanical forces producing dilatation are entirely uterine in origin, whereas those effecting descent are a combination of myometrial contractions plus voluntary expulsive efforts by diaphragmatic and abdominal muscles. Uterine forces can be measured continuously and accurately, as discussed above, but to somewhat better advantage for bedside application is assessment of the end results of these forces as they accomplish the dilatation and descent processes.

This evaluation can be facilitated by relating the changes that occur against the time elapsed from the onset of labor. When plotted against time on a simple square-ruled grid, cervical dilatation will always trace an S-shaped or sigmoid curve in normal labors (Fig. 1-1). For purposes of nomenclatural standardization, certain terms have been applied to the several components of the pattern thus formed.[17] As will be seen, the labor segments to which these terms refer are distinctive in regard to the physiologic events taking place, the kinds of factors affecting them, and the disorders that can arise within them.

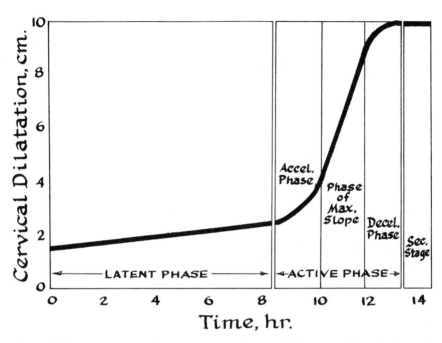

Figure 1-1 Typical pattern of the progression of cervical dilatation in labor for the nulliparous gravida, showing division of the first stage into latent and active phases and further subdivision of the active phase into its distinctive components.

The initial arm or latent phase extends from the onset of regular uterine contractions to the beginning of the active phase characteristically marked by a detectable upswing of the curve. The pattern is seldom symmetrical in that the latent phase usually occupies most of the first stage, leaving only a relatively minor time period for the active phase. Nevertheless, most of the dilatation that will have to occur takes place during the active phase, which can be further subdivided into an initial acceleration phase, a midportion phase of maximum slope, and a terminal deceleration phase. While onset of labor can be defined by most patients on the basis of their subjective appreciation of the discomfort associated with uterine contractions which are occurring with recognizable regularity, it must be accepted that there is nothing truly different, that is, objectively distinguishable, about the events taking place before or afterward. This applies to both the uterine activity as assessed by any currently available means and the condition of the maternal soft tissues. Hendricks et al.[29] correctly pointed out that orderly progressive changes could be documented over the course of the last 4 weeks of pregnancy, preceding the onset of perceived labor. These changes, including some degree of cervical dilatation, continue into the latent phase. Thus, labor begins with the cervix already dilated on average to about 2 cm.

There is, of course, a wide range of dilatation achieved before the onset of labor, some patients beginning labor with a closed, poorly prepared cervix and others with advanced dilatation. It has been shown that the latent phase is inversely correlated with the degree of dilatation at the time labor begins[21,42]; specifically, the greater the dilatation, the shorter the latent phase. This means that one of the principal functions (again speaking teleologically) of the latent phase is to provide the final preparation needed by the cervix before it can begin active phase dilatation. Another important function is the orchestration of the many independent myometrial cellular units into a coordinated muscular structure that is capable of developing strong, effective, polarized contractions to achieve both the dilatation and the descent required of it.

Little is known about the acceleration phase because it is infrequently appreciated, except by hindsight. The transition from latent phase to active phase is not signaled by any special recognizably objective change in the contractility pattern or by alteration in the patient's subjective perception of her status. To identify it requires periodic assessment of cervical dilatation and graphic portrayal to show the changed rate of dilatational progress from that of the latent phase, which is usually very slow or nonexistent, to that of the phase of maximum slope when dilatation is advancing at its most rapid speed. Attempts have been made to identify the onset of the active phase on the basis of the degree of cervical dilatation reached in labor. Peisner and Rosen,[43] for example, showed that women enter the active phase on average at 4.6 cm (calculated from their data), with a range extending up to more than 9 cm. Just half the patients they studied (49.9%) had reached or exceeded 4 cm by this time. Excluding patients who subsequently developed dysfunctional labor patterns (see below), they determined that nearly 90% (88.6%) were in the active phase by the time the cervix was 5 cm dilated. Thus, while it is logical to consider that a parturient whose cervix is 5 cm dilated is probably in the active phase, there is a high proportion of error inherent in the assumption unless the active phase is confirmed by demonstrating the increase in the rate of dilatation expected of the active phase. It is appropriate, therefore, to accept the assertion by Peisner and Rosen[43] that the labor of the patient who is not rapidly dilating her cervix after 5 cm dilatation is probably abnormal and their recommendation that it deserves evaluation, but it is equally appropriate to caution against assuming that an abnormality actually exists in all such cases.

The midportion of the active phase is that part of the labor during which cervical dilatation is proceeding at its most rapid rate, justifying the designation of phase of maximum slope. The graphic tracing of dilatation against time is essentially a straight line under normal circumstances. The inclination of the line reflects the efficiency of the uterine contractions in effecting the dilatation; in other words, it represents an index of the balance between the energy input and the work output. The stronger the contractile forces and the less resistive (more pliant) the soft tissues, the more rapid the dilatation will be. Whereas myometrial contractility alone cannot be used reliably to assess labor progress (see above), its impact on dilatation as shown during this linear component of active labor can.

The linearity of the dilatation process has been challenged. Hendricks et al.,[29] for example, felt that dilatation constantly accelerated during the active phase, that is, its rate kept increasing as dilatation advanced. Their findings confirmed those of Zimmer[60] who in 1951 produced hyperbolic curves of dilatation timed from when the membranes ruptured. Since these curvilinear patterns were produced from digital estimates of dilatation, their accuracy is open to question (just as the straight-line curves can be questioned). Patterns generated by physiologic instruments capable of measuring dilatation somewhat more accurately and continually, however, have verified the linearity of active dilatation.[16,27,34,54] Regardless of whether this is correct or not, active dilatation appears to be close enough to true linearity to be considered acceptable for practical clinical purposes. This acceptance has been the basis upon which all existing graphic systems for following the course of labor have been devised and which has made them useful for clinical application.[2,9,13,15,17,28,32,37,40,41,44,45,53,57–59]

The deceleration phase that concludes the active phase and the first stage of labor is admittedly an artifact. Neither the contractile forces nor the patient's subjective reaction to them is decreasing (if anything, they tend to be enhanced at about this time), yet the rate of dilatation seems to be slowing. This apparently results from the cervix being retracted in a cephalad direction (relative to the mother) around and alongside the fetal head. As it nears full dilatation, the cervix is no longer being dilated in a coronal fashion so that the former rapid rate of dilatation of the phase of maximum slope decelerates even though the cervix is still being retracted at about the same speed as before by the contracting, shortening myometrium of the upper uterine segment (by the process of brachystasis). This portion of the labor pattern is ordinarily quite short in normal labors and easily missed if examinations are not done in timely fashion. Perhaps because of this transiency, some deny the very existence of the deceleration phase[29] and others find it unduly complicating and insufficiently worthy of consideration for clinical practice.[44,45] Since it can be a useful marker for aberrant labor (see below), this omission is unfortunate.

FETAL DESCENT

Just as the relation of cervical dilatation to time can be used as a means for assessing the course of labor, so can the function of fetal descent with time serve a similar purpose. The descent pattern and its close association with the dilatation curve are well established[23,24] and thus far unchallenged. Some descent precedes labor. Engagement of the fetal presenting part deeply into the pelvis several weeks before term (so-called lightening) is a well recognized event in most nulliparas. Even in multiparas, a degree of descent may occur, but it is much less dramatic. It may advance slowly over the span of the month before labor begins.[29] Once labor starts, little if any further descent will be detectable, except perhaps for a small amount in association with rupture of the membranes and loss of forewaters, permitting the presenting part to become more closely adapted to the lower uterine segment and cervix.

This static condition of the descent process will generally prevail during the entire course of the latent phase of the dilatation pattern. Not until the dilatation accelerates into the active phase will descent become active, typically reaching its maximum slope at about the time the dilatation curve enters the deceleration phase. From this point on, the descent pattern tends to be linear as the fetal presenting part accommodates itself to the pelvic architecture (by the classic cardinal movements of flexion and internal rotation) and advances downward at a constant rate through the birth canal until the leading edge abuts the perineum. This straight-line descent normally progresses without interruption or deviation throughout the deceleration phase and most of the second stage (except for the perineal component during which caudad descent slows as the fetal head undergoes extension over the perineum to effect delivery).

For consistency and uniformity in graphing the descent pattern, use of a centimeter scale is strongly recommended for designating fetal station. Measure and record the distance (in centimeters) of the lowermost advancing edge of the fetal presenting part cephalad (negative values) or caudad (positive values) relative to the plane of the ischial spines (designated zero station) as determined by careful assessment by vaginal examination. The fetus thus transverses the normally formed pelvis from about −5 station at the true inlet to +5 station at the outlet (bulging perineum). Such station designations based on vaginal evaluations of the fetus are intended as substitutes for estimates of the level of the biparietal diameter within the maternal pelvis; the station of the biparietal diameter is much more important for determining true descent, but it is just inaccessible to the examining hand. The problem with use of the forward leading edge assessment is the error introduced by caput formation and especially by deformational molding. This shortcoming can be overcome somewhat by periodically verifying that any descent being detected is actually occurring by means of suprapubic palpation of the base of the fetal skull.[11,44] The external examining hand should be able to ensure that the fetal head is becoming progressively more deeply engaged as the forward leading edge advances (if not, one should suspect that the lower station reflects molding rather than real descent).

ABNORMAL LABOR

Pictorial representation of the dilatation and descent patterns, as described, serves as the basis for defining normal labor in quantitative terms derived from objective, timed observations of cervical dilatation and fetal station. These observations require no special equipment; they can be entered on the coordinates of a graph with minimal skill; and interpretation of the tracings that evolve can be learned quickly and disseminated easily. Brief experience with graphing labors in progress will confirm the evolution of the normal patterns and verify the constant interrelationship between the dilatation and the descent phenomena. Recognition of abnormal patterns (Figures 1-2 and 1-3) requires acquisition of some basic information about the nature of the patterns in the gravid population at large. Distinctive differences are recognized to exist in the labor process among nulliparas as contrasted with multiparas, the latter typically advancing at a more rapid rate. It is clear, therefore, that different criteria should apply according to parity. While most of the studies that have examined this issue confirm the parity differential, some insist that the course of labor is about the same for nulliparas as for multiparas,[29,42] while others feel that whatever difference does exist is not important enough to take into account.[40,44,57] Some patient attributes, such as race, do not appear to affect the labor pattern,[12,18] but age does, although only to a limited extent.[10,25] When the different component phases of the cervical dilatation and fetal descent patterns are measured in large numbers of cases, they can be characterized quantitatively on the basis of the distribution around the mean value for each.[17] Analysis of such bell-shaped (normal or gaussian) distribution curves of data for populations of gravidas, stratified by parity, yields useful information that can be translated into clinically applicable signals

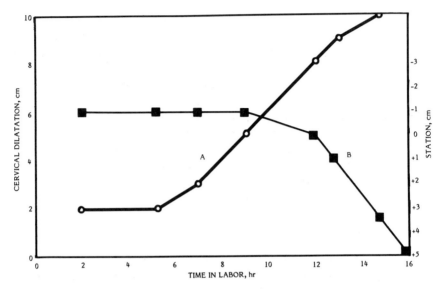

Figure 1-2 Protraction disorders. Protracted active phase dilatation pattern (**A**) is characterized by its abnormally low maximum slope of dilation, while protracted descent (**B**) is recognized by a comparably low rate of descent.

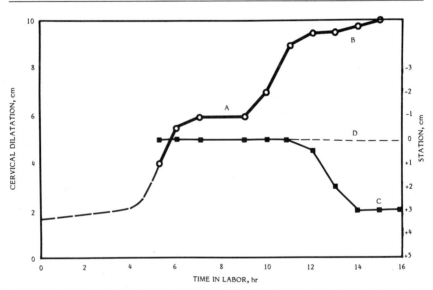

Figure 1-3 Arrest disorders. Secondary arrest of dilation; (**A**), prolonged deceleration phase (**B**), and arrest of descent (**C**) occurred in sequence in this case. Failure of descent (**D**) would have been present if descent had not begun and proceeded actively from the beginning of the deceleration phase of dilation.

for identifying abnormalities. Based on convention, the 5% of the population that falls into the "tails" of the distribution can be deemed sufficiently deviant to be considered likely to be abnormal. Thus, ascertaining the measurement levels (or cut-points) at which these individuals can be identified establishes the criteria for diagnosis. While these cut-points are admittedly arbitrary, they do logically define a subset of cases that warrant clinical attention. Although designated as abnormal by this means, these cases do not necessarily require active intervention for delivery, but rather astute evaluation and targeted management (see below).

Conceptually, the principle applied here is exactly the same as that invoked whenever any new laboratory test is introduced for study of a given phenomenon in an institution or laboratory. The latent phase in nulliparas, for example, averages 6.4 hr in duration with a central tendency described by a standard deviation of 5.1 hr. Since the distribution is somewhat skewed, one cannot satisfactorily use the usual statistical technique for gaussian distributions (namely 2 standard deviations from the mean) to define the 5th and 95th percentiles. It is necessary instead to determine them from the actual distribution curves. When this is done, one finds that the duration of most latent phases in nulliparas is less than 20 hr. Comparable analysis of multiparous labor shows the latent phase cut-point to be 14 hr. These values define normality in practical terms.[19] They have recently been independently confirmed by Peisner and Rosen.[42]

Patients with latent phase durations exceeding these limits can be considered abnormal; they are affected by a disordered labor pattern descriptively termed *prolonged latent phase*. As will be seen, it is quite common and generally innocuous if managed circumspectly. Yet failure to appreciate its true character and significance (especially its distinctive difference from other more serious abnormalities) in the past has given rise to the mistaken impression that it represented a labor aberration requiring operative intervention. Thus, those commonly used labor evaluations that ignore the latent phase[29,40,44,57] risk overlooking this problem to the potential disadvantage and detriment of the patients being followed.

In a similar manner, limits of normal can be derived for the rate of progression of cervical dilatation and fetal descent. Studies have shown that most nulliparas have a maximum slope of dilatation in the active phase of more than 1.2 cm/hr (1.5 cm/hr for multiparas) and a maximum slope of descent toward the end of the first stage and continuing through the second stage of 1.0 cm/hr (2.0 cm/hr in multiparas). Gravidas falling below these defined cut-points can be deemed to be abnormal with protracted dilatation or protracted descent. The disorder is quite different

in its potential impact on mother and fetus (see Chapter 15) than prolonged latent phase, clearly warranting differentiation. While there is no
dispute concerning the fact that the rate of dilatation accelerates abruptly
in active labor, there is some disagreement as to choice of cut-point for
defining the limit of normal. As aforementioned, parity differences have
been denied.[29,42] Abnormality has been ascribed to dilatation rates as low
as 0.4 cm/hr.[55] and 0.6 cm/hr[12], but most round off the clinically relevant
value to 1.0 cm/hr.[2,13,28,29,37,39–41,43,53] In practical terms, recent investigation examining the fetal impact of the range of active phase dilatation
rates has confirmed that labors with slopes below 1.2 cm/hr in nulliparas
and 1.5 cm/hr in multiparas were significantly associated with adverse
outcomes,[18] verifying their inherent value.

Another type of disorder is one that can be recognized on the basis of a
deviation of the deceleration phase from normal, using similar data on
distribution around the mean for large gravid populations. Even those
who feel the deceleration phase does not ordinarily exist acknowledge it
is abnormal when prolonged.[29] It is generally limited to 3 hr in nulliparas
and 1 hr in multiparas in normal labors; those exceeding these limits are
affected by a prolonged deceleration phase labor disorder. This abnormality appears to be related to impeded retraction of the cervix around
the fetal presenting part just prior to full dilatation, often in association
with poor or absent descent. Indeed, bony impediment in the form of
cephalopelvic disproportion is not uncommon, being encountered in
about half the cases. It is this relationship that makes prolonged deceleration phase so important in clinical practice.

Three other patterns are identifiable on the basis of the dilatation and
descent curves, namely, secondary arrest of dilatation, arrest of descent,
and failure of descent. All are easily appreciated and quickly confirmed in
any given case, particularly if the graphs are constructed in an ongoing
fashion as labor evolves. In the course of active phase dilatation, the
pattern of normal progression is expected to be linear; if progress ceases
before the cervix reaches the deceleration phase, *secondary arrest of dilatation* becomes obvious. The diagnosis requires two vaginal examinations,
preferably by the same observer, spaced at least 2 hr apart for confirmation. *Arrest of descent* can be diagnosed in the same way if linear descent is
interrupted (after it has reached its maximum slope in deceleration phase
of dilatation and in the second stage) for at least 1 hr. *Failure of descent*
refers to the situation in which the descent process does not begin at the
time it is expected to be in full progress in late active phase or second
stage.

The three aberrations described above, collectively termed *arrest disorders*, share common clinical features with prolonged deceleration phase

and can be considered variants of the same mechanism, especially as related to cephalopelvic disproportion. The 2 hr definition of secondary arrest has been questioned as perhaps too long and a 1 hr limit has been proposed instead.[4] This suggestion has much merit. While there is no doubt that a more liberal cut-point will serve to detect all cases with arrest of progress destined to extend to 2 hr, however, it will also flag many cases in which the arrest is likely to resolve spontaneously or in which the diagnosis is factitious because not enough time has been allowed to elapse to determine if progress is actually being made (given the innate inaccuracy of digital estimates of cervical dilatation).

Among abnormally slow or arrested labors, therefore, there are only these seven definable aberrant patterns, all of which can be logically grouped into three general types: the prolonged latent phase disorder; the two protraction disorders (protracted dilatation and protracted descent); and the four arrest patterns (prolonged deceleration phase, secondary arrest of dilatation, arrest of descent, and failure of descent). It must be reemphasized that their presence merely signals that the labor process falls outside expected limits, thus alerting attendant personnel to the need for special evaluation and care. The patterns themselves do not diagnose the underlying problem or abnormal mechanism, if any, although certain kinds of problems are common (but not universal) to them. They do not give license to routinized practices of aggressive intervention without prior assessment to disclose problems justifying such intervention.

MANAGEMENT

A number of programs of management have been formulated for these several labor disorders based on experiential observations with good outcome results.[17,26] Cases with prolonged latent phase, for example, have been determined to respond best to therapeutic rest. Use of narcotic analgesic agents, such as morphine sulfate, in doses large enough to provide sleep and stop uterine contractions, proves especially beneficial. Most patients (up to 85%) awaken after 6 to 10 hr and are found to have progressed well into the active phase. They generally proceed to delivery without further problems. Some of them (10%) are out of labor when the analgesia wears off; in retrospect, they were likely to have been in false labor earlier. The therapeutic trial has thus differentiated between true and false labor. The remaining patients (5%) who continue in their nonprogressive pattern after they awaken can be subjected to uterotonic stimulation, usually progressing thereafter in a satisfactory manner.

This approach has the singular advantages of helping to differentiate true labor from false on an objective basis and averting unnecessary cesarean section for "failure to progress" in patients who may never have actually experienced a trial of true labor.[33] Indeed, it has been shown that cesarean section is rarely needed in the latent phase,[42] and it is never indicated in the latent phase for abnormal labor progress.[17] Some have advocated merely defining labor as existing only if there is documentation of progressive dilatation,[29,41] such as occurs normally in the active phase of the first stage. This definition does, of course, avoid the issue of diagnosis and management of any latent phase disorder, but by ignoring it, many needy patients are left without consistent help. Some who accept the responsibility for caring for patients in the latent phase feel there is room for individualization of that care.[5,35,53] They recommend oxytocin for the multipara in latent phase with a favorable cervix and therapeutic rest for the nullipara who may be exhausted well before the limits of normal latent phase are reached. These tailored approaches have potential merit in expediting management, although the lack of any data on benefit and risk leaves them open to question.

The course of labor in gravidas with protraction disorders does not appear to respond to stimulation by oxytocin or amniotomy.[20] Therefore, after cephalopelvic disproportion has been ruled out, they are preferentially managed by supportive measures, such as encouragement, fluids, and electrolytes, as needed. Since insurmountable bony obstruction is present in about one-third of these cases, it is essential to ensure adequate pelvic capacity to accommodate the fetus. If disproportion is found, cesarean section is justified; if not, labor should be permitted to proceed while minimizing the inhibitory effects of analgesic agents and conduction anesthesia, and maintaining continuous surveillance of fetal status. Care should be taken to avoid forceps procedures for delivery in these cases because of their apparently adverse effects on infant outcome, even when carried out in exemplary fashion.[18] Some propose a trial of oxytocin in all such cases[39–41,46] in an effort to distinguish those with disproportion from those with ample pelvis, utilizing response in the form of further dilatation or descent as an index of effectiveness. Given the current limitations of fetal monitoring techniques to anticipate excessive intracranial mechanical stresses, however, uterotonic stimulation may expose the fetus to hazard because it is not yet possible to determine acceptable limits of deformational molding beyond which damage is likely to occur.

Since up to one-half of the cases of arrest disorder are associated with major degrees of cephalopelvic disproportion,[22] the first step in evaluation must be a careful assessment of the cephalopelvic relationships.

Even though the frequency of bony dystocia may be as low as 18% in some populations,[3] cesarean section is clearly indicated unless disproportion can be ruled out with reasonable certainty. This does not give license to undertaking operative intervention in all patients whose labor progress halts. On the contrary, many can be expected to deliver safely and uneventfully by the vaginal route. The poor fetal results[18] do nonetheless stress the importance of determining adequacy of the maternal pelvis before allowing labor to proceed. This applies especially before any use of oxytocin, which is otherwise quite appropriate as a means for enhancing uterine contractility for an arrest of labor (in any of its several forms) occurring in a patient with no evidence of disproportion.

Despite the cautionary statements, there are authorities who currently advocate uterine stimulation with oxytocin on a more or less routine basis except for those cases with overt evidence of pelvic distortion or gross disproportion.[3,46,53] The argument posited above concerning the potential risk of stimulation in an obstructed labor has been partially answered for cases with arrest of labor by the good results reported by Bottoms et al.[3]; their response, albeit somewhat encouraging, must be considered incomplete thus far owing to the absence of long-term follow-up outcome data. Moreover, close perusal of their published data suggests (but admittedly does not prove) increased neurologic abnormalities (2.3% vs. 1.5%) and need for neonatal intensive care (9.9% vs. 7.5%) among infants delivered vaginally after an arrest disorder, whether or not oxytocin was used; they also show a significantly increased need for intensive care among offspring after arrest disorder managed with oxytocin (15.1% vs. 7.8%), especially if delivered abdominally (20.3% vs. 9.9%). Until safety can be better assured, therefore, it is prudent to exercise caution in stimulating arrested labors with oxytocin unless disproportion can be ruled out first.

It thus becomes important to differentiate among the three types of disorders because management of each is distinctive. In general, latent phase prolongation is best managed with rest, protraction disorders with expectancy and support, and arrest disorders with either cesarean section (for disproportion) or uterotonic stimulation. Unless it is clear which abnormality is present in a given case, any single form of routinized management, such as oxytocin, may prove to be inappropriate. Early recognition, by plotting the labor curve, permits prompt assessment and corrective measures. Moreover, knowledge about the type of labor aberration directs the type of evaluation and alerts one to the potential for adverse maternal or fetal outcome. In this way, one can intelligently consider available options, such as seeking consultation, instituting fetal surveillance, or even relocating the patient to a tertiary care center before delivery in the interest of optimizing outcome.

REFERENCES

1. Arulkumaran S, Gibb DMF, Ratnam SS, Lun KC, Heng SH: Total uterine activity in induced labour: An index of cervical and pelvic tissue resistance. *Br J Obstet Gynaecol* 1985;92:393–397.

2. Beazley JM: Use of partograms in labour. *Proc R Soc Med* 1972;65:700.

3. Bottoms SF, Hirsch VJ, Sokol RJ: Medical management of arrest disorders of labor: A current overview. *Am J Obstet Gynecol* 1987;156:935–939.

4. Bottoms SF, Sokol RJ, Rosen MG: Short arrest of cervical dilatation: A risk for maternal/fetal/infant morbidity. *Am J Obstet Gynecol* 1981;140:108–116.

5. Bowes WA Jr: Clinical aspects of normal and abnormal labor, in: Creasy RK, Resnik R (eds): *Maternal-Fetal Medicine: Principles and Practice*. Philadelphia, WB Saunders, 1984, pp 449–489.

6. Caldeyro-Barcia R: Uterine contractility in obstetrics. *Deux Cong Int Gynecol Obstet* 1958;1:65.

7. Calkins LA: On predicting the length of labor: I. First stage. *Am J Obstet Gynecol* 1941;42:802–811.

8. Calkins LA: Second stage of labor: The descent phase. *Am J Obstet Gynecol* 1944;48:798–803.

9. Cardozo LD, Gibb DMF, Studd JWW, Vasant RV, Cooper DJ: Predictive value of cervimetric labour patterns in primigravidae. *Br J Obstet Gynaecol* 1982;89:33–38.

10. Cohen WR, Neuman L, Friedman EA: Risk of labor abnormalities with advancing age. *Obstet Gynecol* 1980;55:414–416.

11. Crichton D: A reliable method of establishing the level of the fetal head in obstetrics. *S Afr Med J* 1974;48:784–788.

12. Duignan NM, Studd JWW, Hughes AO: Characteristics of normal labour in different racial groups. *Br J Obstet Gynaecol* 1975;82:593–601.

13. Earn AA: The partographic labor board: An alternative for earlier decisions regarding management during labor. *Am J Obstet Gynecol* 1982;144:858–859.

14. Frey E: Die Bedeutung der Wehentafel für die Physiologie und Pathologie der Geburt beim vorzeitigen Blasensprung. *Schweiz Med Wochenschr* 1929;59:613–618.

15. Friedman EA: Graphic analysis of labor. *Am J Obstet Gynecol* 1954;68:1568–1575.

16. Friedman EA: Cervimetry: An objective method for the study of cervical dilatation in labor. *Am J Obstet Gynecol* 1956;71:1189–1193.

17. Friedman EA: *Labor: Clinical Evaluation and Management*. New York, Appleton-Century-Crofts, 1978.

18. Friedman EA, Neff RK: *Labor and Delivery: Impact on Offspring*. Littleton, MA: PSG Publishing, 1987.

19. Friedman EA, Sachtleben MR: Dysfunctional labor: I. Prolonged latent phase in the nullipara. *Obstet Gynecol* 1961;17:135–148.

20. Friedman EA, Sachtleben MR: Dysfunctional labor: II. Protracted active phase dilatation in the nullipara. *Obstet Gynecol* 1961;17:566–578.

21. Friedman EA, Sachtleben MR: The determinant role of initial cervical dilatation on the course of labor. *Am J Obstet Gynecol* 1962;84:930–935.

22. Friedman EA, Sachtleben MR: Dysfunctional labor: III. Secondary arrest of dilatation in the nullipara. *Obstet Gynecol* 1962;19:576–591.

23. Friedman EA, Sachtleben MR: Station of the fetal presenting part: I. Pattern of descent. *Am J Obstet Gynecol* 1965;93:522–529.

24. Friedman EA, Sachtleben MR: Station of the fetal presenting part: III. Interrelationship with cervical dilatation. *Am J Obstet Gynecol* 1965;93:537–542.

25. Friedman EA, Sachtleben MR: Relation of maternal age to the course of labor. *Am J Obstet Gynecol* 1965;91:915–924.

26. Friedman EA, Sachtleben MR: Dysfunctional labor: VII. A comprehensive program for diagnosis, evaluation and management. *Obstet Gynecol* 1965;25:844–847.

27. Friedman EA, Von Micsky LI: Electronic cervimeter: A research instrument for the study of cervical dilatation in labor. *Am J Obstet Gynecol* 1963;87:789–792.

28. Hall R, Krins A: The partograph in obstetrics. *Aust Fam Phys* 1981;10:107–112.

29. Hendricks CH, Brenner WE, Kraus G: Normal cervical dilatation pattern in late pregnancy and labor. *Am J Obstet Gynecol* 1970;106:1065–1082.

30. Huey JR Jr, Al-Hadjiev A, Paul RH: Uterine activity in the multiparous patient. *Am J Obstet Gynecol* 1976;126:682–686.

31. Huey JR Jr, Miller FC: The evaluation of uterine activity: A comparative analysis. *Am J Obstet Gynecol* 1979;135:252–256.

32. Hunter DJS, Enkin MW, Sargeant EJ, Wilkinson J, Tugwell P: The outcome of prolonged labor as defined by partography and the use of oxytocin: A descriptive study. *Am J Obstet Gynecol* 1983;145:189–192.

33. Iams JD, Reiss R: When should labor be interrupted by cesarean delivery? *Clin Obstet Gynecol* 1985;28:745–751.

34. Kok FT, Wallenburg HCS, Wladimiroff JW: Ultrasonic measurement of cervical dilatation during labor. *Am J Obstet Gynecol* 1976;126:288–290.

35. Koontz WL, Bishop EH: Management of latent phase of labor. *Clin Obstet Gynecol* 1982;25:111–114.

36. Krapohl AJ, Myers GG, Caldeyro-Barcia R: Uterine contractions in spontaneous labor: A quantitative study. *Am J Obstet Gynecol* 1970;106:378–382.

37. Melmed H, Evans MI: Predictive value of cervical dilatation rates: I. Primipara labor. *Obstet Gynecol* 1976;47:511–515.

38. Miller FC, Yeh SY, Schifrin BS, Paul RH, Hon EH: Quantitation of uterine activity in 100 primiparous patients. *Am J Obstet Gynecol* 1976;124:398–405.

39. O'Brien WF, Cefalo RC: Abnormalities of the active phase: Recognition and treatment. *Clin Obstet Gynecol* 1982;25:115–122.

40. O'Driscoll K, Stronge JM, Minogue M: Active management of labor. *Br Med J* 1973;3:135–137.

41. O'Driscoll K, Foley M, MacDonald D: Active management of labor as an alternative to cesarean section for dystocia. *Obstet Gynecol* 1984;63:485–490.

42. Peisner DB, Rosen MG: Latent phase of labor in normal patients: A reassessment. *Obstet Gynecol* 1985;66:644–648.

43. Peisner DB, Rosen MG: Transition from latent to active labor. *Obstet Gynecol* 1986;68:448–451.

44. Philpott RH, Castle WM: Cervicographs in the management of labour in primigravidae: I. The alert line for detecting abnormal labour. *Br J Obstet Gynaecol* 1972;79:592–598.

45. Philpott RH, Castle WM: Cervicographs in the management of labor in primigravidae: II. The action line and treatment for abnormal labor. *Br J Obstet Gynaecol* 1972;79:599–602.

46. Ross MG, Hayashi R: How can we use oxytocin more effectively? *Contemp Ob Gyn* 1984;24:139–147.

47. Rossavik IK: Relation between total uterine impulse, method of delivery and one minute Apgar score. *Br J Obstet Gynaecol* 1978;85:847–851.

48. Schauberger CW: False labor. *Obstet Gynecol* 1986;68:770–772.

49. Schulman H, Romney SL: Variability of uterine contractions in normal human parturition. *Obstet Gynecol* 1970;36:215–220.

50. Seitchik J, Castillo M: Oxytocin augmentation of dysfunctional labor: II. Uterine activity data. *Am J Obstet Gynecol* 1983;145:526–529.

51. Seitchik J, Chatkoff ML: Intrauterine pressure wave form characteristics in hypocontractile labor before and after oxytocin administration. *Am J Obstet Gynecol* 1975;123:426–434.

52. Seitchik J, Chatkoff ML: Intrauterine pressure wave form characteristic of successful and failed first stage of labor. *Gynecol Invest* 1977;246:8–16.

53. Sheen PW, Hayashi RH: Graphic management of labor: Alert/action line. *Clin Obstet Gynecol* 1987;30:33–41.

54. Sokol RJ, Zador I, Rosen MG: Slowing of active labor associated with internal fetal monitoring. *Am J Obstet Gynecol* 1976;124:764–765.

55. Steer PJ, Carter MC, Beard RW: Normal levels of active contraction area in spontaneous labour. *Br J Obstet Gynaecol* 1984;91:211–219.

56. Steer PJ, Carter MCC, Beard RW: The effect of oxytocin infusion on uterine activity level in slow labour. *Br J Obstet Gynaecol* 1985;92:1120–1126.

57. Studd JWW: Partograms and nomograms of cervical dilatation in management of primigravid labour. *Br Med J* 1973;4:451–455.

58. Studd JWW: The partographic control of labour. *Clin Obstet Gynaecol* 1975;2:127–151.

59. Studd J, Clegg DR, Sanders RR, Hughes AO: Identification of high risk labours by labour nomogram. *Br Med J* 1975;2:545–547.

60. Zimmer K: Die Muttermundseröffnung bei den Schädellagen im Wegzeit-Diagramm. *Arch Gynaekol* 1951;179:35–42.

2

The Pelvic Division of Labor

Wayne R. Cohen

The pelvic division of labor encompasses the portion of parturition during which descent of the fetus through the birth canal occurs. It thus includes the terminal aspects of cervical dilatation, as well as the second stage of labor during which maternal expulsive efforts generally reinforce contractile activity of the uterus. The pelvic division includes and culminates in the thrilling and dramatic events of delivery.

Accurate observation and sagacious interpretation of variations in patterns of fetal descent is an often ignored but vital aspect of labor management. Scrupulous attention to the progress of descent is necessary to make the most appropriate judgments about the need for intervention during the second stage. It should be recognized, however, that interpretations of the progress of fetal descent must be made in the context of other clinical events. The development of progressive molding of the cranial bones, inadequate rotation, malpositions, and other abnormalities distinguishable by examination are equally important and must be integrated into the assessment of each labor.

GRAPHIC LABOR ABNORMALITIES

A dilatational abnormality may occur in the pelvic division (see Chapter 1). A *prolonged deceleration phase* is generally associated with a poor prognosis for vaginal delivery.[42] It frequently follows abnormalities of the phase of maximum slope (protracted active phase dilatation or arrest of dilatation), and should alert the obstetrician to the possibility of serious aberrations of fetal descent. In fact, one may view the terminal portion of cervical dilatation as a milestone in descent. The cervix probably has a

19

limited ability to retract completely around the presenting part without some degree of descent having occurred.

The curve of fetal descent versus elapsed time in labor has a latent phase similar to that of the curve of dilatation. There is generally little or no progress in descent from the onset of labor until the phase of maximum slope of dilatation has been reached. At that time, descent usually enters a phase of acceleration, and by the time the deceleration phase of dilatation has commenced, descent should have become linear. Once active descent has thus evolved, the fetal presenting part will normally descend at a constant rate until it reaches the pelvic floor. Descent then slows as the head extends under the symphysis pubis, and delivers across the perineum. This terminal slowing of descent gives the descent curve a sigmoid shape analogous to that of dilatation. However, these terminal events are rarely plotted graphically in the clinical setting.

Considerable descent may occasionally occur in the latent phase of labor, particularly in multiparas. Nevertheless, it is quite normal for little or no descent to have occurred until nearly full cervical dilatation has been reached. Thus, judgments about the prognosis for vaginal delivery cannot be made based solely upon a lack of apparent descent prior to the deceleration phase of dilatation. The rate at which the fetus descends through the birth canal is influenced by several factors, including uterine contractile force, voluntary maternal expulsive efforts, fetal size, position and attitude, pelvic architecture, and, terminally, the configuration and tone of the pelvic floor.

Three distinct disorders of fetal descent can be distinguished clinically.[42] *Failure of descent*, an uncommon disorder, is diagnosed when there has been no fetal descent by the time the deceleration phase of labor has begun. This disorder is associated with a very high likelihood of cephalopelvic disproportion, particularly when it occurs in the presence of oxytocin stimulation. *Protracted descent* occurs when, having entered the active portion of the descent curve, progress continues in a linear manner at a rate slower than the accepted limits of normal (1 cm/hr in nulliparas and 2 cm/hr in multiparas). An *arrest of descent*[43] is defined as lack of progress, preferably determined by the same examiner, over a 1-hr period after the active phase of descent has commenced. Protraction and arrest anomalies of descent are associated with the same factors that tend to accompany the analogous protraction and arrest patterns of dilatation. The possibility of cephalopelvic disproportion should always be anticipated in these situations, and appropriate clinical and/or radiologic cephalopelvimetry should be performed. Malpositions in the absence of true disproportion may also predispose to disorders of the pelvic division. Excessive anesthesia, amnionitis, or myometrial abnormalities may reduce contractile efficiency and also result in these labor abnormalities.

CEPHALOPELVIMETRY

The assumption that the anatomic characteristics of the bony pelvis influence progress during labor is ingrained in obstetric thought and is readily demonstrable[15,18,35]; but data concerning pelvic size and shape are of limited value when considered alone. Although there is no doubt that decreasing pelvic capacity is associated with increasing probability of instrumental or cesarean delivery, most cesarean sections for the diagnosis of dystocia are done in women with normal bony dimensions.[35] This is because many other factors (enumerated above) influence labor progress. However, clinical dystocia occurs rarely in the presence of average size babies and adequate pelves, suggesting that bony disproportion is a real cause of dysfunctional labor,[35,36] particularly as regards descent disorders.

Our clinical concepts regarding human pelvic architecture were crystallized by the thorough observations of Caldwell and Moloy in the 1930s.[15–18] Their work and the widespread availability of pelvic radiography spawned a generation of obstetricians that regarded knowledge of the mechanical fundamentals of obstetrics and interpretation of x-ray pelvimetry to be essential in the management of labor.

These attitudes have changed recently for several reasons. Deemphasis on the importance of midcavity forceps operations, liberal use of cesarean section, dissatisfaction with and concerns regarding the safety of x-ray pelvimetry, and an emphasis on more esoteric and technology-oriented issues in residency training have all served to reduce attention to the importance of understanding fetopelvic relationships for optimal obstetric management. Some contemporary schemata for treatment of dystocia emphasize liberal use of oxytocin without regard for evaluation of pelvic characteristics.[117] This is regrettable, in part because it denies the obstetric attendant the satisfaction that comes with an understanding of the beauty and logic of the mechanism of labor, but also because ill-considered use of uterotonic agents may be hazardous for mother and fetus.

A review of the extant controversy relating to x-ray pelvimetry was presented in the first edition of this book,[78] and the reader is referred to that source for details. Much evidence supports the idea that *in utero* exposure to diagnostic abdominal or pelvic x-rays in late pregnancy results in an increase in the risk of childhood cancer, but this has not been a universal finding. The U.S. Food and Drug Administration recommended in 1982[38] that radiographic pelvimetry be used only in situations in which the benefit to be derived clearly exceeds the risks. In practical terms, this technique is now used only in special situations, such as breech presentation or determination of lie or position when clinical examination and ultrasonography are not definitive. Possibly, more advanced radiologic techniques, including computed tomography and magnetic resonance imaging, may in the future provide accurate pelvic assessment with minimal fetal risk.

Fortunately, in the absence of radiography, much useful information is obtained from careful clinical cephalopelvimetry. In one sense, the most lamentable result of the abandonment of x-ray pelvimetry is that the student of the pelvis has no standard by which to judge the accuracy of clinical assessment. Keen observation of the mechanism of labor that accompanies pelvic types is necessary for proper self-education. After every delivery clinical pelvimetry should be performed and the findings related to the mechanism of labor. In this way, a library of information will be accumulated in the mind's eye to serve as a source for future examinations.

Whether one considers evaluation of the pelvis to be useful depends on the information expected from it. The term "cephalopelvic disproportion" is used frequently in conjunction with pelvimetry. In truth, pelvimetry is no more likely to predict the need for operative delivery than any other technique (including graphic analysis of labor) when applied in a clinical vacuum. The mechanism of labor is influenced by many other factors, including fetal size, ability of the fetal head to mold, distensibility of pelvic joints, uterine contractility, pelvic soft tissue factors, degree of flexion of the fetal head, and fetal axis. Only by combining and interpreting information from these sources intelligently can keen judgments be made. Knowledge of pelvic architecture and cephalopelvic relationships allows one to explain the observed normal or abnormal mechanism of labor, to judge the effects of the labor on the fetal skull, and thus to assess the *probability* of the need for operative intervention. When this assessment is integrated with those obtained from evaluation of cervical dilatation and fetal descent, uterine activity, and fetal condition, a decision can be made concerning the advisability of uterine stimulation and operative delivery. This approach is preferable to administering oxytocin in every case of labor dysfunction and allowing the compressibility of the fetal head to dictate the route of delivery.

Based on extensive study of museum collections of pelves and of stereoroentgenograms of living subjects, Caldwell and Moloy identified four pure pelvic types, now familiar to all obstetricians: gynecoid, android, anthropoid, and platypelloid.[15,17] They recognized that examples of these archetypes are rare, and that most pelves share characteristics of two or more types. The basic form of the pelvis should be described in terms of the shape of the posterior segment of the inlet[15]; but a detailed assessment of the entire pelvic conformation is necessary to predict labor mechanisms.

A thorough and systematic method of digital examination of the pelvis should be cultivated. Although the inlet shape is not usually discernible without radiographs, many other features of the pelvis may be evaluated. The characteristics listed in Table 2-1 should be ascertained on each examination.

Palpation of a gothic subpubic arch, forward sacrum, short dense sacrospinous ligament, and prominent ischial spines suggests a predominantly android configuration. A wide arch, and large diameters with straight sidewalls and subtle ischial spines with average or backward sacral inclination is found in gynecoid pelves. If the diagonal conjugate is long and transverse diameters relatively narrow with a long sacrospinous ligament, the pelvis has anthropoid features; a short diagonal conjugate with wide transverse space above and below the ischial spines are platypelloid features.[17] Precise measurement of diameters and accurate identification of the parent pelvic type is sometimes useful, but an appreciation of the architectural variations in various portions of the pelvis is more important.

In addition to pelvic evaluation, examination of the fetal head for the presence of excessive degrees of caput succedaneum, molding, and positional or attitudinal abnormalities provides clues to the suitability of the

Table 2-1 Modified Stander Classification

Retropubic angle	Wide	Moderate	Narrow
Subpubic arch	Wide	Moderate	Narrow
Pubic rami	Straight (gothic)	Curved (norman)	
Pubic symphysis	Forward	Average	Backward
Sidewalls	Divergent	Straight	Convergent
Ischial spines	Blunt	Average	Prominent
Sacral curve	Straight	Average	Hollow
Sacral inclination	Forward	Average	Backward
Terminal sacrum/coccyx	Forward	Average	Backward
Lateral bore	Straight	Convergent	Divergent

pelvis. The Müller-Hillis maneuver may be useful in this regard.[62] With the cervix at least 5 cm dilated, firm (but gentle) fundal pressure is applied during a contraction while a vaginal examination is done to assess descent, flexion, and rotation of the presenting part.

The aggregate of ascertainable clinical information concerning cephalopelvic relationships is very useful as part of the dynamic evaluation of labor. Failure of descent is commonly the result of inlet disproportion. Absence of descent despite near complete cervical dilatation, poor responsiveness to oxytocin stimulation, and occurrence at high fetal stations suggest mechanical obstruction. The likelihood of vaginal delivery after this labor disorder is small, and early intervention is indicated if cephalopelvimetry suggests disproportion. For example, android characteristics of the midpelvis, and a molded head impinging on the crest of the symphysis pubis in the presence of failure of descent make the probability of safe vaginal delivery remote. Similarly, an engaged posterior head in a midpelvis with prominent spines (resisting anterior rotation) and a forward lower sacrum (not allowing sufficient compensatory space for descent in the posterior position) is ominous.[30] However, when failure of descent (or other pelvic division aberration) occurs in the presence of a well-flexed unmolded head in a pelvis that seems ample, causes other than insurmountable bony disproportion are likely. In these situations vaginal delivery is more probable and oxytocin infusion is safer and more efficacious.

Arrest of descent and protracted descent are associated with several obstetric features, including malpositions, excessive sedation or anesthesia, insufficient uterine contractility, chorioamnionitis, and cephalopelvic disproportion. Thorough evaluation of each factor is important when confronted with these labor dysfunctions. When the likelihood of disproportion seems high, one should avoid uterine stimulation, or be very judicious about its use. For example, arrest of descent often occurs in the midpelvis with transverse positions of the occiput. This may be an entirely appropriate position in a pelvis with quite ample transverse space throughout and straight or divergent sidewalls. If the lower sacrum is straight or inclined backward and/or if the forepelvis is wide, oxytocin may be given, and one may expect continued descent in the transverse position until internal rotation occurs low in the pelvis. Similarly, stimulation is likely to be successful if the upper pelvis will accommodate anterior rotation and the lower pelvis will allow further descent in an anterior position; however, transverse arrests that occur in a pelvis with features that are unlikely to permit further descent easily, particularly if the head shows asynclytism, or marked molding, are best terminated by cesarean section without a trial of oxytocin.

SECOND STAGE DURATION

An issue of critical importance in the clinical management of the pelvic division of labor concerns the appropriate duration of the second stage. In fact, most controversies regarding this aspect of labor relate directly or indirectly to notions regarding acceptable time limits for the second stage.[17] Decisions to use oxytocin, forceps, episiotomy, and to accept alternative maternal postures or bearing-down techniques depend on the perceived need to shorten the second stage.

Common practice in the United States has been to make preparations for expedient delivery after about 2 hr have elapsed in the second stage, unless spontaneous delivery seems imminent. The origins of this notion are diverse. Obstetric literature has for several generations emphasized the fact that fetal and maternal outcomes were often poor when the second stage was prolonged. However, limits far in excess of 2 hr were considered acceptable prior to the era of safe cesarean section and the popularity and relative ease of instrumental delivery. Contemporary advocates of the 2-hr "rule" cite concerns about development of fetal acidosis or trauma if the second stage is prolonged beyond this limit.

The development of obstetric forceps in the 18th century provided a new means to terminate labor. The "prophylactic" use of forceps was given impetus by Joseph DeLee[29] in the 1920s. Based on his extensive experience, DeLee recommended a pattern of delivery that included use of the dorsal lithotomy position, elective episiotomy, and forceps delivery. The latter two techniques were aimed at limiting the length of the second stage and at preventing excessive pressures on the fetal head. Although these techniques became commonplace in American obstetrics, no objective data were accumulated that proved their superiority to normal spontaneous delivery. The lack of such quantifiable data does not, of course, mean these techniques are without merit, and many obstetricians will attest to their virtues.

The first study of the risks of a prolonged second stage performed in recent times was published in 1952 by Hellman and Prystowsky.[60] They studied a large series of infants and found there was a direct correlation between the duration of second stage labor and the risk of infant mortality, as well as of maternal infection and hemorrhage. It was reasonable to assume, based on this information, that the 2-hr rule made clinical sense. Further corroboration was obtained from clinical studies of fetal and maternal acid-base status during the second stage that suggested the risk of fetal acidosis increased considerably as second stage duration lengthened.[70] However, data obtained more recently do not support these concepts.

In a 1977 study, Cohen[25] evaluated the relationship between the duration of the second stage of labor and measures of perinatal morbidity and mortality, as well as maternal puerperal morbidity. In a series of 4,403 nulliparas no significant increase was observed in perinatal mortality rates with progressive lengthening of the second stage (Table 2-2). This was true regardless of delivery type, the presence of preexisting maternal disease, or of abnormal labors. There was also no obvious trend toward increased neonatal death rates with long second stages. A progressive rise in the frequency of low 1-min Apgar scores was observed with long second stages; however, this phenomenon did not occur in those patients managed with continuous electronic fetal heart rate monitoring. The risk of low 5-min Apgar scores was not related to second stage duration either.

This study did show a rather dramatic increase in the risk of puerperal hemorrhage and maternal febrile morbidity, particularly when the second stage exceeded 3 hr. The excess hemorrhage rate was accounted for by more common use of midforceps procedures after very long second stages. Similarly, the increase in infections was related to the more frequent use of cesarean section in these situations. The study showed, therefore, that there was no direct effect of the duration of second stage of labor on either immediate measures of perinatal outcome or on maternal morbidity.

Several lines of evidence support this conclusion. Roemer et al.[108] indicated that second stage duration was not associated with increased risk of poor immediate outcome as long as the fetal heart rate pattern did

---

Table 2-2 Perinatal Outcome by Duration of Second Stage

Duration (min)	No.	Perinatal mortality (per 1,000)	Neonatal mortality (per 1,000)	Low 1-min Apgar[a] (%)	Low 5-min Apgar (%)
0–29	623	6.5	0.0	3.2 (4.4)	0.6
30–59	1,257	4.8	2.4	3.1 (4.2)	0.7
60–89	1,007	3.0	1.0	3.5 (2.7)	0.3
90–119	599	0.0	0.0	3.7 (4.3)	0.2
120–149	425	2.4	0.0	4.5 (5.9)	0.0
150–179	237	0.0	0.0	6.3 (3.3)	0.8
180 +	255	3.9	0.0	7.1 (5.7)	1.6
Total	4,403	3.4	1.8	3.8 (4.3)	0.5

[a]Distribution of data for total series is statistically significant ($\chi^2_H = 15.6, p < 0.025$), but the relative rates of depressed neonates among monitored patients (in parentheses) are not ($\chi^2_H = 3.9, p > 0.05$).

not evidence distress. Other investigators have similarly failed to find a relation between neonatal outcome and second stage duration.[74,82,88] Analysis of data from the Collaborative Perinatal Project revealed no relationship between length of the second stage and measures of long-term cognitive and neurologic follow-up of children studied at 3 years of age.[95]

Regrettably, the conclusions of these studies have been misinterpreted occasionally to imply that it never matters how long the second stage lasts. This unfortunate inference has resulted in justification of extraordinarily long second stage labors that would be the envy of Pheidippides, sometimes to the detriment of mother and baby. (Thankfully, the outcome of most such marathon second stages is less tragic than that which befell the original marathoner.) The data indicate only that a decision to terminate labor purely because an arbitrary period of time has elapsed is not appropriate. Rather, that decision should be based on a careful evaluation of maternal and fetal condition and of progress in descent. Some fetuses may descend at a normal rate and take several hours to deliver, and to subject such patients to potentially traumatic operative procedures merely because they have not delivered within 2 hr after the second stage has begun should be decried. A long second stage, however, should not be ignored. On the contrary, it may signify an important labor disorder that must be evaluated, and neglecting to diagnose and treat an arrest or failure of descent may have serious consequences.

Kadar et al.[73] showed recently that the probability of spontaneous delivery according to time spent in the second stage is related to birth weight and maternal age. Women who have not delivered by the end of 3 hr are unlikely to do so subsequently, unless the mother is young and the fetus is small (< 3 kg). This is useful information for the practitioner. Perhaps the explanation is that most second stages longer than 3 hr are accompanied by labor disorders associated with a high probability of disproportion. Those without disproportion (small babies) may have had some other explanation for delayed descent. The influence of maternal age is more difficult to explain.

Fetal Oxygenation in the Second Stage

Fetal blood pH is normally stable or diminishes slowly during the first stage of labor and then falls more rapidly during the second stage, accompanied by an increase in fetal base deficit and P_{CO_2}. A drop in fetal oxygen saturation of about 10% also occurs during the second stage.[70] Nevertheless, although a relative fetal respiratory acidosis develops, the amount of metabolic acidosis that occurs during normal labor is probably minimal.[70,76] Many studies of fetal pH during the second stage contain observations only during the first 30 to 60 min. One may conclude (not entirely facetiously) from these studies that if fetal pH fell during the entire second stage at the rate it has been said to fall during the first 60 min, no fetus would survive more than 2 hr of maternal expulsive efforts. As this is obviously not the case, and inasmuch as most babies born after long second stages are normal and vigorous, we must conclude that a continuous decrement in fetal oxygenation during the pelvic division of labor does not occur inevitably. In fact, in the presence of a normal fetal heart rate pattern and attention to maternal hydration and position, progressive fetal asphyxia need not be of concern. It may be that more harm than good has been done by well-intentioned attendants who have resorted to operative vaginal delivery or cesarean section on the basis of specious concerns about fetal status in these situations.

The decrease in fetal pH during the second stage is probably caused by a combination of increased uterine contractility and maternal expulsive efforts. Humphrey et al.[66] studied 35 women with term pregnancies assigned to receive either ritodrine infusion or a placebo in a double-blind fashion beginning at full dilatation. The placebo group had the expected time-dependent fall in cord blood pH, Po_2, oxygen saturation, and a rise in Pco_2. These changes were not present in the ritodrine group. However, the decrease in umbilical artery pH in the placebo group was small, and was not statistically significant. The control group had a respiratory acidosis, perhaps related to strong second stage contractions, which were abolished by ritodrine in the experimental group.

Pearson and Davies[98] studied the effect of peridural anesthesia on maternal acid-base balance. They showed that maternal metabolic acidosis and lactic acidemia occurred during the second stage in control patients who labored without anesthesia; however, this acidosis—the severity of which was correlated directly with the length of the second stage—was abolished in a group of patients who had epidural anesthesia and did not push. Although this study, conducted with mothers in the dorsal position, suggests that expulsive efforts do result in progressive maternal acidosis, the lack of fetal data makes it difficult to determine the significance of these changes. The fact that many studies of both maternal and fetal acid-base status during the second stage of labor were conducted with the mother in the dorsal or supine position tends to vitiate their conclusions now that the potential hazards of that position are recognized.

Humphrey et al.[64] attempted to address this problem by comparing the immediate neonatal outcome of babies whose mothers labored in the dorsal position with those whose mothers were in 15 degrees of lateral tilt during the second stage. There were no significant differences in Apgar scores or cord pH between the two groups, but those few babies in the study with low Apgar scores and acidosis were delivered of mothers who had been in the dorsal position. The authors concluded that there may be a small group of parturients who benefit from the lateral position. The small number of patients and the absence of fetal heart rate information and time-dependent data render the validity of these conclusions uncertain. However, this study did emphasize the possible effect of maternal position during the second stage on neonatal outcome, and the need to study the association systematically. In a similarly designed recent study, Johnstone et al.[71] studied cord blood pH in 58 women assigned randomly to undergo the second stage in supine or in lateral tilt position. They found a progressive metabolic acidosis in the supine group if the second stage lasted more than 15 min. One may conclude that existing data suggest that undergoing the second stage in a dorsal position may enhance the development of fetal acidosis, particularly if the second stage is long.

Wood et al.[122] suggested that the terminal events in second stage and delivery may have an important bearing on fetal blood pH at delivery. They studied fetal acid base changes by obtaining fetal scalp blood during the second stage and at the time the caput appeared at the introitus, and cord blood at delivery. Women with uncomplicated term pregnancies were allocated randomly to a normal spontaneous delivery group, or to one in which delivery was hastened by the use of episiotomy, forceps, and encouragement to push. All labors and deliveries were conducted with the mother in the supine position, and thus it is unknown whether these data are applicable to other situations. They showed that umbilical arterial pH was significantly better in the fast delivery group (7.28 vs. 7.23). This difference seems related to the fact that they found a drop in fetal pH during the second stage of 0.003 pH u/min, a rate of fall that was enhanced during the process of delivery. They did not indicate, however, whether this acidosis was primarily respiratory or metabolic in nature. Although it would seem reasonable not to delay delivery any longer than necessary, this study did not prove that hastening parturition by the techniques mentioned above is necessarily associated with better long- or short-term outcome.

In another study, also conducted with patients supine, Wood et al.[121] determined there was no relationship between the time taken for the delivery and Apgar scores; furthermore, there was no correlation found between the duration of the second stage of labor and umbilical arterial or venous pH. Nevertheless, there was a correlation between umbilical arterial base deficit and pH and the time from original extension of the perineum to completion of the delivery. This would imply that enhancement of delivery by the use of episiotomy might be beneficial; but the rate of fall in pH was slow, and even those patients with long delivery times did not have pH values less than 7.20 (although some with shorter birth times did). This study did show that slow delivery may affect neonatal pH; whether this is of clinical significance during normal labor is uncertain.

Roemer et al.[108] studied the correlation between fetal acid-base balance and the duration of the second stage as well as that part of the second stage associated with active bearing down efforts. They showed no clear correlation of Apgar scores or acid-base variables with the length of the second stage among patients whose fetuses were evaluated using continuous electronic fetal heart rate monitoring.

Fetal Heart Rate Patterns in the Second Stage

The attainment of full dilatation is sometimes heralded by the appearance of variable decelerations in the fetal heart rate. In fact, the second stage of labor is frequently accompanied by changes in fetal heart rate patterns,[79] and erroneous interpretation of these patterns may lead to unnecessary intervention. It is likely that the heart rate decelerations that are seen so often in the second stage are caused by a combination of factors. Descent and rotation probably increase the likelihood of cord entrapment; compression of the fetal head and its attendant chemoreceptor stimulation can produce decelerations as well. In addition to these mechanical factors, uterine blood flow may be diminished by a combination of increasing uterine activity and maternal bearing-down efforts. In a study of a large series of second stage fetal heart rate patterns, Schlotter et al.[113] noted that decelerations superimposed on normal baseline heart rates occurred in 48% of patients. Nevertheless, these were generally benign, only 8.3% of them having been accompanied by significant fetal acidosis. Although fetal heart rate variability was not considered in this study, the authors were able to conclude that the magnitude and duration of the fetal heart rate decelerations in the second stage were not a reliable means of predicting fetal acidosis. Rather, all aspects of the fetal heart rate pattern must be taken into account. The presence of good short-term variability in the fetal heart rate has as important a predictive value in the second stage of labor as it does in the first stage.[48,49]

The interpretation of fetal heart rate patterns in the second stage should not differ from that at other times during labor; that is, the presence of a particular abnormality in the heart rate should not alter notions of pathogenesis or severity of accompanying fetal compromise. Nevertheless, abnormal heart rate patterns may spur different treatment plans in the second stage than they would earlier in labor. For example, the presence of recurrent late decelerations accompanied by diminished variability or progressive fetal acidosis would demand delivery at any time during labor; however if safe vaginal delivery (spontaneous or outlet forceps) can be anticipated to occur promptly, one need not resort to cesarean section.

Prolonged bradycardias are very common in the second stage, probably a result of the various physiologic factors noted above. They should be treated according to the principles outlined in Chapter 10. These include assessment of fetal reserve and of the etiology of the deceleration, as well as fetal blood sampling, when indicated.

Techniques of intrauterine resuscitation are important in the second stage (see Chapter 10). In addition to the usual maneuvers designed to maximize uterine blood flow (lateral position, decreasing oxytocin, and hydration), decreasing maternal expulsive efforts may be important to enhance recovery from fetal heart rate abnormalities. In addition, a special emphasis on position is required. Variable decelerations, particularly when they are accompanied by rapid descent of the fetus, may sometimes be modified by placing the patient in Trendelenberg position. Assumption of the upright posture or knee-chest position may also be valuable to improve abnormal heart rate patterns in the second stage.

If the use of fetal pH becomes necessary, timing of the sample is particularly important during the second stage. Variable decelerations are often accompanied by a transient respiratory acidosis, which improves shortly after the termination of the deceleration. Therefore, when using fetal scalp pH to determine intervention strategies in the presence of recurrent variable decelerations, it is vital that a sample be obtained immediately prior to a contraction. In this way the likelihood of being misled by a temporary respiratory acidosis is minimized, and one has a pH value that is an adequate reflection of fetal condition and reserve.

Although fetal pH normally decreases more rapidly during the second stage than the first, the rate of developing acidosis probably varies considerably among individual fetuses. Therefore, frequent sampling to determine trends in the fetal acid-base milieu is vital. The selection of the method of delivery when fetal hypoxia or acidosis is clearly present requires keen judgment. In general, when spontaneous or low forceps delivery is obtainable within the same time frame as it would take to perform cesarean section, vaginal delivery is preferred. The use of midforceps operations in the presence of fetal hypoxia or acidosis is fraught with risk. There may be some synergy between the adverse effects of hypoxia and of trauma from midforceps delivery.[22] Nevertheless, the obstetrician must judge whether the advantages of midforceps delivery performed expeditiously outweigh the risk of waiting for cesarean section if the latter cannot be accomplished immediately.

EPIDURAL ANESTHESIA

Some practitioners advocate extradural anesthesia be continued throughout the second stage of labor, but others prefer to allow the anesthetic to abate. They argue that descent and rotation may be delayed by inhibition of uterine contractions and relaxation of the pelvic floor, respectively. This could result in increased need for operative delivery, prolonged second stages, and perhaps increased fetal acidosis.

Many obstetric services have enhanced instrumental delivery rates among parturients with epidural anesthesia. Kaminski et al.[75] recently reported considerably increased need for low and midforceps procedures in women even with segmental epidural block, compared to unanesthetized controls. This was not attributable to larger fetal size or to more malpositions in the epidural group. This has not been a universal finding and some studies have not documented a lengthening of the second stage related to epidural block.[72,99] A double-blind study was reported in which women were given a continuous epidural infusion of lidocaine or saline during the second stage. Interestingly, there was no difference between the groups in duration of second stage or operative delivery rate.[21]

Proponents of the notion that peridural anesthesia retards second stage progress suggest it may do so by suppressing uterine activity. Indeed, this type of anesthesia may reduce uterine activity in first or second stage,[5,105] but this effect is usually transient, limited to the first 30 min after the dose.[105] More profound effects usually occur only if excessive amounts of anesthetic have been administered.

It is likely that much of the controversy over the influence of anesthesia relates more to obstetric attitudes than to documentable adverse effects of anesthetics. It is possible that epidural block does slow descent in some patients; but these inhibitory effects can generally be overcome with oxytocin.[52] More importantly, if the conservative approach to management of the second stage described herein is used, excessive rates of operative delivery are avoidable. Maresh et al. randomly assigned women with epidural anesthesia to exert expulsive efforts throughout the second stage, or to delay pushing until they felt a strong urge to do so.[82] The second stage was considerably longer (up to 4 hr) in the delayed pushing groups, but was not associated with more low Apgar scores, acidosis, or fetal heart rate abnormalities. The rate of forceps delivery was, however, lower.

MATERNAL POSTURE DURING THE SECOND STAGE

Considerable disagreement exists concerning which maternal positions will result in the most efficient and comfortable second stage of labor. Some variation of upright posture (standing, sitting, or squatting), has been used by many cultures since antiquity. In fact, references to use of a type of chair designed for both labor and delivery are found in early obstetric literature from many cultures; but upright postures were generally eschewed by Western obstetrics, particularly with the advent of operative deliveries. Mauriceau suggested in the mid-18th century that a recumbent posture was desirable because it facilitated delivery with obstetric forceps. The dorsal lithotomy position, introduced in the U.S. by DeWees in the 19th century, was the standard position for delivery in this country until recently. In Britain, the lateral position was popularized at about the same time. In many nonindustrialized societies today, the upright posture is still used during labor. Despite trends to the contrary, some American obstetricians even in this century have advocated the use of upright posture, or the lateral position.[68,83]

Although many reviews[86,107] strongly advocate use of the upright posture, preciously little information is available concerning either the theoretical or actual benefits of it. Several have emphasized that upright posture makes labor more efficient because it maximizes the benefits of gravity in dilating the cervix and the birth canal. Although this theory remains to be tested by appropriate physical experiments, it is doubtful that gravity plays a large role. The geometric relationship of the pelvis to the hind limb is the same in humans as in quadrupeds. The upright posture of humans is accomplished primarily by angulation of the lumbosacral spine at the sacrum. Thus, when upright, the abdominal and pelvic cavities are almost perpendicular to each other.[28] Upright posture would therefore not direct the fetus down the birth canal. In fact, in the lithotomy position, the inlet of the pelvis is perpendicular to the floor, and in line with the abdominal cavity. From the standpoint of creating the most direct passage for the fetus, the lithotomy position would be preferable to standing. Nevertheless, standing or squatting may have other benefits.

The fact that pelvic joints may relax somewhat during pregnancy is known to most obstetricians, particularly in the form of pathologic separation of the symphysis pubis.[124] Few have considered normal changes in the pelvic articulations as they may influence the progress of descent. In fact, the geometry of the pelvis may change considerably during pregnancy and labor as a consequence of increased elasticity and flexibility of the symphysis pubis and the sacroiliac synchondroses. These alterations in pelvic dimensions are influenced considerably by maternal position. For example, Russell[111] showed that the interspinous diameter may increase by as much as 1.5 cm when a woman moves from supine to a squatting position (Figure 2-1). Similarly, some positions increase the sagittal diameter of the outlet, including dorsal recumbent position with the hips and knees partially flexed.[9] This may also apply to squatting. In addition, it is possible that during squatting, posterior rotation of the iliac bones at the sacroiliac joints might increase the diameter of the pelvic outlet. The squatting position may further enhance descent by rotating the entire pelvis so that the abdominal and pelvic cavities are in line with one another, and thus perhaps reduce soft tissue and bony resistance. Also, during squatting voluntary contraction of the levator sling is inhibited, and insofar as such contractions would inhibit the terminal aspects of descent, they may be minimized by this posture.

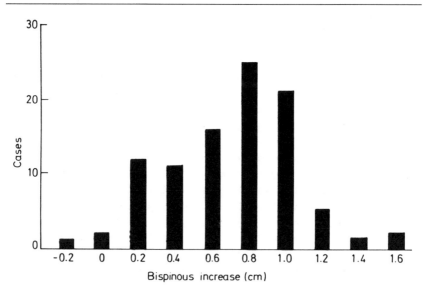

Figure 2-1 The distribution of increases in the interspinous diameter on assuming a squatting position from a supine position. These changes in pelvic dimensions may confer an advantage to squatting for some women in the second stage of labor. *Source:* Reprinted with permission from *British Journal of Obstetrics & Gynaecology* (1969;76:817–820), Copyright © 1969, Blackwell Scientific Publications Ltd.

In addition to these anatomic advantages, upright postures may make bearing-down efforts maximally effective. Mengert and Murphy demonstrated that the greatest rise in intra-abdominal pressure that resulted from voluntary bearing-down efforts occurred when women were in a sitting position.[89,93] Standing and squatting were also much more effective than semisitting or horizontal positions. These observations, made in nonpregnant women, were given clinical credence by Chen et al.[20] They demonstrated that sitting during second stage labor resulted in a rise in the baseline intrauterine pressure and maximal pressure during pushing compared to the supine position. Patients who sat had shorter second stages.

Few scientifically controlled studies of the effect of posture on labor have been performed. McManus and Calder[87] studied the effect of upright posture on labor by randomly assigning 40 patients matched for age, height, and condition of the cervix to have labor induced, and to maintain a recumbent or upright posture. They found no differences in the amounts of uterotonic agents, duration of labor, or type of delivery between the two groups, and concluded that upright posture showed no particular advantage. They noted that in the upright group, multiparas and nulliparas chose to remain out of bed 62% and 34% of the time, respectively. Flynn et al.[37] studied the effects of ambulation in the first stage of labor in 68 women who were randomly assigned to labor upright or recumbent. There seemed to be some disadvantages to recumbency insofar as those women had longer labors, needed oxytocin more frequently, and had more late fetal heart rate decelerations. However, the myriad factors that might influence duration of labor and need for oxytocin (e.g., pelvic architecture, fetal size and position), were not controlled.

Other studies indicate that uterine contractility, as measured by summation of intrauterine pressure recordings, may be greater in upright than in recumbent positions.[106] Nevertheless, an increase in pressure does not necessarily correlate with increased rates of cervical dilatation or fetal descent.

Humphrey et al.[65] studied the effects of dorsal supine versus the left lateral tilt position for the second stage of labor on fetal acid-base status. They noted that among those patients with second stages shorter than 30 min, there was a time-dependent decrease in fetal pH during the second stage in the supine patients, but not in the patients in the lateral position. During longer second stages up to a maximum of 60 min, however, there was no further fall in pH. Although few today would advocate the use of the supine position during the second stage, this study did not clarify whether the lateral position is clearly of benefit to the fetus.

Thus, considerable uncertainty still exists concerning the influence of maternal posture on labor progress.[81] However, much data support the notion that variants of upright posture, including sitting and squatting may optimize descent in the second stage by enlarging some pelvic diameters and maximizing the efficiency of voluntary bearing-down efforts. No information suggests any adverse implications of upright positions, and they should probably be encouraged during the pelvic division of labor, particularly if abnormal descent is present or anticipated.

Closely related to the question of optimal maternal position during the second stage is that of the most appropriate style of pushing. In most obstetric services the second stage is managed in "cheerleader" style. The mother is encouraged to bear down during most of the contraction with sustained Valsalva maneuvers of about 10 sec each. During these efforts she is exhorted to progressively greater feats of strength and endurance by a cacophony of cheers and approbations from her partner, nurse, obstetrician, and sometimes other onlookers.

A more urbane approach has been advocated that involves the mother pushing only when she feels an overwhelming urge to do so. Bearing-down efforts are exerted for a relatively short time with a partially open glottis, and sometimes considerable time may pass between attainment of full cervical dilatation and the urge to push.

Absent the obvious stylistic differences, can one ascribe a clear benefit to either approach? The Valsalva maneuver results in a decrease in distal aortic pulse pressure,[4] and may diminish uterine blood flow, although this has not been measured directly. Adverse effects of prolonged pushing on fetal acid-base balance have also been suggested.[14] Nevertheless, most women deliver normally oxygenated fetuses even if they have been pushing in the traditional manner for prolonged periods. Repeated prolonged Valsalva maneuvers should be avoided in patients with fetal distress and in those with a medical indication to avoid the dramatic fluctuations in blood pressure that accompany the maneuver. Continuous fetal heart rate monitoring should reveal early signs of deterioration if fetal oxygenation is diminished.

It would appear that either style of pushing is reasonable and safe for most women. It does, however, seem that occasionally heroic bearing-down efforts are necessary to effect spontaneous vaginal delivery. Intermittent brief pushing efforts may result in a longer second stage, but this should not generally be a concern. The choice of methods in the absence of abnormal fetal heart rate patterns should depend on the preference of the patient and, to a lesser extent, her caretakers.

SHOULDER DYSTOCIA

Few events that occur during parturition test the delivery attendant's mettle and sang-froid as does shoulder dystocia. It is a complication that is not always predictable or preventable, and that has potentially grave consequences. Although fetal or maternal adversity may occur despite expert obstetric management, optimal outcome in an individual case is possible only if the obstetrician or midwife understands the nature of the disorder and has a system of management to employ without delay.

Risk Factors

A number of studies have identified obstetric features that appear to be associated with an increased likelihood of shoulder dystocia. These include fetal macrosomia,[1,6,50,85] dysfunctional labor (arrest and protraction disorders),[1,2,63] long second stage,[6] midcavity delivery,[6,55,63,85,116] post-term pregnancy,[63] and maternal diabetes mellitus,[1] among others. Although the presence of one or more of these risk factors should alert the attendant to the possibility of shoulder dystocia (and sometimes lower the threshold for cesarean delivery), the majority of labors with these disorders are not compromised by difficult shoulder delivery. Acker et al.[1,2] have emphasized that approximately half of the cases of shoulder dystocia do not occur in large babies, and Gross et al. used multiple discriminant analysis to show that only about 15% of cases of shoulder dystocia can be predicted through knowledge of abnormal labor patterns and various maternal and obstetric variables.[56]

The data concerning the impact of a prolonged second stage of labor (usually defined as more than 2 hr in a nullipara and more than 1 hr in a multipara) are difficult to evaluate. It may seem logical that this would be a risk factor because large babies tend to have longer second stages; but most studies have not specified whether the long second stages involved descent disorders; nor have they discriminated the influence of the length of the second stage from the type of delivery in which it terminated. Indeed, virtually all studies of shoulder dystocia that have included instrumental midpelvic delivery as a variable have concluded that it is a major risk factor for the development of shoulder impaction at delivery.[6,24,55,63,85,116] It seems likely that avoiding midpelvic delivery when the second stage is long, and managing dysfunctional labor according to accepted paradigms, will help minimize difficult shoulder problems.

Mechanism of Shoulder Dystocia

During the normal mechanism of labor in a gynecoid pelvis, the fetal head engages and descends to the midcavity in a transverse position. As internal rotation and delivery of the fetal head occurs, the shoulders engage in the inlet, generally in an oblique diameter (although this is quite variable).[10] As the fetus descends through the birth canal and the head undergoes the cardinal movements, a process of shoulder "molding" probably occurs.[92] This term refers to the gradual way in which the shoulders and trunk accommodate to the conformation of the birth canal during descent; this process serves to ensure proper engagement of the shoulders. The posterior shoulder is then able to negotiate the sacral promontory, the anterior shoulder stems beneath the symphysis and emerges under the subpubic arch.

Several factors may, individually or in combination, confound the normal shoulder mechanism. These may relate to the fetus, to the bony pelvis, or to the rate of descent.

Fetal Factors

When the fetus is very large, the shoulders may be too broad to engage normally, and both may remain trapped at the inlet as the head delivers. More commonly, the posterior shoulder traverses the promontory, but the anterior shoulder becomes impacted behind the symphysis pubis. Fetal macrosomia is particularly problematic with regard to shoulder delivery in fetuses of diabetic mothers. The common clinical observation that shoulder dystocia is especially frequent in such fetuses was explained by Modanlou et al.[90] They showed that the bisacromial diameter in macrosomic babies of diabetic mothers was disproportionately large in relation to head size when compared to equal weight babies of nondiabetic mothers. Most of the babies in their study (with or without maternal diabetes) who experienced shoulder dystocia had these large shoulder measurements, and the authors recommended ultrasound evaluation of all suspected large for gestational age fetuses. They suggested cesarean section be considered if the difference between the chest and head circumference is more than 1.6 cm. Unfortunately, these measurements (and body weight estimation itself) are seldom made easily in the large fetus, and this approach is not in common use.

Pelvic Factors

The role of pelvic architecture in the development of shoulder dystocia has not been studied thoroughly. Seigworth reviewed 51 cases of shoulder dystocia.[116] In 9 of his cases pelvic roentgenograms were available. One-third of these had a narrowed anteroposterior (AP) diameter. Clinical pelvimetry in all 51 cases revealed only 4 with obvious contractions and 10 with a forward projecting coccyx. Clearly, difficult shoulder delivery can occur in a normal gynecoid pelvis, particularly if the fetus is very large. Unfavorable bony conformation probably plays a more important role when difficulties are encountered in the smaller fetus.

Both inlet and outlet architecture may be important. When the AP diameter of the inlet is narrowed, normal engagement of the shoulders may be impeded or prevented. Lack of engagement of both shoulders results in the most difficult (and sometimes insurmountable) problems. Most of the maneuvers used commonly to correct shoulder dystocia are ineffective unless at least one shoulder (usually the posterior) has negotiated the inlet successfully.

A steeply inclined or unusually long pubic symphysis favors impaction of the anterior shoulder, particularly if associated with a foreshortened inlet diameter. Contraction of the midpelvis is not generally a problem, although a laterally narrowed midplane may impede rotation of the bisacromial diameter, and an unusually flattened sacrum may inhibit descent of the posterior shoulder.

Outlet abnormalities may also hinder shoulder delivery. When present in isolation they rarely result in serious dystocia; but they frequently accompany other bony aberrations. A narrow subpubic arch prevents anterior shoulder delivery unless the other shoulder can be directed deeply into the posterior portion of the pelvis. If, in addition the lower sacrum and coccyx are directed anteriorly, delivery will be difficult. Sometimes even soft tissues of the perineum appear to impede the posterior shoulder, but adequate perineotomy should preclude or correct this factor.

Labor Factors

The influence of labor progress on the probability of difficult shoulder delivery is not well understood. Arrest and protraction disorders are indications of possible fetopelvic disproportion, and as such may suggest a large fetus, or at least one too large for the patient's pelvis.

It is the author's observation that many cases of shoulder dystocia, particularly when fetal size is not excessive, accompany precipitate descent. In these situations inadequate time for normal shoulder mechanisms may result in the bisacromial diameter remaining in the AP diameter of the inlet when the head has delivered. It is possible that the same process explains the frequent association of instrumental midpelvic delivery and shoulder impaction. By accelerating the rate of descent artificially, sufficient time for bisacromial conformation to the pelvis results in the shoulders being in an abnormal position or attitude at the time of their expected engagement. This may result in shoulder dystocia even when cephalopelvic disproportion is unlikely; when it is present, the problem is compounded and traumatic delivery is common.

Clinical Management

Several methods to manage shoulder impingement are in common use (Figure 2-2). Not all are appropriate for every circumstance. The obstetrician should have a standard and logical strategy to confront the problem; a repertoire of accessory maneuvers should be called upon in particularly resistant cases. One suggested scheme is presented in Figure 2-2. When the diagnosis of shoulder dystocia is made, a vaginal examination should be performed promptly to assess the position of the bisacromial diameter and the degree of descent of the posterior shoulder. In unusual circumstances a fetal anomaly may be identified to explain the failure of descent of the trunk. Rarely, the cervix may be felt over the anterior shoulder[61]; if present, an attempt to reduce it gently should be made. If the posterior shoulder is at or below the ischial spines in the hollow of the sacrum and the bisacromial plane is AP, the shoulders should be rotated into an oblique dimension. This is most easily accomplished by rotating the posterior shoulder ventrally by pressure behind the scapula. Some suprapubic pressure designed to push the posterior shoulder dorsally helps. Often these maneuvers are sufficient, especially if the pelvis is gynecoid and the fetus not unusually large. Some advocate awaiting the next uterine contraction before attempting efforts to release shoulder impaction.[67]

Whatever maneuvers are utilized to treat this disorder, several principles should be paramount. Despite the urgency of the situation, avoid the temptation to use very intense fundal or suprapubic pressure. They are helpful rarely and may result in fetal damage or in uterine rupture. In

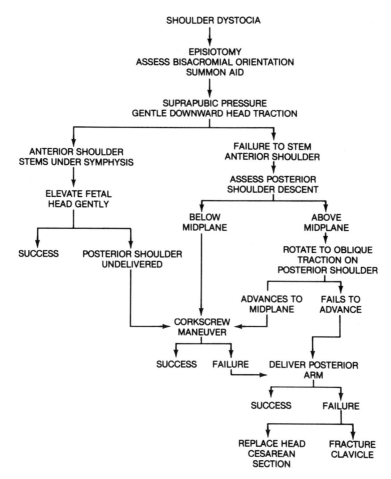

Figure 2-2 Paradigm illustrating a method of management of shoulder dystocia. *Source:* Adapted by permission from "Shoulder Dystocia" by WR Cohen in *Obstetrical Decision Making* by EA Friedman (Ed), BC Decker Inc, Toronto, © 1982.

addition, forsake persistent attempts to deliver the anterior shoulder by traction on the head and neck. It is remarkable how little force is sometimes necessary to produce brachial plexus injury. Finally, a large episiotomy is necessary to eliminate soft tissue resistance to delivery and to allow sufficient room for intravaginal or intrauterine manipulation. Several approaches are acceptable, but one should never hesitate to perform episioproctotomy to provide maximal space in this situation.

Many obstetricians use McRoberts' maneuver early in the course of shoulder impaction management.[51] By flexing the mother's hips against her abdomen the pelvis is rotated anteriorly, reducing the angle of inclination of the symphysis and sometimes allowing the impacted anterior shoulder to emerge between the pubic rami.

In 1943, Woods[123] described a maneuver that has remained the hallmark of management. All involved with obstetric delivery should be familiar with the principles and performance of this potentially lifesaving technique. Woods elegantly described the pelvis as a continuous inclined plane, or screw, with threads represented by the sacral promontory, pubic symphysis and coccyx. To deliver the shoulders the posterior shoulder should be rotated 180 degrees to the anterior position. This will allow it to stem under the symphysis. In most cases this maneuver is effective when attempts to deliver the anterior shoulder directly are not.

None of the manipulations described above is likely to succeed if the posterior shoulder has not engaged spontaneously. If this is determined on initial evaluation, the posterior shoulder should be pulled into the sacral hollow with fingers inserted posteriorly into the axilla. Slight rotation from an AP into an oblique position may be helpful. Once the shoulder is engaged, Woods's maneuver is often beneficial.

Another tactic that is used often, and may be beneficial even if the posterior shoulder is high, is delivery of the posterior arm.[84] With the anterior shoulder arrested against the symphysis, the operator inserts a hand along the ventral surface of the fetus and locates the posterior arm, which is usually extended. A maneuver analogous to that described by Pinard for delivering the extended legs during breech extraction can be used: The arm is flexed at the elbow, drawn across the fetal chest, and delivered. Once the arm is thus extracted, the other shoulder usually delivers easily. If not, application of the Woods maneuver is almost always effective.

Two other radical approaches to shoulder dystocia have been advocated for situations that do not resolve with traditional methods. Subcutaneous symphysiotomy has been utilized frequently and effectively in some parts of the world, but has never achieved acceptance in the U.S. or Europe. It seems extreme and potentially hazardous, but has enthusiastic supporters.[59] Recently, the Zavanelli maneuver was described.[112] It involves pushing the head back into the vagina and delivering the fetus by cesarean section. Only a few anecdotal cases have been reported, but the technique deserves evaluation as a method of last resort. Intentional fracture of the clavicle is often mentioned as a tactic for managing arrested shoulders. Although doubtless it is helpful, it is practiced rarely and may be categorized as more easily said than done. If resorted to in desperation, the force should be exerted with the operator's thumb. Injury to the subclavian vessels or entry into the pleural space may occur, and some have suggested its use be restricted to dead fetuses.[115]

A discussion of shoulder delivery problems would not be complete without allusion to the possible impact of maternal posture on this complication. Although controlled data are lacking, votaries of alternative positions for delivery claim that hinderance of shoulder delivery is encountered rarely when women deliver in upright postures.[19] Squatting for delivery has several theoretical advantages in this regard: voluntary expulsive efforts are maximized; the pelvis is rotated anteriorly, as in the McRoberts maneuver; the midpelvis may be widened; and the outlet may be enlarged by tension from the hip adductors.[115] Surely the putative advantages of squatting deserve evaluation insofar as it may prevent or be useful to treat shoulder dystocia.

EPISIOTOMY

Surgical incision of the perineum was first introduced as a discrete procedure in Europe in the middle of the 18th century. It was brought to the attention of Americans in the latter part of the next century, and obtained considerable popularity somewhat later as hospital delivery became commonplace in this country. Pomeroy[102] emphasized that episiotomy could prevent pelvic tissue damage during delivery and suggested considering its routine use for all nulliparas. There is a paucity of good scientific research that has been brought to bear on this issue. This is perhaps because episiotomy seems such a banal operation. This viewpoint is unfortunate because the commonness of the procedure makes it a considerable contributor to discomfort and morbidity in the gravid population.[8,53]

As forceps delivery became standard of care in the United States, episiotomy became quite important. In fact, DeLee[29] advocated routine episiotomy as an adjunct to prophylactic forceps delivery, and by the 1940s both were practiced widely. As trends away from operative (and hospital) deliveries have evolved more recently, the necessity for episiotomy has been once again called into question,[23,34,58,114] but the procedure is still performed in more than 60% of vaginal deliveries in the U.S.[47,118] Although there is much debate about the necessity and protective value of episiotomy, it has been subjected to very little systematic investigation.

There is some evidence that episiotomy may be associated with increased morbidity in terms of major lacerations (extensions) and sepsis,[34,96] but there is no unanimity of opinion in this regard.[13] Most data are consistent with the conclusion that rectal sphincter and mucosal lacerations are more common if episiotomy is used than if it is not, and that episiotomy probably does not prevent these major perineal disruptions in most circumstances.[12,119] Unfortunately, most studies of these phenomena are retrospective, and it cannot be determined whether the women who did not have episiotomies were at intrinsically lower risk for laceration because they had smaller babies, more favorable outlet architecture, or more elastic tissues. Recently, Thorp et al. reported a prospective nonrandomized study that supported the episiotomy per se as a risk factor for third- and fourth-degree lacerations, and they suggested that episiotomy be used only for operative vaginal delivery or fetal distress.[119] Much evidence does, however, suggest the potential benefits of episiotomy.

The application of local heat or oils for the massage of the perineum during labor has been advocated to reduce the likelihood of laceration. These techniques do indeed result in a reduced risk of perineal tears. Nevertheless, even if these are effective procedures, it is uncertain whether delivery over an intact perineum that has been distended to the extreme is a desirable virtue. As noted, little objective information exists in this regard. The pelvic floor is an extremely complex musculofascial structure that plays an important role during parturition by guiding the course of the fetal head.[103] Damage to the pelvic floor is quite common after vaginal delivery, but systematic and controlled studies of this phenomenon and of obstetric techniques designed to minimize pelvic floor trauma do not exist. Nevertheless, the collective experience of generations of obstetricians and midwives has provided some guidelines with regard to minimizing genital trauma.

Damage to the attachment of the vaginal walls to the underlying endopelvic fascia is especially significant as a precursor of pelvic relaxation later in life. The fascia and connective tissues supporting the bladder and the rectum may be damaged as the vaginal tube stretches during passage of the fetus. Of particular importance in this regard seems to be the elongation of the vagina that develops as the fetal head crowns.[46] Obstetric trauma in these supporting fascial areas will result in cystocele, rectocele, or enterocele. In addition, the levator ani muscles and urogenital diaphragm are less likely to be damaged if the vagina is not stretched excessively.

Gustafson[57] made several suggestions to reduce the development of cystocele after vaginal delivery. These included the avoidance of overdistension of the bladder, maternal bearing down prior to complete dilatation of the cervix, extremely rapid labors, and injudicious use of forceps. He also indicated, as have other authors,[33,46] that in order to minimize this kind of trauma, early episiotomy should be accomplished before excessive stretching of the vaginal and surrounding fascial tissues has occurred.

Gainey[45] examined 1,000 consecutive patients at their postpartum visits for evidence of pelvic tissue damage resulting from delivery. Among primiparas who had episiotomy and repair, laceration and repair, or neither laceration nor episiotomy, there was no significant difference in the frequency of damage to the upper pelvic floor and the pelvic diaphragm (pubococcygeus, ileococcygeus, and coccygeus with their enveloping endopelvic fascia). However, the anovaginal portion of the urogenital trigone was spared trauma in those patients who had episiotomies. Although this was not a controlled or randomized study, it did suggest that episiotomy was helpful in this manner.

In another study, a large series of patients delivered by low forceps with routine episiotomy was compared to a group of patients in which episiotomy was done only if laceration seemed imminent; the routine episiotomy group in general had much less damage.[46] There was a 27% incidence of total levator atrophy in the indicated episiotomy group, but only 11.2% in the routine group. Similarly, there was almost a three times higher frequency of cystocele in the indicated compared to the routine group.

Nugent[96] studied 202 term primiparas in whom episiotomy was performed only when a second-degree or greater laceration was expected. Although the total morbidity in the episiotomy group was higher and the episiotomy was done after the perineum had been thoroughly massaged and thinned manually, he found that there was a considerably increased risk of pelvic tissue damage ranging from minor degrees of relaxation to more major failures of integrity of the pelvic supports in the group with no episiotomies. He also noted that at the 6-week postpartum examination, patients who had incurred a spontaneous laceration had less apparent damage than those who delivered without any. In addition, more damage occurred in the spontaneous group as maternal age increased. Although this was a small, nonrandomized series, and the patients were not evaluated by a disinterested observer, it does suggest that pelvic floor integrity is enhanced by the use of episiotomy.

It would thus seem that if indeed trauma to pelvic fascia and to the pelvic floor can be avoided by episiotomy, this procedure will need to be accomplished prior to the considerable distension and elongation of the vaginal tube that occurs during crowning of the fetal head. It would be ideal, of course, to have a means to assess the likelihood of perineal laceration and other pelvic trauma prior to descent, but no such ability exists. If the anterior segment of the pelvic outlet is contracted, delivery of the head will occur at the expense of the posterior segment,[110] and a pelvis with this kind of architecture would require episiotomy, or at least a very thorough ironing out of the perineal tissues. With narrowing of the posterior portion of the outlet, injury to perineal soft parts is less likely. It could be argued, however, that in patients with a narrow posterior outlet, episiotomy might reduce trauma to anterior structures, particularly the tissues adjacent to and supporting the bladder and urethra. Current consumer trends have brought considerable pressure on obstetricians to eschew the use of routine perineotomy in vaginal delivery. It has been suggested both that spontaneous lacerations tend to be smaller and heal more readily than episiotomies, and that a skillful birth attendant can massage the perineum and the lower posterior vagina sufficiently so that trauma to these structures can be minimized or avoided completely.

Indeed, careful massage of the perineum during the second stage using sterile oils or standard water-soluble lubricant can reduce frictional shearing forces between the fetal head and the vagina and thus reduce the frequency and severity of perineal lacerations. Whether the advantages of this approach in terms of reducing immediate trauma and discomfort will be offset by an increase in long-term problems of pelvic relaxation remains to be seen, and should be studied systematically.

One of the major difficulties of interpreting the effects of a procedure such as episiotomy is that the most serious effects of maternal birth trauma are sometimes not visible until many years after the delivery. Although visible lacerations at parturition and evidence of pelvic tissue relaxation at a postpartum visit are important signs, they rarely indicate the more significant but invisible damage that can occur during delivery. Separation of the vaginal tube from its supporting fascial structures probably results in various degrees of uterine and vaginal prolapse, and descent of the bladder and rectum in later life. The extent to which routine incision of the perineum can avoid these problems is uncertain, and the logistical problems inherent in designing a study to test the hypothesis that routine perineal incision prevents pelvic relaxation are daunting. It has been suggested by Nichols and Randall[94] that in addition to overstretching and tearing of vaginal supports, slow progress in labor can result in prolonged pressure on the vagina and cause focal necrosis in the connective tissues supporting it. If this is indeed so, it is unlikely that episiotomy would reduce it, except insofar as it shortens the terminal portions of labor.

Clearly, the use of episiotomy is a relatively new phenomenon in the history of human birth. It has been suggested that increased longevity of the population has enhanced the likelihood that late problems from parturitional trauma will manifest themselves clinically. In addition, it may be that the generally sedentary lifestyles characteristic of Western civilization may reduce the strength and elasticity of the pelvic floor muscles and thus predispose both to trauma at birth and to late complications from it. None of these speculations has been tested scientifically. It does seem clear, however, that positioning the patient during delivery so that her thighs are not abducted and flexed excessively (thus avoiding stretching the perineal tissues) will allow a greater degree of distention and a lower risk of trauma as the fetal head encounters the pelvic floor. When patients are delivered in the semisitting position without stirrups, it is often helpful to extend the thighs slightly as the head is delivered, rather than having them flexed tightly toward the abdomen, as is customary. This will often allow some relaxation in the perineal structures, and lessen the likelihood of trauma.

The proper timing of an episiotomy is another matter of concern. General practice has been to make the incision as the fetal head is crowning when it becomes obvious that the alternative (spontaneous delivery) will result in lacerations. This approach will certainly limit the number of episiotomies performed, and if one's goal is to prevent the second-degree perineal tears (and the more common small periurethral lacerations) that accompany attempts at delivery over an intact perineum, late episiotomy is reasonable. But once the head is crowning and the perineum stretched maximally, most of the damage to the lower vaginal and perineal tissues has probably already occurred. Episiotomy prior to extreme distension of the perineum would seem to have the greatest likelihood of reducing the severity of permanent damage. As noted, the available data do not allow us to confirm or to negate the notion that early routine perineotomy clearly reduces these risks.

Of concern regarding long-term problems with uterine descensus is the duration of the second stage of labor. It is a generally held concept that long second stages predispose to later pelvic relaxation, perhaps a result of either overstretching of the fascial supports of the vagina or of factors relating to local tissue damage and necrosis mentioned above. In this regard, it is important to remember that although the author advocates that the second stage should not be terminated after an arbitrary period of time has elapsed, it should be terminated for certain definable abnormalities of labor. Whenever maternal bearing-down efforts occur without some progress in fetal descent, the efforts result in descent of the entire uterus and potential damage to its supporting structures.

The debate concerning the use of episiotomy will continue until some controlled studies with long-range follow-up are performed. In the meantime, for those who wish to avoid this procedure, gradual stretching of the perineal tissues during the second stage of labor seems to be important to minimize the risk of lacerations. To this end, the use of some lubricating oil or gel seems beneficial. In addition, the use of a delivery position that tends to stretch the perineal tissues laterally should be avoided. Thus, the dorsal lithotomy position leads to episiotomy being required more often because the tension that flexion and abduction of the thighs produces on the perineal tissues will make them less able to stretch as the fetal head crosses them.

When episiotomy is performed, it would seem that it is done to best advantage prior to extreme stretching of the perineal tissues. Nevertheless, if a spontaneous laceration seems imminent even a late episiotomy is worth doing. It allows the repair to take place in tissues that are strong, namely, the median raphe of the perineum. Although spontaneous laceration theoretically occurs along tissues that offer the least resistance, and results in less strong results when repaired, most spontaneous perineal lacerations occur in the midline.

Midline episiotomy is almost always the technique of choice, unless a major extension seems inevitable because the perineum is very short, the subpubic arch narrow, or there is a malposition or very large baby. Although advocates of routine mediolateral episiotomy exist, it seems difficult to justify that approach.

Whatever incision is used, it is wise to remember that the perineum is a complex structure, and failure to perform a proper surgical repair can result in considerable (and sometimes permanent) misery for the patient.

A standard midline episiotomy traverses the perineal and vaginal skin, and the midline tendonous attachments of the bulbocavernosus, the superficial and deep transverse perineal, and the levator ani muscles, as well as the urogenital diaphragm and the rectovaginal expanse of the endopelvic fascia. Each structure should be repaired anatomically with fine absorbable suture material, and each tissue layer should be approximated accurately with minimal tension.

Several studies to compare the efficacy of different suture materials and techniques for episiotomy repair have been published. Most favor the use of synthetic polyglycolic acid material,[69] but at least one investigator[12] found that this material was associated with more pain and delayed return to sexual function. Probably results are more related to the technique and care with which the perineal wound is repaired than to the nature of the suture. The author prefers 3-0 and 4-0 chromic catgut sutures for this purpose. Although somewhat more reactive in tissue than synthetic absorbables, catgut has the advantage of being resorbed more quickly. Prolonged presence of sutures in this type of wound may be a disadvantage and delay return of suppleness to the tissue. Placing sutures in the skin should be avoided generally, as this results in considerable edema and postoperative pain. The author uses interrupted 4-0 sutures to close the tissue immediately beneath the dermis. This brings the skin edges together to within 1 mm of each other; when the mother's legs are brought together, the wound edges are coapted and heal rapidly and with minimal discomfort.

A thorough knowledge of the functional anatomy of the pelvic floor and meticulous surgical technique are necessary to provide optimal results. The consequences of poor repair (prolonged or permanent dyspareunia) are considerable. The importance of attention to this detail of obstetric care cannot be overemphasized. In addition to the surgical issues, the psychosocial implications of the procedure must be considered. Kitzinger[77] has pointed out the emotional impact of this genital incision, and the sense of violation it can engender. Clearly, an explanation of episiotomy and an exploration of the patient's attitudes and preconceptions about it are important elements of prenatal care.

It is wise to remember that episiotomy involves severing the supporting fascial structures of the lower vagina. It is uncertain how many rectoceles are produced by inadequate or improper repair of episiotomies, but this is probably a factor. Scrupulous care should be taken to repair the defects anatomically. In particular, the perivaginal fascia must be closed.

FORCEPS DELIVERY

Obstetric forceps were introduced in the 17th century, and were eventually used routinely in obstructed labors. Although it was recognized that their injudicious use could result in serious maternal and fetal trauma, they were employed because the alternative, cesarean section, was associated with a formidable maternal mortality rate until the late 19th century. In the 1920s in this country, the use of elective forceps operations was popularized for all routine vaginal deliveries.[29] The avowed goal of this approach was to shorten the second stage of labor (long second stages were then thought to be associated with increased risk), and to reduce the compressive force exerted on the fetal head during delivery.

Forceps operations employed today include low forceps and midforceps procedures. When the instruments are applied after the fetal skull is visible between the labia without a contraction and the sagittal suture is in the anteroposterior diameter of the pelvis, delivery may be considered a low forceps operation. Those procedures performed when these criteria are not met, and when the biparietal diameter has negotiated the inlet, are considered midforceps. High forceps operations should never be performed because of their acknowledged high rates of mortality and morbidity.

Low forceps operations are part of traditional obstetric practice in many areas of the U.S. Nevertheless, their use has diminished in some institutions recently. This relates both to changes in anesthetic technique (more continuous epidural than spinal procedures), as well as to changes in attitudes of consumers and some health care providers and institutions. Although low forceps operations have been criticized by many, there is no evidence that when performed properly, they are associated with any increased risk. For example, Niswander and Gordon[95] analyzed the results of low forceps procedures using data from the Collaborative Perinatal Project. They identified a cohort of nearly 30,000 spontaneous and low forceps deliveries and found that there was no difference between the two groups in the frequencies of neonatal death, low Apgar scores, or 4-year follow-up of intelligence quotient (IQ) and motor activity evaluations. (In fact, there was a nonsignificant trend toward better outcome in the forceps group.) This study strongly suggested that low forceps operation is a safe procedure. In another large retrospective study, Nyirjesy and Pierce[97] showed no difference in perinatal mortality between babies delivered spontaneously or by low forceps operations.

Some studies suggest potential benefits of low forceps delivery, including increased umbilical oxygen tension.[109] However, all studies concerning the potential benefits of the low forceps operation suffer from flaws in experimental design, most pertinently in regard to the general absence of control groups or to consideration of potentially confounding variables. Because the compressive forces of forceps are probably greater than those in normal spontaneous delivery[91] it could be argued that their use always carries the potential for trauma. However, a number of factors other than compressive force are important in the development of fetal cranial injury. Satisfactory studies do not exist that compare the traction forces exerted during forceps operations to the expulsive forces of normal delivery. Moreover, the condition of maternal tissues, the mechanical deformability of the fetal head, the course of labor prior to delivery, and other factors influence the likelihood of trauma.

It seems reasonable to conclude that low forceps operations are usually safe procedures. Whether, when used routinely, they indeed provide improved outcome in comparison to spontaneous delivery is uncertain.

A review of the literature concerning the potential hazards of midforceps operations is more disturbing. In Chapter 17, a detailed evaluation is presented of the available information concerning the hazards of midforceps procedures, and the reasons why their use should generally be avoided in modern obstetrics.[39,41] Some details of this issue as they relate to management of the second stage are presented here.

Only a few studies have compared the outcome of midcavity delivery to the alternatives of cesarean section or spontaneous delivery. Chiswick and James[22] studied 86 consecutive attempts at delivery with Kielland's forceps, and compared these results to those of 86 spontaneous vaginal deliveries that occurred in the same year, and that were matched for age, parity, class, gestational age and frequency of induced labor, but not for complications of pregnancy. There were three neonatal deaths in the study group, but none in the control group. All the deaths were related to tentorial tears, and all of these babies had abnormal fetal heart rate patterns. Two of the three were delivered by cesarean section after a failed forceps procedure. There was a significant increase in the frequency of delayed onset of respiration, birth trauma, and abnormal neonatal neurologic behavior in the midforceps group. Even when the asphyxiated babies were excluded, 14.3% of the study group versus 1.4% of the control group had abnormal neurologic behavior in the newborn period. All of these abnormalities were transient, and there was no long-term follow-up of these infants. The explanation for the increased trauma in association with abnormal heart rate patterns could be that mechanical and asphyxial damage were synergistic, or perhaps that asphyxia leads to undue haste on the part of the obstetrician. Interestingly, in this study there was no significant difference found in the frequency of neonatal problems between the group of Kielland's forceps deliveries said by the obstetrician to be difficult, compared with those that were said not to be.

In a study of 71 midforceps operations performed at term compared to a group of similar patients delivered by cesarean section, Bowes and Bowes[11] found maternal morbidity rates were similar whether infants born after second stages of more than 2 hr were delivered by cesarean section, midforceps, or vacuum extraction. Neonatal morbidity was much lower after cesarean section (5%) than after midforceps or vacuum delivery (each about 20%).

Dierker et al.[31,32] studied immediate and long-term outcomes among babies delivered by midforceps operations and matched them with a control group delivered by cesarean section for similar indications. They found no adverse influence of the forceps delivery per se. The rate of midcavity delivery in their series was 0.8%, and most procedures did not involve major degrees of rotation.

It is possible that some of the recent evidence that has failed to document major degrees of risk from midforceps delivery results from their more judicious application than in times past. The risk of trauma associated with delivery from the midcavity appears to be proportional to the degree of rotation required, and the height in the pelvis from which the delivery is begun.[44] If one confines attempts at these deliveries to anterior or oblique positions with the head at station +3 or lower, and if each forceps application is considered a trial and abandoned if difficult, risks will be minimized. Whether they will be eliminated is unlikely. Even recent studies that show similar rates of complications for babies delivered by cesarean section with or without preceding trial of forceps reveal fetal trauma that resulted from the attempt at instrumental delivery.[80,120] It is difficult to be doctrinaire and to advise against all midpelvic deliveries because there are still clinical situations in which they may be warranted. Careful selection of cases, avoidance of major degrees of traction and rotation, and a skillful obstetrician may serve to minimize trauma.[27] This notwithstanding, the number of cases in which midcavity delivery is applicable is extremely small if the principles of second stage management described above are followed. Most often, allowing more time to pass with careful monitoring will result in spontaneous or outlet instrumental delivery. When a choice must be made between midcavity delivery and cesarean section, the latter is most often chosen, unless it is clear that the risks of cesarean delivery outweigh those of midpelvic instrumentation.

The use of the obstetric vacuum extractor is popular in some areas of the U.S. and in many other parts of the world. Advocates of the vacuum extractor point out that it is capable of producing great traction forces, but only a fraction of the amount of compressive force developed during a forceps delivery.[100] Studies evaluating the vacuum extractor are poorly controlled, and have not really been designed to show whether the instrument is safer than forceps. Most[3,54,100,104] but not all data suggest the frequencies of trauma and other complications with this instrument are roughly comparable to those of midforceps operations. Maternal perineal lacerations are less frequent with the vacuum extractor than with forceps, but trauma to fetal skin, including large cephalohematomas, does occur with some frequency.[101] The vacuum extractor is a safe instrument when used by trained individuals, but it is capable of producing undesirable results, including fatal hemorrhage in some instances. One possible danger of the technique is that the uninitiated may be tempted to apply it prior to complete cervical dilatation or at high fetal stations, or in situations in which attempts to effect vaginal delivery are inappropriate and potentially hazardous.

SUMMARY

Based on the information presented here, a method for managing the second stage of labor has evolved (Figure 2-3). The condition of the mother should be monitored with standard clinical techniques. If her medical status does not mandate termination of labor, consideration is given to fetal and obstetric problems. The routine use of continuous fetal heart rate monitoring (and intermittent fetal blood sampling, if indicated) is desirable. This is certainly so with prolonged second stages because

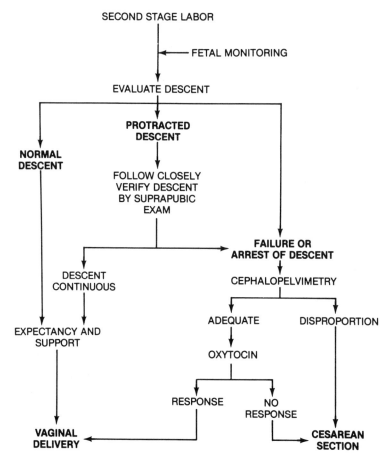

Figure 2-3 Paradigm illustrating a method of management of second stage labor. *Source:* Adapted by permission from "Management of Second Stage" by WR Cohen in *Obstetrical Decision Making* by EA Friedman (Ed), BC Decker Inc, Toronto, © 1982.

there does seem to be an increased risk of low Apgar scores in these situations. As long as there is no evidence of fetal hypoxemia, there is no *fetal* indication for intervention no matter how long the second stage.

There may, nevertheless, be an *obstetric* indication for intervention. The progress of labor in terms of dilatation and descent should be evaluated by the graphic means described previously. If descent is normal, and there is no other suggestion of fetopelvic disproportion, labor may be allowed to progress without interference. In the presence of abnormal descent patterns, clinicians should adhere to the paradigms described in Chapter 1 for guides to delivery and management techniques. Delivery by midforceps procedures should generally be avoided because of its potential for fetal and maternal trauma. This is particularly true of delivery from high stations after abnormal descent patterns.

Attention to measures of maternal comfort and emotional support are vital in the management of very long second stages. Some benefit may accrue from emphasis on the use of upright postures for pushing. The use of episiotomy should be based on the evaluation of the progress of labor and an estimate of the likelihood of maternal trauma. Careful attention to accepted principles of labor management and fetal monitoring can help avoid complications of long second stages, minimize the need for cesarean section, and optimize maternal comfort and fetal safety.

REFERENCES

1. Acker DB, Sachs BP, Friedman EA: Risk factors for shoulder dystocia. *Obstet Gynecol* 1985;66:762–768.

2. Acker DB, Sachs BP, Friedman EA: Risk factors for shoulder dystocia in the average weight infant. *Obstet Gynecol* 1986;67:614–618.

3. Baerthlein WC, Moodley S, Stinson SK: Comparison of maternal and neonatal morbidity in midforceps delivery and midpelvic vacuum extraction. *Obstet Gynecol* 1986;67:594–597.

4. Bassell GM, Humayun SG, Marx GF: Maternal bearing down efforts—another fetal risk? *Obstet Gynecol* 1980;56:39–41.

5. Bates RG, Helm CW, Duncan A, Edmonds DK: Uterine activity in the second stage of labour and the effect of epidural analgesia. *Br J Obstet Gynaecol* 1985;92:1246–1250.

6. Benedetti TJ, Gabbe SG: Shoulder dystocia. A complication of fetal macrosomia and prolonged second stage of labor with midpelvic delivery. *Obstet Gynecol* 1978;52:526–529.

7. Beynon CL: The normal second stage of labor: A plea for reform in its conduct. *J Obstet Gynaecol Br Commonw* 1957;64:815–820.

8. Beynon CL: Midline episiotomy as a routine procedure. *J Obstet Gynaecol Br Commonw* 1974;81:126–130.

9. Borell U, Fernstrom I: The movements at the sacro-iliac joints and their importance to changes in the pelvic dimensions during parturition. *Acta Obstet Gynecol Scand* 1957;36:42–57.

10. Borell U, Fernstrom I: Radiographic studies of the rotation of the foetal shoulders during labor. *Acta Obstet Gynecol Scand* 1958;37:54–61.

11. Bowes WA, Bowes C: Current role of the midforceps operation. *Clin Obstet Gynecol* 1980;23:549–557.

12. Buchan PC, Nicholls JAJ: Pain after episiotomy—a comparison of two methods of repair. *J R Coll Gen Pract* 1980;30:297–300.

13. Bueken P, Lagasse R, Dramaix M, Wollast E: Episiotomy and third degree tears. *Br J Obstet Gynaecol* 1985;92:820–823.

14. Caldeyro-Barcia R, Giussi G, Storch E: The bearing-down effects on fetal heart rate, oxygenation, and acid-base balance. *J Perinat Med* 1981;9(suppl 1):63–67.

15. Caldwell WE, Moloy HC: Anatomical variations in the female pelvis and their effect in labor with a suggested classification. *Am J Obstet Gynecol* 1933;26:479–505.

16. Caldwell WE, Moloy HC, D'Esopo DA: Further studies on the pelvic architecture. *Am J Obstet Gynecol* 1934;28:482–500.

17. Caldwell WE, Moloy HC, D'Esopo DA: The more recent conceptions of the pelvic architecture. *Am J Obstet Gynecol* 1940;40:558–565.

18. Caldwell WE, Moloy HC, D'Esopo DA: Studies on pelvic arrests. *Am J Obstet Gynecol* 1938;36:928–961.

19. Carter V: Another technique for resolution of shoulder dystocia. *Am J Obstet Gynecol* 1986;154:964 (letter).

20. Chen S-Z, Aisaka K, Mori H, Kigawa T: Effects of sitting position on uterine activity in labor. *Obstet Gynecol* 1987;69:67–73.

21. Chestnut DH, Bates JN, Choi WW: Continuous infusion epidural analgesia with lidocaine: Efficacy and influence during the second stage of labor. *Obstet Gynecol* 1987;69:323–327.

22. Chiswick ML, James DK: Kielland's forceps: Association with neonatal morbidity and mortality. *Br Med J* 1979;1:7–9.

23. Cogan R, Edmunds EP: The unkindest cut? *J Nurse-Midwifery* 1978;23:17–21.

24. Cohen AW, Otto SR: Obstetric clavicular fractures. A three-year analysis. *J Reprod Med* 1980;25:119–122.

25. Cohen W: Influence of the duration of second stage labor on perinatal outcome and puerperal morbidity. *Obstet Gynecol* 1977;49:266–269.

26. Cohen WR: Shoulder dystocia, in Friedman EA (ed): *Obstetrical Decision Making*. Trenton, NJ, BC Decker, 1982, pp 182–183.

27. Danforth DN, Ellis AH: Midforceps delivery—a vanishing art? *Am J Obstet Gynecol* 1963;86:29–37.

28. Davies JW: Man's assumption of the erect posture—its effect on the position of the pelvis. *Am J Obstet Gynecol* 1955;70:1012–1020.

29. DeLee JB: The prophylactic forceps operation. *Am J Obstet Gynecol* 1920;1:34–44.

30. D'Esopo DA: The occipitoposterior position. Its mechanism and treatment. *Am J Obstet Gynecol* 1941;42:937–957.

31. Dierker LJ, Rosen M, Thompson K, Debanne S, Lynn P: The midforceps: Maternal and neonatal outcomes. *Am J Obstet Gynecol* 1985;152:176–183.

32. Dierker LJ, Rosen M, Thompson K, Lynn P: Midforceps deliveries: Long-term outcome of infants. *Am J Obstet Gynecol* 1986;154:764–768.

33. Editorial: Pain after birth. *Br Med J* 1973;2:565.

34. Fischer SR: Factors associated with the occurrence of perineal lacerations. *J Nurse-Midwifery* 1979;24:18–26.

35. Floberg J, Belfrage P, Ohlsen H: Influence of pelvic outlet capacity on labor. A prospective pelvimetry study of 1429 unselected primiparas. *Acta Obstet Gynecol Scand* 1987;66:121–126.

36. Floberg J, Belfrage P, Ohlsen H: Influence of the pelvic outlet capacity on fetal head presentation at delivery. *Acta Obstet Gynecol Scand* 1987;66:127–130.

37. Flynn AM, Kelly J, Hollins G, Lynch PF: Ambulation in Labor. *Br Med J* 1978;2: 591–593.

38. Food and Drug Administration. Selection of patients for x-ray examination. *HEN-FDA* 1982;80-8104:9–10.

39. Friedman EA, Niswander KR, Sachtleben MR: Dysfunctional labor. XI. Neurologic and developmental effect on surviving infants. *Obstet Gynecol* 1969;33:785–791.

40. Friedman EA, Niswander KR, Sachtleben MR, Naftaly N: Dysfunctional labor. X. Immediate results to infant. *Obstet Gynecol* 1969;33:776–784.

41. Friedman EA, Sachtleben MR, Bresky PA: Dysfunctional labor. XII. Long-term effects on infant. *Am J Obstet Gynecol* 1977;127:779–783.

42. Friedman EA: *Labor: Clinical Evaluation and Management*, 2nd ed. New York, Appleton-Century-Crofts, 1978.

43. Friedman EA, Sachtleben MR: Station of the fetal presenting part. VI. Arrest of descent in nulliparas. *Obstet Gynecol* 1976;47:129–132.

44. Friedman EA, Neff RK: *Labor and Delivery, Impact on Offspring*. Littleton, MA, PSG Publishing, 1987.

45. Gainey HL: Post-partum observation of pelvic tissue damage. *Am J Obstet Gynecol* 1943;45:457–466.

46. Gainey HL: Post-partum observation of pelvic tissue damage: Further studies. *Am J Obstet Gynecol* 1955;70:800–809.

47. Gass MS, Dunn C, Stys SJ: Effect of episiotomy on the frequency of vaginal outlet lacerations. *J Reprod Med* 1986;31:240–244.

48. Gaziano EP, Freeman DW, Bendel RP: FHR variability and other heart rate observations during second stage labor. *Obstet Gynecol* 1980;56:42–47.

49. Gilstrap LC, Hauth JC, Toussaint S: Second stage fetal heart rate abnormalities and neonatal acidosis. *Obstet Gynecol* 1984;63:209–213.

50. Golditch IM, Kirkman K: The large fetus. Management and outcome. *Obstet Gynecol* 1978;52:26–30.

51. Gonik B, Stringer CA, Held B: An alternate maneuver for management of shoulder dystocia. *Am J Obstet Gynecol* 1983;145:882–884.

52. Goodfellow CF, Studd C: The reduction of forceps in primigravidas with epidural analgesia—a controlled trial. *Br J Clin Pract* 1979;33:287–288.

53. Grant A: Repair of episiotomies and perineal tears. *Br J Obstet Gynaecol* 1986; 93:417–419.

54. Greis JB, Bieniarz J, Scommengna A: Comparison of maternal and fetal effect of vacuum extraction birth forceps or cesarean deliveries. *Obstet Gynecol* 1981;52:571–577.

55. Gross SJ, Shime J, Farine D: Shoulder dystocia: Predictors and outcome. A five-year review. *Am J Obstet Gynecol* 1987;156:334–336.

56. Gross TL, Sokol RJ, Williams T, Thompson K: Shoulder dystocia: A fetal-physician risk. *Am J Obstet Gynecol* 1987;156:1408–1418.

57. Gustafson GW: The prevention and treatment of cystocele in the reproductive age. *Urol Cutan Rev* 1940;44:160–161.

58. Harrison RF, Brennan M, North PM, Reed JV, Wickham EA: Is routine episiotomy necessary? *Br Med J* 1984;288:1971–1975.

59. Hartfield VJ: Subcutaneous symphysiotomy—time for a reappraisal? *Aust NZ J Obstet Gynaecol* 1973;13:147–152.

60. Hellman LM, Prystowsky H: The duration of the second stage of labor. *Am J Obstet Gynecol* 1952;63:1223–1233.

61. Heery RD: A method to relieve shoulder dystocia in vertex presentation. *Obstet Gynecol* 1963;22:360–361.

62. Hillis DS: Diagnosis of contracted pelvis. *Ill Med J* 1938;74:131–134.

63. Hopwood HG: Shoulder dystocia: Fifteen years' experience in a community hospital. *Am J Obstet Gynecol* 1982;144:162–166.

64. Humphrey M, Hounslow D, Morgan S, Wood C: The influence of maternal posture at birth on the fetus. *J Obstet Gynaecol Br Commonw* 1973;80:1075–1080.

65. Humphrey MD, Chang A, Wood ED, Hounslow D: A decrease in fetal pH during the second stage of labor when conducted in the dorsal position. *J Obstet Gynaecol Br Commonw* 1974;81:600–602.

66. Humphrey M, Chang A, Gilbert M, Wood C: The effect of intravenous ritodrine on the acid-base status of the fetus during the second stage of labor. *Br J Obstet Gynaecol* 1975;82:234–245.

67. Iffy L: Comment, in Gross TL, Sokol RJ, Williams T, Thompson K: Shoulder dystocia: A fetal-physician risk. *Am J Obstet Gynecol* 1987;156:1416.

68. Irwin H: Practical considerations for the routine application of left lateral Sims' position for vaginal delivery. *Am J Obstet Gynecol* 1978;131:129–133.

69. Isager-Sally L, Legarth J, Jacobsen B, Bostofte E: Episiotomy repair—immediate and long-term sequelae. A prospective randomized study of three different methods of repair. *Br J Obstet Gynaecol* 1986;93:420–425.

70. Jacobson L, Rooth G: Interpretative aspects on the acid-base composition and its variation in fetal scalp blood and maternal blood during labor. *J Obstet Gynaecol Br Commonw* 1971;78:971–980.

71. Johnstone FD, Aboelmagd MS, Harounty AK: Maternal posture in second stage and fetal acid base status. *Br J Obstet Gynaecol* 1987;94:753–757.

72. Jouppila R, Jouppila P, Karinen J-M, Hollmen A: Segmental epidural analgesia in labour: Related to progress of labour, fetal malposition and instrumental delivery. *Acta Obstet Gynecol Scand* 1979;58:135–139.

73. Kadar N, Cruddas M, Campbell S: Estimating the probability of spontaneous delivery conditional on time spent in the second stage. *Br J Obstet Gynaecol* 1986;93:568–576.

74. Kadar N: The second stage, in Studd J (ed): *The Management of Labour*. Oxford, Blackwell Scientific Publications, 1985, p 271.

75. Kaminski HM, Stafl A, Aiman J: The effect of epidural analgesia on the frequency of instrumental obstetric delivery. *Obstet Gynecol* 1987;69:770–773.

76. Katz M, Lunenfeld E, Meizner I, Bashan N, Gross J: The effect of the duration of second stage of labour on the acid-base state of the fetus. *Br J Obstet Gynaecol* 1987;94:425–430.

77. Kitzinger S: Episiotomy, body image and sex, in Kitzinger S, Simkin P (eds): *Episiotomy and the Second Stage of Labor.* Seattle, Pennypress, 1984, pp 103–108.

78. Klapholz H: Evaluation of Fetopelvic Relationships, in Cohen WR, Friedman EA (eds): *Management of Labor*, Rockville, MD, Aspen Publishers, 1983, pp 25–40.

79. Krebs HB, Petres RE, Dunn LJ: Intrapartum fetal heart rate monitoring v. fetal heart rate patterns in the second stage of labor. *Am J Obstet Gynecol* 1981;140:435–439.

80. Lowe B: Fear of failure: A place for the trial of instrumental delivery. *Br J Obstet Gynaecol* 1987;94:60–66.

81. Lupe PJ, Gross TL: Maternal upright posture and mobility in labor—a review. *Obstet Gynecol* 1986;67:727–734.

82. Maresh M, Choong K-H, Beard RW: Delayed pushing with lumbar epidural analgesia in labor. *Br J Obstet Gynaecol* 1983;90:623–627.

83. Markoe JW: Posture in obstetrics. *Bull Lying-In Hosp NY* 1917;11:11–26.

84. Mazzanti GA: Delivery of the anterior shoulder. A neglected art. *Obstet Gynecol* 1959;13;603–607.

85. McFarland LV, Raskin M, Daling JR, Benedetti TJ: Erb-Duchenne's palsy: A consequence of fetal macrosomia and method of delivery. *Obstet Gynecol* 1986;68:784–788.

86. McKay SR: Maternal position during labor and birth. *J Obstet Gynecol Neonat Nurs* 1980;9:288–291.

87. McManus TJ, Calder AA: Upright posture and the efficiency of labor. *Lancet* 1978;1:72–74.

88. McQueen J, Mylrea L: Lumbar epidural analgesia in labour. *Br Med J* 1977;1:640–641.

89. Mengert WF, Murphy DP: Intra-abdominal pressures created by voluntary muscular effort. II. Relation to posture in labor. *Surg Gynecol Obstet* 1933;57:745–751.

90. Modanlou HD, Komatsu G, Dorchester W, Freeman RK, Bosu SK: Large-for-gestational-age neonates: Anthropometric reasons for shoulder dystocia. *Obstet Gynecol* 1982;60:417–423.

91. Moolgaoker AS, Ahamed SOS, Payne PR: A comparison of different methods of instrumental delivery based on electronic measurements of compression and traction. *Obstet Gynecol* 1979;54:299–309.

92. Morris WIC: Shoulder dystocia. *J Obstet Gynaecol Br Emp* 1955;62:302–305.

93. Murphy DP, Mengert WF: Intra-abdominal pressures created by voluntary muscular effort. I. Technique of measurement by vaginal balloon. *Surg Gynecol Obstet* 1933;57:487–493.

94. Nichols DH, Randall CL: *Vaginal Surgery.* Baltimore, Williams & Wilkins, 1976.

95. Niswander KR, Gordon M: Safety of the low-forceps operation. *Am J Obstet Gynecol* 1973;117:619–630.

96. Nugent FB: The primiparous perineum after forceps delivery. *Am J Obstet Gynecol* 1935;30:249–255.

97. Nyirjesy I, Pierce WE: Perinatal mortality and maternal morbidity in spontaneous and forceps vaginal deliveries. *Am J Obstet Gynecol* 1964;89:568–578.

98. Pearson JF, Davies P: The effect of continuous lumbar epidural analgesia on maternal acid-base balance and arterial lactate concentration during the second stage of labor. *J Obstet Gynaecol Br Commonw* 1973;80:225–229.

99. Phillips KC, Thomas TA: Second stage of labour with or without extradural analgesia. *Anaesthesia* 1983;38:972–976.

100. Plauche WC: Vacuum extraction. Use in a community hospital setting. *Obstet Gynecol* 1978;52:289–293.

101. Plauche WC: Fetal cranial injuries related to delivery with the Malstrom vacuum extractor. *Obstet Gynecol* 1979;53:750–757.

102. Pomeroy RH: Shall we cut and reconstruct the perineum for every primipara? *Am J Obstet Gynecol* 1918;78:211–219.

103. Power RMH: The pelvic floor in parturition. *Surg Gynecol Obstet* 1946;83:296–311.

104. Punnonen R, Aro P, Kuukankorpi A, Pystynen P: Fetal and maternal effects of forceps and vacuum extraction. *Br J Obstet Gynaecol* 1986;93:1132–1135.

105. Raabe N, Belfrage P: Epidural analgesia in labor. IV. Influence on uterine activity and fetal heart rate. *Acta Obstet Gynecol Scand* 1976;55:305–310.

106. Read JA, Miller FC, Paul RH: Randomized trial of ambulation versus oxytocin for labor enhancement: A preliminary report. *Am J Obstet Gynecol* 1981;139:669–672.

107. Roberts J: Alternative positions for childbirth. *J Nurse Midwifery* 1980;25:13–17.

108. Roemer VM, Buess H, Harms K: Zum Problem der Leitung der Austreibungs-und pre-periode. *Arch Gynaek* 1977;222:29–43.

109. Romney SL, Kaneoka T, Gabel PV: Perinatal oxygen environment. II. Influence of maternal anesthesia and type of delivery upon oxygen tension of umbilical cord blood and amniotic fluid. *Am J Obstet Gynecol* 1962;84:32–36.

110. Rongy AS: Discussion, in Gainey HL: Postpartum observation of pelvic tissue damage. *Am J Obstet Gynecol* 1943;45:457–466.

111. Russell JGB: Moulding of the pelvic outlet. *J Obstet Gynaecol Br Commonw* 1969;76:817–820.

112. Sandberg EC: The Zavanelli maneuver: A potentially revolutionary method for the resolution of shoulder dystocia. *Am J Obstet Gynecol* 1985;152:479–484.

113. Schlotter CM, Jager E, Wossner G, Scheub A: Fetale keryfrequenzmuster der austreibungs-und press-periode-typische muster, häufigkeit, aydoserisko und befundung. *Arch Gynecol* 1979;227:55–70.

114. Schrag K: Maintenance of pelvic floor integrity during childbirth. *J Nurse Midwifery* 1979;24:26–31.

115. Schwartz BC, Dixon DM: Shoulder dystocia. *Obstet Gynecol* 1958;11:468–471.

116. Seigworth GR: Shoulder dystocia. Review of 5 years' experience. *Obstet Gynecol* 1966;28:764–767.

117. Sheen PW, Hayashi RH: Graphic management of labor: Alert/action line. *Clin Obstet Gynecol* 1987;30:33–41.

118. Thacker SB, Banta D: Benefits and risks of episiotomy: An interpretive review of the English language literature, 1860-1980. *Obstet Gynecol Surv* 1983;38:322–338.

119. Thorp JM Jr, Bowes W, Brame RG, Cefalo R: Selected use of midline episiotomy: Effect on perineal trauma. *Obstet Gynecol* 1987;70:260–262.

120. Traub AI, Morrow RJ, Ritchie JWK, Dornan KJ: A continuing use for Kielland's forceps? *Br J Obstet Gynaecol* 1984;91:894–898.

121. Wood C, Ng KH, Hounslow D, Benning H: The influence of differences of birth times upon fetal condition in normal deliveries. *J Obstet Gynaecol Br Commonw* 1973;80:289–294.

122. Wood C, Ng KH, Hounslow D, Benning H: Time—An important variable in normal delivery. *J Obstet Gynaecol Br Commonw* 1973;80:295–300.

123. Woods CE: A principle of physics as applicable to shoulder delivery. *Am J Obstet Gynecol* 1943;45:796–804.

124. Young J: Relaxation of the pelvic joints in pregnancy: Pelvic arthropathy of pregnancy. *J Obstet Gynaecol Br Emp* 1940;47:493–524.

3

The Third Stage and Postpartum Hemorrhage

Wayne R. Cohen

Although in some respects the third stage of labor seems banal in comparison to the arduous and exhilarating events of the first and second stages, any obstetrician or midwife who has dealt with severe postpartum uterine bleeding approaches the third stage and immediate puerperium with respect. Postpartum hemorrhage occurs overall in 2% to 10% of deliveries.[18,20] Severe hemorrhage occurs in less than 1% of deliveries and is a major determinant of maternal mortality.[17,51]

Separation of the placenta is generally thought to result from mechanical shearing forces that occur when the uterine wall contracts underlying the broad placental bed. This is a reasonable but, perhaps, simplistic explanation. No studies of other anatomic or biochemical influences on separation have been performed, and the precise mechanisms remain uncertain.

Once separation has been completed, expulsion of the placenta occurs. The time course of these events is probably quite variable, and has not been investigated thoroughly. Placental separation occurs in most women very promptly after delivery of the fetus, as soon as the uterus contracts.[1] The signs ascribed to placental separation in most textbooks (bleeding, descent of the umbilical cord, contraction of the globular uterus) are more likely signs of placental descent. Under almost all circumstances, delivery of the placenta involves some intervention by an attendant. This may be an artifact of our general use of recumbent postures for delivery. If birth occurs in an erect position gravity (and perhaps minimal gentle assistance from mother or attendant) might result in more spontaneous expulsions.[33]

Because of our penchant for intervening in third stage events, and because of the difficulty in differentiating clinically the processes of placental separation and expulsion, it is difficult to assign normal limits to the third stage. Recommendations for intervention to deliver a placenta retained abnormally range from 15 min to 2 hr. The most useful data in this regard are those of Fliegner and Hibbard.[17,18,27] When minimal manipulation of the fundus was performed, and the placenta was expressed by fundal pressure after signs of descent were in evidence, 90% of placentas delivered by 15 min, and by 30 min, only 2% to 3% were still retained. From an operational standpoint, therefore, it is reasonable to refrain from active attempts at placental delivery before 30 min of the third stage have elapsed. Obviously, this approach must be tempered by the presence of excessive bleeding or other factors that mitigate against waiting. In fact, there is direct relation between duration of the third stage and the risk of accompanying postpartum hemorrhage.[17]

The definition of postpartum hemorrhage is as elusive as that of the duration of the normal third stage. The clinician might opine that puerperal hemorrhage is one of those events that requires no precise definition, because you know it when you see it. There is more than a grain of truth to this pragmatic view, but some more rigorously objective definition is necessary if we are to interpret the existing literature and to learn the best approach to third stage problems from the collective experience of our specialty.

Generally, postpartum blood loss in excess of 500 ml is considered abnormal,[20,51] and sometimes, for the purpose of retrospective studies, a drop in hematocrit of more than 5% from intrapartum to postpartum values is a useful guide.[12] However, the former is confounded by the well-known difficulty in the clinical estimation of blood loss, and the latter by major fluid shifts that occur in the first few days after delivery. Gahres et al.[19] used radiolabeled erythrocytes to estimate blood loss at delivery and found it normally not to be in excess of 500 ml for vaginal delivery. Pritchard,[40] who used a similar technique, concluded that the average blood loss at vaginal delivery was about 500 ml and that at cesarean section it was about 1,000 ml. About 7% of women who delivered vaginally had losses in excess of 1,000 ml, and a few had extremely small losses. Thus, the broad range of postpartum blood loss encountered normally and the difficulty in estimating blood loss accurately in the operating or delivery room make the diagnosis of postpartum hemorrhage imprecise and somewhat subjective. Most identified cases probably have hemorrhage considerably in excess of 500 ml.

Several features of obstetric history or of the progress of labor predispose to postpartum hemorrhage. Advanced age and parity and a history of postpartum hemorrhage in a previous pregnancy are risk factors. Dewhurst and Dutton showed that if a third stage problem occurred in a previous pregnancy, there was more than a 20% likelihood that one would occur in a subsequent pregnancy.[14] Conditions that result in excessive uterine distention during pregnancy (polyhydramnios, multiple gestation, macrosomia), that might interfere with uterine contractility (chorioamnionitis, inversion, leiomyomata, magnesium therapy), or that are associated with coagulation abnormalities (acquired or inherited) result in an increased likelihood of excessive postpartum bleeding.[20,42,51] Both prolonged and precipitate labors also predispose, for reasons less apparent. The increased risk of postpartum hemorrhage after a long second stage is accounted for by the frequent use of cesarean section and midforceps delivery in this situation.[12] Both operative delivery techniques may result in excessive blood loss from intentional (large episiotomy, uterine incision) or unanticipated (lacerations) trauma to the birth canal. The presence of certain factors that generally predispose to antepartum hemorrhage (such as placenta previa and abruptio placentae) also may be associated with excessive postpartum blood loss.

In the presence of any of these risk factors, the obstetrician can make certain preparations in anticipation of postpartum hemorrhage. Plans for delivery in an institution with the personnel and resources to deal with massive hemorrhage, an active approach to minimizing puerperal bleeding, and a plan for management of third stage complications are important in this regard. This preparation will help to minimize the consequences of postpartum hemorrhage if it occurs. Unfortunately, despite such preparations, hemorrhage cannot be avoided, but only managed more efficiently. Moreover, at least two-thirds of cases of postpartum hemorrhage occur in the absence of predisposing factors.[27]

MANAGEMENT OF THE THIRD STAGE

General Approach

There is a spectrum of opinion and practice regarding proper routine management of the third stage of labor. Advocates of active intervention prefer attempts to deliver the placenta within a few minutes of delivery, and generally use pharmacologic adjuvants to enhance uterine contractility and to expedite placental separation and expulsion. For example, it has been suggested[17,18,27] that an ergot derivative be given at the time of delivery of the anterior shoulder. Once the baby is delivered and the uterus contracted, controlled traction on the umbilical cord in combination with the Brandt maneuver[3] usually results in prompt placental delivery. In comparing this approach with experience at their institution during a previous time period in which less active management of placental delivery was employed, Fliegner and Hibbard concluded that active intervention reduced the frequency of postpartum hemorrhage from about 5% to 2%. The significance of this observation is uncertain because of the subjective nature of assessing postpartum hemorrhage and the possibility of bias when historical controls are used.

Objections to this proactive enhancement of placental expulsion are that it might result in uterine inversion, retained secundines, or cord avulsion. All of these are uncommonly the consequence of active third stage management, but when they occur they may cause considerable morbidity. A more rare but extremely serious risk of early intervention in the third stage is the potential compromise of an undiagnosed second twin. Also, the sustained contraction of the lower uterine segment caused by ergot derivatives might in fact retard expulsion and make manual removal difficult, although it is not clear to what extent this is a real problem.[1]

Sorbe[46] compared the outcome in two groups of women given either oxytocin or ergometrine at the delivery of the shoulders to that of a third group who received no uterotonic drugs until after placental delivery. The duration of the third stage was similar in all three groups, suggesting that pharmacologic treatment per se may not enhance placental expulsion. The women who did not receive the ecbolic agent until the end of the third stage did have more atony, but the excess blood loss averaged only about 100 ml.

Existing data do not demonstrate a clear benefit from active intervention to expedite placental delivery, except perhaps for reducing postpartum blood loss somewhat. It is unlikely that encouraging immediate uterine contractility with drugs or expediting placental expulsion manually reduces the incidence of severe postpartum hemorrhage. A reasonable approach, based upon available literature and experience is to allow delivery of the fetus and then to assess the condition of the uterus and placenta. Contrary to the opinion that there is a lull in uterine contractility immediately after delivery,[17] there is intense contractility documentable that probably occurs in most labors at this time,[25] making exogenous uterotonics superfluous. If bleeding is not excessive, and no other factors require prompt placental delivery, the Brandt maneuver (transabdominal pressure on the lower segment to push the uterus cephalad) with very modest tension on the umbilical cord should be performed periodically. If performed gently, these maneuvers will result in placental delivery in most instances. Absent hemorrhage or other serious complication, there is no reason to hurry. Vigorous traction may liberate the cord from its placental moorings. In addition to causing embarrassment, this event usually results in the requirement that the patient incur the potential morbidity of manual removal of the placenta.

Additional maneuvers have been recommended to expedite placental delivery. The placenta can be exsanguinated via the umbilical vessels. This is a harmless maneuver touted by some to ease placental separation or expulsion, but it has never been tested in a clinical trial. Recently, the infusion of 10 U of oxytocin into the umbilical vein was suggested to be beneficial by Golan et al.[21] After 30 min of the third stage without placental delivery, they infused 10 U of oxytocin diluted in 20 ml of saline into the umbilical vein in ten patients. This maneuver appeared to precipitate placental delivery. However, when the technique was applied 5 min after delivery, or with retained placenta,[9,32] it did not show any advantage over the injection of saline alone. It is still unclear whether injecting a volume of fluid into the umbilical vein will speed placental separation and delivery.

Use of medication to enhance uterine contractility prior to placental delivery is probably not necessary and, as noted, may entail some risks for questionable benefits. Administration of such drugs after placental delivery is almost universal if they have not been given before. Oxytocin is better suited to this purpose than ergot derivatives, which may cause significant hypertension.[22] The risk of oxytocin for this purpose is negligible, and therefore the practice is probably reasonable; however, it is not necessary in the majority of patients. An acceptable approach is to use oxytocin after placental delivery only in those women with a risk factor for postpartum hemorrhage. Nipple stimulation has been suggested as a replacement for pharmacotherapy in the management of the third stage,[30] and may be as effective, but its precise role in management remains uncertain.

Retained Placenta

Failure of placental delivery may have several causes: (a) separated placenta with contracted lower uterine segment preventing expulsion, (b) failure of separation of a normally implanted placenta, (c) placenta accreta. Of these possibilities the first is most common and generally easily remedied by manual removal of the placenta. Usually minimal analgesia or anesthesia is required, but at times uterine relaxant anesthesia (or a beta-mimetic drug) may be necessary to relax the myometrium and allow entry of the examining hand. Attempts to dislodge a still implanted placenta are more difficult and pose greater risks.

Sometimes expulsion may be delayed by inadequate contractions and to the extent that this mechanism is operative, oxytocin or ergot derivatives may be salutary. Their advantages must be weighed against the fact that manual uterine exploration and placental extraction may be more difficult with a firmly contracted lower uterine segment.

When the placenta has not separated and remains in the uterine cavity, a pathologic state is often present. Sometimes the placenta per se has separated, but adherence of membranes to the surrounding decidua may prevent expulsion.[33] Also, unusually broad, flat placentas or those with accessory lobes may not separate in a timely manner. In these and related circumstances (most of which are idiopathic), a cleavage plane can easily be identified by the hand exploring the uterine cavity, and the placenta removed manually. Manual extraction of the placenta must always be done with great care to ensure the placenta is completely removed and to minimize patient discomfort and the risk of genital tract trauma. Uterine rupture, although rare, can result from careless attempts at placental removal.[1]

Rarely, the placenta implants without an intervening layer of decidua spongiosum, and is attached directly to, or invades the myometrium. Various degrees of placenta accreta occur in about 1 in 2,000 deliveries. This results in a retained placenta. When the entire placental bed is involved, no plane of separation can be found. Sometimes focal areas are involved, and these tend to result in the most severe hemorrhage, as persistent attempts to remove the placenta are made. Hysterectomy is usually necessary, but sometimes can be avoided if the accreta is focal, blood loss is not excessive, and bleeding is controllable by other measures.[41] The definitive diagnosis of placenta accreta can be made only histologically, but the problem should be presumed to exist whenever a distinct cleavage plane cannot be developed between the placenta and the uterine wall. There is an apparent association of placenta accreta with placenta previa, especially when the latter occurs overlying a previous uterine incision. The dramatic increase in the number of cesarean sections done during the last decade will probably increase the frequency with which placenta accreta occurs.[41]

POSTPARTUM HEMORRHAGE

Early postpartum hemorrhage, the subject of this section, is usually defined as a blood loss of more than 500 ml in the first 24 hours after delivery. The most common sources of postpartum hemorrhage are genital tract trauma, retained placental tissue, and uterine atony. Less commonly, inherited or acquired coagulation defects may cause or contribute to these problems.[2] Coagulation abnormalities require treatment for replacement of specific deficient blood components.

A careful and systematic inspection of the birth canal should be done after every delivery to search for trauma. Lacerations of the cervix and vagina are most common after dysfunctional labor or operative vaginal delivery, but may occur under any circumstances. Much subsequent trouble can be avoided by detection and proper repair of lacerations of the lower genital tract before the patient leaves the delivery room. Uterine rupture is an uncommon, but obviously a very serious cause of postpartum hemorrhage. Sometimes patients with rupture present with abdominal pain and signs and symptoms of catastrophic hemorrhage. When disruption occurs in a previous transverse cesarean section scar in the lower uterine segment, bleeding may be minimal and symptoms less pronounced.

Retained secundines may take several forms, from complete retention of the attached or separated placenta to stubborn fragments of cotyledons or membranes that remain behind after placental delivery. When bleeding is due to the retention of the entire placenta or to normally implanted segments of it, uterine bleeding may be heavy, sometimes accompanied by atony. Curettage or manual removal is usually curative. Before attempting manual separation of a retained placenta, it is prudent to be sure that a large-bore intravenous line is in place for fluid administration, blood is available for transfusion, and a skilled anesthesiologist is in attendance. Unwitting attempts to remove a placenta accreta can result in hemorrhagic shock that evolves with startling rapidity.

Heavy uterine bleeding may sometimes occur in the absence of atony and without evidence of genital trauma or of a coagulopathy. This bleeding is commonly from the lower uterine segment, particularly if it has been the site of placental implantation. Bleeding from the lower segment may persist despite good fundal contraction, perhaps because the lower segment is thinner and inherently less contractile, and thus unable to provide hemostasis in the generously vascular placental bed. Bleeding from discrete areas in the corpus or fundus may also occur in the presence of a contracted uterus.[43] The etiology and source of such bleeding is usually difficult to define.

Uterine atony accounts for as much as 75% of cases of postpartum hemorrhage[51] and for about 40% of hysterectomies done for obstetric hemorrhage.[11] Several factors predispose to postpartum uterine atony. Whenever an overdistended uterus or dysfunctional labor precedes delivery or there is a history of previous third stage problems, the use of oxytocin immediately after placental delivery is important, as is gentle massage of the uterine fundus. Also, one should be sure that blood for transfusion is readily available, and that the anesthesiologist is aware of a potential problem.

If there is no response to oxytocin (which must be administered at a rate of at least 50 mU/min for effect) the administration of an ergot derivative such as ergonovine or ergometrine should be considered. Intramuscular administration will result in less of a rise in blood pressure than if the drug is given intravenously. Ergot derivatives should probably not be used if the patient is hypertensive or otherwise hemodynamically unstable.

Failure to respond to standard massage and to oxytocin and/or ergot mandates exploration of the birth canal. Even if the vulva, vagina, and cervix have already been examined, they should be rechecked to rule out lacerations as the source of hemorrhage. Uterine exploration should then be done with a gauze-covered hand or a large curette. This is an important step because even if the placenta appears to be intact, retained fragments or accessory lobes are surprisingly common. Moreover, for mysterious reasons, curettage sometimes provokes uterine contraction even if no retained secundines are removed. Obviously, anesthesia will be necessary for this procedure, and careful communication with the anesthesiologist regarding the need to avoid deep anesthesia and uterine relaxant drugs is pertinent, as well as an explanation of the current status of blood loss, and of fluid and electrolyte balance.

If bleeding continues after curettage, and the uterus is atonic, further pharmacotherapy is required. The development of a 15-methylated analogue of prostaglandin $F_2\alpha$ ($PGF_2\alpha$) has added a new dimension to the management of postpartum hemorrhage. The drug is more potent and has a longer duration of action than its parent compound, and is approved for injection into skeletal muscle, although intramyometrial administration has been used effectively. Whether the latter approach results in more rapid onset of contractility is unknown. In several studies 60% to 85% of patients with uterine atony unresponsive to standard therapy were treated successfully with 15-methyl $PGF_2\alpha$.[7,23,48] The usual dose is 250 µg IM. Most patients who have responded to the drug have done so after one or two doses. Repeated injections can be made at 15- to 90-min intervals, depending on the clinical situation. In one study of intramyometrial injection,[5] a second dose was given within 5 min of the first without adverse reaction.

Side effects of 15-methyl $PGF_2\alpha$ include a 10% to 25% frequency of gastrointestinal symptoms, and about a 5% incidence of pyrexia. Hypertension occurs rarely.[7] The drug is contraindicated in women with cardiovascular or pulmonary disease because of its potential hypertensive and bronchoconstrictor effects. Peak blood levels occur 15 to 60 min after intramuscular injection. As experience with this drug grows, it is possible that it will be used early in the treatment of uterine atony to achieve maximal effectiveness.

If uterine massage, curettage, and uterotonic therapy are to no avail, surgical or angiographic approaches are the next resort. The choice between the two depends on the clinical situation, in particular the rate of blood loss and the stability of the patient. There are still advocates of uterine packing,[26] but most authorities agree that this is helpful infrequently and carries considerable risks, not the least of which is providing a false sense of security that can be disastrous because hemorrhage may continue unobserved.

Angiographic Embolization

Angiographic management of otherwise uncontrollable postpartum uterine hemorrhage has achieved the status of standard therapy.[4] When bleeding is persistent but slow enough so that the patient is hemodynamically stable and can tolerate a 1- or 2-hr procedure, angiography is the management of choice. This obviously presupposes that skilled personnel and facilities for selective angiography and arterial embolization are available. When retention of reproductive potential is a high priority or when anesthesia is relatively contraindicated, angiography should be strongly considered. A catheter is advanced cephalad along one femoral artery and an arteriogram is performed to locate the bleeding site. The catheter can then be advanced distally into the offending vessels and blood flow stopped by embolization[5] or by infusion of vasopressin.[43] If specific distal bleeding branches cannot be identified, the anterior division of each internal iliac artery can be embolized. If bleeding continues after this or if angiography is being undertaken after surgical internal iliac artery ligation has already been performed, feeding collateral branches can be individually identified and occluded.[37] In this respect, selective angiography can even be useful after surgical therapy has failed; but it is performed most easily and is most likely to be efficacious if done prior to operative intervention. Angiography is even potentially useful in postpartum hemorrhage from vulvar or vaginal trauma with hematomas not amenable to surgical therapy.[24]

Surgical Treatment

In some cases of obdurate uterine atony, laparotomy must be resorted to. Surgical procedures involve either hysterectomy or reduction of uterine blood flow by selective ligation of pelvic arteries. Ligation procedures should generally be attempted first, although prompt hysterectomy may sometimes be necessary.

In 1952, Waters[49] suggested ligation of the uterine artery within the broad ligament to manage postpartum hemorrhage. This procedure was given a renaissance by O'Leary,[36] who described a simple, rapid, and safe procedure for ligating the ascending branch of the uterine artery adjacent to the lateral border of the uterus. Because it is so readily accomplished, this kind of uterine artery ligation should generally be done as the primary procedure. In addition, interruption of the ovarian artery contribution to uterine blood flow (which may be considerable during pregnancy) is straightforward and should be accomplished along with uterine artery ligation.

The ovarian arteries can be located readily in the mesovarium and ligated adjacent to the utero-ovarian ligament.[13] Alternatively, but surgically inelegant, a large ligature can be placed including within it the utero-ovarian ligament, ovarian artery, and adjacent myometrium, with the surgeon being careful to avoid compromising the fallopian tube or injuring the adjacent large venous anastomoses between the uterine and ovarian vessels. The surgeon should avoid ligating the ovarian vessels more proximally at the infundibulopelvic ligament lest the devascularization results in loss of the ovaries if hysterectomy proves necessary. If combined uterine and ovarian ligation is not successful in controlling uterine hemorrhage, occlusion of the internal iliac arteries may be attempted. This procedure was probably first described for massive pelvic hemorrhage by Baumgartner in 1888.[45] Despite the fact that it is successful (defined as no need for subsequent hysterectomy) in only 40% to 50% of cases,[10,16] it is a worthwhile procedure because the only other available alternative at this point is hysterectomy.

Internal iliac artery ligation works to control uterine hemorrhage by decreasing pulse pressure and blood flow in the pelvis dramatically.[6] The uterine arterial inflow loses its pulsatile quality and becomes hemodynamically more like a venous circulation, in which hemostasis occurs more readily. The effect of the ligation procedure is primarily ipsilateral. Ligation of one artery may be useful if the source of the bleeding is known to be on that side; but in most cases bilateral ligation is necessary. The collateral arterial circulation of the pelvis is so rich that uterine blood flow remains adequate to support normal pregnancy even after ligation of both internal iliac and both ovarian arteries.[34]

It is important to stress that internal iliac artery ligation should not be attempted by a surgeon unfamiliar with retroperitoneal dissection in this area or with the management of the most serious complication of the operation, namely, large vessel injury, most commonly to the iliac veins. It is useful to have a set of surgical instruments designated for iliac artery ligation available in the delivery suite. The safety of the operation is facilitated if suitable instrumentation and suture material is readily at hand for surgery and management of complications.

The presence of a large postpartum uterus may make exposure of the operative field difficult. It is therefore especially important to proceed cautiously and to verify anatomic landmarks. The artery is best approached by incising the parietal peritoneum over the surface of the psoas major muscle, a landmark identified easily. By reflecting the cut edge of the peritoneum medially, the external iliac artery and usually the genitofemoral nerve are identified readily. Gentle traction on the peritoneal flap will expose the ureter, which may be pulled out of harm's way by a retractor placed in the superior angle of the peritoneal incision. Dissection should take place cephalad along the anterior surface of the external iliac artery until the bifurcation is reached. This is usually identified by the presence of a subtle bulge in the diameter of the vessel. The internal iliac artery is directed posteriorly, and dissection should continue on its anterior surface for a distance of approximately 1 cm. It is important to maintain the plane of dissection on the anterior surface of the arteries in order to avoid injury to the underlying relatively fragile external and internal iliac veins. A ligature should be placed around the internal iliac artery with care. Although some stress the importance of placing this ligature distal to the posterior division of the artery, this probably makes little practical difference in outcome. Use of absorbable suture allows subsequent canalization of vessels,[15] but even if permanent suture is used, ultimate uterine blood flow is not compromised. If bilateral ligation of uterine, ovarian, and internal iliac arteries has not diminished bleeding sufficiently, hysterectomy is the only remaining recourse. Although total hysterectomy is usually preferred, this is a situation in which supracervical hysterectomy is often sufficient therapy, and may be useful when the patient is hemodynamically unstable and operating time must be minimized.

Uterine Inversion

Acute puerperal inversion of the uterus is an uncommon cause of severe postpartum hemorrhage, and sometimes of shock. The patient usually complains of pain, and bleeding may be sudden and profuse. The inverted fundus often presents as a mass visible at the introitus or, less commonly, may be discovered on routine examination of the cervix after delivery.[2] Inversion is sometimes iatrogenic, the result of overzealous traction on the umbilical cord during the third stage.[39,50] Some cases, however, occur in the presence of uterine atony or without apparent cause or provocation. Prompt replacement of the fundus is important to minimize bleeding and to prevent or reduce hypotension, which is said to be sometimes out of proportion to the blood loss, perhaps the result of a vasovagal response.

The traditional approach to this disorder has been to attempt replacement of the fundus under general anesthesia using the method of Johnson.[28] With uterine relaxant anesthesia, the palm of the hand is placed over the dome of the inverted fundus and the uterus is elevated into the abdominal cavity. Firm and persistent pressure at the uterine-cervical junction by the examining hand puts tension on the uterine ligaments and in 3 to 5 min the fundus usually begins to recede. If this maneuver fails, laparotomy and surgical reversion are advocated. Fortunately, surgery is rarely necessary.

Modern obstetric drugs have led to a new method of management that seems to be highly efficacious. When the inversion is identified, a tocolytic drug is given to relax the uterus. The Johnson maneuver[28] is then used and the fundus replaced with relative ease, sometimes without the requirement for anesthesia.[8,31,47] After replacement of the fundus, 15-methyl $PGF_2\alpha$ is given to induce firm myometrial contraction and to prevent reinversion. Ritodrine or terbutaline has been used as a uterine relaxant for the treatment of uterine inversion,[31,47] but Catanzarite et al.[8] prefer magnesium sulfate. Beta-mimetic drugs may potentiate hypotension if the patient has become volume depleted, and this would probably be less problematic with magnesium.

Management of Shock

Hemorrhagic shock can be a consequence of many obstetric procedures. It is beyond the scope of this chapter to review the management of this disorder in detail, but several features are pertinent to emphasize in this context.

As in most acute medical illnesses, to be forewarned is to be forearmed, and insofar as postpartum hemorrhage can be anticipated by attention to prevailing risk factors, therapy will be facilitated. Every obstetric unit should be prepared to deal with unexpected massive hemorrhage. Successful management of exsanguinating postpartum bleeding depends heavily on smooth collaboration among all members of the team, including nurses, obstetrician, and anesthesiologist. The general principle of therapy is to identify hypovolemia promptly and begin rapid fluid replacement while attempts are made to treat the source of the hemorrhage. The more profound and long-lasting the hypovolemia, the more severe are the associated manifestations of shock, including hypoxemia, acidosis, and disseminated intravascular coagulation.

Initial fluid resuscitation usually should consist of large volumes of crystalloid solution. When hemorrhage is massive, more than one intravenous line is necessary, as well as a pressure apparatus to administer fluids rapidly. Placement of a central venous pressure catheter is very useful to help monitor fluid therapy. The use of colloid preparations is controversial, but some individuals believe they are beneficial to help rapidly expand plasma volume. Blood replacement can generally be accomplished with packed red blood cells once initial volume deficits are treated.

When very large volumes of fluid replacement are necessary, dilution of clotting factors may occur and exacerbate the bleeding tendency. Moreover, shock may provoke disseminated intravascular coagulation. One unit of fresh frozen plasma should be given for each 5 U of transfused red blood cells to help sustain levels of clotting factors that are absent in banked blood. Platelet concentrates are also useful and should be given as necessary. Other specific blood component therapy for inherited or acquired coagulation defects is appropriate. Profound hypofibrinogenemia complicates placental abruption and other causes of obstetric hemorrhage. Fresh frozen plasma and cryoprecipitate are the most concentrated sources of fibrinogen for replacement.

In the presence of serious bleeding, use of medical or military antishock trousers (MAST suit) may prove useful in preparation for surgery or, in extreme situations, when surgical intervention has proved fruitless in staunching hemorrhage.[38] MAST trousers consist of inflatable leggings and a circumferential abdominal binder. When inflated, the device raises blood pressure, probably primarily by increasing total peripheral resistance. The result is the preservation of blood flow to vital upper body organs at the expense of the lower body. The MAST suit has proved lifesaving in several kinds of obstetric and gynecologic bleeding, including postpartum hemorrhage.[9,38,44] A concern about the possibility of inducing an air embolism when the suit is used in women with uterine bleeding was raised,[35] but subsequent experience has not confirmed this.

Fortunately, most women with massive obstetric bleeding are otherwise healthy. Anticipation and early recognition of excessive bleeding with prompt attention to volume replacement and identification of the source of the bleeding are critical features of management. Intervention with the appropriate pharmacologic, angiographic, or surgical procedure results in a gratifying outcome most of the time.

REFERENCES

1. Aaberg ME, Reid DE: Manual removal of the placenta. *Am J Obstet Gynecol* 1945;49:368–377.

2. Bell JE, Wilson GF, Wilson LA: Puerperal inversion of the uterus. *Am J Obstet Gynecol* 1953;66:767–780.

3. Brandt ML: The mechanism and management of the third stage of labor. *Am J Obstet Gynecol* 1933;25:662–667.

4. Brown BJ, Heaston DK, Poulson AM, Gabert HA, Mineau DE, Miller FJ Jr: Uncontrollable postpartum bleeding: A new approach to hemostasis through angiographic arterial embolization. *Obstet Gynecol* 1979;54:361–364.

5. Bruce SL, Paul RH, Van Dorsten JP: Control of postpartum uterine atony by intramyometrial prostaglandin. *Obstet Gynecol* 1982;59:47S–50S.

6. Burchell RC: Physiology of internal iliac artery ligation. *J Obstet Gynaecol Br Commonw* 1968;75:642–651.

7. Buttino L Jr, Garite TJ: The use of 15 methyl F2x prostaglandin (prostin 15M) for the control of postpartum hemorrhage. *Am J Perinatol* 1986;3:241–243.

8. Catanzarite VA, Moffitt KD, Baker ML, Awadalla SG, Argubright KF, Perkins RP: New approaches to the management of acute puerperal uterine inversion. *Obstet Gynecol* 1986;68:75–105.

9. Chestnut DH, Wilcox LL: Influence of umbilical vein administration of oxytocin on the third stage of labor: A randomized, double-blind, placebo-controlled study. *Am J Obstet Gynecol* 1987;157:160–162.

10. Clark SL, Phelan JP, Yeh S-Y, Bruce SR, Paul RH: Hypogastric artery ligation for obstetric hemorrhage. *Obstet Gynecol* 1985;66:353–356.

11. Clark SL, Yeh S-Y, Phelan JP, Bruce SR, Paul RH: Emergency hysterectomy for obstetric hemorrhage. *Obstet Gynecol* 1984;64:376–380.

12. Cohen WR: Influence of the duration of second stage labor on perinatal outcome and puerperal morbidity. *Obstet Gynecol* 1977;49:266–269.

13. Cruikshank SH, Stoelk EM: Surgical control of pelvic hemorrhage: Method of bilateral ovarian artery ligation. *Am J Obstet Gynecol* 1983;149:724–725.

14. Dewhurst CJ, Dutton WAW: Recurrent abnormalities of the third stage of labor. *Lancet* 1957;2:764–767.

15. Dubay ML, Holshauser CA, Burchell RC: Internal iliac artery ligation for postpartum hemorrhage: Recanalization of vessels. *Am J Obstet Gynecol* 1980;136:689–691.

16. Evans S, McShane P: The efficacy of internal iliac artery ligation in obstetric hemorrhage. *Surg Gynecol Obstet* 1985;160:250–253.

17. Fliegner JR: Third stage management: How important is it? *Med J Aust* 1978;2:190–193.

18. Fliegner JR, Hibbard BM: Active management of the third stage of labour. *Br Med J* 1966;2:622–623.

19. Gahres EE, Albert SM, Dodek SM: Intrapartum blood loss measured with Cr^{51} tagged erythrocytes. *Obstet Gynecol* 1962;19:455–462.

20. Gilbert L, Porter W, Brown VA: Postpartum hemorrhage—a continuing problem. *Br J Obstet Gynecol* 1987;94:67–71.

21. Golan A, Lidor AL, Wexler S, David MP: A new method for the management of the retained placenta. *Am J Obstet Gynecol* 1983;146:708–709.

22. Hacker NF, Biggs JS: Blood pressure changes when uterine stimulants are used after normal delivery. *Br J Obstet Gynecol* 1979;86:633–636.

23. Hayashi RH, Castillo MS, Noah ML: Management of severe postpartum hemorrhage with a prostaglandin F2α analogue. *Obstet Gynecol* 1984;63:806–808.

24. Heffner LJ, Mennuti MT, Rudoff JC, McLean GK: Primary management of postpartum vulvovaginal hematomas by angiographic embolization. *Am J Perinatol* 1985;2:204–206.

25. Hendricks CH, Eskes TK, Saameli K: Uterine contractility at delivery, and in the puerperium. *Am J Obstet Gynecol* 1962;83:890–906.

26. Hester JD: Postpartum hemorrhage and reevaluation of uterine packing. *Obstet Gynecol* 1975;45:501–504.

27. Hibbard BH: The third stage of labour. *Br Med J* 1964;1:1485–1488.

28. Johnson AB: A new concept in the replacement of the inverted uterus and a report of nine cases. *Am J Obstet Gynecol* 1949;57:557–562.

29. Kaback KR, Sanders AB, Meislin HW: MAST suit update. *JAMA* 1984;252:2598–2603.

30. Kim YM, Tejani N, Chayen B, Verma U: Management of the third stage of labor with nipple stimulation. *J Reprod Med* 1987;32:1033–1034.

31. Kovacks BW, DeVore GR: Management of acute and subacute puerperal uterine inversion with terbutaline sulfate. *Am J Obstet Gynecol* 1984;150:784–786.

32. Kristiansen FV, Frost L, Kaspersen P, Moller BR: The effect of oxytocin injection into the umbilical vein for the management of the retained placenta. *Am J Obstet Gynecol* 1987;156:979–980.

33. Leff M: Management of the third and fourth stage of labor. *Surg Gynecol Obstet* 1939;68:224–229.

34. Mengert WF, Burchell RC, Blumstein RW, Daskal JL: Pregnancy after bilateral ligation of the internal iliac and ovarian arteries. *Obstet Gynecol* 1969;34:664–666.

35. McBride G: One caution in pneumatic anti-shock garment use. *JAMA* 1982;247:1112.

36. O'Leary JL, O'Leary JA: Uterine artery ligation for control of postcesarean section hemorrhage. *Obstet Gynecol* 1974;43:849–853.

37. Pais SO, Glickman M, Schwartz P, Pingoud E, Berkowitz R: Embolization of pelvic arteries for control of postpartum hemorrhage. *Obstet Gynecol* 1980;55:754–758.

38. Pearse CS, Magrina JF, Finley BE: Use of MAST suit in obstetrics and gynecology. *Obstet Gynecol Surv* 1984;39:416–422.

39. Platt LD, Druzin ML: Acute puerperal inversion of the uterus. *Am J Obstet Gynecol* 1981;141:187–190.

40. Pritchard JA: Changes in the blood volume during pregnancy and delivery. *Anesthesiology* 1965;26:393–399.

41. Read JA, Cotton DB, Miller FC: Placenta accreta: Changing clinical aspects and outcome. *Obstet Gynecol* 1980;56:31–34.

42. Reece EA, Fox HE, Rapoport F: Factor VIII inhibitor: A cause of severe postpartum hemorrhage. *Am J Obstet Gynecol* 1982;144:985–987.

43. Sachs B, Palestrandt A, Cohen WR: Internal iliac artery vasopressin infusion for postpartum hemorrhage. *Am J Obstet Gynecol* 1982;143:601–603.

44. Sandberg EC, Pelligra R: The medical antigravity suit for management of surgically uncontrollable bleeding associated with abdominal pregnancy. *Am J Obstet Gynecol* 1983;146:519–525.

45. Smith DC, Wyatt JF: Embolization of the hypogastric arteries in the control of massive vaginal hemorrhage. *Obstet Gynecol* 1977;49:317–322.

46. Sorbe B: Active pharmacologic management of the third stage of labor. *Obstet Gynecol* 1978;52:694–697.

47. Thiery M, Delveke L: Acute puerperal uterine inversion: Two-step management with a β-mimetic and a prostaglandin. *Am J Obstet Gynecol* 1985;153:891–892.

48. Toppozada M, El-Bossaty M, El-Rahman HA, El-Din AHS: Control of intractable atonic postpartum hemorrhage by 15-methyl prostaglandin F2x. *Obstet Gynecol* 1981;58:327–330.

49. Waters EG: Surgical management of postpartum hemorrhage with particular reference to ligation of uterine arteries. *Am J Obstet Gynecol* 1952;64:1143–1148.

50. Watson P, Besch N, Bowes WA Jr: Management of acute and subacute puerperal inversion of the uterus. *Obstet Gynecol* 1980;55:12–16.

51. Weekes LR, O'Toole DM: Postpartum hemorrhage. A five-year study at Queen of Angels Hospital. *Am J Obstet Gynecol* 1956;71:45–50.

4

Obstetric Analgesia and Anesthesia

Scott Fisher, Gerard Ostheimer, and Thomas M. Warren

MAJOR PHYSIOLOGIC CHANGES IN PREGNANT WOMEN

In order to provide appropriate analgesia and anesthesia, the anesthetist must have a thorough knowledge of the physiologic changes that occur during pregnancy, labor, and delivery. The same quality of care that is available in the operating room must be available in the labor and delivery area for the parturient and her fetus or newborn.[165]

Alterations in Gastric Emptying

During pregnancy, progesterone decreases gastrointestinal motility and relaxes the gastroesophageal sphincter. At term the gravid uterus mechanically obstructs the duodenum and increases intragastric pressure during labor. There may be an increase in gastric acidity secondary to enhanced stimulation of the parietal cells by gastrin. During labor, there is a diminution in gastric emptying with the accumulation of gastric juice and gas. These conditions greatly increase the risk of regurgitation and aspiration. Approximately 30% of maternal anesthesia-related deaths are caused by vomiting and aspiration.

In 1946 Mendelson described the clinical syndrome of aspiration pneumonitis.[146] He injected human stomach contents into the lungs of rabbits. When the injected liquids were chemically neutralized, pneumonitis could not be produced. Unaltered human gastric contents, however, produced lung lesions similar to those found during autopsies on people who had aspirated gastric contents and subsequently died. The same pathologic changes were produced by injecting dilute hydrochloric acid solution into the lungs of animals.

Later, Teabeaut[207] found that hydrochloric acid solutions and liquid vomitus must have a pH less than 2.5 in order to produce pneumonitis. Teabeaut also reported that partially digested foods at various pH levels recovered from the stomachs of human volunteers produced pneumonitis in experimental animal lungs. Peptic activity and bacterial infection played no part in producing the aspiration lesions. These observations suggest that gastric fluid containing particulate matter or having a pH less than 2.5 can produce aspiration pneumonitis.

Roberts and Shirley[183] studied 146 patients in labor and demonstrated that 1 in 4 was at risk of acid aspiration. They defined the at risk patient as one who had at least 25 mL of gastric juice of pH less than 2.5 in the stomach at delivery. The use of oral antacids during labor reduces the number of patients at risk. However, the particles in some antacid emulsions may also be hazardous.[89] At least 30 min of elapsed time is necessary for adequate gastric mixing and acid neutralizing with regular antacids.[101]

Glycopyrrolate, a quarternary ammonium compound, decreases salivary activity and gastric secretion. Only minute quantities cross the placenta. Premedication with glycopyrrolate results in gastric pH greater than 2.5 in almost all parturients undergoing elective cesarean delivery.[8]

Recent investigations have focused on the use of clear antacids (sodium citrate) and parenteral medications that decrease gastric emptying time (metoclopramide) or decrease gastric acidity and secretion (cimetidine and ranitidine). Sodium citrate is commercially available in a variety of preparations. Thirty milliliters of 0.3 M sodium citrate given prior to induction of anesthesia neutralizes gastric acidity effectively in the parturient.[76,87] However, the drug must be given within 60 min of induction[71,168] to be maximally effective.

Metoclopramide increases pressure in the lower esophageal sphincter and the gastric fundus, increases the peristaltic contractions of the esophagus, gastric antrum, and small intestine, and increases coordination of mechanical activity of various gut segments. These effects hasten esophageal clearance, accelerate gastric emptying, and shorten transit through the small bowel. Atropine and opioids (especially those with vagolytic activity) have been implicated in decreasing the activity of metoclopramide.[192] However, several other studies have not substantiated this concept when metoclopramide is used in combination with antacid[157] or histamine (H-Z) antagonists.[137,138,203] Therefore, it is appropriate to administer metoclopramide to increase gastric emptying during labor. No adverse effect on the newborn has been documented.[34]

Cimetidine reduces gastric acidity and secretions in patients undergoing elective[47,64,98,112,135] and emergency[73,111] surgery and in parturients undergoing elective cesarean delivery.[111] Placental transfer occurs, with a fetal/maternal ratio of about 0.5. Initial newborn assessments have not documented any effect on the neonate.[106] Cimetidine has not yet been approved by the Food and Drug Administration (FDA) for use in obstetrics. Ranitidine is as effective as cimetidine in decreasing gastric acidity and has the advantage of a longer duration of action.

The following clinical measures are recommended to reduce the risk of aspiration pneumonitis in parturients who require anesthesia:

1. Give the patient nothing by mouth preoperatively for 8 hr or during labor.
2. Administer 30 mL of sodium citrate immediately prior to the induction of anesthesia.
3. Favor regional anesthesia.
4. If general anesthesia is necessary, provide a rapid induction utilizing mandatory preoxygenation, cricoid pressure (Sellick's maneuver) to occlude the esophagus, and endotracheal intubation.
5. Consider administering cimetidine or ranitidine the night before and the morning of the procedure plus a clear antacid 1 hr prior to the induction of general anesthesia for cesarean delivery.
6. Consider metoclopramide if the patient has eaten recently.

Alterations in the Vascular System

From the 6th to 12th week of gestation, maternal plasma and erythrocyte volumes begin to increase. By term the plasma volume has increased by 40% to 50% and the red blood cell volume by 20%, resulting in an overall increase in blood volume of 25% to 40%. These increments facilitate the transport of gases and enable the parturient to withstand blood loss better at delivery. Because plasma volume and erythrocyte mass increase at different rates, a "physiologic anemia" develops during pregnancy. The minimum normal hemoglobin in pregnancy is 11 to 12 mg/dl, and the hematocrit about 35%.

Pregnancy is associated with a decline of serum cholinesterase activity to 60% of normal during the first trimester, that is maintained until term. It is not associated with any structural malfunction of the enzyme, and it is doubtful that the reduction in activity of the normal enzyme leads to prolonged neuromuscular blockade in the absence of other factors.

Cardiac output increases during pregnancy, reaching a level of 30% to 50% above the nonpregnant state. The increase in cardiac output is the result of increases in both heart rate and stroke volume. The increase in stroke volume is greater in the lateral than in the supine position as term approaches because of the decrease in venous return resulting from aortocaval compression in the supine position. The rise in cardiac output results in an increased glomerular filtration rate.[72]

Arterial blood pressure decreases somewhat because of a decrease in peripheral resistance. Venous pressure remains normal except caudad to the venous obstruction produced by the gravid uterus, where the pressure is increased. Cardiac output increases during labor, and each contraction augments cardiac output further.[200]

AORTOCAVAL COMPRESSION

Aortocaval compression was first recognized in 1942 by Hansen.[95] He reported faintness and a marked decrease in brachial blood pressure in seven third trimester parturients when they were supine on the examination table during prenatal visits (Figure 4-1). When these women were turned to the left side, their symptoms disappeared and blood pressure returned to normal (Figure 4-2).

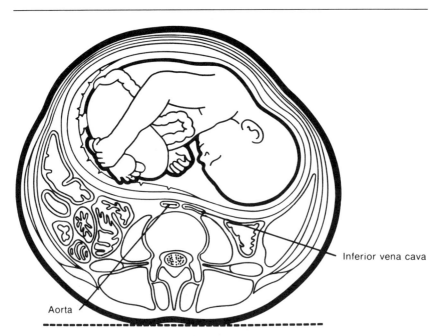

Inferior vena cava

Aorta

Figure 4-1 The pregnant uterus compressing the aorta and the inferior vena cava (aortocaval compression). Patient in supine position.

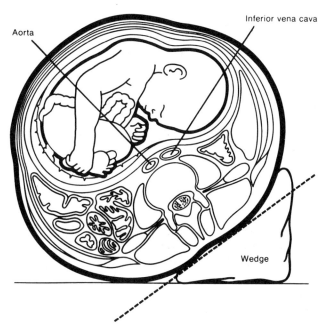

Figure 4-2 Uterine displacement with wedge under hip to relieve aortocaval compression.

In 1953, Howard et al.[105] reported that acute hypotension associated with increased pulse, decreased femoral venous pressure, sweating, and pallor occurred in 10% of parturients in the last trimester when they were supine for 3 to 7 min. This acute hypotension was duplicated experimentally by ligation of the inferior vena cava below the level of renal veins in the pregnant dog. When the ligatures were divided, there was a rapid return of blood pressure to control values. This postural hypotension probably explains why many pregnant women near term feel uncomfortable in the supine position.

In 1964 Kerr et al.[119] studied term pregnant women with venography in the supine position and reported complete obstruction of the inferior vena cava at the level of the bifurcation in 10 of 12 cases. The venous return was redirected via collateral channels, principally the azygous and vertebral venous systems. The authors advised the use of the lateral position to relieve this obstruction.

Bieniarz et al.[13] evaluated aortoplacental blood flow by injecting radiopaque contrast media into 70 parturients in late pregnancy and labor. When the patients were in the supine position, the subrenal part of the aorta was displaced laterally and was less densely opacified at the region of the lumbar lordosis (L4-L5). In 64 patients, aortic displacement was to the left. It was displaced to the right in only three; in three women no change in aortic position was found. During uterine contractions, aortic displacement and narrowing were increased, and the right common iliac artery was frequently occluded.

The hemodynamic changes that occur during aortocaval compression include decreased venous return, stroke volume, and cardiac output. Heart rate may increase initially, but then falls, as does blood pressure. The following methods may be employed to minimize the hypotension that results from aortocaval compression:

1. Patients should be acutely hydrated with 1,000 mL of crystalloid solution immediately before initiation of major regional anesthesia for vaginal delivery. For cesarean delivery, administer 1,500 mL before the block and up to 2,000 mL in the interim until the delivery. Lactated Ringer's or normal saline solution is preferable to glucose containing solutions because hyperglycemia in the mother can cause fetal acidemia[37] and neonatal hypoglycemia.[147]
2. The use of a wedge (usually placed under the right hip) to displace the uterus laterally helps avoid the occlusive pressure of the uterus on the aorta and the inferior vena cava (see Figure 4-2).
3. Before induction of anesthesia, blood pressure should be taken in the supine and lateral positions. Marked supine hypotension may be a contraindication to the use of a major regional technique.
4. Although hypotension can usually be treated with fluids for volume expansion, vasopressor drugs are sometimes necessary. In a study of pregnant ewes Ralston et al.[180] showed that ephedrine is the best vasopressor to use because maternal blood pressure is elevated with the least effect on uterine blood flow.

Ephedrine treatment of hypotension produces significant increases in the fetal heart rate and beat-to-beat variability. These changes are dose related and are not associated with any evidence of fetal hypoxia or acidosis, as judged by fetal capillary pH or Apgar scores.[149]

Datta et al.[61] used ephedrine to treat maternal hypotension as soon as it was detected after the initiation of spinal anesthesia in parturients undergoing cesarean section. They showed that such aggressive care prevents a further decrease in blood pressure. Fetal homeostasis is thus maintained during delivery and the incidence of maternal nausea and vomiting, which is probably a manifestation of cerebral hypoxemia, is reduced markedly.

At term, the placental vasculature is usually maximally dilated. Therefore, systemic perfusion pressure changes are the major determinant of uteroplacental blood flow. Any decrease in uteroplacental perfusion may cause fetal hypoxia and acidosis. Principal causes of decreased uteroplacental perfusion include aortocaval compression, hypotension following the onset of sympathetic block of regional anesthesia, maternal hemorrhage, and certain pharmacologic agents.

High concentrations of inhaled anesthetic agents, such as halothane and enflurane, decrease uterine blood flow. However, halothane and perhaps enflurane may increase uterine blood flow in selected instances, such as a tetanic contraction, in which uterine muscle relaxation and a decrease in uterine vascular resistance is essential.

Increased uterine activity from drugs such as oxytocin, norepinephrine, phenylephrine, methoxamine, and ketamine (in doses above 1 mg/kg) may cause a decrease in uteroplacental perfusion. Maternal hyperventilation, if excessive, may reduce uterine blood flow.[119] In addition, severe hypocarbia can compromise fetal oxygenation by causing constriction of the umbilical vessels and a shift to the left in the maternal hemoglobin-oxygen dissociation curve.[153] Maternal stress and anxiety can cause catecholamine release, which decreases uterine blood flow in sheep.[132] It is uncertain what role stress plays in influencing human uteroplacental blood flow.

Alterations in the Respiratory System

During pregnancy there is capillary engorgement throughout the respiratory tract. Changes in the shape of the chest and the elevated position of the diaphragm are caused by the growing uterus. Ventilation during labor and delivery is increased further by pain, anxiety, and apprehension or by voluntary hyperventilation by the parturient trained in natural childbirth techniques. Changes in pulmonary volumes and function occur, and are indicated in Tables 4-1 and 4-2. All of the factors mentioned above contribute to increased efficiency of gas transfer between alveolar air and maternal blood. Moreover, the increased pulmonary ventilation in conjunction with the concomitant decrease in functional residual capacity permits rapid changes in the concentration of gases in the lungs. The parturient is more likely to incur rapid changes in respiratory gas concentrations during respiratory complications than is the nonpregnant patient. Hypoventilation produces hypoxia, hypercarbia, and respiratory acidosis more readily in the gravida than in the nonpregnant woman. Conversely, hyperventilation can quickly yield carbon

Table 4-1 Changes in Pulmonary Volumes and Capacities during Pregnancy

	Nonpregnant (mL)	Change	Pregnant (mL)
Total lung capacity	4,200	↓	4,000
Tidal volume	450	↑ ↑	600
Respiratory capacity	2,500	↑	2,650
Expiratory reserve volume	700	↓ ↓	550
Residual volume	1,000	↓ ↓	800
Inspiratory reserve volume	2,050	—	2,050
Functional residual capacity	1,700	↓ ↓	1,350
Vital capacity	3,200	—	3,200
Diaphragm position		↑ ↑	

dioxide levels as low as 10 torr and pH values as high as 7.68.[18] In addition, the normal chronic respiratory alkalosis of pregnancy promotes renal excretion of biocarbonate, resulting in a compensatory metabolic acidosis to maintain normal pH. Arterial P_{CO_2} averages 32 to 36 torr at term.

Skin and Mucous Membranes

The increased extracellular fluid characteristic of pregnancy creates dependent and often generalized edema. Leg and arm edema may be bothersome, but edema of the upper airway may be life-threatening. This is particularly likely in pregnancy induced by hypertension, with pro-

Table 4-2 Respiratory Changes Occurring during Pregnancy

	Approximate increase at term (%)
Respiratory rate	10
Tidal volume	40
Minute ventilation	50
Alveolar ventilation	60

is particularly likely in pregnancy induced by hypertension, with prolonged use of the Trendelenburg position, and with the use of tocolytic agents.

The mucous membranes become extremely friable in late pregnancy, and severe nosebleeds may occur secondary to insertion of a nasal airway and a nasogastric or nasotracheal tube. In the obese parturient with a short neck, laryngoscopy may be difficult. The use of a short-handled laryngoscope can be extremely helpful in these patients.[63]

Central Nervous System

The central nervous system of the pregnant woman is exposed to a dramatic change in hormonal activity. Many pregnancy hormones have central nervous system (CNS) activity. An increased emotional lability is seen in pregnancy, and it may be exacerbated by the stresses of a painful birth. For this reason, the parturient should be treated in as supportive and respectful an environment as possible, and allowances made for mood alterations.

In general, decreased doses of all anesthetic drugs are required in pregnancy. The minimal alveolar concentration of inhaled anesthetic is decreased, a fact attributable to increased progesterone levels.[173] This decrease may also result from the increased plasma endorphin levels found in pregnancy. The dose of local anesthetic required for both epidural and spinal block decreases to a variable extent, probably due to changes in the spinal canal caused by vascular congestion, the altered neuronal sensitivity to local anesthetics, and the effect of progesterone.

Musculoskeletal System

The elaboration of relaxin by the placenta leads to generalized ligamentous relaxation. This produces an increased lumbar lordosis and may make the administration of an anesthetic in the lumbar area difficult. This relaxation, combined with the altered body kinetics resulting from the increased size of the uterus, commonly produces back pain and sometimes sciatica in pregnancy. These conditions are not contraindications to regional anesthesia. The pelvis widens more than the shoulders during pregnancy, producing a head-down tilt when the parturient assumes the lateral decubitus position. Compensation should be made for this alteration in position when performing spinal and epidural anesthesia.

TYPES OF PAIN RELIEF

Prepared Childbirth

The concept of natural childbirth was first proposed by Dick-Read, who claimed that the pain of childbirth was induced by fear and tension and could be completely relieved by antepartum preparation and appropriate intrapartum care. The psychoprophylactic method of Lamaze[19] teaches the parturient to breathe in a specific pattern during contractions. Unfortunately, if used improperly, excessive hyperventilation may occur, resulting in a marked decrease in maternal PCO_2 and lowered fetal PO_2.[153] Maternal stress during labor may increase the level of circulating catecholamines, especially norepinephrine,[126,127] and perhaps decrease uterine blood flow.[199] In addition, bearing-down efforts in the second stage of labor can decrease uterine blood flow.[9] Thus, the combination of excessive hyperventilation, stress, and prolonged pushing might jeopardize the fetus.

Its potential problems notwithstanding, prepared childbirth rarely results in fetal compromise. It is apparent from well-controlled studies that excellent results can be achieved with or without medication.[160,193] All pregnant women can probably benefit from the educational and psychologic preparation afforded by prepared childbirth classes.

Parenteral Medications

Barbiturates

Secobarbital, pentobarbital, and amobarbital have lost popularity since their prolonged depressant effects on the neonate became known.[23] These sedative hypnotics possess no analgesic properties and, in agitated patients with pain, may produce an antianalgesic effect, and management problems.

Tranquilizers

Promethazine, hydroxyzine, propiomazine, and promazine are used commonly in some institutions to relieve anxiety during labor. Chlorpromazine and prochlorperazine are less frequently used because of the propensity for their alpha-adrenergic effects to cause hypotension.

Extensive investigation of diazepam has been carried out. This drug rapidly crosses the placenta so that fetal levels equilibrate with maternal levels within a few minutes. Several investigators have reported fetal drug concentrations in excess of the mother's with diazepam. The metabolism of diazepam in the newborn is quite slow.

Diazepam and its active metabolite are detectable in significant concentrations in the newborn for up to 8 days after birth.[57,64,131,139] Neonates whose mothers received large doses of diazepam demonstrated hypotonia, lethargy, diminished suckling, hypothermia, and diminished ability to respond to environmental stimuli.[57,169] Small doses (2.5–10 mg) work well as a calming agent during anesthesia for cesarean delivery, although babies delivered in these situations evidence decreased muscle tone in the first 4 hrs of life.[184]

Ketamine

Ketamine is an intravenous agent that produces intense analgesia and a dissociative state similar to sleep. Controversy surrounds the use of this drug in obstetrics. It is an excellent induction agent for general anesthesia in cases in which cardiovascular stability must be maintained, for example, hemorrhage resulting from abruptio placentae or placenta previa. It has been advocated as a powerful analgesic for pain relief at the time of delivery. Use is technically difficult, however, and may produce general anesthesia, with its inherent problems of regurgitation and aspiration. Ketamine does not preserve the laryngeal and pharyngeal reflexes in the obtunded or anesthetized parturient.[175] Hallucinations and delirium on emergence from anesthesia are common in unpremedicated patients.

Ketamine crosses the placenta rapidly and produces increasing neonatal depression in maternal doses over 1 mg/kg.[79,115] This depression has not been demonstrated with low dosage schedules of ketamine.[2,115] In studies comparing induction agents for general anesthesia, infants whose mothers received ketamine scored better on neurobehavioral tests than those who received thiopental.[97,100] Because ketamine produces its dissociative state by excitation of the central nervous system, it is possible such stimulation in the newborn infant is responsible for the more favorable scores in contrast to thiopental.

Scopolamine

Scopolamine is a belladonna alkaloid with less vagolytic action than atropine. It crosses the blood–brain barrier and the placenta rapidly. In the parturient, it produces amnesia and some sedation. However, it does not possess any analgesic properties.

When used in the presence of pain, it often results in severe agitation, excitement, and loss of control on the part of the parturient. In the fetus it produces loss of beat-to-beat variability and fetal tachycardia. Although widely used in the past, scopolamine has no place in contemporary labor and delivery management because of its unpleasant and potentially hazardous side effects, and because it precludes maternal participation in the delivery process. In situations in which sedation is desirable, tranquilizers produce a more satisfying and safe course than scopolamine.

Narcotics

Narcotics are still the primary form of pain relief used in obstetrics. Adverse maternal effects may include respiratory depression, orthostatic hypotension, nausea and vomiting, decreased gastric motility and inhibition of labor during the latent phase. Fetal effects include loss of heart rate variability, increased time to sustained respiration, decreased Apgar score, decreased minute volume with respiratory acidosis, and neurobehavioral abnormalities. Meperidine is the most popular narcotic analgesic used during labor. Others that have been used are morphine, alphaprodine, pentazocine, and fentanyl.

Morphine,[171] which can be administered in doses of 5 to 10 mg IM or 2 to 3 mg IV, is not as popular as meperidine because, at equianalgesic doses, it is thought to produce more neonatal respiratory depression. This, however, has not been confirmed objectively.[217,219] Alphaprodine,[83] a compound with a more rapid onset of action, has a similar effect. It was recently withdrawn from the market.

Pentazocine has not achieved extensive popularity because of its psychomimetic effects.[117] Fentanyl, given in a dose of 50 to 100 μg IM or 25 to 50 μg IV, is also not widely used, probably because of the rapid onset of respiratory depression and its shorter duration of action compared to meperidine.[80]

Butorphanol, a narcotic agonist-antagonist, can be administered in doses of 1 to 2 mg IM or IV during labor. It has no clear advantages over meperidine, except possibly for less respiratory depression in the 3 to 4 mg range.[179] However, some obstetricians have found that the combination of butorphanol, 1 mg IM and 1 mg IV, produces the desired effect of narcosis plus some tranquilization that otherwise could be achieved by combining a narcotic and a tranquilizer. The effect of butorphanol may be reversed readily by naloxone, if necessary.

Nalbuphine, another narcotic agonist-antagonist, can be given in doses of 10 to 15 mg IM or 5 to 10 mg IV. It also has been claimed to cause less respiratory depression than meperidine, although this probably does not occur until the administered dose is greater than 20 mg.[185] Caution must be observed when a conventional narcotic is followed by administration of a narcotic agonist-antagonist due to the possible adverse interactions.

Meperidine is commonly administered in doses of 50 to 100 mg IM or 10 to 50 mg IV. The peak analgesic effect occurs 40 to 45 min after intramuscular injection and 5 to 10 min after intravenous injection. Titration of dose is the key to successful intravenous use. The duration of action is 2 to 4 hr. Meperidine crosses the placenta rapidly; maternal and fetal equilibrium occurs within six minutes after intravenous injection. The metabolites of meperidine, principally normeperidine, also cross the placenta rapidly. These metabolites may have a greater neonatal respiratory depressant effect than meperidine itself.[152] This may explain the observation that minimal newborn respiratory depression is seen when delivery occurs less than one or more than six hours after intramuscular injection. Respiratory depression is most frequent if the baby is born 2.5 to 3 hr after maternal intramuscular administration.[195]

Neonatal hypercapnia from meperidine has been noted up to 5 hr and neurobehavioral changes have been observed as late as 60 to 72 hr after birth.[99,122] The half-life of the drug is 23 hr in the neonate and approximately 4 hr in the parturient.[36] Meperidine has been found in the neonate up to 6 days after delivery.[30,48,198]

Neonatal depression from a narcotic can be reversed by the administration of naloxone, a pure narcotic antagonist. The dose is 0.01 mg/kg neonatal body weight IM. It is not recommended to administer naloxone to the mother just prior to delivery in an attempt to prevent neonatal depression from maternal narcotic administration. This will only reverse maternal analgesia at a time when it is needed most. Also, reversal of neonatal narcotic depression is unpredictable. Thus, naloxone should be administered to the neonate after delivery only if clinically indicated.[165]

INHALATIONAL TECHNIQUES

Inhalation analgesia refers to the administration of low concentrations of the inhalation anesthetics (nitrous oxide, halothane, enflurane, isoflurane, and methoxyflurane) to provide partial relief of pain. The parturient remains awake with intact laryngeal reflexes so that the risk of aspiration is minimized. Inhalation anesthesia is the administration of higher concentrations of inhalation agents to produce maternal unconsciousness.

Inhalation Analgesia

Inhalation analgesia is rarely used for laboring women because of the possibility of unrecognized transition from the analgesic into the anesthetic stage with its attendant risk of aspiration. Factors that make this transition likely in the parturient are a decrease in the minimal alveolar concentration of agents needed to produce sleep,[107] a decrease in functional residual capacity, and an increase in the rate of alveolar ventilation. Inhalation analgesia should be administered only by a trained anesthetist who can assess changes in maternal consciousness rapidly and can intubate the trachea skillfully if consciousness is lost.

Inhalation Anesthesia

Inhalation anesthesia is used rarely today for vaginal delivery. Situations that might require general inhalation anesthesia for vaginal delivery exist when uterine relaxation is needed (e.g., manual extraction of a placenta, complete breech extraction, internal podalic version, and replacement of an inverted uterus) or when immediate delivery is required for acute fetal distress. Inhalation anesthesia utilizing endotracheal intubation may be necessary in institutions in which there are limited resources for regional block anesthesia or for situations in which patients cannot be given conduction anesthesia (because of some contraindication) or refuse it.

Technique of General Anesthesia for Delivery

The patient is placed on the operating table with head slightly elevated and pelvis tilted to the left by a wedge under the right hip. The abdomen or perineum is prepared as a sterile field and draped. Maternal blood pressure and electrocardiogram are monitored. After acute oxygenation of the patient for three minutes, or, in an emergency, four deep breaths,[35,86] anesthesia is induced rapidly with thiobarbiturate and succinylcholine utilizing cricoid pressure applied by an assistant during intubation with a cuffed endotracheal tube. Anesthesia is maintained until delivery with nitrous oxide/oxygen in a ratio of 50%/50%. A volatile agent (enflurane, halothane, or isoflurane) is added to provide amnesia.[76] A succinylcholine infusion provides adequate muscle relaxation.[154] The volatile agent is discontinued at delivery and, after the cord is clamped, the ratio of N_2O/O_2 is changed to 70%/30%. Narcotics or other intravenous adjuvants are administered as needed. Care must be taken at the termination of the procedure and during extubation to avoid hypoxia and guard against possible aspiration, as with any general anesthetic.

The time interval from induction to delivery (I-D) is important and all efforts should be made to deliver the newborn infant as rapidly as possible, consistent with safety. Marx et al.[143] have shown that I-D intervals in excess of 15 minutes may result in depression of the newborn when nitrous oxide is used. When the I-D or uterine incision to delivery (UI-D) intervals are long or newborn depression is present, the neonate should be given 100% oxygen to breathe immediately after delivery to decrease the concentration of nitrous oxide rapidly.[140] Recent investigations have demonstrated that the UI-D interval is as important as the I-D interval. UI-D intervals greater than 3 min may lead to newborn depression due to altered uteroplacental perfusion.[66]

Both maternal hypercapnia and hypocapnia should be avoided. Hypercapnia leads to fetal carbon dioxide retention and respiratory acidosis. Hypocapnia usually results from excessive positive pressure ventilation. This can impair fetal oxygenation by direct uterine vasoconstriction, a leftward shift of the maternal oxygen-hemoglobin dissociation curve, and increased mean intrathoracic pressure with a resultant decrease in cardiac output.

Anesthetic Agents

Thiopental is the most common induction agent used today. It crosses the placenta rapidly, with the peak umbilical vein concentration occurring 1 min after maternal administration. When the dose is limited to 4 mg/kg, fetal outcome, as measured by Apgar score, is not adversely affected.[123] In addition, delivery should not be delayed in an attempt to allow redistribution of the thiopental because the fetal brain is exposed to only very small amounts. The concentration reaching the fetal brain is kept low as a result of thiobarbiturate extraction from umbilical venous blood by the fetal liver and dilution by blood returning from the fetal viscera and lower extremities.[80]

Succinylcholine is highly ionized and has low lipid solubility. Therefore, it does not cross the placenta in significant amounts.[156] In addition, succinylcholine is rapidly metabolized by both maternal and fetal plasma pseudocholinesterase.[16,130] Respiratory depression in the newborn has been observed in infants who have atypical pseudocholinesterase, indicating that some human placental transfer probably does occur.[170]

The halogenated anesthetic agents (halothane, enflurane, and isoflurane) are used frequently as supplements to nitrous oxide. They decrease maternal recall of intraoperative events, allow administration of higher concentrations of oxygen, and increase uterine blood flow.[215] Because of the dose-related decrease in uterine contractility, these agents can be associated with increased postpartum blood loss, although this is not generally a problem with either halothane or enflurane used at cesarean section.[45,85]

In moderate doses, halothane and isoflurane have no effect on Apgar scores or fetal acid-base balance.[51,172] Methoxyflurane, in low to moderate doses, also has minimal effects on the fetus. Its use has become unpopular, however, because of its potential nephrotoxicity.[56]

LOCAL ANESTHETICS

Considerable information has been obtained concerning the placental transfer of local anesthetics and their effect on the fetus and newborn. Maternal, placental, fetal, and neonatal factors determine the exposure of the baby to medications administered to the parturient.

Maternal Factors

Absorption of local anesthetic from various sites of administration may vary somewhat depending on the regional blood flow, but peak blood concentrations usually occur within 20 min. The concentration of free drug in the maternal circulation determines how much drug is available for transplacental passage. Free drug levels are dependent on maternal circulatory factors (regional blood flow and blood volume), plasma protein binding, hepatic metabolism, and renal excretion of the drug and its metabolites.

Placental Factors

Uterine blood flow at term is approximately 20% of the cardiac output. Placental blood flow determines the availability of the drug in the intervillous space. This important factor may be altered by maternal hypotension or vascular lesions in the placenta itself.

Fetal and Neonatal Factors

The concentration of free drugs in the fetal circulation is determined by the fetal blood volume, plasma binding, metabolism by the liver, and renal excretion of the drug and its metabolites. The role of amniotic fluid in fetal pharmacology is still relatively unknown.

The most important factors determining placental transfer are the amount of nonionized and unbound drug in the maternal circulation to the placenta, the lipid solubility of the agent, and the uptake of the drug by fetal tissues. The higher the plasma protein binding of the drug, the higher is the lipid solubility. It has been postulated that the higher the maternal plasma protein binding, the less toxic the drug may be for the fetus. However, because of the markedly increased lipid solubility of such agents as bupivacaine and etidocaine, increased fetal tissue uptake may neutralize the potential benefits of decreased transfer.[55] Fetal plasma protein binding of the amide local anesthetics is less than the binding in maternal plasma.

Metabolism and Excretion

The basic differences between the ester and amide local anesthetic compounds relate to their metabolism and their allergenic properties. The ester derivatives of benzoic acid are hydrolyzed in the plasma by pseudocholinesterases. The amide compounds undergo enzymatic degradation in the liver. The benzoic acid metabolites of procaine, tetracaine, and 2-chloroprocaine are responsible for the allergic reactions seen with these agents. Reports of allergic responses to amide agents are very rare. There is no apparent cross-sensitivity between the esters and the amides.

The kidney is responsible for excretion of the local anesthetics and their metabolic products. The potential toxicity of local anesthetics and their metabolites may be very important in choosing a particular local anesthetic for a specific purpose.[15,43,81,124,166,167,182]

Pain Pathways in Parturition

The pain of uterine contractions and cervical dilatation is transmitted by afferent fibers that pass to the spinal cord by way of the posterior roots of the 11th and 12th thoracic nerves with some fibers from the 10th thoracic and 1st lumbar nerves. The pain resulting from distention of the birth canal, vulva, and perineum is conveyed by afferent fibers of the posterior roots of the second, third, and fourth sacral nerves. These are the pathways (Figure 4-3) that must be blocked to achieve satisfactory analgesia for the parturient during labor and vaginal delivery.

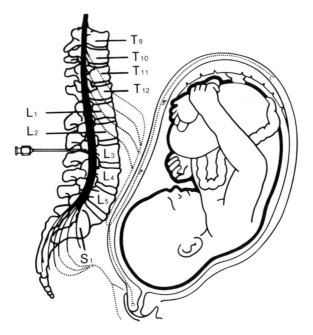

Figure 4-3 Pain pathways during parturition.

Local Infiltration and Pudendal Block

Local infiltration and pudendal block are the most common forms of local pain relief used in obstetric practice (Table 4-3). Few controlled studies have evaluated the placental transfer of local anesthetics during these blocks.

Brown et al.[31] measured the concentration of lidocaine in mothers and their term newborns at delivery following local infiltration of the perineum, bilateral pudendal nerve blocks, or both, with 1% lidocaine. All newborns had Apgar scores above 7 at 1 and 5 min of age. The highest maternal vein concentrations were found in those parturients who received both pudendal block and local infiltration. The fetal concentration increased as the injection to delivery interval increased, averaging 0.69 μg/ml when this interval was over 9 min and 0.42 μg/ml when less than 9 min. The average fetal/maternal concentration ratio was highest after local infiltration (0.74). In some cases, the umbilical vein concentration after these local procedures exceeded the average found after continuous maternal epidural block.

Zador et al.[226] evaluated pudendal block with 200 mg of lidocaine during the second stage of labor. Lidocaine was detected in fetal scalp

Table 4-3 Local Anesthetics and Dosages for Pudendal Block[a]

Local anesthetic	Dosage/injection site[b]		Onset of action (min)	Duration of action (min)
	mL	mg		
Bupivacaine, 0.25%–0.5% (Marcaine)	10–15	25–75	5–15	60–180
2-Chloroprocaine, 1%–2% (Nesacaine)	10–15	100–300	3–5	45–90
Lidocaine, 0.5%–1.0% (Xylocaine)	10–15	50–150	5–15	60–120
Mepivacaine, 0.5%–1.0% (Carbocaine)	10–15	50–150	5–15	60–120

[a]Total milligram dose of the local anesthetic should not exceed manufacturer's recommendations.
[b]Dosages do not include anesthetic solution used to create skin wheals and to infiltrate the area of the anterior perineum. Double the dosage for bilateral pudendal block.

blood within 5 min after injection, and peak levels were reached within 20 min. With the addition of epinephrine, peak levels were 30% lower in maternal blood and 20% lower in fetal blood. An occasional decrease in uterine activity was observed and was more pronounced when epinephrine was used. There was a prolongation of the second stage of labor with increased fetal acidosis at delivery. The peak levels of lidocaine averaged 1.1 μg/ml without epinephrine and 0.8 μg/ml with epinephrine.

Belfrage et al.[10] measured bupivacaine concentrations after pudendal block using 0.25% bupivacaine with 1:200,000 epinephrine for vaginal delivery. The average maternal bupivacaine concentration was 0.22 μg/ml and the umbilical cord concentration was 0.05 μg/ml. The fetal/maternal ratio was 0.25. All babies except one had an Apgar score of 8 or more at 5 min. Their conclusion was that long duration of action and a good fetal/maternal ratio make bupivacaine a suitable agent for pudendal block in obstetrics.

Paracervical Block

Fetal bradycardia after paracervical block (PCB) can be a persistent and troublesome problem. Teramo and Widholm[209] were first to observe a transient decrease in fetal pH after PCB. This finding, together with a prolonged bradycardia, suggests that the fetus is becoming asphyxiated. Teramo[208] recommended that PCB should be used only when continuous fetal heart rate monitoring and ability to assess fetal acid-base balance are available. Greiss et al.[93] demonstrated that intravascular local anesthetics can decrease uterine blood flow in gravid ewes by stimulating vasoconstriction and myometrial contractility. Cibils[41] and Gibbs and Noel[88] postulated that the bradycardia found after PCB is due to uterine artery spasm, causing decreased intervillous space blood flow and fetal hypoxia. Morishima et al.[151] demonstrated that the fetal bradycardia subsequent to PCB is caused in part by a decrease in oxygen availability, a result of increased uterine activity and its consequence, reduced uteroplacental perfusion.

Continuous electronic fetal heart rate monitoring is mandatory if PCB is administered. If signs of fetal distress appear, they should be evaluated and treated appropriately (see Chapter 10). In the vast majority of instances, a previously healthy fetus will tolerate the asphyxia that may accompany PCB. Thus, a conservative and considered approach is vital when evaluating fetal status in these situations.

Subarachnoid Block

Subarachnoid block is still a commonly used major regional technique for obstetric patients.[52,54] Its advantages are simplicity, speed, reliability, minimal fetal drug exposure, and decreased risk of maternal aspiration relative to inhalation anesthesia. Disadvantages of subarachnoid block are the high incidence of hypotension with nausea and vomiting, and the possibility of headache following dural puncture. Contraindications to subarachnoid block include infections at the puncture site, coagulopathy, acute neurologic disease, extreme hypovolemia, and those cardiac disorders in which hypotension may initiate or increase right-to-left shunt.[60]

Subarachnoid block for vaginal delivery is usually given during the second stage of labor when the fetal head is on the perineum. The obstetrician then allows the parturient to push the baby out or may aid delivery of the fetal head by forceps. Ravindran et al.[181] showed that bearing down after subarachnoid block does not increase the incidence of postdural puncture headache. Subarachnoid anesthesia can also be given earlier in the second stage if a midforceps delivery is necessary.

The classical saddle block subarachnoid anesthetic is achieved by blocking dermatome segments S2–S4. This provides anesthesia of the perineum, but it does not inhibit the pain of uterine contractions and may prove inadequate for a midforceps delivery. If such a delivery is contemplated, a modified saddle block is used to anesthetize segments T10–S4. For cesarean delivery the upper level of spinal segment blockade should extend to the T4 dermatome.

Lumbar puncture is performed at the L2-L3 or the L3-L4 interspace with the patient in the right lateral decubitus position. After injection of the anesthetic, the patient is turned supine immediately and a wedge is placed under the right hip. Sprague[204] showed that this is the most effective technique to ensure adequate bilateral blockade of the upper dermatomes while maintaining effective left uterine displacement. Oxygen by mask is administered from the time of induction until the infant is delivered. After delivery, narcotics and tranquilizers are given, if necessary.

Hypotension is the most common complication of subarachnoid anesthesia. Ueland et al.[211] showed an average decrease in blood pressure from 124/72 to 67/38 torr when the patient was moved from lateral position to supine. Cardiac output decreased 34%. Stroke volume decreased 44% and heart rate increased 17%. These hemodynamic changes following subarachnoid anesthesia result from blockade of sympathetic vasomotor activity, causing an increase in venous capacitance and a decrease in venous return to the right heart. When the patient is supine, inferior vena caval compression by the gravid uterus accentuates these changes.

Marx et al.[51,142] demonstrated that maternal hypotension following subarachnoid anesthesia is associated with lower Apgar scores, prolonged time to sustained respiration, and fetal acidosis. Therefore, efforts to avoid maternal hypotension are necessary to ensure fetal well-being. Two techniques that should be employed routinely to prevent maternal hypotension are lateral uterine displacement and acute intravascular volume expansion. Uterine displacement with either a blanket roll, wedge, or mechanical device helps to minimize the decrease in venous return caused by sympathetic blockade and aortocaval compression by the gravid uterus. Uterine displacement is, however, not always completely effective in preventing maternal hypotension. Acute volume expansion with at least 1,500 mL of Ringer's lactate solution should be given within 15 to 30 min prior to induction.[42] In combination with left uterine displacement, this decreases the incidence of hypotension.[50,62,118,196] If blood pressure begins to fall despite these measures, ephedrine[221] should be administered intravenously in 10-mg increments to restore the blood pressure to normal. Administering ephedrine immediately after the first decrease in blood pressure is extremely effective in minimizing the incidence of persistent hypotension with nausea and vomiting.[61]

The incidence of headache following dural puncture is directly related to the diameter of the needle. If a 25- or 26-gauge needle is used, the incidence of postlumbar puncture headache will be low. The incidence of dural puncture headache is about 7% to 8% after spinal anesthesia, but is much higher if the dura is perforated with the large needle used for epidural techniques (Table 4-4).

Another minor complication of subarachnoid block is urinary retention. All types of anesthesia predispose the patient to develop urinary retention for a brief time. Normal bladder function usually resumes within 6 to 12 hr.

The most severe complication of subarachnoid block is excessive cephalad spread of local anesthetic, resulting in total spinal anesthesia. This complication is heralded by severe nausea, hypotension, and dyspnea, and is often accompanied by cardiac and respiratory arrest. Intubation of the trachea is required as there is a risk of aspiration and ventilatory insufficiency. Standard cardiopulmonary resuscitation must be provided as necessary.

Rare complications include paralysis (from dural puncture above the L2 level resulting in spinal cord injury), and meningitis, which may result from contamination of the subarachnoid space if the lumbar puncture is

Table 4-4 Frequency of Dural Puncture Headache

Year	No.	Dural Puncture	Headache
		Subarachnoid block	
1985–1986	997	—	79(7.9%)
1984–1985	857	—	59(6.9%)
1983–1984	962	—	76(7.9%)
		Epidural Block	
1985–1986	4,818	75(1.6%)	53(71%)
1984–1985	4,264	81(1.9%)	52(64%)
1983–1984	3,599	48(1.3%)	24(50%)

Source: Data courtesy of Brigham and Women's Hospital, Boston.

done in the presence of septicemia or local skin infection, or with contaminated equipment.

Local anesthetics used in subarachnoid block most likely have no direct effect on the fetus. They can, however, affect the fetus indirectly by altering maternal hemodynamics and decreasing placental blood flow.[72,164] Fetal distress in human pregnancy is well documented following prolonged hypotension. During epidural anesthesia, late decelerations consistently occur when maternal systolic blood pressure is less than 100 torr for 5 to 7 min.[103] During subarachnoid block, fetal bradycardia is the rule if maternal systolic blood pressure falls to less than 70 torr; bradycardia almost never occurs if the blood pressure is maintained above 100 torr.[50] If maternal hypotension is avoided, fetal heart rate and oxygenation at birth are no different with subarachnoid block than with general anesthesia or any other form of regional anesthesia.[92] During the period immediately following delivery, however, infants delivered with subarachnoid block are better oxygenated and require less resuscitation than those delivered with general anesthesia. Marx et al.[143] found no differences in umbilical artery pH, carbon dioxide tension, and base deficit in babies whose mothers had subarachnoid block without hypotension when compared to a group delivered with general anesthesia. When hypotension did occur with subarachnoid block, there was a significant increase in base deficit. Datta and Brown[64] found even more striking correlation between maternal hypotension and fetal acidosis in diabetic parturients following subarachnoid block. Finster and Poppers[82] determined that a prolonged I-D interval during general anesthesia is often associated with a depressed Apgar score. Unlike general anesthesia, the I-D interval is not important with subarachnoid blocks, provided that maternal hypotension is avoided. A UI-D interval greater than 3 min, however, is associated with fetal acidosis and depressed Apgar scores.[66]

In summary, subarachnoid block is a simple, reliable technique which, when given to a normovolemic obstetric patient by an experienced anesthetist, causes few maternal complications. In addition, fetal outcome is normal as long as maternal hypotension is avoided. The following list illustrates the key points in the management of subarachnoid block in the pregnant patient:

1. Provide adequate acute hydration (about 1,000 mL for vaginal delivery; at least 1,500 mL for cesarean delivery).
2. Induce anesthesia with patient in right lateral position, especially for cesarean delivery.
3. Use 25- or 26-gauge needle.

4. Avoid aortocaval compression.
5. Treat hypotension immediately.
6. Administer ephedrine in increments of 10 mg IV as needed.
7. Minimize induction-to-delivery and uterine incision-to-delivery intervals during cesarean delivery. Effects on fetus are related to the duration of hypotension and altered uteroplacental perfusion.

EPIDURAL ANESTHESIA

A single-dose lumbar epidural block that provides anesthesia from the level of T10–S5 may be used during the final stages of labor and during delivery if the local anesthetic agent has sufficiently long duration of action. It is particularly suitable for patients in whom anesthesia is indicated for the delivery but in whom general anesthesia is undesirable (e.g., presence of hypertension, diabetes, or pulmonary, cardiac, renal, or hepatic disease). A single-dose block may also be used for cesarean delivery. As with any anesthetic technique, the obstetrician and the patient should be made aware of the risks and advantages of lumbar epidural anesthesia.[67] A continuous lumbar epidural block allows the anesthesiologist to provide pain relief during all three stages of labor and during vaginal delivery (Table 4-5), as well as anesthesia and motor block for forceps or cesarean delivery (Table 4-6).

During the first stage of labor, the anesthesiologist can produce a segmental block of the lower three thoracic and upper lumbar segments. This eliminates pain due to cervical dilatation. During the second and third stages of labor, anesthesia can be extended to the sacral innervation, thus blocking the pain that results from distention of the birth canal, vulva, and perineum. Should forceps or cesarean delivery become necessary, the continuous technique facilitates administration of a concentration of anesthetic sufficient to produce motor block as well as perineal and abdominal relaxation.

When the outcome of vaginal delivery is in doubt, a patient who has a segmental epidural block can be given uterotonic stimulation with oxytocin administration, if indicated. The block can be extended in these cases to facilitate a subsequent cesarean delivery. Anesthesia may sometimes benefit abnormal labors.[136] Lumbar epidural block is contraindicated in patients with blood coagulation deficiencies, septicemia, active central nervous system demyelinating disease, or an infection at the intended puncture site.

Brown et al.[30] found detectable levels of lidocaine and mepivacaine in the newborn for 8 and 24 hr after birth, respectively. Pharmacokinetic

Table 4-5 Local Anesthetics and Dosages for Continuous (Intermittent) Epidural Block for Vaginal Delivery

Local Anesthetic[a]	Dosage[b]				Onset of action (min)	Duration of action (min)	Time between top-up doses (min approx)
	First dose[c]		Top-up dose[d]				
	mL	mg	mL	mg			
Bupivacaine[e], 0.125%–0.5%	6–15	7.5–75	6–10	7.5–50	5–10	45–180	Depends on concentration
2-Chloroprocaine, 2%–3%	6–15	120–450	6–10	120–300	3–5	40–60	45
Lidocaine, 1%–2%	6–15	60–300	6–10	60–200	5–10	45–75	60
Mepivacaine, 1%–2%	6–15	60–300	6–10	60–200	5–10	45–75	60

[a]All without epinephrine.
[b]Total milligram dose of the local anesthetic should not exceed manufacturer's recommendations.
[c]Dose range depends on patient's height.
[d]The top-up dose range depends on patient's height. The top-up dose is approximately two-thirds of the first dose if the initial dose resulted in a satisfactory level of analgesia and if this level is to be maintained.
[e]Bupivacaine 0.0625%–0.25% has been used for continuous infusions.

Table 4-6 Local Anesthetics and Dosages for Continuous (Intermittent) Epidural Block for Cesarean Delivery

| Local Anesthetic[a] | Dosage[b] | | | | Onset of action (min) | Duration of action (min) | Time between top-up doses (min, approx) |
| | First dose[c] | | Top-up dose[d] | | | | |
	mL	mg	mL	mg			
Bupivacaine[e], 0.5%	20–30	100–150	8–12	40–60	5–10	90–120	90
2-Chloroprocaine, 3%	12–20	360–600	8–12	240–360	3–5	40–60	45
Lidocaine, 2%[e]	12–20	240–400	8–12	160–240	5–10	60–90	60
Mepivacaine, 2%	12–20	240–400	8–12	160–240	5–10	60–90	60

[a]All without epinephrine.
[b]Total milligram dose of the local anesthetic should not exceed manufacturer's recommendations.
[c]Dose range depends on patient's height.
[d]The top-up dose is approximately two-thirds of the first dose if the initial dose resulted in a satisfactory level of analgesia and if this level is to be maintained.
[e]With or without epinephrine 1:200,000.

models revealed that the long-term rate of disappearance of mepivacaine was approximately three times that of lidocaine.[145] Computed half-time duration averaged 3 hr for lidocaine and 9 hr for mepivacaine.

Etidocaine was evaluated for vaginal delivery utilizing 0.5% to 1% solutions without epinephrine. The quality of pain relief was considered unsatisfactory in most of the parturients and supplemental spinal anesthesia was required in some. As a result of this discouraging evaluation, etidocaine cannot be recommended for vaginal delivery. Etidocaine 1.5% with 1:200,000 epinephrine for epidural anesthesia seems to offer satisfactory sensory and excellent motor blockade for cesarean deliveries; however, the profound motor block has been disturbing to patients, further limiting the role for this drug.

The best drug for obstetric epidural analgesia is one that produces maximal sensory and minimal motor blockade. Bromage[24] suggested that bupivacaine approaches the ideal local anesthetic agent; however, 2-chloroprocaine and lidocaine offer significant advantages in certain situations.

CONTINUOUS EPIDURAL INFUSION

Epidural analgesia can be provided via a continuous, rather than intermittent, infusion of local anesthestic.

Once a stable epidural block at approximately the T10 level has been established with 0.25% bupivacaine, the continuous infusion can be initiated. A large syringe or empty sterile plastic bag is filled with 0.0625% to 0.25% solution of bupivacaine and attached via high-pressure tubing to the epidural catheter. The pump is adjusted to deliver the desired dose, the usual administration being up to 30 mg of bupivacaine per hr.

Patients should be positioned initially in the 30 degree head-up position with left uterine displacement. The block must be checked at least hourly to assure uniformity, rule out subarachnoid or intravascular migration of the catheter, assess adequacy of analgesia, monitor fetal well-being, and check the level of local anesthetic in the reservoir syringe.

Possible Problems

Asymmetric Sensory Block

If a patient lies continuously on one side, the level of sensory block may become asymmetric. The situation should be corrected by repositioning the patient, disconnecting the pump, administering 3 to 5 ml of 0.5% bupivacaine, and then restarting the infusion. The patient should be encouraged to turn from side to side, always with sufficient uterine displacement.

Diminishing Analgesia

Progressive diminution of sensory block and loss of anesthetic effect may be due to a number of factors. Proper assessment requires rechecking the infusion set-up and then testing to determine where the tip of the catheter is positioned. The pump must be disconnected to test for appropriate catheter placement. After aspiration, a 3-mL test dose of 0.5% bupivacaine with 1:200,000 epinephrine is injected. If there is no response, an attempt is made to reestablish the block with incremental 3- to 5-mL doses of 0.5% bupivacaine. Alternatively, a 3-mL test dose of 1.5% to 2% lidocaine with epinephrine can be used. The addition of 1:200,000 epinephrine to either agent should identify intravascular injection. If the block cannot be reestablished or if aspiration and testing indicate intravascular migration of the tip, the catheter must be removed. Depending on the clinical circumstances, either another catheter may be inserted via a second placement or alternative analgesia may be initiated. At the above infusion rates, 0.25% bupivacaine will not produce symptoms from intravascular injection. The only clue may be diminishing analgesia.

Dense Motor Block

Patients given a continuous infusion of 0.25% bupivacaine usually exhibit mild to moderate motor blockade of the lower extremities. If a progressively dense motor effect resembling subarachnoid block ensues, the catheter must be disconnected immediately and carefully aspirated to rule out subarachnoid migration. Suspicion of subarachnoid migration after testing mandates withdrawal of the catheter and reinsertion at another site, if indicated.

Patchy Block

If a spotty or patchy block occurs, one should attempt to solidify the block by disconnecting the pump, aspirating to determine catheter placement, and injecting 3 to 5 mL of 0.5% bupivacaine or 1.5% to 2.0% lidocaine, with or without epinephrine. Then the pump is reconnected.

Miscellaneous

If a patient requires an acute change in the character of the block for cesarean delivery, simply increasing the infusion rate is inadequate to effect the required change in the level of analgesia. The pump must be disconnected from the patient, correct catheter placement verified, and the patient given 0.5% bupivacaine, 2% lidocaine, or 3% 2-chloroprocaine to achieve the desired level of sensory anesthesia.

Often, 0.25% bupivacaine does not provide adequate perineal analgesia. At the time of delivery, the patient may require an additional increment of drug to provide sufficient analgesia for forceps delivery or episiotomy. Placing the parturient in the semi-Fowler's position for pushing also helps achieve a more complete perineal block.

Local Anesthetic and Narcotic Infusion

A loading dose of local anesthetic to establish the epidural block using 0.25% to 0.5% bupivacaine plus a continuous infusion of 0.125% to 0.25% bupivacaine with 2.5 mg of fentanyl per milliliter of local anesthetic solution has outstanding potential for excellent pain relief with minimal motor block. The utilization of continuous infusion epidural analgesia with or without narcotic should virtually eliminate unintentional intravascular or subarachnoid injections of local anesthetic.

EPIDURAL BLOCK AND NEONATAL OUTCOME

In a group of 360 monitored fetuses, Schifrin[191] found that the frequency of late decelerations was highest in those whose mothers received the combination of epidural anesthesia and oxytocin stimulation. Control of oxytocin infusion and correction of hypotension were usually accompanied by improvement in these fetal heart rate patterns.

McDonald et al.[132] evaluated the effect of epidural analgesia on fetal heart rate, acid-base status, and Apgar score. There was an increase in late decelerations after epidural block despite low lidocaine dosages and the absence of hypotension. Unless second stage problems or hypotension occurred, no significant deterioration of the acid-base status was noted. The greatest incidence of late decelerations was noted when epidural analgesia was combined with oxytocin, findings consistent with those of Schifrin.

Brown et al.[32] reported four newborns with a pH below 7.24 in umbilical vein blood who showed an elevated fetal/maternal concentration ratio of local anesthetic, possibly demonstrating trapping of a weak base in the fetus. This differential phenomenon has been demonstrated for gastric contents and urine relative to blood. It is unwise, therefore, to use prolonged epidural block with lidocaine or mepivacaine in situations in which fetal acidosis is likely or already exists.[12]

Wallis et al.[213] evaluated lumbar epidural anesthesia in normotensive pregnant ewes. Some ewes received the anesthesia with 1:100,000 epinephrine and others without it. The sensory level of anesthesia was between the umbilicus and xiphisternum. Except for a transient 14% decrease in uterine blood flow in the ewes receiving 2-chloroprocaine with epinephrine, uterine blood flow remained near control values and was sufficient at all times to maintain stable fetal acid-base and blood gas values. Provided blood pressure and uterine blood flow were stable, the percentage of uterine blood flow distributed to the placenta in the absence of uterine contractions was not altered by epidural anesthesia or by addition of epinephrine to the anesthetic solution.

The use of lumbar epidural analgesia with bupivacaine during uncomplicated labor was assessed by Belfrage et al.[10] Fetal scalp blood pH remained within normal limits and no pathologic fetal heart rate alterations were demonstrated after the block, although there was a temporary decrease in the fetal heart rate baseline in 20% of the cases. A similar decrease in baseline fetal heart rate was reported by Hehre et al.[96] who suggested this was probably due to the effect of the local anesthetic on the fetal myocardium.

Ideally, epidural block should be initiated during the acceleration phase of labor. If started earlier, inhibition of labor progress into the active phase may occur. Segmental lumbar block can be used to block the pain of uterine contractions and cervical dilatation. However, perineal pain relief for the delivery (block of S2–S4) cannot be guaranteed by this approach. If the anesthesia cannot be extended sufficiently, it may require local infiltration, pudendal block, or low subarachnoid block. More extensive epidural block (T10–S5) can provide complete pain relief, but the incidence of hypotension is higher than with segmental block.

Uterine contractions that immediately follow an unintentional intravascular injection seem to cause increased discomfort. This may be due to the fact that high concentrations of local anesthetics can produce uterine hypertonus,[151,190] and the increased intensity of the uterine contraction causes the parturient more discomfort.

Caudal block has been used less often in recent years because the technique requires a higher dose of local anesthetic than epidural block.

However, sometimes a caudal block is the only way to provide adequate analgesia for delivery because of problems such as prior back surgery or upper back deformity.

COMPLICATIONS OF EPIDURAL ANESTHESIA

Massive Subarachnoid Injection

Subarachnoid injection of anesthetic agents may occur when an epidural needle or catheter is placed unintentionally in the subarachnoid space, or when an epidural catheter penetrates the dura after having been placed in the epidural space. Massive subarachnoid injection of drug is followed by rapid onset of total spinal anesthesia with unconsciousness, apnea, hypotension and, occasionally, cardiac arrest.

Subarachnoid puncture can usually be avoided by careful technique and good needle control by an experienced hand. If clear fluid does appear in the hub of the needle, a glucose reagent strip can be used to determine if the fluid is indeed cerebrospinal fluid. In such instances, the epidural needle should be removed, and reinserted in another interspace if epidural anesthesia is still desired. Alternatively, a subarachnoid block can be administered using an appropriate agent in correct dosage.

Treatment of massive subarachnoid injection should be directed to supporting the patient until the effects wear off. If unconscious, she should be intubated immediately to avoid aspiration and, if apneic, ventilated with oxygen until adequate spontaneous respirations return. Adequate fluid should be infused intravenously to counteract hypotension. The uterus should be displaced immediately by placing the patient in the lateral decubitus position to avoid aortocaval compression and altered uteroplacental perfusion. If fluid load and uterine displacement are inadequate to prevent hypotension, ephedrine sulfate in increments of 10 mg should be injected intravenously. If the patient does not become unconscious or apneic, management should be the same as with a high spinal anesthetic (oxygen, fluids, ephedrine, and much reassurance).

Massive Subdural Injection

Between the dura mater and the pia and arachnoid membranes lies a potential subdural space.[17] During insertion of the epidural needle, the dura may be partially punctured with subsequent injection of anesthetic or unexpected placement of a catheter into the subdural space. There is some evidence that injection of an anesthetic into this space may result in a massive epidural block. Injected anesthetic solutions spread extensively, primarily cephalad along the dorsal aspect of the space. Subdural injection, like that of massive subarachnoid injection, can usually be avoided by meticulous technique, good needle control, and avoiding superfluous movement of the needle once it has been positioned in the epidural space. Treatment of this complication is similar to that of massive subarachnoid injection.

Central Nervous System Toxic Reaction

Rapid intravascular injection of local anesthetic results in convulsion and cardiovascular collapse. In regional anesthesia it is important to conduct certain tests to ensure that bolus doses of local anesthetic are not administered into the vascular system.

Cannulation of an epidural vein during administration of epidural anesthesia in labor occurs with an incidence of 1%.[25] It is more likely if the puncture is made in the lateral aspect of the epidural space where the veins are more densely clustered than they are in the midline. As noted previously, there may be occlusion of the inferior vena cava at term causing increased collateral flow in the epidural plexus and azygous veins. Azygous flow is likely to rise in proportion to the degree of caval obstruction; this is greatest when the parturient is lying supine.[19] Epidural venous injections travel quickly and reach the heart as a bolus, allowing small quantities of injected local anesthetic to produce quite extensive effects. The vertebral venous plexus is a valveless, thin-walled, distensible system of veins in which blood is free to flow in any direction, influenced only by pressure gradients and, perhaps, by blood volume.[78] This may account for the more immediate onset of the central nervous system toxic response, in contrast to the more delayed effect ordinarily seen from peripheral vein injection.

To prevent these complications, certain precautions should be observed. The catheter should be inserted in the midline rather than in the lateral portions of the epidural space. The anesthetist should aspirate carefully through the needle and then through the catheter before taping it in place. A test dose should be injected through the needle and/or the catheter, and the catheter should be aspirated before every subsequent dose. Reinforcement doses should be injected in increments of 5 mL or less, with the mother in the lateral position whenever possible.

In the event that intravenous injection does take place, the anesthetist should be alerted by the following symptoms: a feeling of faintness, dizziness, nausea, or anxiety; paresthesias or tingling in the lips or hands; a metallic taste in the mouth; tinnitus; and prodromal twitching of the hands or feet. Diplopia and nystagmus may also occur before the grand mal seizure.[69,156]

When convulsions do occur, the treatment strategy has as its ultimate goal adequate oxygenation of the maternal-fetal unit. Therefore, immediate therapy should consist of the following steps:

1. Ventilate with oxygen by bag and mask. If unconsciousness occurs, rapid intubation facilitated by succinylcholine (1 to 1.5 mg/kg) must be accomplished, with cricoid pressure to prevent aspiration.
2. Turn the parturient into the lateral decubitus position to avoid aortocaval compression.
3. Give IV thiopental (50–75 mg) or diazepam (5–10 mg) to terminate the convulsion, if needed.
4. Administer vasopressor therapy with ephedrine sulfate if arterial hypotension supervenes or persists even with the patient in the lateral decubitus position.
5. Ensure adequate intravenous fluids. (A functioning intravenous infusion is mandatory before any regional block.)
6. Take maternal vital signs as often as necessary until blood pressure stabilizes.
7. Connect the fetal monitor immediately and evaluate the fetal heart rate and uterine contractions for signs of uteroplacental insufficiency.
8. Although ideally it is preferable to support the patient until the local anesthetic is cleared from the fetus and symptoms abate,[150] prepare for possible immediate vaginal or abdominal delivery.
9. In case of cardiovascular collapse, institute the standard protocol of cardiopulmonary resuscitation immediately.[202] A major regional block should never be initiated unless full resuscitative equipment is available. Raising the patient's legs and displacing the uterus laterally will maximize venous return during cardiopulmonary resuscitation (CPR).
10. Cesarean delivery may sometimes increase the likelihood of survival during resuscitation (see Chapter 19).

The Test Dose

The original use of an epidural test dose was to detect unintentional subarachnoid injection. Lidocaine and mepivacaine, both of which gave sensory changes upon subarachnoid injection within 1 to 2 min were often used. However, with the introduction of bupivacaine in the United States in 1973, it became apparent that one could not always determine if the test dose was subarachnoid because sensory changes did not reliably occur for several minutes.

The present consensus is that the utilization of an epinephrine test dose during local anesthetic blocks for surgery is essential. However, the issue is not resolved in obstetrics. Hood et al.[104] demonstrated that epinephrine in a test dose can decrease uterine blood flow in the gravid ewe. Advocates of a test dose of local anesthetic with epinephrine during the initiation of an epidural block for the parturient point out the decrease in uterine blood flow demonstrated in this study is similar to the changes seen with a uterine contraction. Whether the concurrence of a contraction and the test dose would result in a decrease in uterine blood flow sufficient to result in fetal jeopardy is uncertain.

Cartwright et al.[39] further questioned the utility of the test dose in obstetrics in their report that heart rate changes that occur normally in women during labor may obscure the heart rate changes seen with the intravascular injection of epinephrine used as a test dose. Furthermore, if one used a test dose before every top-up dose, a significant amount of epinephrine could be given that might diminish the force of contractions and impair the progress of labor.[144] The authors use an epinephrine-containing test dose for elective cesarean delivery because a larger mass of drug is given over a short period of time and there usually are no contractions.

Two milliliters of a 1.5% or 2.0% hyperbaric lidocaine solution with 15 mg epinephrine as a test dose for epidural anesthesia injected in the subarachnoid space will produce sensory blockade at the second sacral dermatome within 2 min, with spread to approximately the ninth thoracic dermatome. Epidural administration results in sensory changes in approximately 9 min at the second sacral dermatome.[1]

The difficulty with the test dose of isobaric bupivacaine 0.5% with 1:200,000 epinephrine as presently manufactured is that it will not reproducibly produce sensory changes in less than 2 min. Therefore, it is our practice that an epinephrine test dose of 15 mg should be used in all major blocks for cesarean delivery. The best test dose is perhaps a 3-mL injection of 1.5% to 2.0% lidocaine with 1:200,000 epinephrine.

Most importantly, we never give more than 5 mL of local anesthetic at any one time, and we wait 30 to 60 s before injecting another incremental dose. Equipment for cardiopulmonary resuscitation and electrocardiography is immediately available.

INTRASPINAL OPIOIDS IN OBSTETRIC ANALGESIA AND ANESTHESIA

Although subtle transient neonatal neurobehavioral effects attributable to local anesthetics can be demonstrated, the predominant detrimental and/or unwanted effects of this technique result from sympathetic blockade and from degrees of motor blockade in labor patients. In an effort to maximize the desired analgesic effects and minimize sympathetic and motor blockade, a great deal of recent investigational interest has involved the administration of opioid substances into the subarachnoid and epidural space.[33]

Mechanisms of Action

Opiate substances have been used to provide pain relief in childbirth for thousands of years; however, only recently has the site and mechanism of action of these compounds begun to be understood.[141] Opioid receptors were identified in the mammalian central nervous system in the early 1970s. In 1975, Hughes et al.[109] described enkephalins, naturally-occurring peptides with opiate-like characteristics. Yaksh, Kitahata, and others further elucidated these concepts, leading a new approach to the physiology of analgesia.[120,222–224] It is believed that both exogenous opioids and endogenous enkephalins alter the central release of neurotransmitters from afferent nerves and interfere with efferent pathways extending to the spinal cord from higher centers. They thereby interfere with the first level of sensory integration and modify the subjective interpretation of pain. The fact that this is a peripheral phenomenon is supported by the observation that following administration of morphine, even patients with complete spinal cord transection show diminution of the withdrawal response to a noxious stimulus below the level of transection.

Following the identification of opiate receptors, the potent analgesic action of opioids was demonstrated.[53,214,224] These effects were reversed by naloxone.

Further study of spinally mediated analgesia revealed several types of opiate receptors, each characterized by its affinity for specific agents. The actions of a narcotic are determined by its ability to stimulate or inhibit each of the various types of opiate receptors.[174] The first receptor identified was termed the mu-receptor, since it was stimulated readily by morphine to produce analgesia, miosis, and respiratory depression, as well as other symptoms. Ketocyclazocine and related compounds specifically stimulate a second receptor which was termed the "kappa"-receptor. The effects of kappa-activation included analgesia as well, but seemed more specific for visceral pain as compared with the somatic analgesia of the mu-receptor, and produced less respiratory depression. Drugs with strong affinity for this receptor group, such as butorphanol, nalbuphine, and pentazocine, are called "agonist-antagonists," because their stimulation of kappa-receptors is balanced by a weak antagonistic effect on mu-receptors.

Pharmacology

There are similarities in molecular weight, pKa, and lipid solubility between opioids and local anesthetics. In fact, very high concentrations of meperidine produce profound peripheral nerve block.[216] Many of the pharmacologic determinants of local anesthetic action also govern the mechanisms of intraspinal opioid analgesia. The degree of ionization at physiologic pH and the degree of lipid solubility are very important in explaining the variation in effect of different opioid substances.

Increasing pKa, protein binding, and lipid solubility all decrease the accumulation of free drug within the cerebrospinal fluid. Morphine, for example, an opiate with very low lipid solubility and relatively low pKa, remains highly ionized within the cerebrospinal fluid (CSF). This explains both its long duration of action (about 24 hr following a single dose) as well as its potential for rostral spread and delayed respiratory depression. In contrast, fentanyl and sufentanil, being more highly lipid-soluble, exhibit lower CSF solubility and a higher affinity for spinal cord structures. As expected from their physicochemical characteristics these agents exhibit much shorter duration of action and considerably less rostral spread with much less propensity for respiratory depression.[26,125] In addition, the low lipid solubility of morphine results in a very slow onset of action (45–60 min), whereas fentanyl and sufentanil have an onset within 10 to 15 min even following epidural administration.[158,222] While water and lipid solubility are crucial variables in predicting the spinal effects of opioid substances, other factors, such as receptor binding affinity and molecular shape,[149] play important roles as well. An agent with high lipid solubility such as fentanyl and strong receptor affinity might provide the long duration of morphine without the inherent risk of respiratory depression that results from morphine's poor lipid solubility.

Analgesia for Labor

In 1979, Yaksh et al. reported analgesia produced by intrathecal morphine in pregnant rats.[224] Early reports of this technique applied to humans were quite favorable;[3,29] however, despite consistent reports of adequate analgesia for the pain of early uterine contractions and cervical dilatation, a majority of patients reported inadequate pain relief for the second stage of labor.[7,194] In addition, many patients experienced side effects, including somnolence, nausea, vomiting, and severe pruritis. Brookshire et al.[29] reported these side effects could be reduced with intravenous naloxone without diminishing analgesic effects.

Administration of epidural opioids[84] is complicated by the need for the drug to cross the dura and by the presence of a rich venous plexus which absorbs the drug.[162,176] Several investigators have demonstrated an increase in meperidine absorption from the epidural space in pregnant women, compared with nonpregnant controls.[58,94,110]

Furthermore, the brief analgesia provided by epidural meperidine appeared to correlate with measured plasma levels,[110] suggesting the drug was effective only after vascular uptake and distribution. Similarly disappointing results were seen following epidural administration of morphine for labor analgesia,[21,111,113,114,134] although the lack of apparent efficacy may have been due to the very slow onset of action of epidural morphine and evaluation prior to its peak effect. By contrast, fentanyl can provide good epidural analgesia for postcesarean delivery pain[38,220] with plasma levels well below those known to be analgesic. This suggested a direct spinal analgesic mechanism with a slow absorption of fentanyl by epidural veins, probably due to the affinity of the drug for lipid-containing structures, including epidural fat.

Compared to the efficacy of intrathecal morphine,[20] epidural opioids[14] seemed unreliable, especially in comparison to the success rate of epidural bupivacaine, which is greater than 95%. In 1982 Justins et al.[116] tested the hypothesis that epidural opioid added to a small amount of local anesthetic might improve the efficacy of the anesthetic without added risk. In a double-blind study they added 80 µg fentanyl to 3 mL of 0.5% bupivacaine and found analgesia had a more rapid onset, a longer duration, and was perceived by the patient as more complete than that achieved in the control group with bupivacaine alone. Several investigators have since evaluated various combinations of fentanyl and bupivacaine reporting better labor analgesia than the local anesthetic alone.[6,201,212,225]

Cohen et al.[44] studied four groups of laboring women with varying concentrations of fentanyl and bupivacaine. They found analgesia with 0.068% bupivacaine combined with 100 µg of fentanyl was similar to that of their control group of 0.20% bupivacaine alone. They saw no maternal or fetal/neonatal side effects other than mild transient pruritis, which did not require treatment. Two of their fentanyl groups demonstrated a shorter duration of labor which they suggested was related to inhibition of maternal catecholamines that might inhibit uterine contractility.[127,161] However, with respect to analgesia, side effects, duration of labor, and neonatal effects they felt the addition of epidural fentanyl to bupivacaine did not result in a statistically significant improvement in analgesia when compared with the local anesthetic alone. It is important, however, that fentanyl in this study was administered only with the initial dose of local anesthetic. All subsequent reinforcement doses consisted of 0.25% bupivacaine. Also, the initial and all subsequent doses were preceded by a test dose of 3 mL of 1% lidocaine with epinephrine. The dilute local anesthetic effect could have influenced the findings.

Hughes et al.[109] reported results in 1,700 patients who received epidural morphine and demonstrated excellent, long-lasting analgesia with a very low rate of serious side effects. Four patients had a decrease in respiratory rate below 10 breaths per min. Only one of these experienced significant ventilatory compromise. She was readily treated with oxygen and naloxone and suffered no long-term effects. This suggests an incidence of serious respiratory depression significantly less common than with conventional opioid therapy; however many of us remain concerned that the long gap between administration of the drug and the onset of compromise may predispose to a false sense of security, especially on busy nursing units where these patients may not be able to receive sufficiently close observation. With this in mind, in our institutions we prefer to use the more lipid-soluble agents unless the patient is going to be kept in a recovery room or intensive care setting in which close observation is expected for 24 hr following subarachnoid or epidural morphine administration.[59] The kappa-specific agents show promise in providing good analgesia without respiratory depression,[159] but produce a high incidence of unwanted sedation. The development of a mu_1-specific agonist with potent analgesic properties, but without the respiratory depression that accompanies stimulation of mu_2-receptors would provide ideal properties.

Potential Toxicity

Respiratory depression, as noted, is the major complication related to intraspinal opioid administration.[68,74,90,163] Factors other than the nature of the narcotic used that may predispose to respiratory depression following epidural or intrathecal morphine include: concomitant parenteral administration of other opioids or sedatives, high doses of opioids, and lack of tolerance to opioids. Obstetric patients tend to be young and healthy with little preexisting respiratory disease. Investigations are underway to evaluate whether the ventilatory stimulation of pregnancy may further protect against the potential respiratory depression of spinal narcotics.

Nausea and vomiting is caused by stimulation of the chemoreceptor trigger zone and also is more common with intrathecal morphine in higher doses.[6,33,177,194]

Urinary retention results from opioid inhibition of the detrusor muscle and is less common in women than men. Brownridge[33] reported a series of 9,000 injections of 50 mg of epidural meperidine for postoperative analgesia following cesarean delivery without the need for catheterization of the bladder.

Pruritus is a direct effect of opiate receptor stimulation. Reported incidence of pruritus has been as high as 100%;[27] however, the incidence of pruritus requiring treatment is much less. Often patients must be questioned to elicit this side effect since it is usually not troubling, especially accompanying use of the more lipid-soluble agents. When necessary, naloxone reverses pruritus effectively.

Dysphoria and sedation have been reported following intraspinal administration of morphine in volunteers[28,121] but this seems significantly less common following intraspinal opioids compared with other routes such as intramuscular and oral administration. Acute narcotic withdrawal syndrome[218] has been reported following epidural administration of butorphanol, a mixed "agonist-antagonist" narcotic.

The use of intraspinal opioids is one of the most exciting recent advances in obstetric analgesia and anesthesia.[108,128,155,205] Techniques for maximizing efficacy while reducing the incidence of unwanted side effects are currently being evaluated at a number of centers. The existing data suggest significant benefits can be accrued for obstetric patients from both psychologic and physiologic standpoints.

NEUROBEHAVIORAL ASSESSMENT TECHNIQUES

The Apgar score is the traditional method for evaluating effects of obstetric medication.[5,75] Although it is an excellent test for vital functions during the first few minutes of life, it is an imperfect predictor of neurologic outcome[49] and is unlikely to reflect subtle effects of drugs. More sophisticated techniques of neurobehavioral testing of the newborn are more useful in this regard, and several such tests have been devised.[70,91,164,178,186]

Infants whose mothers received anesthesia or analgesia are most accurately described as "recovering patients."[164] Recovery from drug effects begins after delivery when placental circulation ceases and the infant begins to metabolize and eliminate the drugs. A good Apgar score does not rule out the possibility of problems arising subsequently during the first few hours of life.

To study the effects of parturitional epidural anesthesia on the newborn, Scanlon et al.[187–189] devised a neurobehavioral examination that utilizes elements adapted from both Prechtl and Beintema's neurologic examination[178] and Brazelton's scale.[22,23] The scheme for the Scanlon Early Neonatal Neurobehavioral Scale includes an evaluation of the newborn infant's state of consciousness before each individual observation. Habituation to pinprick, resistance against passive motion (pull to sitting, arm recoil, truncal tone, and general body tone), rooting, sucking, Moro responses, habituation to light and sound, placing, alertness, and general assessment are graded on a numerical scale. Finally, a judgment is made on the lability of state exhibited by the newborn during this examination.

Amiel-Tison et al.[4] devised a scoring system to evaluate adaptive capacity and neurologic function in full-term infants. This system is quicker than other examinations, puts more emphasis on neonatal tone, and does not use noxious stimuli. Initial results indicate that it is sensitive and has a high interobserver reliability. More information is necessary to assess the value of this test.

It must be borne in mind that there are few long-term studies available to determine if the findings on neurobehavioral examination correlate with later cognitive and neurologic development. Such information is vital for understanding the effects of anesthetic techniques and other labor and delivery practices.[206]

Neurobehavioral Effects of Local Anesthetics and Regional Block

Conway and Brackbill[46] used four different behavioral and physiologic tests to study 20 infants for 4 weeks after birth. They observed that anesthesia administered to the mother had definite effects on sensorimotor function in newborns, demonstrated by impaired muscular, visual, and neurologic performance. The greatest effect was seen with general anesthesia, but changes were also detectable after regional anesthesia.

Scanlon et al.[188] utilized the Early Neonatal Neurobehavioral Scale to evaluate babies whose mothers had received epidural anesthesia with mepivacaine or lidocaine, and compared them with babies whose mothers received spinal, local, or no anesthesia. The epidural group contained a higher proportion of infants who failed to habituate to certain forms of stimulation. In tests designed to assess muscle strength and tone, the epidural group scored lower than the nonepidural group. In general, the epidural babies were characterized as "floppy, but alert." Subsequently, Tronick et al.,[210] using the Brazelton examination, found that all evidence of diminished muscle tone associated with lidocaine or mepivacaine disappeared within the first 12 hr of life. Possible explanations for the poorer motor tone in the mepivacaine and lidocaine groups are impaired transmission of conducted impulses at the neuromuscular junction, depression of spinal reflex activity, and alteration by the local anesthetics of the contractile mechanism in skeletal muscle.

Scanlon et al.[189] evaluated a group of newborns whose mothers received bupivacaine for epidural anesthesia. The test results of these babies were comparable with the nonepidural group from their original study. In fact, in some of the tests, the bupivacaine group scored better than the control group, although the differences were not statistically significant. The differences between the two studies may be the result of smaller dosage of bupivacaine, the longer time from last injection to delivery, high maternal plasma binding, and subsequent decreased placental transfer.

Hodgkinson and Hussain[99] evaluated newborn infants whose mothers received either lumbar epidural anesthesia with 2-chloroprocaine, thiopental-nitrous oxide, or ketamine-nitrous oxide for vaginal delivery. Lumbar epidural anesthesia with 2-chloroprocaine was associated with the greatest percentage of high scores on both the first and second day for overall assessment, muscle tone, rooting, sucking, Moro response, placing, alertness, and habituation to pinprick. Scores were lowest after thiopental. No relationship was found between neurobehavioral responses and the use of outlet forceps, oxytocin stimulation, parity, or duration of labor. However, no control group was included and the test was first administered between 4 and 24 hr of life. To obtain information concerning drug effects, neurobehavioral assessment should be carried out between 2 and 4 hr of age. It will then coincide with the unresponsive period[70] when the effects of drugs administered to the mother are most likely to be present, and also with the half-life of the amide local anesthetics in the newborn.

Corke[49] compared three groups of neonates: one had no analgesia, another had meperidine and promazine, and a third had bupivacaine epidural. He tested the babies within 4 hr of delivery, and found that infants born to mothers who received meperidine and promazine scored significantly lower than babies of mothers who received no analgesia or lumbar epidural analgesia with bupivacaine. The epidural group scored better than the no analgesia group in all tests except motor tone. However, the differences were not statistically different.

Hodgkinson et al.[97] extended their investigations to elective cesarean section and compared general anesthesia with spinal anesthesia. The latter was associated with the greatest percentage of high scores on both the first and second day. The lowest scores followed thiopental induction; they were intermediate with ketamine, although the differences between these two groups were not significant. McGuinness et al.[133] compared bupivacaine epidural block with tetracaine spinal anesthesia for elective cesarean section and found no difference in discernible neurobehavioral effects. Lund et al.[130] evaluated etidocaine for cesarean section and found no neurobehavioral changes in 40 patients within 2 to 4 hr of birth. Datta et al.[65] evaluated three groups of patients undergoing elective cesarean section under lumbar epidural anesthesia with bupivacaine 0.75%, chloroprocaine 3%, and etidocaine 1%. They found that the neonatal outcomes as determined by Apgar scores and neurobehavioral testing were equal in all groups.

From the preceding review, it is apparent that the currently used amide and ester local anesthetics have been evaluated extensively by neonatal neurobehavioral techniques. A decrease in muscle tone is present in the newborn infant during the first few hours after birth if lidocaine or mepivacaine is used in large doses. By 12 hr of age, however, there are no differences when the groups are compared with controls. Subarachnoid and pudendal blocks produce no significant neurobehavioral alterations. It is apparent that other factors (e.g., decreased uteroplacental perfusion from maternal hypotension, preeclampsia, and so forth) must be considered when depression is observed in a newborn infant whose mother received regional anesthesia.

Corke et al.[50] evaluated the neurobehavior of infants born to mothers with and without hypotension (systolic arterial pressure less than 90 torr) following spinal anesthesia. Hypotension was reflected by acidosis in the infant at delivery even when the hypotension was corrected within 2 to 3 min. When the babies were examined between 2 and 4 hr of age, no neurobehavioral differences were found in either group.

Hollmen et al.[102] studied the effect of epidural anesthesia with 1.5% lidocaine with 1:200,000 epinephrine versus general anesthesia using thiopental, nitrous oxide/oxygen, and succinylcholine on the neurologic activity of newborns following cesarean section. In six patients following epidural anesthesia, mean arterial blood pressure fell below 70 torr. In four of the infants whose mothers had hypotension after epidural anesthesia, pH values were below 7.20 15 min after delivery. There was a significant correlation between maternal hypotension and weak rooting and sucking reflexes in the newborn infants at 1 and 2 days of age. Avoidance of the supine position is important in minimizing hypotension and its adverse effects on the fetus.[63]

All infants of high-risk obstetric patients in this series had abnormal neurologic activity independent of the anesthetic technique used. This work extends that of Corke et al.[50] and confirms the hypothesis that uncorrected maternal hypotension can result in alterations in the infant's neurobehavioral status.

It is obvious that the key to maintaining the best possible intrauterine environment for the fetus is adequate uteroplacental perfusion to prevent fetal acidosis and hypoxia. Even short periods of hypotension can produce altered biochemical and neurobehavioral results for up to 48 hr after delivery.

REFERENCES

1. Abraham RA, Harris AP, Maxwell LG, Kaplow S: The efficacy of 1.5% lidocaine with 7.5% dextrose and epinephrine as an epidural test dose for obstetrics. *Anesthesiology* 1986;64:116–119.

2. Akamatsu TJ, Bonica JJ, Rehmet R, Eng M, Ueland K: Experiences with the use of ketamine for parturition. I. Primary anesthetic for vaginal delivery. *Anesth Analg* 1974;53:284–287.

3. Alper MH: Intrathecal morphine; A new method of obstetric analgesia? *Anesthesiology* 1979;51:378.

4. Amiel-Tison C, Barrier G, Shnider SM: A new neurological scoring system. Abstracts of XI World Congress of Obstetrics and Gynecology, Tokyo, October 1979.

5. Apgar V: A proposal for a new method of evaluation of the newborn infant. *Anesth Analg* 1953;32:260–267.

6. Baraka A, Maktabi M, Noueihid R: Epidural meperidine-bupivacaine for obstetric analgesia. *Anesth Analg* 1982;61:652–656.

7. Baraka A, Noueihid R, Hajj S: Intrathecal injection of morphine for obstetric analgesia. *Anesthesiology* 1981;54:136–140.

8. Baraka A, Saab M, Salem MR, Winnie AP: Control of gastric acidity by glycopyrrolate premedication in the parturient. *Anesth Analg* 1977;56:642–645.

9. Bassell GM, Humayun SG, Marx GF: Maternal bearing down efforts—another fetal risk? *Obstet Gynecol* 1980;56:39–41.

10. Belfrage P, Berlin A, Lindstedt M, Raabe N: Plasma levels of bupivacaine following pudendal block in labour. *Br J Anaesth* 1973;45:1067–1069.

11. Belfrage P, Raabe N, Thalme B, Berlin A: Lumbar epidural analgesia with bupivacaine in labor. *Am J Obstet Gynecol* 121:360–365.

12. Biehl D, Callender K, Shnider SM: The effect of fetal acidosis on lidocaine blood levels. Abstracts of Scientific Papers, American Society of Anesthesiologists Annual Meeting, San Francisco, 1976, p 535.

13. Bieniarz J, Crottogini JJ, Curuchet E: Aortocaval compression by the uterus in late pregnancy. II. An arteriographic study. *Am J Obstet Gynecol* 1968;100:203–217.

14. Binsted R: Epidural morphine post caesarean section. *Anaesth Intensive Care* 1983;11:130–134.

15. Blankenbaker WL, Difazio CA, Berry FA: Lidocaine and its metabolites in the newborn. *Anesthesiology* 1975;42:325–330.

16. Blitt CD, Petty WC, Alberternst EE, Wright BJ: Correlation of plasma cholinesterase activity and duration of action of succinylcholine during pregnancy. *Anesth Analg* 1977;56:78–83.

17. Bloomberg RG: The lumbar subdural extraarachnoid space of humans: An anatomical study using spinaloscopy in autopsy cases. *Anesth Analg* 1987;66:177–180.

18. Bonica JJ: *Principles and Practice of Obstetric Anesthesia.* Philadelphia, FA Davis, 1967.

19. Bonica JJ: *Obstetric Analgesia and Anesthesia.* Amsterdam, World Federation of Societies of Anaesthesiologists, 1980.

20. Bonnardot JP, Maillet M, Colau JC, Millot F, Deligne P: Maternal and fetal concentrations of morphine after intrathecal administration during labor. *Br J Anaesth* 1982;54: 487–489.

21. Booker PD, Wilkes RG, Bryson THL, Beddard J: Obstetric pain relief using epidural morphine. *Anaesthesia* 1980;35:377–379.

22. Brazelton TB: Effect of prenatal drugs on the behavior of the neonate. *Am J Psychiatry* 1970;126:95–100.

23. Brazelton TB: *Neonatal Behavioral Assessment Scale.* Clinics in Developmental Medicine, No. 50. London, Spastics International Medical Publishers, 1973.

24. Bromage PR: An evaluation of bupivacaine in epidural analgesia for obstetrics. *Can Anaesth Soc J* 1969;16:46–56.

25. Bromage PR: *Epidural Analgesia.* Philadelphia, WB Saunders, 1978.

26. Bromage PR: The price of intraspinal narcotic analgesia: Basic constraints. *Anesth Analg* 1981;60:461–463.

27. Bromage PR, Camporesi EM, Chestnut D: Epidural narcotics for postoperative analgesia. *Anesth Analg* 1980;59:473–480.

28. Bromage PR, Camporesi EM, Durant PAC, Nielsen CH: Nonrespiratory side effects of epidural morphine. *Anesth Analg* 1982;61:490–495.

29. Brookshire GL, Shnider SM, Abboud TK, Kotelko DM, Noueihid R, Thigpen JW, Khoo SS, Raya JA, Foutz SE, Brizgys RV: Effects of naloxone on the mother and neonate after intrathecal morphine for labor analgesia. *Anesthesiology* 1983;59:A417.

30. Brown WU, Bell GC, Lurie AO, Weiss J, Scanlon JW, Alper MH: Newborn blood levels of lidocaine and mepivacaine in the first postnatal day following maternal epidural anesthesia. *Anesthesiology* 1975;42:698–706.

31. Brown WU, Scanlon JW, Ostheimer GW, Alper MH: Levels of lidocaine in mother and baby following pudendal and local blocks. *Abstracts of Scientific Papers,* Society for Obstetric Anesthesia and Perinatology Annual Meeting, San Francisco, 1974.

32. Brown WU Jr, Bell GC, Alper MH: Acidosis, local anesthetics, and the newborn. *Obstet Gynecol* 1976;48:27–30.

33. Brownridge PR: Epidural and intrathecal opiates for postoperative pain relief. *Anaesthesia* 1983;38:74–75.

34. Bylsema-Howel M, Riggs KW, McMorland GH, Rurak DW, Ongley R, McErlane B, Price JDE, Axelson JE: Placental transport of metoclopramide: Assessment of maternal and neonatal effects. *Can Anaesth Soc J* 1983;30:438–492.

35. Byrne F, Odura-Dominah A, Kipling R: The effect of pregnancy on pulmonary nitrogen washout: A study of pre-oxygenation. *Anaesthesia* 1987;42:148–150.

36. Caldwell J, Wakile LA, Notarianni LJ: Maternal and neonatal disposition of pethidine in childbirth: A study using quantitative gas chromatography—mass spectrometry. *Life Sci* 1978;22:589–596.

37. Caritis SN, Abouleish E, Edelstone DI, Mueller-Heubach E: Fetal acid-base state following spinal or epidural anesthesia for cesarean section. *Obstet Gynecol* 1980;56:610–615.

38. Carrie LE, O'Sullivan GM, Seegobin R: Epidural fentanyl in labour. *Anaesthesia* 1981;36:965–969.

39. Cartwright PD, McCarrol SM, Antzaka C: Maternal heart rate changes with a plain epidural test dose. *Anesthesiology* 1986;65:226–228.

40. Channing WB: *A treatise on Etherization in Childbirth (Illustrated by 581 Cases)*. Boston, William D. Ticknor, 1848.

41. Cibils LA: Response of human uterine arteries to local anesthetics. *Am J Obstet Gynecol* 1976;126:202–210.

42. Clark RB, Thompson DS, Thompson CH: Prevention of spinal hypotension associated with cesarean section. *Anesthesiology* 1976;45:670–674.

43. Climie CR, McLean S, Starmer GA, Thomas J: Methaemoglobinaemia in mother and foetus following continuous epidural analgesia with prilocaine. *Br J Anaesth* 1967;39:155–160.

44. Cohen SE, Tan S, Albright GA, Halpern J: Epidural fentanyl/bupivacaine mixtures for obstetric analgesia. *Anesthesiology* 1987;64:403–407.

45. Coleman AJ, Downing DW: Enflurane anesthesia for cesarean section. *Anesthesiology* 1975;43:354–357.

46. Conway E, Brackbill Y: Delivery medication and infant income—an empirical study: Effects of obstetrical medication on the fetus and infant. Bowes WA, Brackbill Y, Conway E, (eds). *Meninger Soc. Res. Child Dev.* 1970.

47. Coombs DW, Hooper D, Cotton T: Preanesthetic cimetidine alteration of gastric fluid volume and pH. *Anesth Analg* 1979;58:183–188.

48. Cooper LV, Stephen GW, Aggett PJA: Elimination of pethidine and bupivacaine in the newborn. *Arch Dis Child* 1977;52:638–642.

49. Corke BC: Neurobehavioral responses of the newborn. *Anaesthesia* 1977;32:539–543.

50. Corke BC, Datta S, Ostheimer GW: Influence of hypotension during spinal anesthesia for cesarean section on infant outcome. Abstracts of Scientific Papers, Obstetric Anesthetists Association Meeting, Edinburgh, 1978.

51. Cosmi EV, Marx GF: The effect of anesthesia on the acid-base status of the fetus. *Anesthesiology* 1978;30:238–242.

52. Cousins MJ: Epidural neural blockade, in Cousins MJ, Bridenbaugh PO (eds): *Neural Blockade in Clinical Anesthesia and Management of Pain*. Philadelphia, JB Lippincott, 1980, pp 176–274.

53. Cousins MJ, Mather LE: Intrathecal and epidural administration of opioids. *Anesthesiology* 1984;61:276–310.

54. Cousins MJ, Mather LE, Glynn CJ, Wilson PR, Grahan JR: Selective spinal analgesia. *Lancet* 1979;1:1141–1142.

55. Covino BG, Vassallo HG: *Local Anesthetics: Mechanisms of Action and Clinical Use*. New York, Grune & Stratton, 1976.

56. Creasser CW, Stoelting RK, Krishna G, Peterson C: Methoxyflurane metabolism and renal function after methoxyflurane analgesia during labor and delivery. *Anesthesiology* 1964;41:62–66.

57. Cree JE, Myer J, Hailey DM: Diazepam in labor: Its metabolism and effect on the clinical condition and thermogenesis of the newborn. *Br Med J* 1973;4:251–254.

58. Cummings AJ, Rosankiewicz JR: Comparison of epidural and intramuscular pethidine for analgesia in labour. *Br J Obstet Gynecol* 1981;88:711–717.

59. Danielson DR, Coombs DW, Pageau M, Rippe E: Epidural morphine for post-caesarean analgesia. *Anesthesiology* 1981;55:A323.

60. Datta S, Alper MH: Anesthesia for cesarean section. *Anesthesiology* 1980;53:142–160.

61. Datta S, Alper MH, Ostheimer GW, Weiss JB: Method of ephedrine administration and nausea and hypotension during spinal anesthesia for cesarean section. *Anesthesiology* 1982;56:68–70.

62. Datta S, Alper MH, Ostheimer GW, Brown WU, Weiss JB: Effect of maternal position on epidural anesthesia for cesarean section, acid-base status and bupivacaine concentrations at delivery. *Anesthesiology* 1979;50:205–209.

63. Datta S, Briwa J: Modified laryngoscope for endotracheal intubation of obese patients. *Anesth Analg* 1981;60;120–121.

64. Datta S, Brown WU: Acid-base status in diabetic mothers and their infants following general or spinal anesthesia for cesarean section. *Anesthesiology* 1977;47:272–276.

65. Datta S, Corke BC, Alper MH, Ostheimer GW: Epidural anesthesia for cesarean section. A comparison of bupivacaine, chloroprocaine and etidocaine. *Anesthesiology* 1980;52:48–51.

66. Datta S, Ostheimer GW, Weiss JB: Neonatal effect of prolonged anesthetic induction for cesarean section. *Obstet Gynecol* 1981;58:331–335.

67. David H, Rosen M: Perinatal mortality after epidural analgesia. *Anaesthesia* 1976;31:1054–1059.

68. Davies GK, Tolhurst-Cleaver CL, James TL: Respiratory depression after intrathecal narcotics. *Anaesthesia* 1980;35:1080–1083.

69. de Jong R: Toxic effects of local anesthetics. *JAMA* 1978;239:1166–1168.

70. Desmond MM, Franklin RR, Vallbona C: The clinical behavior of the newly born. I. The term baby. *J Pediatr* 1963;62:307–325.

71. Dewan DM, Floyd HM, Thistlewood JM, Bogard TD, Spielman FJ: Sodium citrate pretreatment in elective cesarean section patients. *Anesth Analg* 1985;64:34–37.

72. Dignam WJ, Titus P, Assali NS: Renal function in human pregnancy I. Changes in glomerular filtration rate and renal plasma flow. *Proc Soc Exp Biol Med* 1958;97:512–514.

73. Dobb GJ: Pulmonary acid aspiration syndrome: Prophylaxis with cimetidine, in Wastell C, Lance P (eds): *Cimetidine: The Westminister Hospital Symposium 1978.* Edinburgh, Churchill Livingstone, 1978, pp 235–245.

74. Downes JJ, Kemp RA, Lambertsen CJ: The magnitude and duration of respiratory depression due to fentanyl and meperidine in man. *J Pharmacol Exp Ther* 1967;158:416–429.

75. Drage JS, Kennedy C, Berendes H, Schwarez BK, Weiss W: The Apgar score: Index of infant morbidity. *Dev Med Child Neurol* 1966;8:141–148.

76. Duffy BL, Woodhouse PC: Sodium citrate and gastric acidity in obstetric patients. *Med J Aust* 1982;2:37–38.

77. Ebner H, Barcohana J, Bartoshok AK: Influence of post-spinal hypotension on the fetal electrocardiogram. *Am J Obstet Gynecol* 1960;80:569–572.

78. Eckenhoff JE: The physiological significance of the vertebral venous plexus. *Surg Gynecol Obstet* 1970;131:72–78.

79. Ellingson A, Haram K, Sagen N, Solheim E: Transplacental passage of ketamine after intravenous administration. *Acta Anaesth Scand* 1977;21:41–44.

80. Finster M, Morishima HO, Mark LC, Perel JM, Dayton PG, James LS: Tissue thiopental concentrations in the fetus and newborn. *Anesthesiology* 1972;36:155–158.

81. Finster M, Perel JM, Hinsvark ON, O'Brien JE: Pharmacodynamics of 2-chloroprocaine (Nesacaine), an estertype local anesthetic, in *Fourth European Congress Anesthesiology.* Amsterdam, Excerpta Medica, No. 330, p 189.

82. Finster M, Poppers PJ: Safety of thiopental used for induction of general anesthesia in elective cesarean section. *Anesthesiology* 1968;29:190–191.

83. Forrest WH, Bellville JW: Respiratory effects of alphaprodine in man. *Obstet Gynecol* 1968;31:61–68.

84. Francis DM, Justins D, Reynolds FJM: Obstetric pain relief using epidural narcotic agents. *Anaesthesia* 1980;35:69.

85. Galbert MW, Gardner AE: Use of halothane in a balanced technique for cesarean section. *Anesth Analg* 1972;51:701–704.

86. Gambee AM, Hertzka RE: Preoxygenation techniques: Comparison of three minutes and four breaths. *Anesth Analg* 1987;77:468–470.

87. Gibbs CP, Spohr L, Schmidt D: Effectiveness of sodium citrate as antacid. *Anesthesiology* 1982;57:44–46.

88. Gibbs CP, Noel SC: Response of arterial segments from gravid human uterus to multiple concentrations of lignocaine. *Br J Anaesth* 1977;49:409–411.

89. Gibbs CP, Schwartz DJ, Wynne JW, Hood CI, Kuck EJ: Antacid pulmonary aspiration in the dog. *Anesthesiology* 1979;51:380–385.

90. Glynn CJ, Mather LE, Cousins MJ, Wilson PR, Graham JR: Spinal narcotics and respiratory depression. *Lancet* 1979;2:356–357.

91. Graham FK, Pennayer MM, Caldwell BM, Hartman AP: Relationship between clinical status and behavior test performance in a newborn group with histories suggesting anoxia. *J Pediatr* 1957;50:177–189.

92. Greene NM: *Physiology of Spinal Anesthesia,* 3rd ed. Baltimore, Williams & Wilkins, 1981.

93. Greiss FC Jr, Still JG, Anderson SG: Effects of local anesthetic agents on the uterine vasculatures and myometrium. *Am J Obstet Gynecol* 1976;124:889–899.

94. Gustafsson LL, Garle M, Johannisson J, Rane A, Stenport J, Walson P: Regional epidural analgesia: Kinetics of pethidine. *Acta Anaesth Scand* 1982;(suppl)74:165–168.

95. Hansen R: Ohnmach and Schwangerschaft. *Klin Wochenschr* 1942;21:241–250.

96. Hehre F, Hook R, Hon E: Continuous lumbar epidural anesthesia in obstetrics. VI. The fetal effects of transplacental passage of local anesthetic agents. *Anesth Analg* 1969;48:909–913.

97. Hodgkinson R, Bhatt M, Kim SS: Neonatal neurobehavioral tests following cesarean section under general and spinal anesthesia. *Am J Obstet Gynecol* 1978;132:670–674.

98. Hodgkinson R, Glassenberg R, Joyce TH, Coombs DW, Ostheimer GW, Gibbs CP: Comparison of cimetidine (Tagamet) with antacid for safety and effectiveness in reducing gastric acidity before elective cesarean section. *Anesthesiology* 1983;59:86–90.

99. Hodgkinson R, Hussain F: The duration of effect of maternally administered meperidine on neonatal neurobehavior. *Anesthesiology* 1982;56:51–52.

100. Hodgkinson R, Marx GF, Kim SS, Miclat MM: Neonatal neurobehavioral tests following vaginal delivery under ketamine, thiopental, and extradural anesthesia. *Anesth Analg* 1977;56:548–553.

101. Holdsworth JD, Johnson K, Mascall G, Roulston RG, Tomlinson PA: Mixing of antacids with stomach contents. Another approach to the prevention of the acid aspiration (Mendelson's) syndrome. *Anaesthesia* 1980;35:641–650.

102. Hollmen AI, Jouppilla R, Koivisto M, Maata L, Pihlajaniemi R, Puukka M, Rantakyla P: Neurologic activity of infants following anesthesia for cesarean section. *Anesthesiology* 1978;48:350–356.

103. Hon EH, Reid BL, Hehre FW: The electronic evaluation of the fetal heart rate. II. Changes with maternal hypotension. *Am J Obstet Gynecol* 1960;79:209–215.

104. Hood DD, Dewan DM, James FM: Maternal and fetal effects of epinephrine in gravid ewes. *Anesthesiology* 1986;64:610–613.

105. Howard BK, Goodson JH, Mengert WF: Supine hypotension syndrome in late pregnancy. *Obstet Gynecol* 1953;1:371–377.

106. Howe JP, McGowan WAW, Moore J, McCaughey W, Dundee JW: The placental transfer of cimetidine. *Anaesthesia* 1981;36:371–375.

107. Hughes J, Smith TW, Kosterlitz HW, Fothergill LA, Morgan BA, Morris HR: Identification of two related pentapeptides from the brain with potent opiate agonist activity. *Nature* 1975;258:577–579.

108. Hughes SC: Intraspinal narcotics in obstetrics. *Clin Perinatol* 1982;1:167–175.

109. Hughes SC, Rosen MA, Shnider SM, Abboud TK, Stefani SJ, Norton M: Maternal and neonatal effects of epidural morphine for labor and delivery. *Anesth Analg* 1984;63:319–324.

110. Husemeyer RP, Cummings AJ, Rosankiewicz JR, Davenport HT: A study of pethidine kinetics and analgesia in women in labour following intravenous, intramuscular and epidural administration. *Br J Clin Pharmacol* 1982;13:171–176.

111. Husemeyer RP, Davenport HT: Prophylaxis for Mendelson's syndrome before elective cesarean section. A comparison of cimetidine and magnesium trisilicate mixture regimens. *Br J Obstet Gynecol* 1980;87:565–570.

112. Husemeyer RP, Davenport HT, Rajasekaran T: Cimetidine as a single oral dose for prophylaxis against Mendelson's syndrome. *Anaesthesia* 1978;33:775–778.

113. Husemeyer RP, O'Connor MC, Davenport HT: Aspects of epidural morphine. *Lancet* 1979;2:583–584.

114. Husemeyer RP, O'Connor MC, Davenport HT: Failure of epidural morphine to relieve pain in labour. *Anaesthesia* 1980;35:161–163.

115. Janeczko GF, El-Etr AA, Younces S: Low dose ketamine anesthesia for obstetrical delivery. *Anesth Analg* 1974;53:828–831.

116. Justins DM, Francis D, Houlton PG, Reynolds F: A controlled trial of extradural fentanyl in labor. *Br J Anaesth* 1982;54:409–414.

117. Kanto J, Erkkola R, Sellman R: Accumulation of diazepam and N-demethylated diazepam in the fetal blood during labour. *Ann Clin Res* 1973;5:375–379.

118. Kenepp NB, Shelley WC, Kumar S, Gutsche BB, Gabbe S, Delivoria-Papadopoulos M: Dextrose hydration in cesarean patients. *Anesthesiology* 1980;53:S304.

119. Kerr MG, Scott DB, Samuel E: Studies on the inferior vena cava in the late pregnancy. *Br Med J* 1964;1:532–533.

120. Kitahata LM, Collins JG: Spinal action of narcotic analgesics. *Anesthesiology* 1981;54:153–163.

121. Knill RL, Clement JL, Thompson WR: Epidural morphine causes delayed and prolonged ventilatory depression. *Can Anaesth Soc J* 1981;28:537–543.

122. Koch G, Wandel H: Effect of pethidine on the post natal adjustment of respiration and acid-base balance. *Acta Obstet Gynecol Scand* 1968;47:27–37.

123. Kosaka Y, Takahashi T, Mark LC: Intravenous thiobarbiturate anesthesia for cesarean section. *Anesthesiology* 1969;31:489–506.

124. Kuhnert BR, Kuhnert PM, Prochaska AL, Gross TL: Plasma level of 2-chloroprocaine in obstetric patients and their neonates after epidural anesthesia. *Anesthesiology* 1980; 53:21–25.

125. Lam AM, Knill RL, Thompson WR: Epidural fentanyl does not cause delayed respiratory depression. *Can Anaesth Soc J* 1983;30:578–579.

126. Lederman RP, Lederman E, Work BA Jr, McCann DS: The relationship of maternal anxiety, plasma catecholamines and plasma cortisol to progress in labor. *Am J Obstet Gynecol* 1978;132:495–500.

127. Lederman RP, Lederman E, Work BA Jr, et al: Anxiety and epinephrine in multiparous labor: Relationship to duration of labor and fetal heart rate pattern. *Am J Obstet Gynecol* 1985;153:870–877.

128. Leicht CH, Hughes SC, Dailey PA, Shnider SM, Rosen MA: Epidural morphine sulfate for analgesia after cesarean section; a prospective report of 1000 patients. *Anesthesiology* 1986;65:A366.

129. Levinson G, Shnider SM, deLorimier AA, Steffenson JL: Effects of maternal hyperventilation on uterine blood flow and fetal oxygenation and acid-base status. *Anesthesiology* 1974;40:340–347.

130. Lund PC, Cwik JC, Gannon RT, Vassallo HG: Etidocaine for cesarean section—effects on mother and baby. *Br J Anaesth* 1977;49:457–460.

131. McCarthy GT, O'Connel B, Robinson A: Blood levels of diazepam in infants of two mothers given large doses of diazepam during labour. *J Obstet Gynaecol Br Commw* 1973;80:349–352.

132. McDonald JS, Bjorkman LL, Reed EC: Epidural analgesia for obstetrics. *Am J Obstet Gynecol* 1954;120:1055–1065.

133. McGuinness BA, Merkow AJ, Kennedy RL, Erenberg A: Epidural anesthesia with bupivacaine for cesarean section: Neonatal blood levels and neurobehavioral responses. *Anesthesiology* 1978;49:270–273.

134. Magora F, Olshwang D, Eimerl D, Shorr J, Katzenelson R, Cotev S, Davidson JT: Observations of extradural morphine analgesia in various pain conditions. *Br J Anaesth* 1980;52:247–252.

135. Maliniak K, Vakil AH: Preanesthetic cimetidine and gastric pH. *Anesth Analg* 1979;58:309–313.

136. Maltau JM, Andersen HT: Epidural anesthesia as an alternative to cesarean section in the treatment of prolonged exhaustive labour. *Acta Anaesth Scand* 1975;19:349–354.

137. Manchikanti L, Colliver JA, Marrero TC, Roush JR: Rantidine and metoclopramide for prophylaxis of aspiration pneumonitis in elective surgery. *Anesth Analg* 1984;63:903–910.

138. Manchikanti L, Marrero TC, Roush JR: Preanesthetic cimetidine and metoclopramide for acid aspiration prophylaxis in elective surgery. *Anesthesiology* 1984;61: 48–54.

139. Mandelli M, Morselli PL, Nordio S: Placental transfer of diazepam and its disposition in the newborn. *Clin Pharmacol Ther* 1975;17:564–572.

140. Mankowitz E, Broch-Utne JG, Downing JW: Nitrous oxide elimination by the newborn. *Anaesthesia* 1981;36:1014–1016.

141. Martin WR: Opioid antagonists. *Pharmacol Rev* 1967;19:463–521.

142. Marx GF, Cosmi EV, Wollman SB: Biochemical status and clinical condition of mother and infant at cesarean section. *Anesth Analg* 1969;48:986–994.

143. Marx GF, Joshi CW, Orkin LR: Placental transmission of nitrous oxide. *Anesthesiology* 1970;32:429–432.

144. Matadial L, Cibils LA: The effect of epidural anesthesia on uterine activity and blood pressure. *Am J Obstet Gynecol* 1976;125:846.

145. Meffin P, Long GJ, Thomas J: Clearance and metabolism of mepivacaine in the human neonate. *Clin Pharmacol Ther* 1973;14:218–225.

146. Mendelson CL: The aspiration of stomach contents into the lungs during obstetric anesthesia. *Am J Obstet Gynecol* 1946;52:191–205.

147. Mendiola J, Grylack L, Scanlon JW: Effects of intrapartum maternal glucose infusion on the normal fetus and newborn. *Anesth Analg* 1982;61:32–35.

148. Merritt JC, Sprague DH, Merritt WE, Ellis RA: Retroental fibroplasia: A multifactorial disease. *Anesth Analg* 1981;60:109–111.

149. Moore RA, Bullingham RSJ, McQuay HJ, Hand CW, Aspel JB, Allen MC, Thomas D: Dural permeability to narcotics; in vitro determination and application to extradural administration. *Br J Anaesth* 1982;54:1117–1128.

150. Morishima HO, Adamsons K: Placental clearance of mepivacaine following administration to the guinea-pig fetus. *Anesthesiology* 1967;28:343–349.

151. Morishima HO, Covino BG, Yeh MN, Stark RI, James LS: Bradycardia in the fetal baboon following paracervical block anesthesia. *Am J Obstet Gynecol* 1981;140:775–780.

152. Morrison JC, Whybrew WD, Rosser SI, Bucovaz ET, Wiser WL, Fish SA: Metabolites of meperidine in the fetal and maternal serum. *Am J Obstet Gynecol* 1976;126:997–1003.

153. Motoyama EK, Rivard G, Acheson F, Cook CD: Adverse effects of maternal hyperventilation on the fetus. *Lancet* 1966;1:286–288.

154. Moya F, Kvisselgaard N: The placental transmission of succinylcholine. *Anesthesiology* 1961;22:1–6.

155. Muller A, Laugner B, Farcot JM, Singer M, Gauthier-Lafaye P, Gandar R: Epidural morphine for obstetrical pain relief. *Anesth Analg (Paris)* 1981;38:35–41.

156. Munson ES, Paul WL, Embro WJ: Central nervous system toxicity of local anesthetic mixtures. *Anesthesiology* 1977;46:179–183.

157. Murphy DF, Gardiner J, Unwin A: Effect of metoclopramide on gastric emptying before elective and emergency cesarean section. *Br J Anaesth* 1984;56:1113–1116.

158. Naulty JS, Ostheimer GW, Datta S, Burger G: Epidural fentanyl for post cesarean delivery analgesia. *Anesthesiology* 1985;31:394–397.

159. Naulty JS, Weintraub S, Ostheimer GW, Datta S: Epidural butorphanol for post cesarean delivery analgesia. *Anesthesiology* 1984;61:A415.

160. Nelson NM, Enkin MW, Saigal S, Bennett KJ, Milner RM, Sackett DL: A randomized clinical trial of the LeBoyer approach to childbirth. *N Engl J Med* 1980;302:655–660.

161. Neumark J, Hammerle AF, Biegelmayer CH: Effects of epidural analgesia on plasma catecholamine and cortisol in parturition. *Acta Anaesthesiol Scand* 1985;29:555–559.

162. Nybell-Lindahl C, Carlsson C, Ingemarsson I, Westgren M, Paalzow L: Maternal and fetal concentrations of morphine after epidural administration during labour. *Am J Obstet Gynecol* 1981;139:20–21.

163. Odoom JA: Respiratory depression after intrathecal morphine. *Anesth Analg* 1982;61:70.

164. Ostheimer GW: Neurobehavioral effects of obstetric analgesia. *Br J Anaesth* 1979;51(suppl):35–40.

165. Ostheimer GW: Newborn resuscitation. *Clin Obstet Gynecol* 1981;24:635–648.

166. Ostheimer GW, Lurie AO, Brown WU: Maternal and newborn concentrations of bupivacaine and 2,6-pipecoloxylidide (PPX) in blood and urine. Abstracts of Scientific Papers, Annual Meeting, American Society of Anesthesiologists, Chicago, 1974, pp 393–394.

167. Ostheimer GW, Lurie AO, Brown WU: Metabolism of lidocaine in mother and newborn. Abstracts of Scientific Papers, Society of Obstetric Anesthesia and Perinatology Annual Meeting, Philadelphia, 1975.

168. O'Sullivan GM, Bullingham RE: Noninvasive assessment by radiotelemetry of antacid effect during labor. *Anesth Analg* 1985;64:95–100.

169. Owens JR, Irani SF, Blair AW: Effects of diazepam administered to mothers during labour on temperature regulation of the neonate. *Arch Dis Child* 1972;47:107–110.

170. Owens WD, Zeitlin GL: Hypoventilation in a newborn following administration of succinylcholine to the mother: A case report. *Anesth Analg* 1975;54:38–40.

171. Paddock R, Beer EG, Bellville JW, Ciliberti BJ, Forrest WH, Miller EV: Analgesic and side effects of pentazocine and morphine in a large population of postoperative patients. *Clin Pharmacol Ther* 1969;10:355–365.

172. Palahniuk RJ, Shnider SM: Maternal and fetal cardiovascular and acid-base changes during halothane and isoflurane anesthesia in the pregnant ewe. *Anesthesiology* 1974;41:462–472.

173. Palahniuk RJ, Shnider SM, Eger EI: Pregnancy decreases the requirement of inhaled anesthetic agents. *Anesthesiology* 1974;41:82–83.

174. Pasternak GW: Opiate, enkephalin, and endorphin analgesia: Relations to a single population of opiate receptors. *Neurology* 1981;31:1311–1315.

175. Penrose BH: Aspiration pneumonitis following ketamine induction for general anesthesia. *Anesth Analg* 1972;51:41–43.

176. Perriss BW: Epidural pethidine in labour: A study of dose requirements. *Anaesthesia* 1980;35:380–382.

177. Perriss BW, Malins AF: Pain relief in labour using epidural pethidine with adrenaline. *Anaesthesia* 1981;36:631–633.

178. Prechtl JFR, Beintema D: *The neurologic examination of the full term infant.* Clinics in Developmental Medicine, No. 12. London, Spastics International Medical Publishers, 1964.

179. Quilligan EJ, Keegan KA, Donahue MJ: Double-blind comparison of intravenously injected butorphanol and meperidine in parturients. *Int J Gynaecol Obstet* 1980;18:363–367.

180. Ralston DH, Shnider SM, deLorimier AA: Effects of equipotent ephedrine, metaraminol, mephentermine and methoxamine on uterine blood flow in the pregnant ewe. *Anesthesiology* 1974;40:354–370.

181. Ravindran RS, Viegas PJ, Tasch MD: Bearing down at the time of delivery and the incidence of spinal headache in parturients. *Anesth Analg* 1981;60:524–526.

182. Reynolds F, Taylor G: Maternal and neonatal blood concentrations of bupivacaine. *Anaesthesia* 1970;25:14–23.

183. Roberts RB, Shirley MA: Reducing the risk of acid aspiration during cesarean section. *Anesth Analg* 1974;53:859–868.

184. Rolbin SH, Wright RG, Shnider SM: Diazepam during cesarean section—effects on neonatal Apgar scores, acid-base status, neurobehavioral assessment and maternal and fetal plasma norepinephrine levels. Abstracts of Scientific Papers, Annual Meeting of the American Society of Anesthesiologists, 1977, pp 449–450.

185. Romagnoli A, Keats AS: Ceiling effect for respiratory depression by nalbuphine. *Clin Pharmacol Ther* 1980;27:478–485.

186. Rosenblith JF: The modified Graham behavior tests for neonates: Test-retest reliability, normative data and hypotheses for future work. *Biol Neonat* 1961;3:174–192.

187. Scanlon JW: Clinical neonatal neurobehavioral assessment: Methods and significance, in Marx GF (ed): *Clinical Management of Mother and Newborn.* New York, Springer-Verlag, 1979, pp 65–83.

188. Scanlon JW, Brown WU Jr, Weiss JB, Alper MH: Neurobehavioral responses of newborn infants after maternal epidural anesthesia. *Anesthesiology* 1974;40:121–128.

189. Scanlon JW, Ostheimer GW, Lurie AD, Brown WU, Weiss JB, Alper MH: Neurobehavioral responses and drug concentrations in newborn after maternal epidural anesthesia with bupivacaine. *Anesthesiology* 1976;45:400–405.

190. Schellenberg JS: Uterine activity during lumbar epidural analgesia with bupivacaine. *Am J Obstet Gynecol* 1977;127:26–31.

191. Schifrin BS: Fetal heart rate patterns following epidural anesthesia and oxytocin infusion during labour. *J Obstet Gynaecol Br Commonw* 1972;79:332–339.

192. Schulze-Delrieu K: Metoclopramide. *N Engl J Med* 1981;305:28–33.

193. Scott JR, Rose NB: Effect of psychoprophylaxis (Lamaze preparation) on labor and delivery in primiparas. *N Engl J Med* 1976;294:1205–1207.

194. Scott PV, Bowen FE, Cartwright P, Rae BCM, Deeley D, Wotherspoon HG, Samren IMA: Intrathecal morphine as sole analgesic during labour. *Br Med J* 1980;281:351–353.

195. Shnider SM: Serum cholinesterase activity during pregnancy, labor and puerperium. *Anesthesiology* 1965;26:335–339.

196. Shnider SM, Levinson G: Anesthesia for cesarean section, in Levinson G, Shnider SM (eds): *Anethesia for Obstetrics,* Baltimore, Williams & Wilkins, pp 254–275.

197. Shnider SM, Levinson G: *Anesthesia for Obstetrics.* Baltimore, Williams & Wilkins, 1979.

198. Shnider SM, Moya F: Effects of meperidine on the newborn infant. *Am J Obstet Gynecol* 1964;89:1009–1015.

199. Shnider SM, Wright RG, Levinson G, Roizen MF, Wallis KL, Rolbin SH, Craft JB: Uterine blood flow and plasma norepinephrine changes during maternal stress in the pregnant ewe. *Anesthesiology* 1979;50:524–527.

200. Skaredoff MN, Ostheimer GW: Physiologic changes during pregnancy: Effects of major regional anesthesia. *Reg Anesth* 1981;6:28–40.

201. Skerman JH, Thompson BA, Goldstein MT, Jacobs MA, Gupta A, Blass NH: Combined continuous epidural fentanyl and bupivacaine in labor: A randomized study. *Anesthesiology* 1985;63:A450.

202. Sladen A: Pharmacologic management of cardiopulmonary resuscitation, in Hershey SG (ed): *ASA Refresher Courses in Anesthesiology*. Philadelphia, JB Lippincott, 1976, pp 113–114.

203. Solanki DR, Suresh M, Ethridge HC: The effect of intravenous cimetidine and metoclopramide on gastric volume and pH. *Anesth Analg* 1984;63:599–602.

204. Sprague DH: Effects of position and uterine displacement on spinal anesthesia for cesarean section. *Anesthesiology* 1976;44:164–166.

205. Srinivasan T: Intrathecal morphine for obstetric analgesia. *Anesthesiology* 1981;55: A298.

206. Stanley K, Soule AB, Copan SA, Duchowny MS: Local-regional anesthesia during childbirth, effect on newborn behavior. *Science* 1974;186:634–635.

207. Teabeaut JR II: Aspiration of gastric contents—an experimental study. *Am J Pathol* 1952;28:51–67.

208. Teramo K: Effects of obstetrical paracervical blockade on the fetus. *Acta Obstet Gynecol Scand* 1976;16(suppl):6–55.

209. Teramo K, Widholm O: Studies of the effect of anesthetics on foetus. Part I. The effect of paracervical block with mepivacaine upon fetal acid-base values. *Acta Obstet Gynecol Scand* 1967;46(suppl):2–39.

210. Tronick E, Wise S, Als H, Adamson L, Scanlon J, Brazelton TB: Regional obstetric anesthesia and newborn behavior: Effect over the first ten days of life. *Pediatrics* 1976;58: 94–100.

211. Ueland K, Gills RE, Hansen JM: Maternal cardiovascular dynamics I. Cesarean section under subarachnoid block anesthesia. *Am J Obstet Gynecol* 1968;100:42–54.

212. Vella LM, Willats DG, Knott C, Lintin DJ, Justins DM, Reynolds F: Epidural fentanyl in labor. *Anaesthesia* 1985;40:741–747.

213. Wallis KL, Shnider SM, Hicks JS, Spivey HT: Epidural anesthesia in the normotensive pregnant ewe: Effects on uterine blood flow and fetal acid-base status. *Anesthesiology* 1976;44:481–487.

214. Wang JK, Nauss LE, Thomas JE: Pain relief by intrathecally applied morphine in man. *Anesthesiology* 1979;50:149–151.

215. Warren TM, Datta S, Ostheimer GW, Naulty JS, Weiss JB, Morrison JA: Comparison of the maternal and neonatal effects of halothane enflurane and isoflurane for cesarean delivery. *Anesth Analg* 1983;62:516–520.

216. Way EL: Studies on the local anaesthetic properties of isonipecaine. *J Am Pharm Assoc* 1946;35:44–47.

217. Way WL, Costley EC, Way EL: Respiratory sensitivity of the newborn infant to meperidine and morphine. *Clin Pharmacol Ther* 1965;6:454–461.

218. Weintraub S, Naulty JS, Datta S, Ostheimer GW: Acute narcotic withdrawal syndrome precipitated by epidural butorphanol. *Anesth Analg* 1985;64:452–453.

219. Whitelaw AGL, Cummings AJ, McFadyen IR: Effect of maternal lorazepam on the neonate. *Br Med J* 1981;282:1106–1108.

220. Wolfe MJ, Davies GK: Analgesic action of extradural fentanyl. *Br J Anaesth* 1980;52: 357–358.

221. Wright RG, Shnider SM, Levinson G: The effect of maternal administration of ephedrine on fetal heart rate and variability. *Obstet Gynecol* 1981;57:734–738.

222. Yaksh TL: Spinal opiate analgesia: Characteristics and principles of action. *Pain* 1981; 11:293–346.

223. Yaksh TL: In vivo studies on spinal opiate receptor systems mediating anti-nociception. *J Pharmacol Exp Ther* 1983;226:303–316.

224. Yaksh TL, Wilson PR, Kaiko RF, Inturissi CE: Analgesia produced by a spinal action of morphine and effects on parturition in the rat. *Anesthesiology* 1979;51:386–392.

225. Youngstrom R, Eastwood D, Patel H, Bhatia R, Cowan R, Sutheimer C: Epidural fentanyl and bupivacaine in labor: Double-blind study. *Anesthesiology* 1984;61:A414.

226. Zador G, Lindmark G, Nilsson BA: Pudendal block in normal vaginal deliveries. *Acta Obstet Gynecol Scand* 1974;34(suppl):51–54.

5

Fetal Oxygenation

Benjamin T. Jackson and George J. Piasecki

"The fetus exists in a chronically hypoxic state." This pronouncement, or one very similar to it, is often made. If the fetal situation is compared with that of the postnatal individual in terms of the arterial partial pressure of oxygen (PO_2), this statement is of course true. The arterial PO_2 of the normal adult or child is approximately 90 torr, whereas that in the carotid artery of the fetus is only about 30 to 35 torr. When viewed in a functional sense, however, because the outcome of most pregnancies is a well-developed, healthy baby, it is unlikely that oxygen deprivation is a feature of normal fetal life. The ensuing discussion is concerned with the way in which an adequate supply of oxygen is delivered to the fetus. An understanding of this system is important in the interpretation of fetal heart rate patterns or blood gas and pH values obtained clinically.

Following a historical review of the investigation of fetal respiration, a substantive discussion of fetal oxygenation is presented in two general sections. The first involves normal mechanisms with an emphasis on the quantitative nature of fetal oxygenation. The second involves the compensatory mechanisms evoked by alterations in the supply of oxygen to the fetus.

HISTORICAL REVIEW

The evolution of thinking leading to the concept of fetal respiration via the placenta, which set the stage for modern concepts of fetal oxygenation, was reviewed in a scholarly article by Barron.[3] Barron's work, along with a review of the historical development of respiratory physiology by Perkins,[56] served as major sources for the following summary.

131

In his *Exercitationes de Generatione Animalium,* published in 1651, William Harvey was intrigued by the observation that babies born prematurely after the seventh month could respire in the manner of full-term infants, yet babies normally survived in utero for a further 2 months without apparent respiration. This suggested the possibility that the placenta might serve as the fetal "lungs."[3] This glimpse of the truth coupled with advances in the basic understanding of respiration from the work of Boyle et al.[56,65] might reasonably have led rapidly to a grasp of the elements of fetal respiration and the role of the placenta. Such was not the case.

The "phlogiston" theory of combustion advanced by Stahl confused the issue of respiration.[56] Phlogiston was believed to be the active principle of combustible materials that was released by heat into the air as fire. Animal respiration (recognized as being analogous to combustion) was therefore believed to involve the removal by the lungs of phlogiston formed within the body. For almost a hundred years, the general understanding of respiration actually regressed. The understanding of fetal respiration could hardly have been expected to move forward independently; it did not. Further advances in this area were to come only after the independent discovery of oxygen by Priestly in 1774 (he called it "dephlogisticated" air) and by Scheele in 1777 (he referred to oxygen as "fire air").[3,56] Stumbling over the phlogiston theory, neither Priestly nor Scheele understood the true nature of oxygen, and it remained for their contemporary Lavoisier to coin the term *oxygine* and to recognize it as an active rather than a passive principle in combustion and respiration.[56]

Armed with the new knowledge of oxygen and aware of the fact that blood brightened to red on exposure to air, Blumeback and Hunter concluded that the blood of the chick in ovo is aerated in its passage through the allantoic circulation.[3] Somewhat later, in 1796, Erasmus Darwin (grandfather of Charles) correctly observed that dark blood carried to the placenta by the umbilical arteries was considerably brightened on exiting in the umbilical vein. He inferred that the placenta functioned as the fetal "lung" and was analogous to the gills of fish as a respiratory organ.

Once again, one would have expected knowledge in this field to have burgeoned. Darwin's conclusions were not widely accepted, however, and there followed a period wherein confusion reigned, largely as a result of incorrect observations by various investigators. For example, shortly after Darwin's work was published, Scheel, an obstetrician, made a large number of clinical examinations in which he failed to observe any meaningful difference in the color of umbilical venous and arterial blood. G.F. Schuz concluded on the basis of a series of animal experiments that oxygen was not transferred from mother to fetus and that the fetus generated no heat.

In the early 1800s, Müller, the famous physiologist, recognized the methodologic problems besetting these studies and proposed that only large animals be used for observations of umbilical arterial and venous blood.[3] Based on experiments in sheep, he correctly concluded that fetal respiration does occur and that it is served by oxygen transfer via the placenta. In later years, in response to conflicting data resulting from inadequate techniques, he disavowed these original conclusions.

The general concept of respiration at that time (ca. 1840) also created significant problems in the understanding of the role of the placenta. The lungs were believed to be the site of utilization of oxygen and formation of carbon dioxide and heat. Respiration was thought to be principally an excretory process. The next phase in the understanding of respiration held that oxidation took place in capillary beds adjacent to the cells where the excretory products of metabolism were formed. It was proposed that the fetus gave up its excretory products at the placenta where oxygen was utilized in their oxidation.

The concept of tissue metabolism, with utilization of oxygen directly in cells, developed gradually as the 19th century progressed. Of particular importance was the work of Liebig, Claude Bernard, and the noted physiologist Pfluger.[56]

During this period (mid-19th century) Schwartz, an obstetrician, apparently accepting the idea of cellular respiration, expressed the view that the fetus must receive and utilize oxygen directly.[3] With brilliant insight, he concluded that the frequent failure by himself and others to observe differences in the color of umbilical arterial and venous blood was a secondary effect of parturition itself. Somewhat later, Schultz and Gusserow, also obstetricians, insisted that the fetus, on the basis of its rapid growth, must have a large requirement for oxygen.

Paul Zweifel, an obstetrician as well, demonstrated for the first time by spectroscopy (just then becoming available) the presence of oxygen in fetal blood and thus proved the transfer of oxygen from mother to fetus via the placenta. Recognizing the methodologic problems that had plagued earlier investigators, he performed very careful experiments in rabbits with the uterus bathed in warm saline. He clearly demonstrated the relatively greater amount of oxygen in the umbilical venous circulation compared with that in umbilical arteries.

The clear establishment by Zweifel of the role of the placenta in oxygen transfer to the fetus paved the way for the modern quantitative study of fetal respiration. This period of investigation, including both laboratory and clinical studies, may be divided into two phases. The earlier phase, extending from the early 1900s to the 1960s, was exemplified by animal experiments performed acutely on exposed fetuses. The later phase, continuing to the present day, has been characterized by a switch from acute to chronic animal experiments performed on fetuses and by advances in the complexity and accuracy of clinical observations.

This modern era in the study of fetal oxygenation began with the work of Huggett in Great Britain.[57] Soon thereafter, Joseph Barcroft,[2] after an outstanding career as a respiratory physiologist, developed a more circumscribed interest in fetal respiratory and circulatory physiology and went on to become the dominant figure in this field of research in the first half of the 20th century. His volume, *Researches on Pre-natal Life*[2] stands as a classic. In later years, Geoffrey Dawes, as Director of the Nuffield Institute, established a strong investigational program in this area. In the United States, S.R.M. Reynolds and Albert Plentl were pioneers in the investigation of fetal respiratory and circulatory physiology. Nicholas Assali was also a powerful force in this field. Donald Barron, after spending a number of years as a close associate of Barcroft, returned to the United States where he made major contributions to the understanding of fetal oxygenation. Many people regard him as the "dean" of fetal physiologists.

The last 15 to 20 years, comprising the second phase of this modern era, have seen a dramatic expansion of interest in the study of fetal respiration, and hosts of investigators from various clinical and scientific disciplines devote their principal efforts to this field. As noted, the studies of Barcroft and his contemporaries and their early successors were conducted in "acute" preparations with the fetus exteriorized and the experimental animal under anesthesia. During the 1950s and 1960s, a number of technical developments contributed to a fundamental change in this experimental approach. In 1954, Reynolds et al.[58] reported a method for cannulating the interplacental vessels in pregnant monkeys without loss of amniotic fluid and without exposure of the fetus. Jackson and Piasecki developed a method for direct lead fetal electrocardiography and for intrauterine fetal operations using a marsupializing incision.[31,33] This operative approach was subsequently applied to the placement of chronic catheters in fetal monkeys.[49,51] Meschia et al.[48] initiated chronic studies in fetal sheep utilizing cannulas placed in the umbilical vessels. The use of intrauterine fetal operations and the performance of chronic experiments days or weeks after surgical preparation of the fetus now represent the state of the art.

Wide availability of complex electronic equipment and new means of quantitating fetal circulatory and respiratory function have contributed measurably to advances in this field. Of particular importance was the development of radionuclide-labeled microsphere technology by Rudolph and Heymann.[61] Many advances have been made in the area of the clinical investigation of fetal respiration. The utilization of fetal electrocardiography by Hon and Hess[28] and others has been of great importance as has the technique of blood sampling from the fetal scalp first described by Saling.[7]

The development of the study of fetal respiration thus proceeded from Harvey to Zweifel, when the questions of the existence of fetal respiration and the role of the placenta as the fetal "lung" were settled, to the first half of the 20th century in which the quantitative study of fetal respiration by Barcroft and others developed, and finally to the present day of intensive investigation of fetal circulatory and respiratory physiology based on numerous technologic advances. The current state of knowledge of fetal oxygenation derived from this long period of study is reviewed in the discussion that follows.

NORMAL OXYGEN TRANSFER TO THE FETUS

Placental transfer of oxygen depends upon the delivery of maternally inspired oxygen to the placenta by the maternal circulation. Quantitatively, this is a function of the rate of maternal blood flow to the placenta and the concentration of oxygen in the mother's blood. Once delivered to the placenta, its transfer to the fetus is dependent upon the balance between the force tending to drive oxygen across the placenta (the maternal-fetal oxygen gradient) and the net forces resisting the release of oxygen from maternal hemoglobin (diffusion across placental membranes and uptake of oxygen by fetal hemoglobin). These simple statements belie the complexity of the steps actually involved in transport of oxygen to the fetus. The more important of these are discussed below in some detail. In pursuing these points, the sequential movement of oxygen in its course from the atmosphere to fetal tissues will be followed.

Oxygen Transport to the Placenta

To reach the fetus, oxygen must first be breathed in by the mother. (This process, encompassed by the major discipline of pulmonary physiology, will not be discussed further, except to note the obvious fact that any significant alteration in maternal pulmonary function is likely to be reflected in the status of the fetus.) Once oxygen has traversed the alveolar membrane into the mother's blood, transport to the fetus is dependent upon the integrity of the maternal circulation. This process is discussed only in terms of its specific application to uteroplacental oxygen delivery.

Oxygen is transported in the mother's blood largely in combination with hemoglobin, each gram of which has the potential of combining with 1.34 mL of oxygen.[16] The percent saturation of hemoglobin with oxygen is determined by the Po_2. At a Po_2 of 100 torr, maternal hemoglobin would be virtually 100% saturated. With a hemoglobin level of 12 g/dL, the total quantity of oxygen carried in a combined state in 100 mL of blood would be 16.08 mL. A small amount of additional oxygen is dissolved in plasma. The solubility of oxygen in plasma at 37° C is approximately 0.00003 mL/mL for each torr Po_2. Hence, the roughly 60 mL of plasma in 100 mL of blood, at a partial pressure of 100 torr, would contain approximately 0.18 mL of oxygen. Under ordinary circumstances the amount of dissolved oxygen is trivial compared with that carried by hemoglobin. Therefore, the quantity of oxygen delivered to the placenta is largely dependent upon the blood flow to the placenta and the hemoglobin concentration in the blood (together defined as the hemoglobin flow rate), and the percent saturation of maternal hemoglobin with oxygen. A certain portion of this oxygen is utilized by placental tissues and does not reach the fetus. This factor is of some quantitative importance but is not considered further, as we follow oxygen along its course.

Oxygen Diffusion across the Placenta

As maternal blood arrives at the placenta, molecular oxygen dissolved in plasma diffuses across the intervening membranes into fetal plasma. The rate of diffusion is dependent on the partial pressure gradient for oxygen between maternal and fetal plasma and the diffusing capacity of the placenta. The latter factor is derived from the surface area of the membrane available for oxygen transfer and the physical characteristics of that membrane. As oxygen moves out of maternal plasma, the Po_2 falls, and oxygen is released into plasma from hemoglobin in maternal red cells. As oxygen moves into fetal plasma, the fetal Po_2 rises and increasing amounts of oxygen are bound to hemoglobin in fetal red cells. This process is continuous, with a steady movement of oxygen from maternal red cells into plasma on the maternal side of the placenta and then transfer across placental membranes into fetal plasma and then into red cells. Although the partial pressure differential between mother and fetus is the factor that drives oxygen across the placenta, it is the quantity of oxygen delivered that is significant in serving fetal metabolic needs. As noted, the transport of significant quantities of oxygen is dependent on binding to hemoglobin. Certain aspects of hemoglobin are of particular pertinence to fetal oxygenation.

The affinity of hemoglobin for oxygen is of basic importance. This characteristic is defined in terms of the hemoglobin-oxygen dissociation curve, and in almost all species is different in the fetus and the adult. Figure 5-1 illustrates the curves for adult and fetal sheep.[46] Although less striking than in sheep, the difference between maternal and fetal hemoglobin-oxygen dissociation curves in humans is significant. For any Po_2 represented along the horizontal axis, the percent saturation of hemoglobin is defined on the vertical axis. The fetal curve falls to the left of that for the adult. Therefore, at any given Po_2, fetal hemoglobin will be more highly saturated than adult hemoglobin and will thus contain a greater total quantity of oxygen than would be true if the fetal dissociation curve were the same as that of the mother.

The basis for the differential in hemoglobin-oxygen affinity between fetus and adult, in spite of considerable study, remained obscure until relatively recently. Fetal blood, even late in gestation, contains predominantly fetal hemoglobin. Because fetal and adult hemoglobin are known to be structurally distinct, it would be natural to assume these distinctive

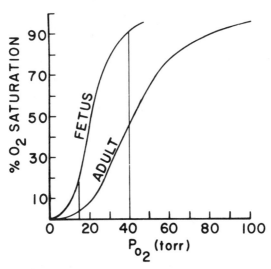

Figure 5-1 Hemoglobin-oxygen dissociation curves for adult and fetal hemoglobin in the sheep. Po_2 expressed in torr is equivalent to mm Hg. *Source*: Reprinted with permission from "Evolution of Thinking in Fetal Respiratory Physiology" by G Meschia in *American Journal of Obstetrics and Gynecology* (1978;132:807), Copyright © 1978, The CV Mosby Company.

oxygen affinity characteristics to be related directly to hemoglobin structure. This is not the case. McCarthy[43] demonstrated many years ago that there is relatively little difference in the dissociation curves of adult and fetal hemoglobin in solution; the differential position of the adult curve to the right of the fetal is present only with intact red cells. The necessary clue to understanding this puzzling phenomenon appeared in 1967 when Benesch and Benesch[6] and Chanutin and Curnish[9] reported that intracellular phosphate compounds, predominantly 2,3-diphosphoglycerate (2,3-DPG), act to decrease the affinity of hemoglobin for oxygen. More recently, it has been shown that 2,3-DPG has a minimal effect on fetal hemoglobin. Therefore, even though the levels of 2,3-DPG in fetal cells are appreciable, there is minimal alteration of the intrinsic hemoglobin-oxygen affinity.[19,52,63,64]

The functional significance of the differential in the affinity of maternal and fetal blood for oxygen has been debated over the years. Battaglia et al.[4] introduced adult blood via exchange transfusions into fetal sheep; there was a marked decrease in the oxygen content of fetal blood when it contained a large proportion of maternal cells. This work obviously supports the concept of a quantitative advantage for the high oxygen affinity of fetal hemoglobin. Forster[24] has expressed a contrary view, stating: "The ultimate purpose of the placenta and circulatory systems of the mother and foetus is to provide oxygen to the foetal peripheral tissue at the required pressure." The authors' intuitive view (data do not exist to prove the point unequivocally) is in keeping with the opinion of Meschia[47] that the high avidity of fetal blood for oxygen yielding a relatively higher concentration of oxygen in fetal blood provides a net advantage for normal development and survival. However, it is known that this special characteristic of fetal blood is not essential for survival of the fetus as attested to by the successful outcome of pregnancies in erythroblastosis fetalis after major replacement of fetal red cells by intrauterine transfusions of adult cells. Perhaps the hemoglobin-oxygen dissociation characteristics of fetal blood provide a margin of safety that only comes into play during fetal stress.

In addition to the inherent difference in hemoglobin-oxygen affinity of maternal and fetal blood discussed above, dynamic events within the placenta tend to enhance further the transfer of oxygen from mother to fetus. The affinity of hemoglobin for oxygen is decreased both by increased partial pressure of carbon dioxide (Pco_2) (the Bohr effect) and H^+ concentration so that the dissociation curve is shifted to the right.[60] Therefore, as fetal blood gives up its excess CO_2 and H^+ to maternal blood in the placenta, the fetal curve shifts progressively to the left enhancing the uptake of oxygen by fetal hemoglobin. As maternal blood takes up CO_2 and H^+ from the fetus, its curve shifts to the right, enhancing the release of oxygen from the mother's hemoglobin.

The hemoglobin-oxygen dissociation characteristics discussed above determine the degree of saturation of hemoglobin with oxygen for any Po_2. For a given degree of saturation, the actual oxygen content of blood is dependent upon the oxygen binding capacity of the blood, and hence the hemoglobin concentration—the more hemoglobin, the more oxygen the blood can carry.

The mother's hemoglobin concentration decreases during pregnancy, thus lowering the efficiency of her blood as a transporter of oxygen.[49] It has been suggested that in humans, as well as certain other species, fetal hemoglobin levels (and hence oxygen carrying capacity) rise with advancing gestation and are higher than in the adult.[17,18,49] This conclusion is based to a large extent on observations in neonates. Being influenced by "placental transfusion" and fluid shifts associated with birth, such data cannot be accepted as indicative of the fetal situation. There is actually strong evidence in humans, monkeys, and sheep to indicate that the fetal hemoglobin concentration is relatively stable in the latter stages of gestation;[32,48,67] data in the monkey suggest that fetal levels are not appreciably higher than in the normal adult animal.[32]

The capacity of the fetus to respond to a hypoxic stress with an elevated rate of erythropoiesis has been demonstrated experimentally in both sheep and monkeys.[32,68] The fact that the normal fetus does not have an exaggeratedly high hemoglobin concentration provides a certain functional proof that the fetus does not exist in a hypoxic state.

As noted, oxygen is believed to cross the placenta by simple diffusion. The capacity for diffusion of a gas is determined by the physical characteristics of the placenta, particularly the solubility of the gas in the tissue, and the thickness and surface area of the membranes separating maternal and fetal circulations. The diffusing capacity of the placenta is relatively stable for each species under normal circumstances. The fact that it may be altered in various pathologic situations makes it clinically important (see Chapter 10).

The physical characteristics of maternal and fetal blood flow through the placenta also have an influence upon the net transfer of oxygen from mother to fetus. In the theoretically most efficient system, maternal and fetal blood streams would move in opposite directions (countercurrent flow). In this way, the maternal blood having the highest Po_2 would come into contact initially with fetal blood that had been enriched with oxygen in its passage through the placenta. The oxygen-poor fetal blood entering the exchange zone would be exposed to maternal blood that had already given up some of its oxygen. In this fashion the gradient between maternal and fetal blood would tend to be maintained at an effective level throughout the entire period of exchange. Fetal blood leaving the exchange zone would have a higher Po_2 than maternal blood exiting at the opposite end and, in fact, would potentially come close to matching the Po_2 of maternal arterial blood. Movement of maternal and fetal blood in the same direction (concurrent flow) would be less efficient in that maternal blood with the highest Po_2 would be exposed initially to fetal blood having the lowest Po_2, and at the end of the passage the most oxygen-enriched fetal blood would be exposed to the most depleted maternal blood so that the effective gradient would be significantly reduced. At best, the oxygen concentrations of fetal and maternal blood leaving the placenta would be equal. It seems highly unlikely that a perfect countercurrent system exists. Inequalities of perfusion on the two sides of the placenta probably exist so that the functional result of maternal-fetal exchange would be expected to vary from what would otherwise be anticipated from any anatomic arrangement. Probably, the functional equivalent, or nearly so, of concurrent flow is present in most species. Experimental evidence is insufficient to reach firm conclusions in this area.[24,26,27]

Distribution of Oxygen by the Fetal Circulation

In this section the course of fully oxygenated fetal blood from the placenta to fetal tissues is traced. A representation of the fetal circulation is seen in Figure 5-2 and may be helpful in this review.[8]

Once the maximally oxygenated fetal blood leaves the placenta, it courses by way of the umbilical vein to the liver. Within the substance of the liver, multiple branches arise from this vessel; they comprise the portal system of the lateral segment of the left lobe of the liver and persist postnatally in that same role. A shunt, the ductus venosus, continues directly from the umbilical vein to the inferior vena cava. In addition, there is a direct connection within the liver between the umbilical vein and the portal vein proper that persists after birth as part of the definitive portal system.[41]

The blood that flows through the ductus venosus retains the same level of oxygen established at the placenta. A certain fraction of umbilical venous blood courses through the portal system of the left lobe of the liver and into the vena cava via the left hepatic vein. This blood presumably loses only a small quantity of its oxygen in its passage through the liver.

The poorly oxygenated portal flow proper coming from the viscera mixes slightly with umbilical venous flow, but largely passes through the

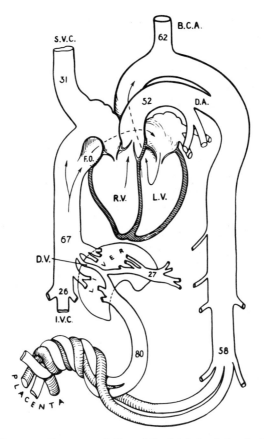

Figure 5-2 Semidiagrammatic representation of the fetal circulation in the sheep. BCA, brachiocephalic artery; DA, ductus arteriosus; DV, ductus venosus; FO, foramen ovale; IVA, inferior vena cava; LV, left ventricle; RV, right ventricle; SVC, superior vena cava. *Source*: Reprinted with permission from *Cold Spring Harbor Symposium on Quantitative Biology* (1954;19:103), Copyright © 1954, Cold Spring Harbor Laboratory.

right lobe of the liver and empties into the vena cava via the right hepatic vein where it joins another stream of relatively deoxygenated blood returning to the heart from the lower body of the fetus.[21] Edelstone and Rudolph[20] reported that the oxygen-rich blood from the ductus venosus and the left lobe of the liver flows preferentially through the foramen ovale into the left atrium; the relatively oxygen-poor blood from the lower body and right lobe of the liver streams to a large extent into the right atrium where it joins another stream of relatively oxygen-poor blood returning from the head via the superior vena cava. The septa dividing the atria are arranged in such a fashion that a large part of inferior vena caval blood, rich in oxygen, flows virtually directly into the left atrium without ever reaching the right ventricle. This system, separating blood of high and low oxygen levels, is remarkably effective so that the blood emerging from the left side of the heart into the aorta will have a P_{O_2} only a few torr below that in the umbilical vein as it leaves the placenta. This relatively oxygen-rich blood supplies the "high-priority" fetal tissues, the heart and the brain.

The blood in the right side of the heart (relatively low in oxygen) is ejected into the pulmonary artery where a small fraction flows through the lungs, and the greater part is shunted through the ductus arteriosus to become enriched with oxygen by blood rounding the arch of the aorta. Thus, the arterial blood that supplies the "low-priority" fetal tissues—the lower body and the viscera—contains an intermediate level of oxygen. As discussed below, the relative priority of fetal tissues defined by the richness of their normal oxygen supply persists when compensatory mechanisms are called into play in the presence of hypoxemic stress.

How successful is this system of oxygen delivery to fetal tissues? Obviously, the fact that the majority of fetuses develop normally indicates that it is quite effective; but going beyond this generalization, the efficacy of fetal oxygenation might reasonably be defined in terms of the transport of oxygen to the heart and brain because they have been identified as "high-priority" organs in the fetus. To illustrate, data obtained from chronically cannulated rhesus monkey fetuses are shown in Figure 5-3.[36] With the mother breathing room air observed values for maternal arterial and fetal carotid arterial P_{O_2} were 89 and 30 torr, respectively. Equivalent oxygen contents were 15 vol% in maternal blood and 11 vol% in fetal blood.[36] The point of fundamental importance is that although the P_{O_2} in fetal blood is much lower than that in maternal arterial blood, the actual quantity of oxygen is only slightly lower in the fetus than in the mother. Thus, with the very high blood flow rate through the umbilical circuit, a large volume of oxygen is delivered to the fetus under normal circumstances. This lends further support to the concept that the fetus is not chronically hypoxic. After all, it is the number of oxygen molecules available to serve as electron receptors that limits metabolic activity. Oxygen must, of course, move from blood into cells before it can be utilized, and it is here that the P_{O_2} is important.

Movement of Oxygen from Blood into Tissues

As recounted above, early in the evolution of the science of physiology, the oxidative or respiratory process was thought to take place in the

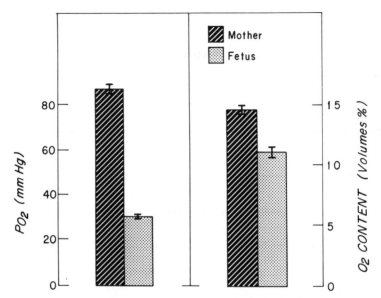

Figure 5-3 Comparison of maternal and fetal P_{O_2} and oxygen content in chronically cannu-lated rhesus monkeys with maternal inspiration of room air.

lungs. Later, this was believed to occur in blood itself. Only late in the 19th century was the cell theory accepted and the direct utilization of oxygen by tissues demonstrated. It is now known that the great majority, if not all, of the utilization of oxygen in the oxidative process takes place in mitochondria.[37] Thus, the final step in oxygen transport to the fetus occurs as the gas diffuses from plasma in capillary beds into the mitochondria of cells. As plasma P_{O_2} falls with loss of oxygen into tissues, additional oxygen is given up by hemoglobin which provides the supply necessary to maintain metabolic processes.

The importance of the oxygen content of fetal arterial blood has been emphasized correctly; however, the P_{O_2} must be given some considera-tion because a certain level is required to maintain the movement of oxygen from blood into cells. Much remains to be learned about this general area of cellular physiology, but experimental work suggests that uptake and utilization of oxygen occur effectively at a very low P_{O_2}. Figure 5-4 shows that oxygen uptake by yeast cells is maintained until the ambient P_{O_2} falls below 1 or 2 torr, depending on the substrate.[37] Isolated mitochondria require a minimum P_{O_2} of only 0.5 torr to sustain normal respiration, and a capillary P_{O_2} of 10 torr in the rat is sufficient to provide such a mitochondrial oxygen level. This information on the P_{O_2} required for tissue respiration applies to adult animals. Although understanding

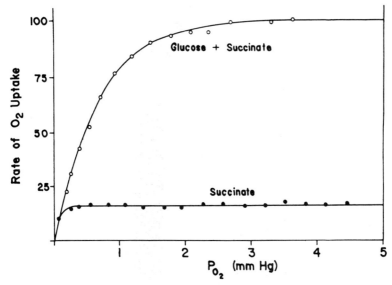

Figure 5-4 Oxygen uptake relative to P_{O_2} in yeast cells. With appropriate substrates, oxygen uptake is maintained even at very low oxygen tensions. *Source:* Reprinted from *Handbook of Physiology, Section 3, Respiration,* Vol 1, by WO Fenn and H Rahn (Eds) with permission of American Physiological Society, © 1964.

of the specific characteristics of equivalent fetal systems is incomplete, it is known that fetal respiratory chain enzymes are deficient by adult standards and that they increase rapidly just before birth.[44] Although the fetus has been regarded as having a particularly high tolerance for oxygen lack,[50] it is not known whether fetal cells are specially adapted to the utilization of oxygen at low partial pressures.

Compensatory Mechanisms in Fetal Hypoxemia

Even though under normal circumstances the fetus receives a generous supply of oxygen, in occasional instances abnormal events supervene, and the fetus is deprived of its usual supply. Fetal hypoxemia may result from a decreased perfusion of the maternal side of the placenta, as might occur with maternal hypotension or heart disease. The volume of oxygen contained in maternal blood perfusing the placenta may under certain circumstances be low, as with maternal pulmonary disease or anemia. The placenta itself may be deficient (e.g., extensive infarction), and fetal complications, such as umbilical cord compression, may also result in a deficiency in the supply of oxygen to the fetus. The temporary reduction in oxygen delivery to the fetus occasioned by the normal uterine contractions of labor are generally of no clinical significance. When the effect of contractions is superimposed on preexisting fetal hypoxemia, or when the contractions are unusually intense, late decelerations in the fetal heart rate may occur and indicate true fetal distress (see Chapter 10). The effects of hypoxemia on fetal heart rate have been studied experimentally in pregnant sheep.[27,29,54] Fetal hypoxemia resulting from decreased uterine blood flow led to late decelerations in fetal heart rate even in previously normal fetuses once the oxygen deprivation was carried beyond a certain threshold. The heart rate response was shown to be due to a vagal reflex medicated by chemoreceptor stimulation. Acute episodes of hypoxia applied against a background of preexisting hypoxemia induced more profound changes, with late decelerations based in this case on a combination of vagally mediated reflex and also on direct hypoxic myocardial depression. These results support the concept of hypoxemia as the cause of late decelerations in fetal heart rate and explain the mechanisms underlying this response. In addition, the applicability to humans of these aspects of fetal physiology investigated in the sheep is demonstrated.

The consequences and potential compensatory mechanisms of fetal hypoxemia will now be considered.

Acute Hypoxia—Maternal Response

Rather striking changes in the maternal circulation occur in the natural course of events as pregnancy advances. Of particular importance are increases in cardiac output and uterine blood flow, which ultimately reach 30% to 35% and 17- to 20-fold, respectively, above nonpregnant levels.[1] However, when the fetus becomes acutely hypoxic, for whatever reason, there are no clearly established maternal physiologic mechanisms to compensate for this fetal deficiency. Indeed, during periods of maternal oxygen deprivation, the preservation of blood flow to the uterus and hence to the placenta seems to be of a relatively low order of priority in the distribution of maternal cardiac output.[1,30,34]

Acute Hypoxia—Fetal Response

There are certain characteristics of the fetus that do play a role in its ability to avoid or withstand a hypoxic stress. The overall mechanism for oxygen transport to the fetus seems to have a margin of safety in the form of excess capacity. This has been shown experimentally in sheep by the observation that reduction of the oxygen content of fetal arterial blood by almost 50%, secondary to diminution of maternal inspired concentration, does not reduce oxygen consumption by the fetus.[55] In this situation fetal arterial oxygen levels are reduced, but the quantitative transport of oxygen to the fetus per unit time remains largely unchanged. This involves an important passive mechanism.[42] When P_{O_2} and oxygen content are decreased in umbilical venous blood going to the fetus, oxygen extraction by fetal tissues continues, and the P_{O_2} and oxygen content are decreased proportionately in the umbilical arterial blood returning to the placenta. As a result, the P_{O_2} gradient between the maternal and fetal sides of the placenta is increased, the driving force for diffusion is maintained and transport of oxygen to the fetus is preserved. The system functions normally in a qualitative sense but at a lower level in terms of fetal arterial P_{O_2}. In a way, fetal reserve (see Chapter 10) may be thought of as the ability of the tissues to extract oxygen from capillary blood even after the arterial P_{O_2} falls below "normal" resting levels. Obviously, when the fetal oxygen supply falls below a certain critical point, this system begins to fail and fetal oxygen consumption is reduced; true hypoxia in a metabolic sense is the result.

Several active changes in cardiovascular function are seen in the fetus in response to hypoxemia. The principal parameters involved include heart rate, blood pressure, and distribution of fetal cardiac output. The timing and the extent of these changes are dependent upon the degree of hypoxemia that occurs in the fetus.

The fetal heart rate is rather labile and may either increase or decrease as a sign of fetal distress. Tachycardia may be seen with relatively mild and bradycardia is seen with more severe hypoxemia. The tachycardia is believed to be due to adrenergic stimulation of the heart[18] and bradycardia may be due both to a vagal reflex,[2,18] and in some instances to a direct effect of hypercapnea and hypoxia on the myocardium.[18,29,54] Experimentally, in sheep the vagal bradycardic response may be elicited with only a moderate degree of fetal hypoxemia (umbilical arterial P_{O_2} 10 to 12 torr).[12] Once established, bradycardia does not tend to progress. Indeed, there is, if anything, a tendency for the fetal heart rate to increase slightly as hypoxemia becomes more severe.[11] Although it has not been specifically defined as such, this vagally mediated response to hypoxemia seems to be an "all or nothing" phenomenon with its effect on heart rate modulated by opposing beta-adrenergic activity.[13] The severity of the hypoxemia is not necessarily directly related to the magnitude of the drop in heart rate. The functional significance of the status of the fetal heart rate is discussed further below.

In experimental studies, fetal hypoxemia has generally been found to be associated with an increase in arterial blood pressure. This elevation in systemic arterial pressure is secondary to a net increase in peripheral resistance and is maintained by the fetus even in the face of quite severe hypoxemia.

In response to a diminished supply of oxygen the fetus could conceivably elevate its cardiac output and thus increase oxygen pickup from the placenta and distribution to tissues. In fact, the fetal heart does not respond in this manner. When subjected to mild to moderate hypoxemia, the fetus increases its cardiac output only modestly or not at all.[12,14] With more profound hypoxemia, the output of the fetal heart decreases significantly.[12] These findings are in keeping with an apparent general overall constraint of the fetal heart to a narrow range of variability in output. This contrasts sharply with the adult heart, which in certain situations may increase its output fivefold.

In the late gestation fetus, this characteristic of cardiac function does not seem to be the result of a lack of active control mechanisms. Both alteration in heart rate and the Frank-Starling mechanism have been shown to play a role in the regulation of the fetal heart, although their relative importance is debated.[40,62] The functional limitation of the fetal cardiac output is apparently due principally to immaturity in myocardial development. This concept is supported by in vitro studies showing the contractile force per unit weight of fetal myocardium to be much less than that of the adult.[40] In a practical demonstration of the limited cardiac reserve of the experimental animal fetus, rapid onset of fetal heart failure and death followed establishment of maternal-fetal parabiosis and exposure of the fetus to the systemic pressure of the mother.[34,35] The provision for a low-pressure fetal vascular system compatible with the capacity of the developing heart may be thought of as one of the vital functions served by the placenta.

Even though only minor adjustments in total output occur, the fetal response to hypoxemia is characterized by a major redistribution of cardiac output.[12,14] This involves an increased blood flow to the heart and the brain (defined above as high-priority tissues) and the adrenal glands (now added to this favored group). With mild to moderate hypoxemia, there is a striking decrease in fetal pulmonary blood flow and a milder and more delayed decrease in blood flow to the viscera, skeletal muscle, and bone. At this level of hypoxemia little change in umbilical blood flow occurs.

As fetal hypoxemia becomes more severe, that is, with an umbilical arterial P_{O_2} in the range of 7 to 10 torr, a point is reached at which there is either no further increase or even a slight decrease in volume blood flow to the heart, brain, and adrenals. Given the decreased content of oxygen carried by the fetal blood, this represents a failure of the compensatory mechanisms to maintain oxygen distribution to these organs. Blood flow to the placenta characteristically undergoes a small to moderate decrease at this level of hypoxemia. There is also a definite further decrease in the blood flow to the low-priority tissues including the viscera and skeletal muscle. This decrease may reach such extreme levels that the flow to these structures virtually ceases.

The cardiovascular responses to hypoxemia in relatively mature fetuses described above are largely the result of combined vagal and sympathoadrenal mechanisms. As far as is known, vagal activation is the principal mechanism responsible for the production of bradycardia. The fetal sympathoadrenal response has been studied rather extensively in sheep, being quantitated both in terms of both peripheral concentrations of epinephrine and norepinephrine and directly measured adrenal secretion.[10,11,15,39] In the fetal peripheral blood, both epinephrine and norepinephrine have an inverse exponential relation to the fetal P_{O_2}, as illustrated in Figure 5-5.[11] The most dramatic increases in these catecholamines are associated with the same low fetal oxygen levels as is the most extreme redistribution of blood flow away from low priority tissues. This suggests that the maximum cardiovascular response to hypoxemia is elicited only by an extreme degree of sympathoadrenal activation.

The fetal cardiovascular mechanisms described above obviously work only for a limited time, but may be of great importance in allowing the fetus to survive a severe hypoxemic stress of short duration.

Chronic Hypoxia

Maternal anemia and pregnancy at high altitude are two primary examples of conditions associated with chronic fetal hypoxia.[49] Maternal anemia is at least partly compensated by an increase in maternal cardiac output. The fetus also responds with an increase in its hemoglobin concentration. At high altitudes with low ambient oxygen, both mother and fetus develop increased hemoglobin levels. In addition, increased uterine blood flow and increased placental diffusing capacity have been found experimentally. The fetus (both experimental animal and human) at high altitude is characteristically subnormal in size. Infants are typically small for gestational age. Interestingly, these fetuses seem to be otherwise relatively normal. This adjustment in fetal size has itself been defined as an adaptive mechanism.

Active Intervention in Fetal Hypoxia

The possibility of beneficial intervention on the part of the practitioner is now considered (see Chapter 10). Any measure taken to improve and/

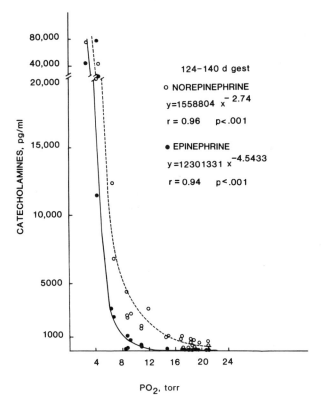

Figure 5-5 Relations between P_{O_2} and plasma epinephrine and norepinephrine in the umbilical artery of the sheep fetus. *Source*: Reprinted with permission from *American Journal of Physiology* (1982;243:R522), Copyright © 1982, American Physiological Society.

or to maintain maternal respiration and generally support the mother's circulation would obviously be of benefit in preserving the delivery of oxygen to the placenta. The administration of oxygen in high concentration to the pregnant woman is one such measure. Although this form of therapy is controversial, the weight of evidence suggests that it does lead to increased oxygen delivery to the fetus, and may thus be of benefit. The basis for this statement is elaborated below.

A number of clinical and experimental studies have reported no change (or even a decrease) in fetal oxygen levels in response to maternal inspiration of pure oxygen.[18,45,59] The suggestion has also been made that the associated high maternal oxygen tension leads to decreased placental perfusion.[45,59] In contrast to this work, a number of studies have demonstrated enhancement of fetal oxygenation by this maneuver.[18,36,46] Moreover, high-quality experimental work in sheep has shown no influence of high maternal levels of oxygen on either uterine or umbilical blood flow.[5] It is true, as has been stated, that the change in fetal P_{O_2} is small in comparison with that in the mother when she breathes oxygen. However, the quantitative gain in oxygen by the fetus is greater than this would imply.

An analysis of data obtained in rhesus monkeys may be helpful in understanding this issue.[36] Figures 5-6 and 5-7 illustrate maternal-fetal relations for P_{O_2} and oxygen content. It is readily apparent that very high maternal arterial oxygen tensions are associated with fetal oxygen tensions that are lower by a factor of 10, whereas maternal and fetal oxygen contents are of the same order of magnitude over the range of experimental results. Numerically (with 100% oxygen breathing) maternal P_{O_2} increased from 87 to 349 torr while fetal P_{O_2} increased from 29 to 34 torr. However, fetal oxygen content increased by 1.2 vol% (a gain of about 10%), which was not significantly different from the maternal increase of 1.4 vol%. Therefore, when the mother inspires a high oxygen concentra-

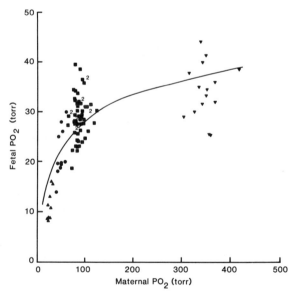

▲ = 10% O_2
● = 15% O_2
■ = air
▼ = 100% O_2

Figure 5-6 Relation between maternal and fetal P_{O_2} with mother breathing 10% O_2, 15% O_2, air, and 100% O_2. *Source:* Reprinted with permission from *American Journal of Physiology* (1987;252:R94–R101), Copyright © 1987, American Physiological Society.

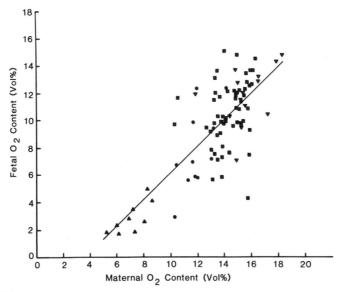

A = 10% O_2
● = 15% O_2
■ = air
▼ = 100% O_2

Figure 5-7 Relation between maternal and fetal oxygen content with mother breathing 10% O_2, 15% O_2, air, and 100% O_2. *Source:* Reprinted with permission from *American Journal of Physiology* (1987;252:R94–R101), Copyright © 1987, American Physiological Society.

tion, the fetus, in spite of its small increase in P_{O_2}, makes about the same quantitative gain in oxygen concentration as the mother.

The disparity between the gain in maternal P_{O_2} and oxygen content, a key point, is readily explained. Because maternal hemoglobin is normally 90% to 95% saturated, only a small quantitative gain in oxygen is realized when saturation is increased to 100% in response to the elevated P_{O_2}. The increment in oxygen dissolved in plasma secondary to the high P_{O_2} is also small. Because the net increase in the oxygen content of maternal blood is small, the high P_{O_2} rapidly falls as placental transfer occurs. Simply, an increase in the amount of oxygen in the mother's blood, no matter what the starting P_{O_2}, leads to a similarly small gain in oxygen by the fetus.

What is seen is that maternal inspiration of oxygen does not affect uterine or umbilical blood flow adversely and that it leads reliably to a small increase in fetal oxygen levels. It is likely that clinical situations occur in which this increase in oxygen delivery to the fetus is beneficial. When flow to the placenta is decreased markedly or placental function is otherwise adversely affected this potential benefit may, of course, not be fully realized. For this reason, simple clinical maneuvers of intrauterine resuscitation described in Chapter 10 should focus primarily on improving uterine and umbilical blood flow. Once maximal flow has been achieved, enhancing oxygen content of maternal blood will lead to increased fetal oxygen availability.

Manipulation of fetal heart rate represents another maneuver that has been considered to have possible use in aiding the distressed fetus. Because moderate to severe fetal distress is usually associated with bradycardia, why not correct the problem by bringing the fetal heart rate back into the "normal" range? In most instances it is possible to block the fetal vagal activity responsible for the bradycardia by maternal administration of atropine.[17,38] Before this approach is embraced, however, a careful evaluation is in order.

Experiments in pregnant sheep have shown that with very mild fetal hypoxemia, fetal cardiac output may be slightly increased when fetal heart rate is increased by the administration of atropine.[25] However, with hypoxemia of increasing severity, cardiac output is either unchanged or moderately decreased when reflex bradycardia is eliminated by atropine treatment.[12,53] This latter point is illustrated in Figure 5-8 in which restoration of heart rate to resting values is seen to have no effect on blood flow in the descending aorta.

At hypoxic levels of sufficient degree to warrant aid for the fetus, elevation of the fetal heart rate is of no benefit in enhancing cardiac output. A further point to consider is whether the elimination of bradycardia with preservation of a normal heart rate might actually be harmful to the fetus. Although there is as yet no direct proof, it may be inferred from certain bits of evidence that the maintenance of a normal fetal heart rate in the face of hypoxemia sufficient to induce a vagal bradycardic response is indeed potentially harmful. It must be assumed that the fetal response to hypoxemia is designed to conserve available oxygen maximally. It is widely accepted that the heart, in terms of oxygen utilization, works more efficiently at a slower rate.[26] There is no reason to believe that this general rule does not hold for the fetus. Consider specifically the diving response in marine mammals (characterized by bradycardia, decreased cardiac output, and redistribution of blood flow), which is in many ways analogous to the fetal response to hypoxia.[22] In the diving response, bradycardia is believed to be a significant element in the efficient use of a limited oxygen supply. For example, in the nutria, prevention of bradycardia by atropine during diving was shown to increase oxygen utilization and to shorten diving time.[23] Given the weight of available evidence, it is deemed injudicious at present to attempt to manipulate the fetal heart rate directly by administration of atropine to the mother. To the contrary,

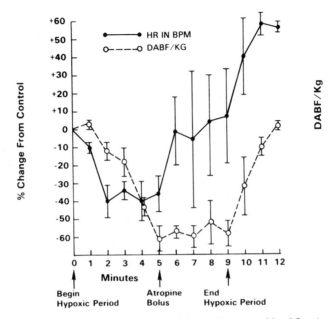

Figure 5-8 Relation between fetal heart rate and descending aortic blood flow in response to experimentally induced hypoxemia in fetal sheep. Note alteration in heart rate by injection of atropine but no change in aortic blood flow, a reflection of cardiac output. *Source:* Reprinted with permission from "The Effect of Fetal Heart Rate on Cardiovascular Function during Hypoxemia" by HE Cohn, GJ Piasecki, and BT Jackson in *American Journal of Obstetrics and Gynecology* (1980;138:1196), Copyright © 1980, The CV Mosby Company.

fetal bradycardia should generally be viewed as an important part of the fetal adaptive response to hypoxia; as such it probably provides important physiologic benefits.

SUMMARY

After hundreds of years of study and thought, the placental transfer of oxygen and its utilization by the fetus was demonstrated unequivocally in the late 19th century. Building on this fundamental observation, the quantitative investigation of fetal oxygenation began in the first half of the 20th century. This has now developed into a major discipline of basic and clinical research and has led to a much broader understanding of this process.

Fetal oxygenation is dependent upon the integrity of maternal respiratory and circulatory function for transport of oxygen to the placenta.

Transfer of oxygen across the placenta occurs by simple diffusion and is determined largely by the diffusing capacity of the placenta and the Po_2 gradient between maternal and fetal plasma. Quantitative transfer of oxygen across the placenta to the fetus is high even though the fetal Po_2 is much lower than that of the mother. This is explained partly by high blood flow rates on both sides of the placenta and by a high affinity for oxygen of fetal (as compared with adult) blood. Actually, the usual concentration of oxygen in fetal blood is in excess of metabolic requirements, as illustrated by the fact that this value can be considerably lowered experimentally without reduction of fetal oxygen consumption. This is based upon the ability of fetal tissues to utilize oxygen effectively for normal metabolic activity at blood concentrations well below normal. The fetus has a further survival advantage in the efficient arrangement of its circulation for delivery of blood with the highest oxygen content to tissues with the highest oxygen requirement (heart and brain) and for delivery of blood with a lower oxygen content to tissues with lesser needs.

When available oxygen does fall below metabolic needs, the fetal circulation usually responds with a vagally mediated bradycardia, a slight increase in blood pressure, a decrease in cardiac output, and a redistribution of blood flow away from the less critical to the more critical tissues, heart, brain, and adrenals. This conservation of available oxygen may be of great benefit to fetal survival in short-term stress, and probably explains why so many fetuses survive oxygen deprivation without evidence of injury (see Chapters 6 to 9). In addition, understanding these mechanisms allows a considered and intelligent approach to the clinical management of fetal hypoxemia (see Chapter 10).

When fetal oxygenation during labor is diminished, uterine and/or umbilical blood flow is often reduced. Improvement of these flows is of fundamental importance in maintaining an oxygen gradient to maximize placental transfer of respiratory gases.

If placental function is intact, the administration of oxygen to the mother leads to a small but definite increase in fetal oxygen levels and may be a clinically useful maneuver in fetal distress. Any attempt to speed up a slowed fetal heart rate directly by maternal injection of atropine, however, is of no demonstrable benefit and may be harmful to the fetus.

REFERENCES

1. Assali NS, Brinkman CR III: The uterine circulation and its control, in Longo LD, Bartels H (eds): *Respiratory Gas Exchange and Blood Flow in the Placenta*. Bethesda, MD, U.S.

Department of Health Education and Welfare, National Institute of Child Health and Human Development, DHEW Publication No. (NIH) 73-361, 1972, pp 121–141.

2. Barcroft J: *Researches on Pre-natal life*. Oxford, Blackwell Scientific Publications, 1946.

3. Barron DH: A history of fetal respiration: From Harvey's question (1651) to Zweifel's answer (1876), in Longo LD, Reneau DD (eds): *Fetal and Newborn Cardiovascular Physiology*. New York, Garland STPM Press, 1978, pp 1–32.

4. Battaglia FC, Bowes W, McGaughey HR, Makowski EL, Meschia G: The effect of fetal exchange transfusions with adult blood upon fetal oxygenation. *Pediatr Res* 1969;3:60–65.

5. Battaglia FC, Meschia G, Makowski EL, Bowes W: The effect of maternal oxygen inhalation upon fetal oxygenation. *J Clin Invest* 1968;47:548–555.

6. Benesch R, Benesch RE: The effect of organic phosphates from the human erythrocyte on the allosteric properties of hemoglobin. *Biochem Biophys Res Commun* 1967;26:162–167.

7. Berg D, Saling E: The oxygen partial pressures in the human fetus during labor and delivery, in Longo LD, Bartels H (eds): *Respiratory Gas Exchange and Blood Flow in the Placenta*. Bethesda, MD, U.S. Department of Health Education and Welfare, National Institute of Child Health and Human Development, DHEW Publication No. (NIH) 73-361, 1972, pp 441–457.

8. Born GVR, Dawes GS, Mott JC, Widdicombe JH: Changes in the heart and lungs at birth. *Cold Spring Harbor Symp Quant Biol* 1954;19:102–108.

9. Chanutin A, Curnish RR: Effect of organic and inorganic phosphates on the oxygen equilibrium of human erythrocytes. *Arch Biochem* 1967;121:96–102.

10. Cohen WR, Piasecki GJ, Cohn HE, Young JB, Jackson BT: Adrenal secretion of catecholamines during hypoxemia in fetal lambs. *Endocrinology* 1984;114:383–390.

11. Cohen WR, Piasecki GJ, Jackson BT: Plasma catecholamines during hypoxemia in fetal lambs. *Am J Physiol* 1982;243:R520–R525.

12. Cohn HE, Piasecki GJ, Jackson BT: The effect of fetal heart rate on cardiovascular function during hypoxemia. *Am J Obstet Gynecol* 1980;138:1190–1199.

13. Cohn HE, Piasecki GJ, Jackson BT: The effect of β-adrenergic stimulation on fetal cardiovascular function during hypoxemia. *Am J Obstet Gynecol* 1982;144:810–816.

14. Cohn HE, Sacks EJ, Heymann MA, Rudolph AM: Cardiovascular responses to hypoxemia and acidemia in fetal lambs. *Am J Obstet Gynecol* 1974;120:817–824.

15. Comline RS, Silver M: The release of adrenaline and noradrenaline from the adrenal glands of the foetal sheep. *J Physiol* 1961;156:424–444.

16. Comroe JH: *Physiology of Respiration*. Chicago, Year Book Medical Publishers, 1965, pp 160–166.

17. Cosmi EV: Fetal homeostasis, in Scarpelli EM (ed): *Pulmonary Physiology of the Fetus, Newborn and Child*. Philadelphia, Lea & Febiger, 1975, pp 61–95.

18. Dawes GS: *Foetal and Neonatal Physiology*. Chicago, Year Book Medical Publishers, 1968.

19. Delivoria-Papadopoulos M, Roncevic NP, Oski FA: Postnatal changes in oxygen transport of term, premature, and sick infants: The role of red cell 2,3-diphosphoglycerate and adult hemoglobin. *Pediatr Res* 1971;5:235–245.

20. Edelstone DI, Rudolph AM: Preferential streaming of ductus venosus blood to brain and heart in fetal lambs. *Am J Physiol* 1979;237:H724–H729.

21. Edelstone DI, Rudolph AM, Heymann MA: Effects of hypoxemia and decreasing umbilical flow on liver and ductus venosus blood flows in fetal lambs. *Am J Physiol* 1980; 238:H656–H663.

22. Elsner R: Asphyxial survival: Diving seals and fetal lambs, in Longo LD, Reneau DD (eds): *Fetal and Newborn Cardiovascular Physiology*. New York, Garland STPM Press, 1978, pp 399–411.

23. Ferrante FL: Oxygen conservation during submergence apnea in a diving mammal, the nutria. *Am J Physiol* 1970;218:363–371.

24. Forster RE II: Some principles governing maternal-foetal transfer in the placenta, in Comline RS, Cross KW, Dawes GS, et al (eds): *Foetal and Neonatal Physiology*, Sir Joseph Barcroft Centenary Symposium. London, Cambridge University Press, 1973, pp 223–237.

25. Green JR, Creasy RK, Heymann MA, Rudolph AM: Effect of atropine on fetal cardiac output during hypoxemia, abstracted. *Gynecol Invest* 1977;8:36.

26. Gregg DE, Fisher LC: Blood supply to the heart, in Hamilton WF, Dow P (eds): *Handbook of Physiology, Section 2: Circulation*. Washington, DC, American Physiological Society, 1963, vol 2, pp 1517–1584.

27. Harris JL, Krueger TR, Parer JT: Mechanisms of late decelerations of the fetal heart rate during hypoxia. *Am J Obstet Gynecol* 1982;144:491–496.

28. Hon EH, Hess OW: Instrumentation of fetal electrocardiography. *Science* 1957; 125:553–554.

29. Itskovitz J, Goetzman BW, Rudolph AM: The mechanism of late deceleration of the heart rate and its relationship to oxygenation in normoxemic and chronically hypoxemic fetal lambs. *Am J Obstet Gynecol* 1982;142:66–73.

30. Jackson BT: Epinephrine effects on uterine blood flow and fetal hemodynamics: Protective effect of dibenamine. *Surg Forum* 1962;13:398–400.

31. Jackson BT, Clark JP, Egdahl RH: Direct lead fetal electrocardiography with undisturbed fetal-maternal relationships. *Surg Gynecol Obstet* 1960;110:687–692.

32. Jackson BT, Cohn HE, Piasecki GJ: Erythropoiesis in the rhesus monkey fetus, abstracted. *Gynecol Invest* 1976;7:59.

33. Jackson BT, Egdahl RH: The performance of complex fetal operations in utero without amniotic fluid loss or other disturbances of fetal-maternal relationships. *Surgery* 1960;48:564–569.

34. Jackson BT, Egdahl RH: Consideration of the fetus in surgery of the pregnant female. *Surgery* 1962;52:165–173.

35. Jackson BT, Piasecki GJ, Novy MJ: Hemodynamic effects of maternal-fetal parabiosis. *Am J Obstet Gynecol* 1974;119:567–569.

36. Jackson BT, Piasecki GJ, Novy MJ: Fetal responses to altered maternal oxygenation in rhesus monkey. *Am J Physiol* 1987;252:R94–R101.

37. Jobsis FF: Basic processes in cellular respiration, in Fenn WO, Rahn H (eds): *Handbook of Physiology, Section 3, Respiration*. Washington, DC, American Physiological Society, 1964, vol 1, pp 63–124.

38. John AH: Placental transfer of atropine and the effect on foetal heart rate. *Br J Anaesth* 1965;37:57–60.

39. Jones CT, Robinson RO: Plasma catecholamines in foetal and adult sheep. *J Physiol* 1975;248:15–33.

40. Kirkpatrick SE, Friedman WF: Myocardial determinants of fetal cardiac output, in Longo LD, Reneau DD (eds): *Fetal and Newborn Cardiovascular Physiology*. New York, Garland STPM Press, 1978, vol 1, pp 369–389.

41. Lind J, Stern L, Wegelius C: *Human Foetal and Neonatal Circulation.* Springfield, IL, Charles C Thomas, 1964.

42. Longo LD: Respiratory gas exchange in the placenta, in Fishman AF, Farhi LE, Tenney SM, Geiger SR (eds): *Handbook of Physiology, Section 3: The Respiratory System, vol 4, Gas Exchange.* Bethesda, MD, American Physiological Society, 1987, pp 351–401.

43. McCarthy EF: Oxygen affinity of human maternal and foetal haemoglobin. *J Physiol* 1943;102:55–61.

44. Mela L, Delivoria-Papadopoulos M, Miller LD: Fetal and neonatal mitochondrial electron transfer chain, in Longo LD, Reneau DD (eds): *Fetal and Newborn Cardiovascular Physiology.* New York, Garland STPM Press, vol 2, 1978, pp 81–88.

45. Meschia G: Normal exchange of respiratory gases across the sheep placenta, in Longo LD, Bartels H (eds): *Respiratory Gas Exchange and Blood Flow in the Placenta.* Bethesda, MD, U.S. Department of Health Education and Welfare, National Institute of Child Health and Human Development, DHEW Publication No. (NIH) 73-361, 1972, pp 229–242.

46. Meschia G: Evolution of thinking in fetal respiratory physiology. *Am J Obstet Gynecol* 1978;132:806–813.

47. Meschia G: Supply of oxygen to the fetus. *J Reprod Med* 1979;23:160–165.

48. Meschia G, Cotter JR, Breathnack CS, Barron DH: The hemoglobin, oxygen, carbon dioxide concentrations in the umbilical bloods of sheep and goats sampled via indwelling plastic catheters. *Q J Exp Physiol* 1965;50:185–195.

49. Metcalfe J: Placental gas transfer. *Anesthesiol* 1965;26:460–464.

50. Mott JC: The ability of young mammals to withstand total oxygen lack. *Br Med Bull* 1961;17:144–148.

51. Novy MJ, Piasecki GJ, Hill JD, Jackson BT: Cardiorespiratory measurements in fetal monkeys obtained by chronic catheters. *J Appl Physiol* 1971;31:788–791.

52. Oski FA, Gottleib AJ, Miller WW, Delivoria-Papadopoulos M: The effect of deoxygenation of adult and fetal hemoglobin on the synthesis of red cell 2,3-diphosphoglycerate and its in vivo consequences. *J Clin Invest* 1970;49:400–407.

53. Parer JT: Effect of atropine on heart rate and oxygen consumption of the hypoxic fetus, abstracted. *Gynecol Invest* 1977;8:50.

54. Parer JT, Krueger TR, Harris JL: Fetal oxygen consumption and mechanisms of heart rate response during artificially produced late decelerations of fetal heart rate in sheep. *Am J Obstet Gynecol* 1980;136:478–482.

55. Peeters LLH, Sheldon RE, Jones MD Jr, Makowski EL, Meschia G: Blood flow to fetal organs as a function of arterial oxygen content. *Am J Obstet Gynecol* 1979;135:637–646.

56. Perkins JF Jr: Historical development of respiratory physiology, in Fenn WO, Rahn H (eds): *Handbook of Physiology, Section 3: Respiration.* Washington, DC, American Physiological Society, 1964, vol 1, pp 1–62.

57. Reynolds SRM: Many slender threads: An essay on progress in perinatal research, in Longo LD, Reneau DD (eds): *Fetal and Newborn Cardiovascular Physiology.* New York, Garland STMP Press, 1978, vol 1, pp 33–45.

58. Reynolds SRM, Paul WM, Huggett AS: Physiological study of the monkey fetus in utero: A procedure for blood pressure recording, blood sampling, and injection of the fetus under normal conditions. *Bull Johns Hopkins Hosp* 1954;95:256–268.

59. Rivard G, Motoyama EK, Acheson FM, Cook CD, Reynolds EOR: The relation between maternal and fetal oxygen tensions in sheep. *Am J Obstet Gynecol* 1967;97:925–930.

60. Roughton FJW: Transport of oxygen and carbon dioxide, in Fenn WO, Rahn H (eds): *Handbook of Physiology, Section 3: Respiration*. Washington, DC, American Physiological Society, 1964, vol 1, pp 767–825.

61. Rudolph AM, Heymann MA: Circulation of the fetus in utero: Methods for studying distribution of blood flows, cardiac output, and organ blood flow. *Circ Res* 1967;21:163–184.

62. Rudolph AM, Heymann MA: Control of the foetal circulation, in Comline RS, Cross KW, Dawes GS, Nathanielz PW (eds): *Foetal and Neonatal Physiology*, Sir Joseph Barcroft Centenary Symposium. London, Cambridge University Press, 1973, pp 89–111.

63. Tyuma I, Shimiza K: Different responses to organic phosphates of human fetal and adult hemoglobin. *Arch Biochem* 1969;129:404–405.

64. Versmold H, Seifert G, Riegal KP: Blood oxygen affinity in infancy: The interaction of fetal and adult hemoglobin, oxygen capacity, and red cell hydrogen ion and 2,3-diphosphoglycerate concentration. *Resp Physiol* 1973;18:14–25.

65. Wilson LG: The transformation of ancient concepts of respiration in the seventeenth century. *Isis* 1960;51:161–172.

66. Yaffe H, Parer JT, Llanos A, Block B: Fetal hemodynamic response to graded reductions of uterine blood flow in sheep. Paper presented at the 29th Annual Meeting of the Society for Gynecologic Investigation, Dallas, March 24–27, 1982.

67. Zaizov R, Matoth Y: Red cell values on the first postnatal day during the last 16 weeks of gestation. *Am J Hematol* 1976;1:275–278.

68. Zanjani ED, Gordon AS: Erythropoietin production and utilization in fetal goats and sheep. *Isr J Med Sci* 1971;7:850–856.

6

Cerebral Palsy, Mental Retardation, and Intrapartum Asphyxia

Nigel Paneth and Raymond Stark

The suspicion that events in the perinatal period might be related to handicaps in adults has long been part of both medical thinking and popular folklore. Assessment of clinical evidence on the subject began with the observations of Little,[33] published in 1862. He noted that children with cerebral palsy were frequently born prematurely, often were the products of difficult deliveries, and had delays in initiating respiration. His classic report is remarkable for its clarity, prescience, and the large number of cases of cerebral palsy assembled. Little concluded that prematurity and perinatal asphyxia were related causally to cerebral palsy.

Objections to Little's hypothesis were raised by Sigmund Freud,[21] whose monograph *Infantile Cerebral Paralysis* was the most comprehensive look at cerebral palsy of its era. Freud acknowledged the association between prematurity and cerebral palsy, but argued that some preexisting condition might predispose to both disorders.

It was not until the early 1950s that the first attempts were made to put the relationship between neurologic abnormalities and labor events onto a firm epidemiologic and physiologic footing. Lilienfeld and others, in a series of papers, used the retrospective case-control method to assess the frequency of abnormalities of pregnancy and labor in children with cerebral palsy and mental retardation compared to their frequency in children free of such disorders.[31,46] In general, their results supported the notion that phenomena associated with oxygen deprivation, as opposed to those capable of causing mechanical injury, were associated with these handicaps. The strong association of cerebral palsy and low birth weight was reaffirmed by these studies and those of Eastman and DeLeon.[16]

Current understanding is that the brain of the fetus can be deprived of oxygen by two major pathogenic mechanisms: hypoxemia and ischemia.

During hypoxemia, the amount of oxygen in the blood supply to the brain is decreased, whereas in ischemia the amount of blood perfusing the brain is diminished. During parturition, hypoxemia and/or ischemia are most often the result of asphyxia, defined as an impairment of the exchange of respiratory gases, both oxygen and carbon dioxide, across the placenta. The term "asphyxia" will be used in this chapter in describing the perinatal condition that is the subject of most of the follow-up studies discussed.

Concurrent with the epidemiologic work of Lilienfeld and colleagues, studies of human umbilical cord blood demonstrated that uncomplicated labor and delivery are normally associated with some degree of asphyxia.[24] Furthermore, it came to be appreciated that one of the initial homeostatic responses of the newborn is recovery from this physiologic asphyxia and the establishment of a normal acid-base state.[58]

The understanding of the factors regulating fetal oxygenation was derived mainly from experiments that utilize chronic animal models with indwelling catheters in the fetal and maternal circulations. Such experiments were greatly facilitated by the development in the 1950s of reliable techniques for measurement of arterial blood gas concentrations and pH levels. As Dawes[10] has demonstrated, the fetus does not develop in a relatively acidotic and hypoxic environment, as had previously been thought.

Experimental studies in several species also defined a relatively greater resistance of fetal and neonatal animals to asphyxial injury.[23,25] In subsequent years the neuropathologic, metabolic, and cerebrovascular aberrations associated with severe perinatal asphyxia have been investigated extensively. These are discussed in detail in Chapters 7 through 9. Perhaps influenced by these epidemiologic and physiologic studies, the obstetric community seems to have settled on a rather strict interpretation of the relationship between perinatal asphyxia and later neurologic deficits. The concept that asphyxia during labor is a major determinant of handicap in the childhood population has become widely prevalent. This concept has done much to enhance the widespread use of fetal monitoring and to prompt various interventions during labor. Consider the following three quotations from leading authorities on both sides of the Atlantic: "Early recognition and elimination of fetal distress should reduce by one-half the incidence of handicapping conditions or mental retardation."[48] "Asphyxia is generally regarded as the major cause of disability in later life."[3] "Perinatal asphyxia is the principal recognized cause of perinatal death and long-term neurodevelopmental handicap in mature infants in the United Kingdom."[2]

In this chapter, evidence that pertains to the relationship of asphyxia in labor to two important handicapping conditions—mental retardation and cerebral palsy—is reviewed.

EPIDEMIOLOGY OF MENTAL RETARDATION

A necessary first condition for placing intrapartum asphyxia in its proper perspective in relation to neurologically handicapping disorders is to understand these conditions, their frequency in the human population, and their other known determinants.

Stein and Susser[53] and, more recently, Kiely[27] have reviewed the epidemiology of mental retardation. Much of what is known of the epidemiology of this condition is derived from the work of Stein and Susser and that of Birch et al.[5]

Although clinicians use multiple criteria to diagnose and classify mental retardation, epidemiologic studies have generally used the results of intelligence quotient (IQ) tests alone as the central criterion. The limitations of IQ tests are well known; they are not free of cultural bias, and they do not test many important aspects of cognitive functioning. Nonetheless, they can serve as a useful numerical standard for population surveys in which one attempts to measure the frequency of severe handicap. Mental retardation is defined as severe if the IQ is less than 50, and mild if it is between 50 and 69. As IQ tests are standardized to a mean of 100 and a standard deviation of 15 on a normal population, it is to be expected that 2% to 3% of the population will have IQs under 70, that is, more than 2 standard deviations from the mean. However, children classified as mildly retarded usually do have school difficulties and often require special classes to make best use of their abilities. The severely retarded require either special schooling or are institutionalized.

Two major features distinguish these two groups of retarded individuals. The first is the presence of clinical features suggestive of brain damage—motor handicap, seizure disorder, or abnormal facies—in almost all severely retarded individuals. These findings are rare in the mildly retarded, particularly in the majority, whose IQs are more than 60. The second is that the two forms of mental retardation have markedly different distributions in the population. The severely retarded are generally found with equal frequency in all social classes. Mild mental retardation, on the other hand, exhibits a pronounced social class gradient, with the bulk of cases coming from the socially most disadvantaged classes, and particularly from the later-born children of large families. These two features have led many authorities to consider the two forms of retardation as etiologically distinct. Severe mental retardation most likely represents a biologic insult to the brain, whereas mild mental retardation most likely represents the effect of environmental deprivation or an insufficiency of the postnatal stimulation necessary for the development of normal mental function.

The prevalence of severe mental retardation is quite similar in different parts of the industrialized world; the remarkable consistency is shown in Table 6-1. In disparate populations sampled at different ages, the prevalence of severe retardation is consistently three to four cases per 1,000 school-age children. Rates for mild mental retardation, however, vary considerably depending on the social class distribution of the population sampled. Mild mental retardation not only varies in frequency, but it is, of course, much commoner. Figure 6-1, from the study of mental retardation by Birch et al.[5] in Aberdeen, Scotland shows how sharply mild mental retardation varies with social class. Note that in social classes I to IIIa (the professional, managerial, and skilled worker classes) no cases of mild mental retardation with IQs 60 to 69 were found, whereas such cases constitute the bulk of mental retardation in the lower social classes.

In many cases of severe mental retardation, it is difficult to determine etiology. Nevertheless, carefully examined series of cases have given reasonable estimates of the breakdown of probable causes. Table 6-2 gives an estimate based on several published series. The dominant role of Down syndrome is apparent, always constituting at least one-third and sometimes as many as one-half of the cases of severe retardation in any given series. All perinatal events taken together are thought to contribute

---

Table 6-1 Selected Estimates of the Prevalence of Severe and Mild Mental Retardation per 1,000 Population of a Given Age

Location	Year of publication	Age group (years)	Rate per 1,000 Severe	Mild
Oregon	1962	12–14	3.3	30.3
Aberdeen, Scotland	1970	8–10	3.7	23.7
Onandaga, New York	1955	5–7	3.6	—
Middlesex, England	1962	9–14	3.6	—
Quebec, Canada	1973	10	3.8	—
Netherlands	1976	19	3.7	31.0
Isle of Wight, England	1970	9–14	—	25.3

Source: Adapted from Public Health and Preventive Medicine, ed 11, by MJ Last (Ed) with permission of Appleton & Lange, © 1980.

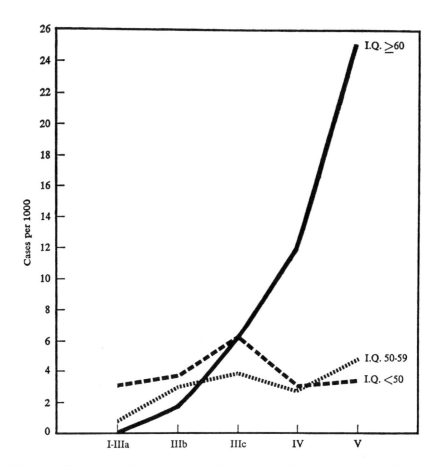

Figure 6-1 Relationship between the prevalence of mental retardation and social class. *Source:* Reprinted from *Mental Subnormality in the Community: A Clinical and Epidemiological Study* (p 56) by HG Birch, SA Richardson, and D Baird with permission of Williams & Wilkins Company, © 1970.

no more than 10% of severe mental retardation. The dominant role of genetic, and particularly chromosomal, disorders in severe mental retardation suggests that amniocentesis is the obstetric procedure most likely to impact favorably upon rates of severe mental retardation in the population.

EPIDEMIOLOGY OF CEREBRAL PALSY

The epidemiology of cerebral palsy has been reviewed by Nelson and Ellenberg,[38] by Alberman and Stanley,[1] and by Paneth.[43] Nelson and

Table 6-2 Estimated Current Distribution of Selected Causes of Severe Mental Retardation in Developed Countries

Cause	Distribution
Chromosomal anomaly (e.g., Down syndrome)	36
Congenital malformation syndromes with recurrence risks (e.g., neural tube defects)	20
Inborn errors of metabolism	7
Prenatal (e.g., intrauterine growth retardation)	8
Perinatal (e.g., birth trauma, asphyxia, hyperbilirubinemia, hypoglycemia)	8
Infections	
Prenatal	2
Perinatal	2
Postnatal	2
Miscellaneous (including lead exposure, trauma, Reye's syndrome) and unknown	15

Source: Adapted from *Public Health and Preventive Medicine,* ed 11, by MJ Last (Ed) with permission of Appleton & Lange, © 1980.

Ellenberg's definition of this disorder is useful: "a chronic disability, characterized by aberrant control of movement and posture, appearing early in life, and not the result of recognized progressive disease." The inciting event is assumed to occur in the pre- or perinatal period, although in any series a small number of children are included whose cerebral palsy has been acquired postnatally (e.g., from meningitis or head trauma). When congenital nervous system anomalies such as spina bifida are excluded, fairly consistent rates of cerebral palsy are seen in the industrialized world, averaging about two cases per 1,000 school-age children.[43]

Although the cause of cerebral palsy in any individual patient is often obscure, a rough estimate of the distribution of causes in the population can be made (Table 6-3). A comparison of Tables 6-2 and 6-3 demonstrates the epidemiologic distinctiveness of these two handicapping conditions.

The most prominent epidemiologic feature of cerebral palsy is its relationship to low birth weight and premature delivery. As noted earlier, this association has been known for over a century and was reconfirmed by Eastman and DeLeon[16] and by Lilienfeld and Parkhurst.[31] The relationship is a very strong one. The risk for an infant weighing less than 1,500 g at birth is about 9%, or 22 times that of infants of normal birth

Table 6-3 Approximate Distribution of Causes in Cerebral Palsy

Low birth weight, preterm birth	35%–40%
Perinatal asphyxia in term infants	25%–30%
Congenital and perinatal infections (CMV, rubella, toxoplasma, neonatal meningitis)	5%–10%
Intrauterine ischemic events	5%–10%
Congenital brain anomalies not evident on clinical examination	5%–10%
Perinatal metabolic conditions other than asphyxia (hyperbilirubinemia, hypoglycemia, hyperosmolarity, amino acid disorders)	5%
Genetic origin	2%–5%

Abbreviations: CMV, cytomegalovirus.

Source: Reprinted with permission from *Pediatric Annals* (1986;15:191–201), Copyright © 1986, Charles B Slack Inc.

weight.[17] Infants weighing 1,500 to 2,500 g at birth have a risk about three to four times higher than that of larger infants. Despite this powerful relationship, it should be remembered that extremely low birth weight is relatively rare, and the majority of cases of cerebral palsy occur in babies of normal weight delivered at or near term. Some data tend to support an association between cerebral palsy and intrauterine growth retardation.[9,17,52]

Only a minority of cases of cerebral palsy can be attributed to birth asphyxia, and some knowledgeable authorities would probably find our estimate of 25% to 30% too high. In some parts of the world the most important cause of cerebral palsy is prenatal iodine deficiency, which produces the triad of spastic diplegia, deaf-mutism, and mental retardation and is termed "neurologic cretinism."

Cerebral palsy and mental retardation overlap to some extent clinically. About 50% of children with cerebral palsy have IQs within the normal range; of the remainder, about one-half are severely retarded. Ten percent to 20% of the severely retarded have cerebral palsy.

Athetoid cerebral palsy, particularly if associated with hearing loss, is known to be associated with high bilirubin levels in the newborn period and presumably kernicteric staining of the brain. This entity has become rare since the development of methods to control bilirubin levels in the newborn and to prevent rhesus hemolytic disease.

Whether cerebral palsy in general is on the decline in the industrialized world is less certain. Despite early optimistic reports from Sweden, evidence is mixed in the several population studies that have been performed since World War II.[44]

NEUROPATHOLOGY AND ANIMAL MODELS

The neuropathologic features of experimental birth asphyxia have been reviewed in detail elsewhere in this volume. The animal studies have confirmed the potential of asphyxia at birth to produce both cerebral palsy and other brain lesions that have been associated with mental retardation. The precise role of the severity and duration of oxygen deprivation in the genesis of brain pathology remains to be defined, as do the more controversial roles of other factors including systemic blood pressure, cerebral blood flow, cerebral edema, and metabolic aberrations (see Chapters 7 and 8).

FOLLOW-UP STUDIES IN HUMANS

Defining Asphyxia in the Clinical Situation

A central difficulty in studies that examine the prognosis of infants with birth asphyxia is the lack of a commonly agreed upon definition of birth asphyxia. Too often the term is used casually, and the medical records of handicapped children frequently contain ascriptions of the handicap to birth asphyxia based on nothing more than a history of minor obstetric complications.

The first generation of follow-up studies, reviewed in 1973 by Gottfried,[22] used simple clinical indicators of birth depression, such as duration of time to first spontaneous breath, as the measure of asphyxia. Studies published in the 1970s, and reviewed by us in detail in the previous edition of this book,[45] focused predominantly on the Apgar score, another clinical marker of birth depression. It is only in recent years that studies have appeared that report on the follow-up findings in infants whose birth asphyxia is defined either biochemically or by its neurologic effects on the neonate.

It may be useful to view birth asphyxia as having three overlapping but discrete components. The first is the asphyxial insult itself—impairment of gas exchange in the fetal-placental unit. The second component is the birth depression that may follow biochemical asphyxia, and the third is the constellation of neurologic signs in the neonate that sometimes follows the first two components.

The biochemical asphyxial insult is very difficult to quantitate. Its best clinically available measure is either umbilical artery or venous pH obtained immediately at birth, or fetal scalp pH obtained during labor. Fetal cardiotocographic abnormalities *when severe* bear some correlation to fetal acidosis, and are often the only available proxy measure for this biochemical insult.

The second component of birth asphyxia is the infant's response to the asphyxial insult, manifest as birth depression, and indicated by low Apgar scores, and difficulty in initiating spontaneous respiration and adequate circulation. Lagercrantz has shown, in a small but provocative study, that infants who respond to an episode of biochemical asphyxia with birth depression have lower serum catecholamine levels than infants in good condition at birth.[28] Thus the condition of the infant at birth may reflect not just the severity of the biochemical asphyxia, but the response of the host to it. This way of conceptualizing asphyxia may help to explain why infants with poor reserve, such as those with intrauterine growth rate (IUGR), are at greater risk of birth depression.

The quantitative relationship between these two components of asphyxia, acidosis and birth depression, has been elucidated in some very useful recent studies. In 1982, Sykes et al. showed, in a large and relatively unselected series of infants, only a weak correlation between umbilical artery pH and depressed Apgar score.[55] However, in their data the risk of having had an umbilical artery pH ≤ 7.1 if the Apgar score was ≤ 3 at 5 min was 3.8 times higher than if the Apgar score were 4 or more. Moreover the risk of having *both* the umbilical artery pH less and the base deficit more than 2 standard deviations from the mean was increased 14-fold in infants with Apgar scores ≤ 3 at 5 min. In this study, only two newborns were found to have neurologic signs thought due to asphyxia, and both of them had both acidosis and birth depression.

DeSouza et al. also found only a weak correlation between umbilical venous pH and Apgar score, although in their data, obtained from a very healthy population (uncomplicated singleton births at 39 to 42 weeks), a modified Apgar score less than 2 at 1 min more than doubled the risk of the umbilical venous pH being ≤ 7.27.[11] In this study as well, the only infants with neurologic problems in the nursery had extreme values *both* for acidosis and for modified Apgar score.

Lissauer et al., restricting their attention to infants requiring intubation at birth who were over 32 weeks and 1,500 g, found that the majority of intubated babies had neither acidosis nor abnormal fetal heart rate patterns.[32] Once again, however, the neurologically abnormal infants all had *both* acidosis at birth and were depressed. In this study, an abnormal fetal heart rate pattern was found in the three children with neonatal neurologic abnormality. Lauener et al. found that Apgar scores ≤ 4 at 1 min were 8.7 times more likely to be associated with umbilical artery pH values $\leq$7.15 than were higher scores.[29] Infants with major neurologic complications were, again, both acidotic and depressed.

Thus, biochemical asphyxia and birth depression overlap in incidence but are not synonymous. The presence of both phenomena together is characteristic, and may even be a necessary feature, of infants who progress to develop neurologic abnormalities in the nursery.

If the first component of asphyxia is the biochemical insult itself, and the second is the immediate host response to the insult, the third component is the evidence of injury to the nervous system. Only a minority of infants who pass through the first two stages ever manifest abnormal neurologic signs.

In the past decade it has come to be widely accepted that a set of neonatal neurologic findings that occur in a relatively fixed sequence and in characteristic combinations can be linked to asphyxia and birth depression.[57] This combination of findings has been termed hypoxic-ischemic encephalopathy (HIE). Although none of the individual component signs is specific to hypoxic-ischemic brain injury, the combination of signs characteristically seen, and especially the time course of their evolution and resolution, bear a reasonably specific relationship to asphyxial insults. Unfortunately, this assumption has not been subjected to critical scrutiny, for example, by studying whether examiners blinded to the birth history can distinguish infants suffering the effects of asphyxia from those with developmental brain abnormalities or metabolic derangements other than asphyxia, or from infants whose neurologic disorder is unknown, but in whose background there is no evidence of biochemical asphyxia.

The neurologic signs seen in HIE have been organized into three grades of severity by Sarnat and Sarnat,[50] and with some variations this classification has been generally accepted. The mildest abnormality consists of a syndrome of hyperalertness and irritability generally with mild changes in tone and some feeding difficulties. Moderate HIE includes depression of the sensorium, along with major tonal abnormalities and seizures, and the most severe grade describes severely obtunded infants who require artificial feeding and ventilation for some time in the neonatal period. The seizures of HIE characteristically appear 6 to 12 hr after birth, and the severity of the neurologic syndrome does not reach a maximum until 24 to 72 hr postnatally. Infants with mild or moderate HIE usually improve neurologically by the end of the first week. Whether the severity of the neurologic syndrome is correlated to the severity of the biochemical asphyxia has not yet been documented.

FOLLOW-UP STUDIES OF ASPHYXIATED INFANTS

In recent years, cohorts of asphyxiated infants have been defined on the basis of each of the three components of asphyxia and followed up prospectively. Unfortunately for the student of biochemical asphyxia, the rarest studies are those that define the asphyxial exposure biochemically or even by the fetal heart rate response. Only five such studies have appeared in the literature, and these are summarized in Table 6-4. A larger number of studies have examined infants whose birth asphyxia is defined by the extent of birth depression, as manifest by delays in onset of spontaneous respiration, poor Apgar scores, need for ventilatory assistance, or cardiac arrest. These studies are summarized in Table 6-5. Studies that use the neurologic state of the infant after a presumed asphyxial insult in utero as the exposure variable are summarized in Table 6-6.

In these tabulations, the outcome we have chosen to focus upon is cerebral palsy. The evidence that asphyxial injury to the nervous system is virtually always manifest in motor damage is very strong.[39] Mental retardation in isolation does not seem to occur as a consequence of asphyxial damage.

Infants with Acidosis or Abnormal Fetal Heart Rate Patterns
(Table 6-4)

Only one study has described the follow-up findings in a cohort of infants defined by having experienced fetal heart rate abnormalities.

Table 6-4 Prevalence of Cerebral Palsy in Infants with Fetal Acidosis or Abnormal Fetal Heart Rate Patterns

Study (no.)	No. infants followed	Criterion	Prevalence of cerebral palsy (%)
D'Souza et al.[13]	43	U_v pH<7.27 (mean = 7.14)	0
Painter et al.[42]	38	Moderately to severely abnormal fetal heart rate patterns	0
Lauener et al.[29]	98	U_a pH <7.15	2
Low et al.[35]	60	U_a buffer base <34.0 mEq/L	13
Lissauer et al.[32]	17	Endotracheal intubation *and* abnormal fetal heart rate pattern	18

Abbreviations: U_a, umbilical artery; U_v, umbilical vein.

Painter et al.[42] reported that among 38 infants with a variety of abnormal patterns of considerable duration (acute intervention was rare as the births took place in the early days of electronic fetal monitoring) only two were neurologically abnormal in childhood (Painter, personal communication). One abnormal child had a major congenital anomaly of the nervous system, and the other had sensorineural hearing loss.

In a recent report on infants intubated endotracheally at birth, Lissauer described a subset of infants with abnormal cardiotocograms in labor, most of whom also had acidosis at birth.[32] In this group of infants with both birth depression and abnormal fetal heart rate patterns, 3 of 17 had cerebral palsy at follow-up. In a normal group of deliveries (uncomplicated, singleton, 39 to 42 weeks gestation), De Souza found the umbilical venous pH at birth to range from 7.0 to 7.55.[11] The 43 infants had more than 1 standard deviation more acidotic than the mean (i.e., <7.27) had an average umbilical venous pH of 7.14, but contributed no infants with permanent neurologic sequelae. Two severely acidotic infants with encephalopathic features in the nursery recovered subsequently.

Low et al. found 8 infants with definite motor abnormalities among 60 infants followed with umbilical artery buffer base less than 34.0 mEq/L.[35] This study included preterm and low birth weight infants and was limited in inference because of the early age at assessment, 12 months.

Lauener et al. followed a consecutive series of 98 surviving infants whose umbilical artery pH had been less than 7.15.[29] Two children had permanent sequelae; although 16 more experienced mild encephalopathy in the nursery, all recovered.

It is unfortunate that in spite of the enormous attention electronic fetal heart rate monitoring has received in the obstetric literature, the data on follow-up findings in infants experiencing fetal heart rate abnormalities are so sparse.

Infants with Birth Depression (Table 6-5)

The majority of follow-up studies of what has been termed "anoxia" or "asphyxia" or perhaps more reasonably "clinical asphyxia" have been studies of infants with depressed cardiorespiratory and neurologic state at birth. As we have seen, only a subset of infants depressed at birth have in fact experienced recent biochemical asphyxia. However, with more severe degrees of birth depression, particularly when bradycardia is a component, the likelihood of preexisting acidosis increases, as does, of course, the risk of subsequent acidosis if resuscitation is delayed or incomplete. Factors other than birth asphyxia, in particular maternal

Table 6-5 Prevalence of Cerebral Palsy in Infants with Varying Degrees of Birth Depression

Study (no.)	No. infants followed	Definition of depression	Prevalence of cerebral palsy (%)
Neligan et al.[37]	221	5 or more min to breathe	1
Peters et al.[47]	647	3 or more min to breathe	1
Thompson et al.[56]	31	Apgar score 0 at 1 min, or <4 at 5 min	6
D'Souza et al.[12]	26	Intensive resuscitation for ≥10 min	11
Mulligan et al.[36]	65	Positive-pressure ventilation for >1 min	15
Steiner and Neligan[54]	22	Cardiac arrest at birth or within 15 min	18
Scott[51]	23	"Fresh" stillbirths or no regular respirations by 20 min	26
Ergander et al.[18]	76	Apgar score ≤3 at 5 min *and* transferred for intensive care	27

medications, can also cause birth depression. Since initiation of respiration is in part a neurologic response, and since two additional components of the Apgar score (grimace, tone) are neurologic functions, infants with anomalously formed central nervous systems frequently show birth depression. These factors should be kept in mind in reviewing studies of the relation of birth depression to later outcome.

Delays of three to five minutes in initiating respirations are associated with low risks of subsequent handicap. In two very large population based series from the United Kingdom, Neligan et al.[37] and Peters et al.[47] found less than a 1% risk of cerebral palsy for this degree of birth depression. With more severe degrees of depression, defined by the need for resuscitation or very low Apgar scores, the risk of cerebral palsy ranged from 6% to 15%.[13,36,56] Between one-fifth and one-quarter of infants with cardiac arrest or prolonged failure to initiate respirations developed cerebral palsy in two small studies.[51,54] The most recently published follow-up study of infants with Apgar scores of 3 or less at 5 min found a relatively high rate of handicap (27%); but all of these infants had the additional selection factor of having been transferred to a regional unit, implying that they continued to manifest symptoms beyond the immediate neonatal period.[18] Most authors have been struck by the fact that even after very severe birth depression, including cardiac arrest and prolonged resuscitation, only a minority of infants experience neurologic sequelae.

Infants with Hypoxic-Ischemic Encephalopathy (Table 6-6)

Follow-up studies of infants with HIE vary in their findings, in part because the proportion of infants with mild, moderate or severe HIE has varied in the several cohorts studied. In general, studies with the highest proportion of severe cases, as, for example, those of Finer et al.,[19] Brown et al.,[6] and Fitzhardinge et al.,[20] include or are limited to infants transported to regional centers.

Criteria for what constitutes a preceding asphyxial insult are very variable in the several studies. Brown et al.[6] include antepartum risk factors such as hemorrhage as evidence of asphyxia, whereas Sarnat and Sarnat[50] restrict their attention to asphyxia as manifest by birth depression. All studies but that of Brown et al. describe only term or normal birth weight infants.

In general, as evident in Table 6-6, HIE is followed by a higher likelihood of subsequent handicap than is either biochemical asphyxia or birth depression. In effect, an abnormal neurologic examination in the nursery, particularly if persistent, is a good predictor of neurologic abnormality later. It is likely that this generalization is true whether or not

Table 6-6 Prevalence of Cerebral Palsy in Infants Who Had Experienced Hypoxic-Ischemic Encephalopathy

Study	No. infants followed	Proportion with moderate or severe encephalopathy (%)	Prevalence of cerebral palsy (%)
De Souza et al.[11]	53	60	2
Bergamasco et al.[4]	371	37	5
Levene et al.[30]	108	29	6
Robertson et al.[49]	167	60	12
Sarnat and Sarnat[50]	19	100	26
Brown et al.[6]	76	80 at least	30
Finer et al.[19]	83	70	30
Fitzhardinge et al.[20]	62	100	42

asphyxia precedes the abnormal neurologic finding. When infants with HIE have been categorized, a clear relationship between severity and risk of handicap is seen.[30,49] Mild HIE seems in these studies to carry little or no risk of subsequent handicap.

Results of the National Collaborative Perinatal Project

Some early results of the National Collaborative Perinatal Project (NCPP) concerning Apgar score and outcome were published almost two decades ago.[14] The final results, however, have become available only relatively recently. These results are important for several reasons. The NCPP is the largest study of its kind ever undertaken. About 50,000 pregnant women, cared for at 12 medical centers in the United States, were enrolled between 1959 and 1966. The infants resulting from these pregnancies received an Apgar rating that was obtained by a specially trained independent observer who recorded the results on a special form at 1 and 5 min. Recording continued at 5-min intervals until 20 min if the Apgar score had not yet reached 8. Although one institution did not participate in the follow-up, over 85% of the remaining children were followed until 7 years of age. The Apgar score and presence or absence of cerebral palsy and mental retardation is thus known for almost 40,000 children. Given the era in which this study took place, there are of course no data concerning the sequelae of fetal acidosis or abnormal fetal heart rate patterns as diagnosed by continuous monitoring. The relevant results of this study are presented in Tables 6-7 to 6-9.

Cerebral Palsy

The rates of cerebral palsy by Apgar scores in the NCPP are shown separately for infants above and below 2,500 g, and are derived from the work of Nelson and Ellenberg[39] (Table 6-7). The trends are actually quite different in the two weight groups. For normal-sized infants, prolongation of low Apgar score is associated with increasingly high rates of cerebral palsy. The rate for infants having a 20-min Apgar score of 3 or less is almost 300 times higher than the rate for infants with a 1-min Apgar score of 7 or higher. Nevertheless, it is important to note that even such severely depressed infants as those with a 10-min Apgar score of 3 or less have a better than 80% chance of being free of cerebral palsy.

Table 6-7 Prevalence of Cerebral Palsy (per 1000 Survivors) by Apgar Score and Birth Weight

Apgar score		2,500 g		<2,500 g		Total
1 min	7–10	6	(3,065)	2	(35,971)	2
1 min	0–3	29	(395)	15	(1,890)	17
5 min	0–3	67	(97)	47	(337)	51
10 min	0–3	37	(34)	167	(80)	126
15 min	0–3	0	(14)	360	(28)	255
20 min	0–3	0	(6)	571	(16)	381

Note: Number of survivors in parentheses.

Source: Adapted with permission from *Pediatrics* (1981;68:36–44), Copyright © 1981, American Academy of Pediatrics.

For infants with birth weights less than 2,500 g, the relationship is much less linear. Although the cerebral palsy rates increase with worsening Apgar scores up to a 5-min Apgar of less than 3, even such severe depression as is manifest in Apgar scores of less than 3 at 10, 15, or 20 min does not seem to add to the risk of cerebral palsy. Of course, at the time of the NCPP, mortality among low-birth-weight infants with these Apgar scores was very high. It is conceivable that under present conditions with advances in neonatal intensive care and improved survival rates for low-birth-weight infants, the impairment rate might be higher. It is also likely, however, that the determinants of cerebral palsy in low-birth weight infants are different from those of term infants and, in particular, are less closely related to birth depression.

The large increments in risk with increasing severity of postnatal asphyxial depression should not obscure the observation that the bulk of cerebral palsy arises in infants who appeared to make a smooth transition to extrauterine life. Fifty-five percent of cases of cerebral palsy in the NCPP occurred in infants with 1-min Apgar scores of 7 or higher.

Since the last edition of this book, Nelson and Ellenberg have published two other relevant analyses of the NCPP data concerning the causes of cerebral palsy. The first of these reported the risk of cerebral palsy for several obstetric complications likely to predispose to asphyxia.[40] Some obstetric risk factors often cited as markers of asphyxia bore little or no relation to risk of cerebral palsy in childhood (Table 6-8). Moreover, in term infants, if the Apgar score at 5 min was not depressed, no significant elevation of the cerebral palsy risk was associated with any

Table 6-8 Risk of Cerebral Palsy with Specific Obstetric Complications

Complications	Frequency in population (%)	Risk of cerebral palsy in infants >2500 g (%)
Placenta previa	0.6	1.9
Breech	2.6	1.0
Abruptio placentae	1.7	0.6
FHR <100	6.3	0.4
Mid or high forceps	8.4	0.4
Meconium	18.4	0.4
Cord prolapse	0.8	0.3
Second stage 1 hr or more	10.1	0.3
Nuchal cord	24.9	0.3
No complications	38.1	0.3

Abbreviations: FHR, fetal heart rate.

Source: Adapted with permission from *Journal of the American Medical Association* (1984;251: 1843–1848), Copyright © 1984, American Medical Association.

of the tabulated complications. The error of the all too common practice of singling out obstetric risk factors as "causes" of handicap in a given child is shown both by the very high prevalence of risk factors such as meconium passage (18%) and nuchal cord (25%), and by the very low risks of cerebral palsy associated with them.

A multivariate analysis of all factors potentially related to cerebral palsy in the NCPP uncovered some surprising new risk factors.[41] Low IQ in the mother proved a significant risk, as did administration of thyroid hormone and estrogen in the pregnancy. Seizure disorder in the mother also proved to increase the risk of cerebral palsy in the offspring. The three most potent risk factors for cerebral palsy in normal birth weight infants turned out to be descriptions of the neonate: prolonged time to first cry, seizures, and presence of a congenital anomaly outside the nervous system. Although the first two factors at times reflect asphyxia, the presence of the third risk factor points to the likelihood that some children with cerebral palsy have brains that are malformed prenatally. All known risk factors together predicted only a minority of cases of cerebral palsy. Clearly much is yet to be learned about the etiology of this important childhood handicap.

Mental Retardation

Broman[7] has published findings concerning the relationship of Apgar scores and other indicators of asphyxia to the results of intelligence test scores at age 7 years (Table 6-9). Unfortunately, IQ data were analyzed differently from those concerning cerebral palsy. The influence of extended Apgar scores was not considered, nor were results reported separately for low- and normal birth weight children. On the other hand, several indicators of perinatal asphyxia were studied, including fetal heart rate, meconium staining, resuscitative efforts, apneic episodes, and respiratory difficulties. An assessment of the overall contribution of these indicators to intelligence tests results was made.

Low 1- and 5-min Apgar scores were associated with somewhat lower IQ scores and a higher frequency of mental retardation in both blacks and whites, with the effect stronger in the latter. Although race, sex, and socioeconomic status were controlled in the analysis of the IQ data, mental retardation rates are reported only by race. In neither analysis can the contribution of other potentially confounding variables, such as birth weight, be assessed from the data presented. However, in a multiple regression equation, all perinatal asphyxia indicators combined contributed less than 1% of the variance in IQ score at age 7. The major factors influencing intelligence test results were maternal characteristics, in particular mother's education, socioeconomic status, and performance on a 20-min oddity discrimination test. As observed with cerebral palsy, the overwhelming majority of infants with quite severe depression at birth (5-min Apgar score of 3 or less) had an IQ score within the normal range.

Table 6-9 Mean IQ at Age 7 by Apgar Score and Race

Apgar score	Mean IQ		IQ <70	
	White	Black	White (%)	Black (%)
Infants free of any anoxic sign	103.39	89.60	1.2	4.9
1-min Apgar, 0–3	99.19	88.22	3.9	9.0
5-min Apgar, 0–3			5.1	10.0

Source: Adapted with permission from *Infants Born at Risk: Physiological, Perceptual & Cognitive Processes* by T Field and A Sostek, Prentice-Hall Inc, © 1979.

SUMMARY AND CONCLUSIONS

Perinatal asphyxia has the potential to cause brain injury and interfere with subsequent development; its role in producing later neurologic impairment should not, however, be overestimated. The evidence from long-term follow-up studies of asphyxiated infants, with asphyxia defined in several ways, does not support the conclusion that perinatal asphyxia is the major cause of cerebral palsy and severe mental retardation. Despite the heterogeneity in their designs, these studies give surprisingly consistent results.

The majority of even quite severely asphyxiated infants who survive the neonatal period do not develop motor handicaps and have intelligence test scores well within the normal range. Nonetheless, a substantial minority of asphyxiated infants do develop chronic brain impairment, which seems to be the result of the asphyxia. Three generalizations can be made about such infants:

1. Their asphyxia and birth depression is likely to have been very severe.
2. They virtually always show abnormal neurologic signs in the neonatal period, such as seizures, uncoordinated feeding, and difficulties with respiratory control.
3. The subsequent handicap is generally severe, often multiple, and almost always involves the motor system.

This last observation suggests a useful clinical principle. In cases of mental handicap in which cerebral palsy is not also present, it is virtually certain that the damage is not due to birth asphyxia.

The apparent dichotomization of the outcomes of perinatal asphyxia— either normalcy or severe handicap—may reflect the considerable recuperative capacities of the developing brain exposed to moderate degrees of birth asphyxia. It may also, however, reflect the limitations of IQ tests in detecting subtle cognitive dysfunction. It should also be noted that asphyxial episodes may occur during gestation, prior to the onset of labor, and may not be reflected in the condition of the infant at birth. There are no reliable means to assess the contribution of such prenatal asphyxial events to later outcome.

What practical principles should the practicing obstetrician derive from this review? First, because many infants with birth asphyxia survive intact, it is incumbent on delivery personnel to be expertly trained in neonatal resuscitation. Vigorous resuscitative efforts should be undertaken at virtually any Apgar score at 1 and 5 min. Second, in counseling the parents of asphyxiated infants, an optimistic prognosis can be given unless the asphyxia has been extraordinarily severe or other adverse features, particularly severe HIE, are present. Finally, the indications for obstetric interventions during labor need to be defined clearly. Interventions during labor play only a limited role in shaping the pattern of mental retardation in the community; nevertheless, neglected perinatal asphyxia can result in cognitive and motor handicaps. A large body of data, not reviewed in this chapter, links indicators of birth asphyxia to fetal and neonatal death and to various manifestations of neonatal morbidity. The desire of obstetricians to lower intrapartum and neonatal mortality and morbidity to their lowest possible frequencies should properly serve as the justification for intensive labor monitoring and prompt intervention when severe and uncorrectable fetal asphyxia is documented during labor.

REFERENCES

1. Alberman E, Stanley F: The epidemiology of the cerebral palsies. *Clin Dev Med* 1984;87:46–56.

2. Archer LNJ, Levene MI, Evans DH: Cerebral artery doppler ultrasonography for prediction of outcome after perinatal asphyxia. *Lancet* 1986;2:1116–1118.

3. Beard RW, Rivers RP: Fetal asphyxia in labor. *Lancet* 1979;2:1117–1119.

4. Bergamasco B, Benna P, Ferrero P, Gavinelli R: Neonatal hypoxia and epileptic risk: A clinical prospective study. *Epilepsia* 1984;25:131–136.

5. Birch HG, Richardson SA, Baird D: *Mental Subnormality in the Community. A Clinical and Epidemiological Study*. Baltimore, Williams & Wilkins, 1970.

6. Brown JK, Purvis RJ, Forfar JO, Cockburn F: Neurological aspects of perinatal asphyxia. *Dev Med Child Neurol* 1974;16:567–580.

7. Broman S: Perinatal anoxia and cognitive development in early childhood, in Field TM, Sostek AM, Goldberg S, Shuman HH (eds): *Infants Born at Risk*. New York, Spectrum Books, 1979, pp 29–52.

8. Brown JK, Purvis RJ, Forfar JO, Cockburn F: Neurological aspects of perinatal asphyxia. *Dev Med Child Neurol* 1974;16:567–580.

9. Commey JO, Fitzhardinge PM: Handicap in the preterm small-for-gestational-age infant. *J Pediatr* 1979;94:779–786.

10. Dawes G: *Fetal and Neonatal Physiology*. Chicago, Year Book Medical Publishers, 1978.

11. De Souza SW, Black P, Cadman J, Richards B: Umbilical venous blood pH: A useful aid in the diagnosis of asphyxia at birth. *Arch Dis Child* 1983;58:15–19.

12. D'Souza SW, McCartney E, Nolan M, Taylor IG: Hearing speech and language in survivors of severe perinatal asphyxia. *Arch Dis Child* 1981;56:245–252.

13. D'Souza SW, Richards B: Neurological sequelae in newborn babies after perinatal asphyxia. *Arch Dis Child* 1979;53:564–569.

14. Drage JS, Berendes HW, Fisher PD: The Apgar scores and four year psychological examination performance, in *Perinatal Factors Affecting Human Development* (Science Publication No. 185). Washington, DC, Pan American Health Organization, 1969.

15. Dweck HS, Huggins W, Dorman LP, Saxon SA, Benton JW, Cassady G: Developmental sequelae in infants having suffered severe perinatal asphyxia. *Am J Obstet Gynecol* 1974;119:811–815.

16. Eastman NJ, DeLeon M: The etiology of cerebral palsy. *Am J Obstet Gynecol* 1955;69:950–961.

17. Ellenberg JH, Nelson KB: Birth weight and gestational age in children with cerebral palsy or seizure disorders. *Am J Dis Child* 1979;133:1044–1048.

18. Ergander U, Eriksson M, Zetterstrom R: Severe neonatal asphyxia. Incidence and prediction of outcome in the Stockholm area. *Acta Paediatr Scand* 1983;72:321–325.

19. Finer NN, Robertson CM, Richards RT, Pinnell LE, Peters KL: Hypoxic-ischemic encephalopathy in term neonates. Perinatal factors and outcome. *J Pediatr* 1981;98:112–117.

20. Fitzhardinge PM, Flodmark O, Fitz CR, Ashby S: The prognostic value of computed tomography as an adjunct to assessment of the term infant with postasphyxial encephalopathy. *J Pediatr* 1981;99:777–781.

21. Freud S: *Infantile Cerebral Paralysis*, Russin LA (trans). Coral Gables, FL, University of Miami Press, 1968, pp 257–259.

22. Gottfried AW: Intellectual consequences of perinatal anoxia. *Psychol Bull* 1973;80:231–242.

23. Himwich HE, Alexander FAD, Fazekas JF: The tolerance of the newborn to hypoxia and anoxia. *Am J Physiol* 1941;133:327–328.

24. James LS, Weisbrot IM, Prince CE, Holaday DA, Apgar V: The acid-base status of human infants in relation to birth asphyxia and the onset of respiration. *J Pediatr* 1958;52:379–394.

25. Kabat H: The greater resistance of very young animals to arrest of the brain circulation. *Am J Physiol* 1940;130:588–599.

26. Kiely J, Paneth N, Stein ZA, Susser MW: Cerebral palsy and newborn care. I. Secular trends in cerebral palsy. *Dev Med Child Neurol* 1981;23:533–538.

27. Kiely M: The prevalence of mental retardation. *Epidemiol Rev* 1987;9:194–218.

28. Lagercrantz H: Asphyxia and the Apgar score (letter). *Lancet* 1982;1:966.

29. Lauener PA, Calame A, Janecek P, Bossart H, Monod JF: Systematic pH-measurements in the umbilical artery: Causes and predictive value of neonatal acidosis. *J Perinat Med* 1983;11:278–282.

30. Levene MI, Grindulis H, Sands C, Moore JR: Comparison of two methods of predicting outcome in perinatal asphyxia. *Lancet* 1986;1:67–68.

31. Lilienfeld AM, Parkhurst E: A study of the association of factors of pregnancy and parturition with the development of cerebral palsy. *Am J Hyg* 1951;53:262–282.

32. Lissauer TJ, Steer PJ: The relation between the need for intubation at birth, abnormal cardiotocograms in labour and cord artery blood gas and pH values. *Br J Obstet Gynaecol* 1986;93:1060–1066.

33. Little WJ: On the influence of abnormal parturition, difficult labor, premature birth, and asphyxia, neonatorum on the mental and physical condition of the child, especially in relation to deformities. *Trans Obstet Soc Lond* 1862;3:293–344.

34. Low JA, Galbraith RS, Muir D, Killen H, Karchmar J, Campbell D: Intrapartum fetal asphyxia: A preliminary report in regard to long-term morbidity. *Am J Obstet Gynecol* 1978;130:525–533.

35. Low JA, Galbraith RS, Muir DW, Killen HL, Pater EA, Karchmar EJ: Factors associated with motor and cognitive deficits in children after intrapartum fetal hypoxia. *Am J Obstet Gynecol* 1984;148:533–539.

36. Mulligan JC, Painter MJ, O'Donoghue PA, MacDonald HM, Allen AC, Taylor PM: Neonatal asphyxia. II. Neonatal mortality and long-term sequelae. *J Pediatr* 1980; 96:903–907.

37. Neligan G, Purdham D, Steiner H: *The Formative Years: Birth, Family and Development in Newcastle-upon-Tyne*. London, Oxford University Press, 1974.

38. Nelson KB, Ellenberg JH: Epidemiology of cerebral palsy, in Schoenberg BS (ed): *Advances in Neurology*. New York, Raven Press, vol 19, 1978, pp 421–435.

39. Nelson KB, Ellenberg JH: Apgar scores as predictors of chronic neurologic disability. *Pediatrics* 1981;68:36–44.

40. Nelson KB, Ellenberg JH: Obstetric complications as risk factors for cerebral palsy or seizure disorders. *JAMA* 1984;251:1843–1848.

41. Nelson KB, Ellenberg JH: Antecedents of cerebral palsy. *N Engl J Med* 1986;315:81–86.

42. Painter MJ, Depp R, O'Donoghue PD: Fetal heart rate patterns and development in the first year of life. *Am J Obstet Gynecol* 1978;132:271–277.

43. Paneth N: The etiology of cerebral palsy. *Pediatr Ann* 1986;15:191–201.

44. Paneth N, Kiely JL: The frequency of cerebral palsy: a review of population studies in industrialized nations since 1950. *Clinic Dev Med* 1984;87:46–65.

45. Paneth N, Stark R. Mental retardation, cerebral palsy, and intrapartum asphyxia, in Cohen WR, Friedman EA (eds): *Management of Labor*. Rockville, MD, Aspen Publishers, 1983, pp 143–161.

46. Pasamanick B, Lilienfeld AM: Association of maternal and fetal factors with development of mental deficiency. I. Abnormalities in the prenatal and perinatal periods. *JAMA* 1955;119:155–160.

47. Peters TJ, Golding J, Lawrence CJ, Fryer JG: Delayed onset of regular respiration and subsequent development. *Early Hum Dev* 1984;9:225–239.

48. Quilligan E: Fetal monitoring: Is it worth it? *Obstet Gynecol* 1976;45:96–100.

49. Robertson C: Term infants with hypoxic-ischemic encephalopathy: Outcome at 3–5 years. *Dev Med Child Neurol* 1985;27:473–484.

50. Sarnat HB, Sarnat MS: Neonatal encephalopathy following fetal distress. *Arch Neurol* 1976;33:696–705.

51. Scott H: Outcome of very severe birth asphyxia. *Arch Dis Child* 1976;51:712–716.

52. Stanley F: Spastic cerebral palsy. Changes in birthweight and gestational age. *Early Hum Dev* 1981;5:167–178.

53. Stein ZA, Susser MW: Mental retardation, in Last MJ (ed): *Public Health and Preventive Medicine*, 12th ed. Norwalk, CT, Appleton-Century-Crofts, 1986, pp 1313–1326.

54. Steiner M, Neligan G: Perinatal cardiac arrest. Quality of the survivors. *Arch Dis Child* 1975;50:696–702.

55. Sykes GS, Molloy PM, Johnson P, Gu W, Ashworth F, Stirrat GM, Turbull AC: Do Apgar scores indicate asphyxia? *Lancet* 1982;1:494–496.

56. Thompson AJ, Searle M, Russell G: Quality of survival after severe birth asphyxia. *Arch Dis Child* 1977;53:620–626.

57. Volpe JJ: Neurology of the Newborn, 2nd ed. Philadelphia, WB Saunders. 1987.

58. Weisbrot IM, James LS, Prince CE: Acid-base homeostasis of the newborn infant during the first 24 hours of life. *J Pediatr* 1958;52:395–403.

7

Acute Perinatal Brain Injury: Hypoxia-Ischemia

Robert C. Vannucci

The brain damage that results from hypoxia-ischemia (asphyxia) is a major cause of perinatal mortality and chronic neurologic disability in infants and children. Statistics suggest an incidence of asphyxia in 2/1,000 to 4/1,000 full-term infants and an incidence that approaches 60% in small premature neonates.[67,137,151,175,210] Between 20% and 50% of asphyxiated infants expire during the neonatal period; of the survivors, up to 25% exhibit permanent neuropsychologic handicaps in the form of cerebral palsy, mental retardation, learning disability, or epilepsy. Given the magnitude of the problem, it is appropriate that health professionals give high priority to the fetus and newborn infant at risk for cerebral hypoxia-ischemia.

DEFINITIONS

Fetal and neonatal hypoxia and asphyxia are well-recognized clinical entities that confront obstetricians and neonatologists almost daily. *Hypoxia* denotes a partial lack of oxygen in the tissues of the body, including the blood-stream (hypoxemia). *Asphyxia* is the state in which pulmonary or placental gas exchange is disrupted, leading in turn to progressive hypoxemia and hypercapnia. Moderate to severe hypoxia leads to metabolic acidosis (lactic acid accumulation), whereas asphyxia is associated with a mixed metabolic and respiratory acidosis. *Ischemia* is a

This work was supported by Grant 09109 and 15738 from The National Institute of Child Health and Human Development and Grant 19190 from The National Heart and Lung Institute.

reduction in or cessation of blood flow that arises from either systemic hypotension or occlusive vascular disease.

NEUROPATHOLOGY

General Considerations

The neuropathologic hallmarks of hypoxic-ischemic brain damage are *selective neuronal necrosis* and *infarction*.[22,192,238] Selective neuronal necrosis relates to tissue injury in which neurons have been destroyed with relative sparing of the supporting glia and blood vessels (Figure 7-1). Infarction occurs when all cellular elements have been affected by the pathologic process (Figure 7-2). The two entities often coexist in the same brain.

The severity and distribution of the neuropathologic lesions arising from hypoxia-ischemia depend on several factors, including (a) the nature and duration of the insult; (b) the gestational age of the fetus or newborn infant, and (c) the presence or absence of superimposed systemic stress, for example, hypoglycemia, sepsis, and undernutrition.[231] Vascular and metabolic factors also play a critical role. In this regard, specific areas of the developing and adult brain are especially sensitive to the damaging effect of hypoxia-ischemia. Such vulnerable regions include portions of the cerebral cortex, hippocampus, brain stem, and the Purkinje cell layer of the cerebellum.[22,192,224]

Vascular factors influence the topography of the pathologic lesions that arise from hypoxia-ischemia[22,192,238] (Figure 7-3). If a nutrient artery to the brain is occluded (focal cerebral ischemia), the brunt of the tissue damage resides within the distribution of that vessel. If global cerebral ischemia arises from systemic hypotension, the resultant tissue injury is limited to or accentuated at so-called "boundary zones" between the major arteries that supply blood to the brain.[21,23]

Pathologic alterations in brain also result from disruption of the venous circulation secondary to hypoxia-ischemia.[139,223] Venous stasis arising from decompensation of heart action may be severe enough in asphyxial situations to compromise brain perfusion, leading ultimately to tissue injury. Lesions, usually infarctional in nature, are located in the distribution of the venous channels draining blood to the major sinuses of the brain. Regions most vulnerable to damage include the posterior aspects of the cerebral hemispheres and the cerebellar hemispheres.[192]

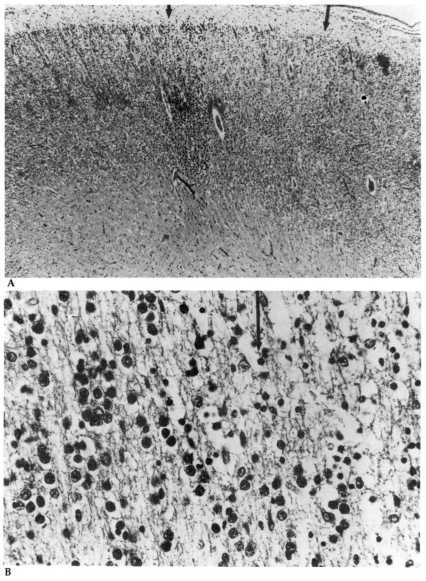

Figure 7-1 A. A coronal section of cerebral cortex from infant delivered at 36 weeks gestation. The infant expired 36 hr following birth. Note the focus of neuronal necrosis (arrows) characterized by tissue pallor. **B.** Higher-magnification view of selective neuronal necrosis shown in (A). Cells on the left are normal and display recognizable nuclear structure; cells on the right are pyknotic and set in a loose, spongy neuropil. Arrow marks separation between the two regions. *Source:* Reprinted from *Pathology of Perinatal Brain Injury* (pp 4–12) by LB Rorke with permission of Raven Press, © 1982.

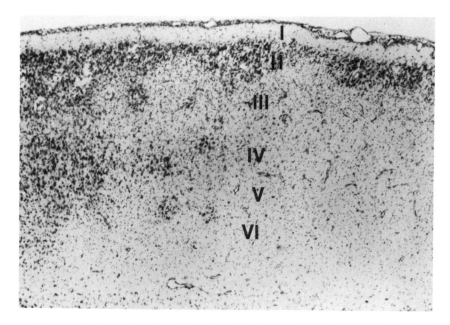

Figure 7-2 Cerebral infarction. Coronal section of cerebral cortex from a term infant who expired at 96 hr of age following severe perinatal asphyxia. Note the total destruction of cerebral cortical layers III and V + VII with slight preservation of layers II and IV.

Human Perinatal Neuropathology

Acute Lesions

In general, pathologic changes reflecting hypoxia-ischemia in full-term infants are located predominantly in the gray matter structures of the brain, including the cerebral cortex, hippocampus, basal ganglia and thalamus, brain stem, and cerebellar hemispheres[1,78,121,138,192,201,238] (see Figures 7-1 and 7-2). In premature infants, the lesions are focused primarily on white matter structures, especially of the cerebral hemispheres.[11,91,122] Acute lesions of the cerebral cortex take the form of selective neuronal necrosis and/or infarction that often has a laminar distribution, that is, areas of tissue destruction aligned parallel to the surface of the brain. Selective neuronal necrosis and/or infarction of other gray matter structures can coincide with the cerebral cortical lesions.[121,192,201]

Acute lesions of white matter range from an early reactive gliosis with relative preservation of axon cylinders to frank infarction.[11,17,77,84,91,119,122,125,192,207] Reactive gliosis denotes the prolifera-

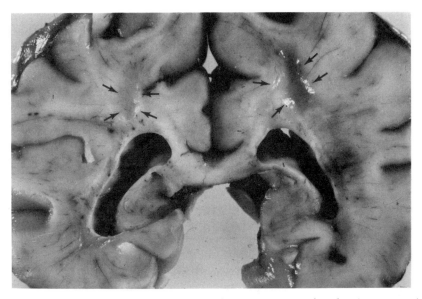

Figure 7-3 A posterior coronal section of brain from a premature infant showing acute peri-ventricular leukomalacia. There is softening of white matter within both cerebral hemi-spheres (arrows). The lateral ventricles are mildly dilated.

tion of glial elements, primarily astrocytes, presumably in response to antecedent hypoxia-ischemia or other insult to brain. The lesions are typically seen in subcortical and periventricular white matter of the cerebral hemispheres as well as in the centrum ovale and corpus callosum. Reactive white matter gliosis is a common finding postmortem in both premature and full-term infants, suggesting the presence of multiple etiologies, including hypoxia-ischemia, perinatal sepsis, intrauterine viral infection, and malnutrition.[11,91,122,192,207] Unlike white matter infarction, the lesions do not appear to follow a vascular distribution and can be found in white matter throughout the brain and spinal cord.[192]

White matter necrosis (infarction) is prominent in infants sustaining hypoxic-ischemic insults to brain.[11,77,91,121,192] In premature infants, the lesions are typically bilateral and situated adjacent to the lateral ventricles of the cerebral hemispheres; hence the term *periventricular leukomalacia* (Figure 7-3). In infants born closer to term, the topography of the necrotic foci shifts from subependymal to subcortical areas, often with associated selective neuronal necrosis or infarction of the overlying cerebral cortex.[11,91,192] The necrotic lesions often contain a hemorrhagic component.

Unlike isolated white matter gliosis, periventricular leukomalacia appears to follow a vascular distribution. In premature infants, prominent arterial boundary zones exist in the periventricular white matter adjacent to the external margins of the lateral ventricles.[53,54,218] These zones are situated 3 to 10 mm from the ventricular wall between the terminal branches of ventriculofugal arteries that course from the choroid plexus peripherally to meet penetrating branches of long parenchymal (ventriculopedal) arteries originating at the surface of the brain. The number of ventriculofugal vessels increases with increasing gestational age; therefore, their relative paucity in the premature infant targets the periventricular white matter as a structure prone to ischemic injury. Sparing of the cerebral cortex from hypoxic-ischemic damage in the premature infant may be related to the presence of rich vascular anastomoses between arteries supplying the meninges and the anterior, middle, and posterior cerebral arteries. These anastomoses are prominent in the immature brain but have essentially disappeared by term.

Prominent brain stem injury with or without involvement of the cerebral cortex and subcortical white matter recently has been reported as a consequence of an acute asphyxial insult to the newborn brain.[1,78,121,192,201,246] The predilection for damage in the brain stem closely mimics the pathologic changes observed in children and adults sustaining cardiac arrest.[20] Sensory nuclei, including the thalamus, lateral geniculate body, and colliculi are the brain stem structures that bear the brunt of the injury, with relative sparing of motor nuclei and white matter. Notably, these lesions do not appear to follow a vascular distribution; they are probably the result of an intrinsic vulnerability of the specific tissues to hypoxic-ischemic damage.

Cerebral Edema

A well-known accompaniment to the brain damage that results from perinatal hypoxia-ischemia is cerebral edema.[77,119,192] Despite the close association between selective neuronal necrosis or infarction and brain swelling, it is not yet known whether edema is simply a by-product of tissue injury or whether edema actually leads to or accentuates brain damage.

Initially, brain edema arising from cerebral hypoxia-ischemia is cytotoxic in origin and results from failure of ionic pumping across the cell membrane and intracellular accumulation of electrolytes and water. Vasogenic edema results from disruption of the blood–brain barrier with secondary free passage of large molecular weight substances and water from blood into brain parenchyma. Vasogenic edema temporally follows cytotoxic edema. Hypoxic-ischemic edema may aggravate brain damage, at least in adults, by increasing tissue volume in a nondistensible skull, thereby compromising the vascular compartment and decreasing cerebral perfusion below critical levels.[72]

Brain edema is a common finding in autopsies of newborn infants sustaining cerebral hypoxia-ischemia.[5,39,179] If the brain damage has been widespread and severe, on gross examination the brain appears swollen, with slitlike lateral ventricles, widening and flattening of the cerebral gyri with associated obliteration of the sulci, and herniation of hippocampal structures.[77,119,192] Lesser degrees of edema are associated with patchy or confluent pallor of the cerebral cortex and deep nuclear structures, often with congestion of the intervening white matter. The existence of edema is readily discernible by rarefaction of the neuropil and separation of neuronal and axonal elements.

Chronic Lesions

Chronic neuropathologic alterations arising from perinatal hypoxia-ischemia are natural extensions of the acute lesions described above.[37,44,77,119,139,192,231] Such lesions include (a) atrophic, laminar, and columnar sclerosis of the cerebral cortex; (b) subcortical and periventricular sclerosis of white matter with or without cyst formation (leukomalacia and porencephaly); (c) status marmoratus of the basal ganglia and thalamus; and (d) degeneration of the brain stem and cerebellum (Figure 7-4). Many of these end-stage lesions often coexist in the same brain.

Status marmoratus of the basal ganglia and thalamus is a characteristic, albeit uncommon, neuropathologic manifestation of perinatal hypoxia-ischemia. Grossly, the basal ganglia and thalamus exhibit a patchy, marbled appearance, which histologically has been identified as areas of hypermyelination.[77,138,192,231] Under the electron microscope, these hypermyelinated areas have been found to represent myelinated astrocytic processes rather than neurons.[16] The lesions typically result from an asphyxial insult in term infants but have also been described in infants in whom insults occurred as late as 3 months following birth.[138]

Occlusive Vascular Disease (Stroke)

Arterial occlusive vascular disease producing cerebral infarction (stroke) occurs in both the fetus and newborn.[12,120,145,215,250] Previously, most if not all cerebral infarcts were assumed to be of hypoxic-ischemic origin, with or without venous occlusion. However, more recent investigations indicate that either embolic or thrombotic occlusion of one or more arteries supplying the brain produces a distinct clinical and pathologic entity. Large, single infarcts predominate in full-term infants,

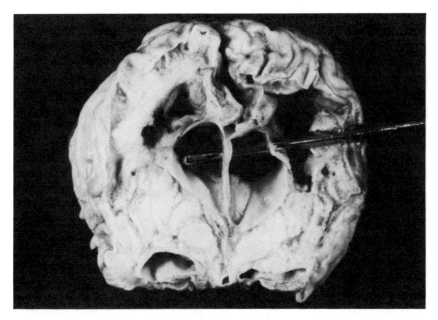

Figure 7-4 Brain of an infant showing ulegyria. The baby, which expired at 2 years of age, previously had sustained both perinatal asphyxia and intraventricular hemorrhage. The porencephalic cyst on the right communicates with the ipsilateral lateral ventricle (rod).

whereas multiple, small infarcts are more common in premature infants. The lesions typically involve the cerebral cortex and subcortical white matter, primarily in the territory of the middle cerebral artery and rarely in the distribution of the basilar artery. Hemorrhage into originally ischemic infarcts is frequent. The etiologies of arterial occlusive vascular disease in the fetus and newborn infant are numerous, with infectious disease and asphyxia the most common[12,145] (Table 7-1).

Antepartum versus Intrapartum Brain Damage

Although physicians tend to focus on the intrapartum period as the time when perinatal hypoxic-ischemic brain damage is most likely, there is overwhelming evidence that acute brain injury can and does occur in the antepartum period.[12,120,141,174] In this regard, it must be emphasized that the brains of fetuses who expire acutely from an intrauterine asphyxial event would be normal, since brain damage is an evolving process requiring hours to days for gross and microscopic verification of tissue injury. It is difficult to envision how a fetus of any gestational age could spontaneously recover from severe asphyxia unless as the direct conse-

Table 7-1 Etiologies of Perinatal Arterial Occlusive Vascular Disease

---

Sepsis
Meningitis
Asphyxia
Disseminated intravascular coagulation (DIC)
Congenital heart disease
Erythroblastosis
Polycythemia (hyperviscosity)
Postnatal hypoxia-acidosis
 (respiratory distress syndrome)
Maternal diabetes
Physical birth trauma
Arterial (temporal) catheterization
Demise of twin fetus (DIC)
Developmental anomaly of carotid, vertebral and/or basilar arteries?

---

quence of a transient maternal hypoxic or hypotensive insult.[120] Intermittent umbilical cord compression might also produce progressive but ultimately reversible fetal asphyxia, although such a situation would be difficult to document. It follows that acute brain injury in surviving but as yet undelivered fetuses most often arises from occlusive vascular disease sparing the heart rather than from systemic hypoxia-ischemia.

The occurrence of in utero hypoxic-ischemic brain damage has been amply demonstrated in the medical literature.[12,120,141,162,172,215,219,246,250] Occasionally there is a history of a catastrophic maternal illness, such as asphyxia, anaphylaxis, or major physical trauma.[120] In other situations the antecedent pathogenetic event is confined to the fetus, with or without an associated abnormality of the uteroplacental unit. Whatever the cause of the cerebral hypoxia-ischemia, the neuropathologic consequence is often devastating. Depending on the age of the lesions at the time of postmortem analysis, the severity of the brain damage may vary from acute infarction to multicystic degeneration of the cerebral cortex and white matter to total destruction of one or both cerebral hemispheres (hydranencephaly). Brain stem and even spinal cord abnormalities can coexist or occur independently.[162,172,219,246] Lesser degrees of remote damage may take the form of ulegyria, polymicrogyria, or porencephaly. These lesions can now be identified by fetal ultrasonography (US), postnatal cranial sonography, or computed tomographic (CT) scanning. Although hypoxic-ischemic brain damage may antedate the intrapartum period, the fact remains that adverse obstetric events during labor and delivery also culminate in brain damage of the newborn infant (see below).

Neuropathology of Experimental Perinatal Cerebral Hypoxia-Ischemia

Animal research has provided important information on the pathogenesis of and neuropathologic responses to perinatal cerebral hypoxia-ischemia. In experimental animals, structural brain damage from hypoxia-ischemia has been produced in immature rats, rabbits, guinea pigs, sheep, and monkeys.[186,191,217,222,248] The fetal and newborn rhesus monkey has been studied extensively because of its similarities to humans with respect to the physiology of reproduction and its neuroanatomy at birth.

Asphyxial Brain Damage

Monkey fetuses asphyxiated at birth to the point of apnea and then reanimated by resuscitation exhibited hypotonia, poor coordinated movements, and a loss of postural righting reflexes following the insult.[186] Neuropathologic examination at 1 to 3 months of age revealed brain damage, predominantly in the brain stem. The neuronal lesions did not appear to follow a specific vascular distribution. If severely asphyxiated animals were reared for 10 months to 8 years, atrophy of the cerebral hemispheres evolved as the prominent neuropathologic feature, with the most severe neuronal loss in the cerebral cortex, thalamus, and basal ganglia.[247]

Interestingly, monkeys with extensive brain damage often appeared fairly normal behaviorally. However, detailed examination revealed a lack of manual dexterity and fine motor coordination as well as a reduced level of spontaneous activity, a description that in many ways resembles that applied to children with attention deficit disorders.

Myers et al. have studied the pattern of brain damage following "prolonged partial asphyxia."[153,204] Fetal monkeys at term were asphyxiated for 0.5 to 3 hr by constriction of the abdominal aorta above the origin of the uterine vessels. Animals who recovered had damage mainly in the cerebral hemispheres. The principal lesions consisted of atrophy of cortical gray matter, sclerosis of white matter, and status marmoratus of the basal ganglia. These lesions are almost identical to those found in humans late after presumed perinatal hypoxia-ischemia.

In an additional investigation, Brann and Myers[18] produced intrauterine "partial asphyxia" by inducing prolonged (2–4 hr) maternal hypotension with halothane. Measurements of fetal oxygen and acid-base balance revealed severe combined (respiratory and metabolic) acidosis and hypoxemia. Following delivery and resuscitation, the animals required prolonged ventilation, developed seizures, and could not be maintained for longer than 96 hr. Neuropathologic analysis at that time showed extensive brain swelling and both pale and hemorrhagic necrosis of the cerebral cortex and subcortical white matter (Figure 7-5). The monkeys with the lowest systemic blood pressure exhibited the most severe brain damage. Since swelling was a prominent feature of the neuropathologic alterations, the investigators speculated that cerebral edema was a primary event, leading in turn to impaired cerebral blood flow and secondary cerebral necrosis.

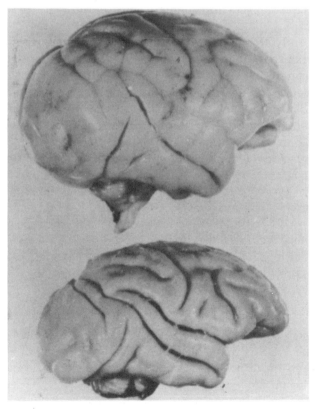

Figure 7-5 The upper brain is that of a monkey subjected to in utero prolonged partial asphyxia at term and who survived the newborn period only for 96 hr. Note brain swelling with flattening of the cerebral convolutions as well as area of softening with small vessel hemorrhage. The lower brain is that of a control newborn monkey, age 6 months, not previously subjected to intrauterine asphyxia. *Source:* Reprinted with permission from *Neurology* (1975;25:327–338), Copyright © 1975, Modern Medicine Publications Inc.

Based on his investigations spanning 15 years, Myers[152] has proposed that the distribution of brain damage seen in the perinatal monkey depends on the severity of the systemic hypoxia and the type and severity of superimposed acidosis. Specifically, monkeys exposed to anoxemia with concurrent respiratory acidosis (total asphyxia) exhibit brain damage that is predominantly or exclusively restricted to brain stem structures. Hypoxemia combined with respiratory and metabolic acidosis (partial asphyxia) leads to widespread cerebral cortical necrosis with associated cerebral edema. Hypoxemia with little or no respiratory acidosis results in cerebral white matter injury. Finally, when hypoxemia is followed by anoxemia, brain injury focuses on the basal ganglia and thalamus. The topography of all these lesions is remarkably similar to that observed in the brains of human infants previously subjected to hypoxic-ischemic stress.

Until recently, Myers appears to have underestimated the role of cerebral ischemia in the pathogenesis of hypoxic brain damage. Indeed, there is a continuing debate among investigators of hypoxic-ischemic brain damage in adult animals and humans whether hypoxia alone is capable of damaging the brain without superimposed cerebral ischemia secondary either to arterial occlusion or systemic hypotension. In all of the studies published by Myers et al. in which systemic blood pressure was monitored, an element of systemic hypotension resulting from hypoxic cardiovascular depression was apparent. Furthermore, the greater the degree of hypotension, the more extensive the neuropathology. That cerebral ischemia is a necessary prerequisite to hypoxic brain injury is supported by observations in perinatal animals of other species. In our own laboratory we have been unable to produce brain damage in newborn rats and dogs subjected either to anoxemia (asphyxia) or to progressive hypoxia with metabolic acidosis. Either the animals die acutely from apnea and cardiovascular collapse or recover without functional deficit or histologic evidence of brain damage. When systemic hypotension does occur during the course of hypoxemia or anoxemia, its duration until death or to recovery by resuscitation apparently is too short to injure the brain permanently. However, when cerebral ischemia is superimposed on hypoxemia by induced systemic hypotension or by arterial occlusion, brain damage inevitably occurs.[191,217] These observations underscore the importance of cerebral ischemia in the pathogenesis of perinatal hypoxic-ischemic brain damage and explain the observation that such brain lesions occur (or are accentuated) only at arterial boundary zones.

Occlusive Vascular Disease

A model of perinatal brain damage resulting from occlusive vascular disease has been developed in the immature rat.[191] The 7-day postnatal rat was chosen for study because at this stage of development the animal's brain is histologically similar to that of the 32- to 34-week human fetus or newborn infant, that is, cerebral cortical neuronal layering is complete, the germinal matrix is involuting, and white matter as yet has undergone little myelination. The rat pups were capable of surviving hypoxia induced by the inhalation of 8% oxygen for 3 or more hr without an appreciable mortality. Measurements of systemic physiologic variables during hypoxia revealed hypoxemia combined with hypocapnia produced by hyperventilation.[243] The hypocapnia compensated for a metabolic acidosis caused by lacticacidemia, such that systemic pH did not change from the control value. Mean systemic blood pressure decreased during hypoxia.

Hypoxic-ischemic brain damage was a near universal finding in immature rats surviving either 2 or 3 hr of systemic hypoxia.[191] By 16 to 50 hr of recovery, damage, restricted to the cerebral hemisphere ipsilateral to the common carotid artery occlusion, was observed in cerebral cortex, subcortical and periventricular white matter, basal ganglia, and hippocampus. Tissue injury took the form of either selective neuronal necrosis (glia and blood vessels spared) or infarction (all elements destroyed). Cerebral cortical damage was often laminar in distribution but also appeared as columns of dead neurons adjacent to columns of preserved neurons oriented at right angles to the pial surface. This pattern of damage has been described in premature infants subjected to repeated bouts of hypoxia-acidosis with hypotension and is proposed to be the early pathologic lesion of ulegyria.[141,161] The evolution of the ischemic cell change and the associated glial reaction appeared more rapid than that found in adults. Thus, at least in the immature rat, hypoxic-ischemic damage involving cerebral cortex, white matter, and deep gray matter structures (basal ganglia and thalamus) coexist and of necessity result from the same hypoxic-ischemic stress. The effect of age and variations in the systemic hypoxic stress (anoxia rather than hypoxia, hypoxia plus respiratory acidosis, hypoxia followed by anoxia) on the severity and distribution of brain damage is still unknown.

The chronic neuropathologic sequelae of perinatal cerebral hypoxia-ischemia in the immature rat also have been elucidated.[234] A spectrum of neuropathologic changes was noted at 30 days of postnatal age in rats previously subjected to cerebral hypoxia-ischemia at 7 days of age. As in the brain specimens analyzed at 15 to 50 hr of recovery, brain damage was characterized by either selective neuronal necrosis or infarction. Selective neuronal necrosis took the form of homogenized nerve cell change (ghost cells) and was most prominent in the hippocampus and the middle cerebral artery territory of the cerebral cortex. The minimal lesion consisted of this type of damage focused on the hippocampus alone. In cerebral cortex, selective neuronal necrosis was often seen in randomly dispersed columns oriented perpendicular to the pial surface and alternating with columns of normal neurons. The columns of damaged neurons were condensed to gliotic strips. Infarction, seen less frequently than selective neuronal necrosis, was most marked in cerebral cortex, basal ganglia, and thalamus, with secondary tissue autolysis such that in a few specimens the cerebral cortex was reduced greatly in size and occasionally to a thin membrane bordering either a clear cystic space or a greatly expanded lateral ventricle. Necrotic neurons and infarcted tissue were frequently calcified, most prominent in basal ganglia and hippocampus. These end-stage lesions mimic closely the neuropathological entities of ulegyria, porencephaly, polymicrogyria, and hemihydranencephaly observed in humans subjected to perinatal cerebral hypoxia-ischemia.

PATHOGENESIS OF PERINATAL HYPOXIC-ISCHEMIC BRAIN DAMAGE

General Considerations

While progressive hypoxemia or asphyxia in adults quickly causes death or permanent brain damage, it has long been recognized that the immature organism is more resistant to similar insults.[24,51,64,69,86] The greater tolerance of developing animals, and presumably human fetuses and newborn infants, to hypoxia-ischemia is inversely proportional to the metabolic requirements of the immature brain[64,221] and directly proportional to the glycolytic capacity of the immature heart.[52,149,212] However, the tolerance to hypoxia-ischemia as measured in survival capability exacts a price in terms of increasing susceptibility to permanent brain damage (Figure 7-6). Specifically, the longer the survival time from onset of the insult to death or resuscitation, the greater the likelihood of irreversible tissue injury in those who recover.

The circulatory and cerebral metabolic events leading to and culminating in overt brain damage arising from hypoxia-ischemia have been examined primarily in adult and to a lesser extent in immature experi-

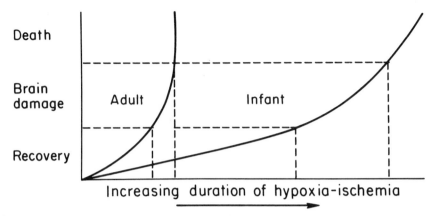

Figure 7-6 The relationship of the duration of hypoxia-ischemia to brain damage or death in developing animals. The longer the animal is capable of surviving hypoxia-ischemia, the greater the likelihood of brain damage if recovery occurs prior to death.

mental animals. The fundamental observation during hypoxia-ischemia has been so-called uncoupling of cerebral blood flow (CBF) from oxidative metabolism[106,185,208] (Table 7-2). Specifically, when blood flow to part or all of the brain is reduced below a critical level, oxygen and substrate (glucose) delivery to the tissue is curtailed (Table 7-2). Within the brain, tissue energy demands must be met to maintain cellular integrity and to generate nerve action potentials. In the absence of oxygen, these metabolic demands depend entirely on the endogenous energy reserves, phosphocreatine and adenosine triphosphate (ATP), and upon the energy derived from anaerobic glycolysis. Glycolytic flux increases five- to ten-fold, which, in the face of an inadequate glucose delivery, results in a depletion of endogenous stores of glycogen and glucose.[64,225,226] In addition, an accumulation of lactic acid, the end-product of glycolysis, leads to a progressive tissue acidosis. Anaerobic glycolysis alone is an inefficient mechanism to generate cellular energy, and eventually the high-energy phosphate reserves are exhausted. The resultant energy failure is associated with a shift of water and electrolytes from the extra- to the intracellular compartment (cytotoxic edema) and an equilibrium of transmembrane ion gradients (transmembrane ion pumping is an energy-dependent process). Also with the energy failure, catabolic processes proceed, including ribosomal disaggregation, protein degradation, and the intracellular liberation of free fatty acids from membrane phospholipids.[106,185,208] All these and probably other metabolic events culminate in cellular disintegration if the circulation and oxygen supply to the brain are not restored promptly and adequately.

Table 7-2 Systemic and Cerebral Responses to Asphyxia

	Early	Intermediate	Late
Cardiovascular	↑ Heart rate ↑ Blood pressure Redistribution of organ blood flows	↑ or ↓ Heart rate ↑ Blood pressure	↓↓ Heart rate ↓ Blood pressure "Shock"
Oxygen and acid-base balance	Hypoxia Hypercapnic acidosis	Anoxia Hypercapnic + metabolic (lactate) acidosis	Anoxia Severe combined acidosis
Cerebrovascular	↑ Cerebral blood flow	↑ or ↓ Cerebral blood flow ↑ Cerebral glucose uptake	↓ or 0 Cerebral ischemia Cerebral glucose uptake
Cerebral metabolism	Energy balance maintained	↑ Glycolytic flux ↑ Lactate	↓ Glycogen + glucose ↑ Lactate ↓ Phosphocreatine + ATP } Nerve cell death

If asphyxia is terminated before death—spontaneously or by resuscitation—cardiovascular function must be established before the cerebral anoxia-acidosis and ischemia are reversed. As systemic blood pressure and arterial oxygen tension rise and arterial carbon dioxide tension falls, the cellular metabolic machinery of the brain is gradually normalized. However, since neurons are selectively vulnerable to hypoxia-ischemia, certain cell populations may already have been irreversibly damaged. Even with recirculation and reoxygenation of the tissue, the metabolic perturbations occurring during the course of the insult may worsen, at least in part because of the rapid development of cerebral edema brought about by osmotic gradients between blood and brain (vasogenic edema). Peroxidation of free fatty acids with the formation of free radicals, an uncoupling of oxidative phosphorylation, the accumulation of cytosolic calcium ions and potentially cytotoxic excitatory neurotransmitters, and a lingering cellular lacticacidosis all enhance the process of cellular destruction.[106,185,208] Whatever the final common denominator of tissue injury, alterations in cerebral perfusion and/or metabolism are the early—and probably late—critical events that ultimately determine the presence and extent of brain damage.

Perinatal Cerebral Blood Flow and Metabolism

Numerous investigations have been conducted over the past several years to elucidate CBF and metabolic responses to perinatal hypoxia-ischemia and asphyxia. As expected, most of these investigations have involved experimental animals. In an early, now classic study, Purves and James[183] measured CBF in term fetal sheep and found that a reduction in umbilical vein arterial partial pressure of oxygen (Po_2) was associated with a 50% increase in blood flow to the cerebral cortex. Notably, blood flow to the subcortical white matter was not increased with this degree of hypoxia. The absence of hyperemia in white matter has been duplicated recently in newborn dogs rendered similarly hypoxic.[34]

Germane to the discussion of the vulnerability of perinatal white matter to hypoxic-ischemic injury is the knowledge that these regions of brain react differently to systemic stress than do gray matter structures. In all animal species, including humans, cerebral blood vessels are sensitive to changes in carbon dioxide (CO_2) tensions of the blood, that is, CBF increases during hypercapnia and decreases during hypocapnia.[182,228] CBF responses to changes in arterial carbon dioxide pressure ($Paco_2$) are less well developed in perinatal animals, and regional differences clearly exist.[65,98,183,188,189,195] In several gray matter structures of newborn dog brain studied independently by Shapiro et al.[205] and by Cavazzuti and Duffy,[34] CBF increased one- to two-fold when $Paco_2$ was increased from 34 to 65 torr by CO_2 inhalation. Subcortical white matter CBF-CO_2 sensitivity was considerably less than that shown for any gray matter region. Furthermore, maximal CBF-CO_2 sensitivity in white matter occurred at lower $Paco_2$ tensions than in gray matter. Since asphyxia by definition involves hypercapnia in addition to progressive hypoxemia, the blunting of white matter CBF-CO_2 sensitivity targets this tissue for injury.

Differences in the CBF responses of gray and white matter structures also exist for other systemic disturbances. CBF autoregulation is the phenomenon whereby the brain is assured of a continuing blood supply during variations in systemic blood pressure.[182,228] That autoregulation is present in fetal and newborn animals, including humans, has been amply demonstrated.[9,97,171,183,253] However, as with asphyxia and hypercapnia, there are regional differences in the ability of the brain to maintain constant blood flow during hypotension. Young et al.[251] produced systemic hypotension in newborn dogs by partial exsanguination. During hypotension, blood flows to all of 12 analyzed gray matter structures was preserved, even at mean arterial blood pressures (MABP) as low as 20 torr. In contrast, blood flows to subcortical and periventricular white matter of the cerebral hemispheres decreased significantly, indicating a selective hypoperfusion (ischemia) of these pathologically vulnerable regions of brain.

Investigations indicate that the compensatory increases in CBF during hypoxemia adequately protect at least the cerebral cortex of the brain unless cerebral ischemia secondary to systemic hypotension is superimposed. Unfortunately, similar studies have yet to be accomplished on a regional basis; therefore, it is not known whether similar degrees of hypotension combined with hypoxemia are required to damage white matter and other brain structures.

Major alterations in CBF and metabolism also occur during acute asphyxiation. Newborn dogs tolerate total asphyxia for up to 15 min without sustaining irreversible brain damage or death.[225] Other perinatal animals exhibit greater or lesser degrees of tolerance, depending on their neurologic maturity at the time of the insult (the lesser the maturity, the greater the anoxic resistance).[24,51,64,69,86] To estimate brain perfusion during asphyxia, Vannucci and Duffy[225] injected colloidal carbon black intravenously into puppies 2.5, 5, 10, and 15 min following respiratory arrest (Figure 7-7). At 2.5 min of asphyxia, the brains appeared uniformly dark, although not as intense in color as control brains. After 5 min of asphyxia, there were areas of pallor throughout the cerebral cortex, and after 15 min the brains were completely pale. Coronal sections of the

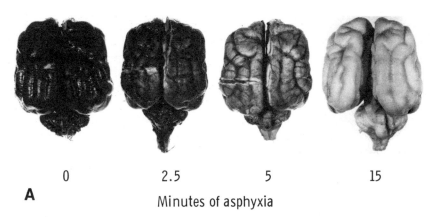

0   2.5   5   15

A   Minutes of asphyxia

Figure 7-7 Cerebral perfusion during asphyxia in newborn dogs. The figure shows the brains of four puppies injected intravenously with carbon black during asphyxia. Note relative pallor of brain of animal perfused after 5 min of asphyxia and virtual absence of carbon black in the brain of the animal injected after 15 min. *Source:* Reprinted with permission from *Annals of Neurology* (1977;1:528–534), Copyright © 1977, Little, Brown & Company.

brains revealed a preferential distribution of carbon black from forebrain to brain stem structures.

The above-described investigation has been extended by more recent studies on the cerebrovascular responses to asphyxia in newborn dogs using an indicator diffusion technique with ^{14}C-iodoantipyrine to measure regional cerebral blood flow (rCBF).[228] Asphyxia elicited dramatic changes in rCBF, including ischemia in forebrain gray and white matter structures and hyperemia in the brain stem. This selective perfusion of the brain stem would be expected to provide at least temporary protection for the vegative centers of respiratory and vasomotor control. Paradoxically, the neuropathologic consequence of acute total asphyxia in the perinatal animal and presumably in the human infant is characteristically one of brain stem rather than cerebral hemispheric injury. Therefore, differences in cellular energy demands and not blood flow per se appear to explain the selective vulnerability of brain stem structures to total asphyxia.

Although the investigations described above provide insight into how CBF and metabolism are altered by systemic hypoxia-acidosis and hypotension, their importance is limited to the extent that a known neuropathologic endpoint was lacking. Indeed, the only studies to date to correlate CBF and metabolism with perinatal hypoxic-ischemic brain damage are those reported by Myers et al. in fetal monkeys and sheep as well as studies in immature postnatal rats and rab-

bits.[18,190,191,222,229,241,243] Myers et al. were the first to correlate alterations in CBF with neuropathologic outcome in a model of perinatal
asphyxia. Brann and Myers[18] produced asphyxial brain damage in term
fetal monkeys by inducing prolonged maternal systemic hypotension
with halothane. In parallel studies, Reivich et al.[190] measured rCBF using
[14]C-antipyrine at the terminus of an asphyxial insult in four fetal
monkeys. Based on their findings, the investigators speculated that brain
edema occurs as a primary event during fetal asphyxia and leads in turn
to impaired CBF and secondary tissue necrosis.

In more recent studies, Ting et al.[222] subjected 38 midgestational fetal
sheep to hypoxemia. Some of the fetuses were rendered concurrently
hypotensive by partial exsanguination. During hypoxemia, the fetuses
developed metabolic acidosis secondary to the accumulation of lactic
acid; this was especially apparent in the hypoxic-hypotensive animals.
Three days following the experimental manipulation, the 38 fetuses were
delivered by cesarean section. Of the survivors, 29% showed evidence of
brain damage with moderate to severe hemorrhagic necrosis (infarction)
of cerebral cortex, subcortical white matter, and basal ganglia. Less frequently, injury involved the hippocampus, thalamus, and brain stem.
The lesions in cerebral cortex were situated primarily in the distribution of
the middle cerebral artery with accentuation at the cortical boundary
zones. All the brain-damaged animals had been significantly hypotensive
during the hypoxic exposure whether or not they were partially exsanguinated, whereas the brains of the fetuses that remained normotensive
during hypoxemia were free of tissue injury. The findings support the
notion that acute perinatal brain damage arises not from hypoxia alone
but rather from cerebral ischemia superimposed on hypoxemia.

The animal model of perinatal hypoxic-ischemic brain damage most
extensively studied thus far is that of the immature rat subjected to
unilateral common carotid artery occlusion combined with systemic
hypoxia.[191] This insult produces brain tissue injury in the vast majority of
animals, and the chronic neuropathologic sequelae closely mimic those of
humans who have suffered perinatal hypoxia-ischemia and/or occlusive
vascular disease. Although the pathophysiologic mechanism to produce
brain damage is not asphyxial in nature, the cerebrovascular and metabolic alterations that precede and accompany the pathologic alterations
are probably identical to those arising from systemic hypoxia-acidosis
with concurrent hypotension.

Using the immature rat model of perinatal hypoxic-ischemic brain
damage, Vannucci et al.[229] have elucidated the rCBF responses of the
perinatal brain during the course of the insult and in the recovery period
when brain tissue injury is evolving. Seven-day postnatal rats were

subjected to unilateral common carotid artery ligation, following which they were rendered hypoxic with 8% oxygen for 3 hr. Before and during hypoxia, the rat pups received ^{14}C-iodoantipyrine to determine rCBF. Blood flows to individual structures of the cerebral hemisphere ipsilateral to the carotid artery ligation were not influenced by vascular occlusion alone. However, hypoxia-ischemia was associated with progressive decreases in rCBF of the ipsilateral hemisphere, such that by 2 hr flows to subcortical white matter, cerebral cortex, basal ganglia, and thalamus were 15%, 17%, 34%, and 41% of control blood flows, respectively. The hierarchy of the blood flow reductions correlated closely with the distribution and extent of ischemic neuronal necrosis and infarction. However, within each major region, the severity of ischemia appeared homogeneous, unlike the pattern of brain damage, that is, laminar and/or columnar cerebral cortical necrosis. From the findings one can conclude that ischemia is the predominant factor that determines the severity and topography of tissue injury to major regions of the perinatal brain, whereas metabolic factors (intrinsic vulnerability) influence the heterogeneous pattern of damage seen within individual structures.

As discussed previously, lingering CBF and metabolic disturbances during early recovery from hypoxia-ischemia may contribute to the presence and extent of brain damage. In this regard, studies have demonstrated that following resuscitation of an adult animal destined to be brain damaged by a prior hypoxic-ischemic insult, there is a transient interval of cerebral hyperemia followed within minutes to hours by hypoperfusion.[46,165,180] It has been assumed that the "delayed hypoperfusion" and its attendant secondary cerebral ischemia promotes and/or accentuates the severity and distribution of ultimate tissue injury. Mujsce et al.[150] recently extended these investigations to the immature rat, in which rCBF was measured sequentially for up to 6 days following cerebral hypoxia-ischemia (unilateral common carotid artery ligation and hypoxia). Neither an early hyperemia nor hypoperfusion was observed. Rather, CBF in both cerebral hemispheres was similar at 30 min and 24 hr of recovery and no different from age-matched controls. At 72 hr, CBF in the ipsilateral hemisphere was 30% of the contralateral hemisphere and 23% of controls, and these CBF alterations persisted for at least 3 more days. Thus an early hypoperfusion does not follow perinatal hypoxia-ischemia, as in adults. Rather, a late delayed hypoperfusion takes place when tissue necrosis is already well advanced. Thus posthypoxic-ischemic hypoperfusion appears to be a consequence rather than a cause of brain tissue injury, at least in the perinatal animal. These findings have clear clinical implications for management of asphyxiated newborn infants.

Cerebral metabolic alterations following perinatal hypoxia-ischemia also have been investigated in the immature rat.[243] As in adults, the metabolic machinery of the tissue is never fully restored in animals whose brains are undergoing damage arising from the prior insult. Such restoration does occur in unscathed perinatal animals, usually within 1 to 2 hr of recovery.[226] The notable features of metabolic failure in the brain-damaged animals include an incomplete recovery of high-energy phosphate reserves, although previously low brain glucose and high lactate levels return to baseline values.[243] These findings, combined with evidence that the tissue is again fully oxidized, suggest that cellular oxidative phosphorylation (the production of ATP from nicotinamide-adenine dinucleotide [reduced form] [NADH] in the presence of oxygen) is uncoupled, that is, heat rather than chemical energy is generated. Such cells have died or will surely die. These experimental observations have direct clinical relevance, as techniques (nuclear magnetic resonance [NMR] and infrared spectrometry) now are available to ascertain the redox and energy states of brain tissue in human infants.

CBF and Metabolism in Human Infants

Modern technology has provided the clinical scientist with several diagnostic tools to ascertain disturbances in CBF and metabolism as well as neuroanatomical alterations in high-risk newborn infants. Computed tomography (CT), cranial ultrasonography (US) and magnetic resonance imaging (MRI) are now readily available at major medical centers throughout the world, and their clinical applicability and utility have been demonstrated. Other techniques, including positron emission tomography (PET) and magnetic resonance (MR) spectroscopy, are still experimental, and their availability is limited to a few institutions in the United States and Europe.

In PET, a short-decay, positron-emitting isotope is either inhaled by or injected intravenously into a subject. The tracer then circulates to the brain (or other organ), the positrons of which collide with electrons of other compounds to form neutrons with the emission of gamma radiation, which is detected on a circular array of gamma counters. In this regard, PET is similar to CT with the exception that CT both externally transmits and detects radiation (x-ray), whereas PET externally detects radiation endogenously generated within the body.

Volpe et al.[239] employed PET to measure rCBF in 17 full-term asphyxiated newborn infants. A consistent decrease in blood flow to the parasagittal region of both cerebral hemispheres was found in the majority of infants. This region of reduced CBF corresponds to the boundary zone between the territories of the anterior cerebral and the middle and posterior cerebral arteries of the brain, an area where hypoxic-ischemic brain damage is known to occur. Presumably, the lower blood flow values seen in the postasphyxial period represent "delayed hypoperfusion" arising as a consequence of tissue injury.[150] The finding confirmed an earlier study of Lou et al.[130] that showed lower than normal CBF in the early postpartum period following perinatal asphyxia, which reflected prior brain damage demonstrated either pathologically or by compromised neurologic development.[131,239]

Regional cerebral glucose utilization (rCGU) also has been investigated with PET following perinatal hypoxia-ischemia. Doyle et al.[56] investigated five newborn infants using [18]fluoro-2-deoxyglucose as the positron-emitting isotope. Localized decreases in CGU were seen, corresponding to areas of hypodensity in cerebral gray and white matter structures noted on CT scans. As with the CBF data, the alterations in rCGU presumably represented corresponding regions of tissue necrosis in which oxidative metabolism had declined below the rate of normal tissue.

Magnetic resonance spectroscopy is a technique whereby the concentration of an organic compound in a tissue can be determined by the realignment of selected molecules with a supraconducting magnet.[123] Almost any substance can be analyzed according to the strength, duration, and other characteristics of the magnetic field. The most commonly examined metabolites are the phosphorus-containing compounds. Thus MR spectroscopy is capable of ascertaining the energy status of brain tissue in vivo under both physiologic and pathophysiologic conditions.

Recent studies using MR spectroscopy in premature and full-term newborn infants have confirmed earlier studies in animals that perinatal hypoxia-ischemia is associated with lingering alterations in the energy state of the brain occurring as a consequence of tissue injury.[30,94,104,252] These metabolic disturbances correlated with evolving abnormalities on CT or US, death, and/or poor neurodevelopmental outcome.

Although the above-described studies in newborn infants are preliminary in scope, it is anticipated that the continued use and sophistication of PET scanning and MR spectroscopy will contribute substantially to our understanding of how and to what extent the perinatal brain is damaged by hypoxia-ischemia. Possibly even more important will be the application of these techniques to the fetus to ascertain blood flow and metabolic alterations before and during the course of hypoxia-ischemia and before overt tissue injury. The early detection of such adverse events in brain should provide more rational methods for preventing or minimizing permanent brain damage.

Acute and Chronic Hypoxemia and Perinatal Brain Damage

As has been emphasized previously, mounting evidence indicates that hypoxia alone does not acutely damage the perinatal brain and that either ischemia alone (occlusive vascular disease) or hypoxia-ischemia is a necessary prerequisite for tissue injury. The question remains whether either acute or chronic hypoxemia without superimposed ischemia can alter the normal developmental processes of the brain to the extent that damage other than necrosis ultimately occurs.

Unfortunately, there are no studies in humans concerning the late neurologic and neuropathologic effects of acute, isolated perinatal hypoxia. The vast majority of survivors of transient episodes of hypoxia (intrauterine asphyxia, near sudden infant death, and so on) are typically neurologically normal. In those few infants who are neurologically compromised, there may have been an undocumented period of systemic hypotension during the hypoxic event, and overt brain damage may actually be present in the form of patchy, widespread selective neuronal or white matter necrosis. Even a normal CT or MRI scan does not exclude neuronal cell loss or gliosis that, if not extensive, might be beyond the resolution of the radiographic technique. Only postmortem examination would confirm or deny the presence of overt neuropathologic abnormalities.

Acute hypoxemia in perinatal animals does not appear to result in overt brain damage, even if the insult is severe enough to cause transient alterations in CBF and metabolism.[221,225,226] Vannucci and Duffy[226] subjected term fetal and newborn rats to anoxia (nitrogen breathing) nearly to the point of death and allowed them to recover into adulthood. Pathologic analysis at that time revealed no brain damage, and the brain growth of the previously hypoxic animals was comparable to that of age-matched controls. One must conclude from these studies that transient hypoxia without superimposed ischemia is relatively innocuous and of no long-term neurologic consequence.

Chronic hypoxemia is another issue. Clinical evidence in support of the brain-damaging potential of chronic hypoxemia is derived from the neuropsychologic maturation of infants suffering from cyanotic congenital heart disease. The blood oxygen concentrations of these infants are readily monitored by arterial blood gas analysis or oximetry. Such children often exhibit poor attention spans, impaired gross and fine motor skills, and low academic achievement, even if they have undergone complete surgical repair of their cardiac malformations.[127,164,209] However, the majority of these infants and children exhibit complications of their congenital heart lesions, including congestive heart failure, stroke, epilepsy, and central nervous system (CNS) infections, any one of which could have acutely injured their brains.[164]

"Chronic fetal hypoxemia" is a widely discussed albeit not well documented entity that presumably arises from placental insufficiency or a reduction in uteroplacental blood flow and results in newborn infants who are "low birth weight for gestational age" (SGA).[33] These infants appear undernourished at birth and are prone to disturbances in systemic homeostasis, including thermoregulatory instability, polycythemia, hypoglycemia, and hypocalcemia. Despite the prior existence of an adverse intrauterine environment and the presence of nutritional and metabolic abnormalities at birth, SGA infants often fare well in long-term neurologic and mental development. Intelligence quotients are usually normal and major neurologic handicaps infrequent unless perinatal asphyxia accompanied the intrauterine growth retardation.[43,66,74,133,237,244]

To what extent human fetuses that ultimately exhibit growth retardation at birth are truly hypoxic remains open to question because of the difficulty of sampling umbilical vein blood for oxygen and acid-base analysis before birth. The numerous systemic metabolic aberrations that exemplify these newborn infants are more likely the result of fetal undernutrition than fetal hypoxemia, although the two conditions potentially coexist. In experimental models of intrauterine growth retardation, lower than normal blood oxygen tensions and glucose concentrations have been observed following partial placental ablation and uterine artery ligation.[35,47,126,154] These alterations in systemic oxygen and glucose homeostasis of fetal animals adversely influence systemic as well as brain growth and differentiation.[25,197,245] The mechanism leading to stunted brain growth is unclear but may reflect cerebral hypoxia and/or insufficient delivery of required nutrients to brain.

To clarify the issue of cerebral hypoxia producing fetal brain growth retardation, Brown and Vannucci[25] subjected pregnant rats to unilateral uterine artery ligation and examined the cerebral metabolic status of their offspring immediately following delivery at term by cesarean section. As in other investigations, the rat pups delivered from the previously ligated uterine horn were physically stunted at birth, and their brains also were affected. However, the substrates (glucose and glycogen) and end-product (lactic acid) of cerebral glycolysis were not altered by the uterine artery ligation, suggesting that anaerobic glycolytic flux was not accelerated in the brains of the growth-retarded fetuses. The high-energy phosphate reserves, ATP and phosphocreatine, were also unaltered by the prior uterine artery ligation. The findings documented the absence of hypoxia to a degree sufficient to disrupt oxidative metabolism and the energy state of the fetal brain. Furthermore, insufficient glucose delivery to brain could not account for the stunted growth, since cerebral glycogen and glucose levels were normal. Whether deficient substrates other than glucose were responsible for the cerebral growth retardation remains to be determined.

Degrees of chronic hypoxemia less than that required to affect cerebral oxidative metabolism adversely might alter brain maturation by inhibiting oxygen-dependent and other biosynthetic processes. In both immature and adult animals, mild hypoxia without systemic hypotension leads to at least transient reductions in brain dopamine, norepinephrine, and serotonin and to impaired synthesis of these monoamine neurotransmitters.[28,49,50,95,96] Reduced rates of synthesis of acetylcholine, cyclic nucleotides, and certain amino acids have also been observed during mild hypoxia in adult animals.[80–83] Since monoamines and possibly other putative neurotransmitters exert a trophic influence on dendritic arborization during cerebral maturation,[45] altered neurotransmitter function during chronic hypoxemia might contribute to the retarded brain development seen in intrauterine growth retardation.[210]

Thus human and experimental investigations do not as yet fully clarify the extent to which the perinatal brain is vulnerable to the untoward effect of chronic hypoxia without superimposed cerebral ischemia. The evidence suggests that the immature brain cannot proceed normally in its maturational processes, even when minimally deprived of oxygen and organic substrates, but the manner in which growth retardation occurs is not completely understood. Certainly, nutrition plays a critical role, because the most prominent biochemical abnormalities observed in the brains of growth-retarded animal and human fetuses involve protein and fatty acid metabolism.[36,47,197,236,245] Fortunately, the undernourished brain appears capable of at least partial recovery once the adverse environmental stress is corrected after birth.[33,249] The capability of the immature brain to "catch up" in its growth and differentiation explains why SGA infants are often normal on long-term neurologic follow-up. Further clinical and experimental investigation should provide additional insight into how hypoxia and undernutrition adversely affect the developing brain and how these aberrant processes can be prevented.

Birth As an Asphyxial Process

The process of birth, whether vaginal delivery or cesarean section, is accompanied by major physiologic and biochemical adjustments that allow the newborn infant to accommodate to the extrauterine environment.[160] During labor and delivery, the already relatively hypoxemic state of the fetus is accentuated, even when intrauterine conditions have been ideal. Blood oxygen tensions in fetal blood decline at least transiently during parturition from their already low values of 25 to 35 torr, and carbon dioxide accumulates to varying degrees.[42,107,112,183,242] In addition, CBF falls momentarily as a large part of the cardiac output is directed to the newly expanded lungs.[136] Since these physiologic changes are essentially universal, it seems unlikely that the alterations in systemic oxygen and acid-base balance and in CBF would adversely affect the brain, unless they were accompanied by antecedent or concurrent hypoxia-acidosis.

Studies from our own laboratory have indicated that the normal process of vaginal birth is associated with metabolic alterations in the perinatal brain equivalent to that of acute asphyxia.[115,227] Vannucci and Duffy[227] measured the concentrations of glycolytic intermediates and high-energy phosphate reserves in newborn rats at sequential intervals following vaginal delivery and compared the results with those in animals delivered by cesarean section. Immediately after birth, brain lactate and the lactate/pyruvate ratio increased fourfold above fetal values. Concurrent with the elevations in lactate and pyruvate, glucose and glycogen decreased in brain, findings that indicate an acceleration of anaerobic glycolytic flux. By 10 min of postnatal life, the lactate/pyruvate ratio had decreased substantially owing to a 400% rise in the tissue pyruvate, presumably reflecting the intracellular oxidation of lactate. Both the lactate concentration and the lactate/pyruvate ratio required 8 hr to return to a stable level. Brain lactate also increased in animals delivered by cesarean section, but only by 30%, and the lactate/pyruvate ratio never changed from the fetal value.

Birth was also associated with changes in the cerebral high-energy metabolites. In the vaginally delivered rat pups, concentrations of ATP and phosphocreatine decreased by 28% and 72%, respectively, immediately after birth but were partially resynthesized by 10 min of postnatal life. New steady-state values were attained by 60 min. In animals delivered by cesarean section, the decrease in phosphocreatine was less striking and ATP never fell. The magnitude of the decreases in ATP and phosphocreatine and the increases in lactate and lactate/pyruvate ratios is analogous to that observed in the brains of perinatal animals subjected to five or more minutes of total asphyxia or isolated cerebral ischemia.[64,225,226] It is evident from the data that any complication of the "normal" process of birth would potentiate an already present asphyxial risk to the fetus.

CLINICAL CORRELATIONS

Obstetrical Antecedents

Obstetricians have long recognized certain abnormalities that pre-dispose the fetus to hypoxia-ischemia either antepartum, during parturi-tion, or in the early postpartum period. These risk factors are categorized in Table 7-3 according to maternal conditions, complications of preg-nancy and delivery, and disturbances arising in the fetus or newborn infant exclusive of adverse environmental events. As anticipated, these conditions overlap somewhat. Whatever the predisposing factors, such high-risk mothers require greater obstetric surveillance than routinely provided to prevent or minimize fetal mortality and neonatal morbidity.

Obstetricians have developed numerous techniques to assess the phys-ical and neurologic well-being of the fetus in the antepartum and intra-partum periods. These techniques include the visualization of fetal size, breathing pattern, posture, tone, and movements by US; monitoring of fetal movements by maternally perceived activity and by elec-tromechanical devices (tocodynamometry); and monitoring of fetal heart rate patterns by external cardiographic monitoring.[76,140,173,177,187] Fetuses shown to be at risk for hypoxia-ischemia are subjected to greater scrutiny during labor and delivery. Procedures presently available to assess the intrapartum status of the fetus include the determination of passage of meconium into the amniotic fluid, external or internal monitoring of fetal heart rate patterns in relation to maternal contrac-tions, and the assessment of fetal oxygen and acid-base status by blood gas analysis.[85,101,134,143,148,254] More recently developed but still experi-mental methods to monitor fetal well-being include transcutaneous anal-ysis of fetal PO_2, PCO_2, and pH as well as fetal electroencephalogra-phy.[6,13,194,211]

These techniques, when applied separately or collectively, provide valuable information on how well the newborn infant can adjust appro-priately to the extrauterine environment and whether transient or even permanent neurologic compromise is likely.

Assessment of the Infant at Birth

Thanks to Virginia Apgar, clinicians have available a rapid and accurate means of determining the functional well-being of the newborn infant immediately following birth. The Apgar score provides a clinical index of the physiologic adaption of the infant to postnatal life and includes

Table 7-3 Conditions That Predispose the Fetus and Newborn Infant to Cerebral Hypoxia-Ischemia

| Prenatal (intrauterine) | | Intrapartum | Neonatal |
Maternal	Obstetric	(labor and delivery)	(extrauterine)
Toxemia (eclampsia)	Abruptio placentae	Abnormal presentation	Prematurity
Diabetes mellitus	Prolapse of umbilical cord	Precipitate delivery	Respiratory distress
Drug addiction	Placenta previa	Prolonged labor	Cardiopulmonary anomalies
Cardiovascular disease	Hydramnios	Difficult forceps delivery	Infectious disease
Infectious disease	Premature rupture fetal membranes	Intrauterine growth retardation	Hemolytic disease
Isoimmunization	Multiple pregnancy	Prolonged pregnancy	Septic or viremic shock
Collagen vascular disease			

measurements of muscular tone, color, respiratory effort, heart rate, and behavioral response to noxious stimuli.[7] The 1-min Apgar score draws immediate attention to the newborn infant requiring resuscitative intervention. However, neither the 1- nor the 5-min score has strong predictive value to assess long-term outcome but rather serves only to identify infants demanding special attention.[178]

Neonatal Neurologic Assessment

The clinical picture of a newborn infant sustaining hypoxia-ischemia depends on the severity and duration of the insult to brain.[27,59,200,238] Aside from monitoring vital signs and determining the Apgar score, little attention is given to the clinical examination immediately following the birth of an asphyxiated infant, since all efforts are directed to resuscitative measures at the moment of delivery. When these procedures have been accomplished and transport to the newborn nursery or intensive care unit expedited, the infant's physical and neurologic status is subjected to greater scrutiny and an appropriate management plan is initiated. Thus the clinical examination focuses on the evolving encephalopathy that follows the asphyxial stress.

Distinctive stages of neurologic dysfunction occur in the early hours following an acute perinatal asphyxial insult.[4,128,200,238] Fortunately, the majority of newborn infants sustaining intrapartum hypoxia or asphyxia appear clinically normal at the time of the first and subsequent examinations; it can be assumed that the brains of these infants did not suffer a metabolic disturbance during the prior systemic stress. In contrast, infants in whom the asphyxia was severe enough to affect brain homeostasis adversely exhibit one or more symptoms and signs that are readily apparent in the early postpartum period. These disturbances in neurologic function have been well described in full-term newborn infants but relatively poorly defined in premature infants.

Sarnat and Sarnat[200] were among the first investigators to categorize asphyxiated full-term infants according to the degree of neurologic deficit apparent at the time of initial examination (see also refs. 4 and 128) (Table 7-4). Infants having suffered a mild asphyxial insult to brain (Stage I) appear alert or even hyperalert with intermittent fussiness and hyperexcitability. Postural tone and phasic muscular tone (resistance to passive motion) are normal or slightly increased, predominantly in the upper extremities. Head lag is present on traction from the supine to the sitting position. Deep tendon reflexes typically are exaggerated, and the complex infantile reflexes of rooting, sucking, and grasping as well as the

Table 7-4 Clinical Staging of Postasphyxial Encephalopathy

	Stage I	Stage II	Stage III
Level of consciousness	Alert	Lethargy	Coma
Muscle tone	Normal	Hypotonia	Flaccidity
Tendon reflexes	Increased	Increased	Depressed or absent
Myoclonus	Present	Present	Absent
Seizures	None	Common	Uncommon
Complex reflexes			
Suck	Active	Weak	Absent
Moro	Exaggerated	Incomplete	Absent
Grasp	Normal to exaggerated	Exaggerated	Absent
Oculocephalic (doll's eye)	Normal	Overactive	Reduced or absent
Autonomic function			
Pupils	Dilated	Constricted	Variable or fixed
Respiratory	Regular	Variations in rate and depth, periodic	Ataxic, apnea
Heart rate	Normal or tachycardia	Bradycardia	Bradycardia
EEG	Normal	Low voltage, periodic and/or paroxysmal	Periodic or isoelectric

Source: Adapted with permission from *Archives of Neurology* (1976;33:695–706), Copyright © 1976, American Medical Association.

Moro response are intact. Cranial nerve function, including pupillary responses to light, oculocephalic (doll's eye) reflexes, and gag reflex are normal. Repetitive visual (bright light), auditory (bell), and somatosensory (pin) stimulation elicits immediate adversive reactions with habituation.[19] Seizures almost never occur in this group of infants, although stimulus-related myoclonus might be present. The electroencephalogram (EEG) typically is normal.

Infants moderately asphyxiated at birth appear lethargic and exhibit diffuse muscular hypotonia (Stage II). The hypotonia is usually more apparent in the upper extremities, with greater weakness in the proximal than in the distal musculature.[238] Popliteal angles are increased, the scarf sign is positive, head lag is prominent, and the Landau response is poor.[63] The infant reacts to sensory stimuli (light, bell, pin), but the reactions are depressed and habituation might not occur. Deep tendon reflexes, including the jaw jerk, are hyperactive, and clonus is easily elicited. Pupillary responses to light and the oculocephalic reflex are present, but the gag reflex is decreased or absent. Other bulbar disturbance leads to an inability to suck and swallow.[238] Seizures are frequent at this stage, and the EEG ranges from low-amplitude slowing to a burst-suppression pattern.

Infants severely asphyxiated at birth are comatose, flaccid, and either minimally reactive or unresponsive to noxious stimuli (Stage III). Deep tendon and all complex reflexes are absent. Bulbar palsy is present. Pupils react poorly or are fixed to light, and the oculocephalic reflex cannot be elicited even with vigorous head turning or body rotation. The oculovestibular (caloric) reflex, normally induced by irrigating one or both ears with ice water, also might not be present. Vital functions often are compromised with systemic hypotension, bradycardia, and irregular respirations or apnea. Seizures are variably present at this stage, and the EEG typically shows a burst-suppression or isoelectric pattern.

The clinical staging of newborn infants asphyxiated at or before birth provides the means to record the severity of the insult to brain accurately and initiate optimal medical management. However, it must be emphasized that the evolution of the postasphyxial encephalopathy is not a static process; therefore, sequential evaluations must be accomplished in the days to weeks following birth. Infants exhibit partial or complete recovery or may deteriorate initially followed by either death or slow recovery. In general, the less severe the degree of encephalopathy at initial staging and/or the more rapid the reversion to or toward normality, the better the long-term neuropsychologic outcome.

The clinical identification of newborn premature infants asphyxiated at birth is more difficult than that of full-term infants because of the functional immaturity of the brain. Thus the very signs clinicians recognize as evidence of CNS depression in the full-term infant might represent the normal maturational level of a premature infant. Specifically, the more immature the infant is at birth, the more prominent is the degree of intrinsic hypotonia and the less well developed are the complex infantile reflexes. However, with the availability of scales of functional neurologic maturation in premature infants,[3,63,199] the clinician can evaluate reasonably accurately alterations in tone and reflex activity out of proportion to those anticipated for a newborn infant of any specific gestational age. Furthermore, most cranial nerve functions are well developed even in small premature infants (26 to 32 weeks). Thus the staging of premature infants according to the severity of the postasphyxial encephalopathy is feasible, although to date a detailed clinical investigation has not been published.

In addition to neurologic dysfunction arising from hypoxic-ischemic encephalopathy, systemic complications of perinatal asphyxia also occur and involve multiple organ systems including the heart, lungs, kidneys, and liver. Continuing hypoxemia, hypotension, and acidosis denote cardiopulmonary insufficiency.[29] Anemia, due to blood loss or hemolysis, places further stress on less than optimal heart action. Persisting metabolic disturbances include hypoglycemia, hypocalcemia, and fluid and electrolyte abnormalities secondary to acute renal failure and/or inappropriate secretion of antidiuretic hormone.[48,92,109,114] Hyperammonemia reflects hepatic dysfunction.[87] The extent to which these systemic derangements contribute to the postasphyxial encephalopathy is unknown, but their presence can only worsen an already compromised brain.

Newborn infants who have sustained cerebral hypoxia-ischemia or occlusive vascular disease prior to parturition typically do not appear asphyxiated at birth. Apgar scores often are in the range of 7 to 9 (points are lost for tone and response to stimuli), and major resuscitation is rarely required. Systemic signs of a recent asphyxial insult are notably absent. Some infants are asymptomatic in the days following birth, but signs of brain damage become increasingly apparent in the weeks to months following discharge from the nursery. Other infants exhibit symptoms and signs of prior brain damage early following birth in the form of lethargy, alterations in muscle tone, attenuation of primitive reflex activity, poor feeding, and seizures.[12,145] Head size may be small for gestational age, reflecting underlying cerebral underdevelopment. Unlike acutely asphyxiated infants, who either deteriorate or at least partially improve, infants suffering more remote cerebral hypoxia-ischemia show fixed neurologic deficits that do not change over time. Thus they exhibit a subacute or chronic rather than an acute encephalopathy. Such infants appear clinically indistinguishable from newborn infants who harbor a congenital anomaly of the brain, who have sustained a congenital viral or parasitic infection, or who suffer a hereditary neurodegenerative disease. Laboratory and radiographic investigations often resolve the diagnostic dilemma and assist the clinician in dating the onset of the insult to brain.

Infants occasionally sustain a hypoxic-ischemic insult to brain that arises from a complication in the newborn period, whether or not it is the consequence of abnormalities during pregnancy, labor, and delivery. Infants at risk for neonatal cerebral hypoxia-ischemia include those who are prematurely born; who harbor a developmental anomaly, especially of the heart and lungs; and who contract a neonatal infection (pneumonia, sepsis, meningitis). The presenting symptoms and signs are similar to those of infants sustaining birth asphyxia, and the onset of the neurologic manifestations is temporally related to the occurrence of the systemic malady. Distinguishing these infants from those who have suffered intrapartum asphyxia is relatively easy because of their neurologic well-being in the immediate newborn period.

Postasphyxial Seizures

Convulsive activity occurs in 50% to 70% of acutely asphyxiated newborn infants and accounts for 30% to 50% of all neonatal seizures.[70,111,193,200,238] The majority of infants exhibit seizure activity within 24 hr following birth; this activity is seen most frequently in infants exhibiting Stage II postasphyxial encephalopathy. These seizures are described as subtle (fragmentary), focal clonic, multifocal clonic, or tonic.[238] They occur either alone or in combination and may be single or repetitive. Unlike the older infant, child, or adult, the newborn infant does not experience tonic-clonic seizures. The absence of such seizure activity probably reflects the morphologic and biochemical immaturity of the perinatal brain.

Radiographic Features

Recently developed radiographic procedures have become invaluable in assessing the nature and extent of damage to the brains of infants sustaining hypoxic-ischemic insults before or following birth. In addition, the evolution of the hypoxic-ischemic lesions can be ascertained by sequentially scanning any individual patient, and, to some extent at least, the interval between the initial radiographic study and the antecedent stress can be documented. The latter capability allows clinicians to determine more accurately whether tissue injury occurred or began before or during labor and delivery.

Computed Tomography

Abnormalities, readily apparent on CT scans performed 24 to 72 hr following an asphyxial insult in newborn infants, consist of focal or diffuse areas of decreased attenuation in gray and/or white matter structures of the cerebral hemispheres.[73,75,147,202] These hypodensities are presumed to represent either focal ischemic infarcts or areas of cerebral edema (Figures 7-8 and 7-9). Such radiographic interpretations appear to be well-founded because, at least in full-term infants, the presence and location of hypodensities on CT correlate with the finding of either ischemic brain injury (infarction) or diffuse brain swelling at autopsy in infants who expired early following the insult.[75] The presence of slitlike or obliterated lateral ventricles in association with hypodensities on CT supports the radiographic diagnosis of cerebral edema with or without associated tissue infarction. Unlike in full-term infants, there is a poor

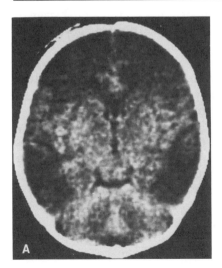 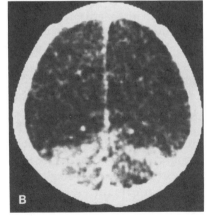

Figure 7-8 CT scan of a term newborn who had intrapartum asphyxia. **A.** Hypodensities involving both gray and white matter of the parieto-occipital and the frontal lobes are apparent. **B.** Taken at a higher level, this CT scan shows widespread hypodensity in both cerebral hemispheres.

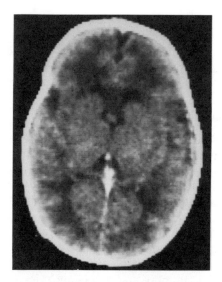

Figure 7-9 CT scan of a 34-week infant who exhibited antepartum and intrapartum asphyxia. Note diffuse hypodensities involving periventricular and subcortical white matter of both cerebral hemispheres. The cerbral cortex is relatively preserved.

correlation between CT and postmortem findings in premature infants[75] because certain features on CT in these infants reflect a normal stage of brain development. Specifically, periventricular hypodensities in the frontal and occipital lobes of the cerebral hemispheres, originally assumed to represent edema or infarction, actually represent areas where nerve fibers were relatively unmylineated.[176,184] These hypodensities typically disappear with increasing brain maturation.

In contrast to areas of decreased attenuation (hypodensities) on CT as representative of tissue infarction or edema, areas of increased attenuation are characteristic of hemorrhage, specifically hemorrhagic infarction (Figure 7-10). In full-term infants such hyperdense areas typically involve cerebral cortex and subcortical white matter of the posterior aspects of the cerebral hemispheres. Occasionally, a hyperdense area (hemorrhage) is surrounded by an area of reduced attenuation (edema). Such hemorrhagic infarcts are most likely the result of venous stasis and thrombosis.

Late abnormalities on CT reflect the anticipated chronic neuropathologic sequelae of hypoxic-ischemic brain damage (Figure 7-11). Varying degrees of cerebral cortical and subcortical atrophy are often seen with prominent sulci and an expanded subarachnoid space with or without compensatory dilatation of the lateral, third, and/or fourth ventricles. Cystic degeneration of the parenchyma of the cerebral hemispheres is

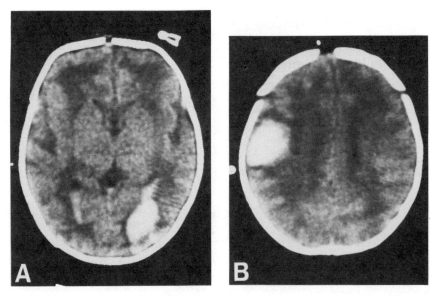

Figure 7-10 CT scans of a term asphyxiated infant, showing large parenchymal hemorrhagic infarcts involving the right occipital **(A)** and left frontotemporal **(B)** regions. Hypodensities of both gray and white matter noted predominantly in the frontal regions.

readily apparent, and if a large cerebral infarction has previously occurred, a porencephalic cyst is radiographically visible. If the brain damage has been catastrophic, hydranencephaly results with little or no residual cerebral tissue apparent on CT.

Cranial Ultrasonography

Cranial ultrasound has become increasingly useful as an adjunct to CT in diagnosing anatomical alterations of the brain following perinatal hypoxia-ischemia. Using the anterior fontanelle as the acoustic window, real-time US is capable of visualizing primarily the midline structures of the immature brain, including the entire ventricular system, the basal ganglia and thalamus, and periventricular white matter. Imaging of the cerebral cortex, hippocampus, and subcortical white matter is difficult. Numerous published reports have documented the presence and evolution of the ultrasonic abnormalities arising from perinatal hypoxia-ischemia in both premature and full-term infants.[31,90,93,124,142,163]

Unlike in CT, hypoxic-ischemic lesions are seen early as areas of increased echogenicity in the gray and white matter structures adjacent to the lateral and third ventricles (Figure 7-12). Studies correlating ultrasonic and postmortem abnormalities have revealed that the hyperdense

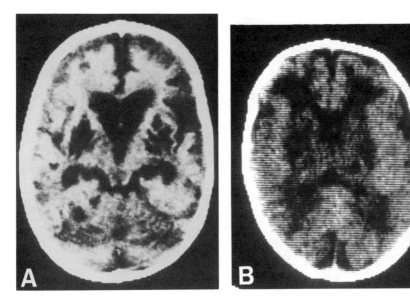

Figure 7-11 CT scans of two infants showing late abnormalities, reflecting prior cerebral hypoxia-ischemia. **A.** Scan of a term asphyxiated infant, performed at 3 months of postnatal age. Note widespread cerebral cortical and subcortical atrophy, more prominent on the right. Cystic degeneration of basal ganglia is also apparent. There is compensatory enlargement of lateral ventricles and basal cisternes. **B.** CT scan of premature infant, performed at 4 months of age. Note widespread hypodensities largely restricted to periventricular and subcortical white matter of both cerebral hemispheres with relative preservation of cerebral cortex.

areas represent either hemorrhage alone, ischemic infarction alone, or hemorrhage combined with infarction (hemorrhagic necrosis).[93,99,163,216] Furthermore, US alone cannot distinguish these individual lesions. Adjunct CT is required to make the distinction. However, the age of appearance and the location of the echoic areas aid in determining the nature of the lesion, especially in premature infants. Hyperdense areas inferolateral to the anterior horns of the lateral ventricles and adjacent to the caudate nuclei most likely represent primary hemorrhage into the germinal matrix (see Chapter 8). In contrast, echoic areas superolateral to the anterior horns, body, trigone, and/or posterior horns of the lateral ventricles most likely represent ischemic or hemorrhagic infarction of periventricular white matter (Figure 7-12). Furthermore, areas of increased echogenicity that appear within days following birth are likely the result of primary hemorrhage or hemorrhagic necrosis, whereas echoic lesions appearing late (days to weeks) probably represent ischemic

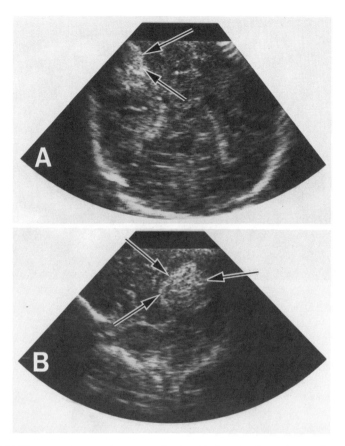

Figure 7-12 Ultrasound scans of a term asphyxiated infant. **A.** Coronal scan showing large echogenic area in left parieto-occipital region (arrows). Lateral ventricles are not well visualized. **B.** Left parasagittal scan showing same echogenic area (arrows) as in (A), which presumably represents a hemorrhagic infarct.

(nonhemorrhagic) infarction.[163] The time-specific appearance of the echodense lesions of hemorrhagic or nonhemorrhagic nature is consistent with the evolution of the brain damage seen pathologically.[122]

Increased echogenicity also has been observed in the basal ganglia and thalamus, especially of full-term infants suffering cerebral hypoxia-ischemia. As with periventricular lesions, such ultrasonic abnormalities presumably represent areas of ischemic or hemorrhagic infarction, as confirmed by CT or postmortem examination.[118,206]

The evolution of hypoxic-ischemic lesions noted on US in newborn infants has been well documented (Figure 7-13). In infants who survive

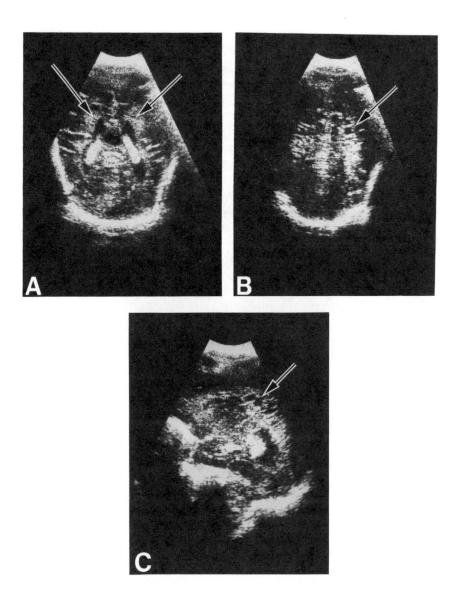

Figure 7-13 Ultrasound scans of a premature asphyxiated infant. **A.** Coronal scan showing increased echogenicity adjacent to both lateral ventricles (arrows). **B.** Horizontal scan showing bilateral echogenic areas with microcyst formation apparent on right (arrow). **C.** Right parasagittal scan showing microcyst formation superior to lateral ventricle (arrow).

the initial hypoxic-ischemic insult, the original hyperdense areas slowly either resolve completely or more typically are replaced by one or more cystlike hypodense areas. These abnormalities most certainly represent the development of cystic periventricular leukomalacia or porencephaly.[31,60,90,124] Lateral ventricular enlargement is often an associated finding, especially in the presence of extensive leukomalacia or porencephaly.

The incidence of ultrasonic abnormalities in distressed premature infants is well known because many medical centers routinely scan all newborn infants below a certain gestational age or birth weight. In a retrospective study of 2,056 newborn infants weighing less than 2,000 g at birth, periventricular echodensities greater than 1 cm in size were observed by US in 75 (4%).[93] The lesions were classified as either extensive, that is, involving most of the periventricular region, or localized. The vast majority of the lesions were associated with intraventricular hemorrhage, and typically the periventricular hyperdense areas were restricted to the cerebral hemisphere exhibiting greater ventricular enlargement owing to the presence of blood clot. Smaller, more symmetrical areas of periventricular leukomalacia might exist in a larger population of premature infants, their lesions being beyond the resolution of present-day US.

MANAGEMENT

Obstetric Intervention

Management of the hypoxic fetus and newborn infant entails both obstetric and neonatal care. Therapeutic endeavors are based on objective clinical and laboratory evidence of progressive systemic and CNS dysfunction. Once clinical deterioration of the infant is documented, intervention must be prompt and judicious if a medical catastrophe is to be avoided. Decisions for obstetric intervention of the compromised fetus are based on abnormalities in heart rate patterns and blood acid-base status.[38,85,103,117,134,148,254] The goal of these procedures is to detect early fetal hypoxia and thereby to attempt to prevent any adverse consequences of the metabolic derangement. Fetal heart rate abnormalities that suggest fetal distress arising from hypoxia have been correlated with fetal acidosis, low Apgar scores at birth, neonatal death, and adverse short- and long-term neurologic sequelae in survivors.[38,110,117,134,137,166,168] However, not all abnormal fetal heart rate patterns correlate with a poor outcome, and the extent to which obstetric intervention reduces or prevents permanent brain damage in the acutely asphyxiated fetus requires investigation.

An acutely deteriorating course as determined by fetal heart rate monitoring and/or acid-base analysis usually necessitates immediate termination of pregnancy by cesarean section. If labor is active but delivery is not imminent, continued labor is fraught with danger because of the risk of superimposing elevated transcephalic pressures on an already metabolically disturbed brain. An additional potential risk of vaginal birth is intracranial trauma brought about by the instrumentation employed to expedite the delivery.

When cesarean delivery is to take place, anesthesia for the mother must be chosen carefully to avoid aggravating an already compromised situation. General anesthesia employing combinations of analgesic agents with muscle relaxation is usually preferred.[156] Supplemental oxygen is always administered, and maternal blood glucose concentrations are maintained well above 100 mg/dl.

Following birth, immediate attention is given to the status of the newborn infant's cardiopulmonary system, and endotracheal intubation and closed cardiac massage are performed when required (see Chapter 10). Once an adequate heart rate and ventilation have been established, the infant is transported to the intensive care unit without further delay.

Table 7-5 Laboratory Studies to Evaluate Perinatal Hypoxia-Ischemia

---

Indicated
  Complete blood count; urinalysis
  Blood glucose, blood urea nitrogen, calcium, phosphorus, magnesium, electrolytes
  Arterial blood gases
  Blood, CSF, and other cultures
  Lumbar puncture and CSF analysis
  Chest x-ray
  Ultrasound and/or CT scan
  EEG

Elective (When Condition Other than Asphyxia Suspected)
  Serum immunoglobulins and TORCH antibody studies
  Viral cultures
  Blood and urine metabolic studies, including lactate, ammonia, and so on
  Skull and spine x-rays

Neonatal Management

Upon arrival in the intensive care nursery, the infant is promptly and thoroughly examined to ascertain the extent of systemic and neurologic dysfunction resulting from the prior asphyxial insult. In addition, coexisting metabolic, structural, or infectious disturbances must be identified by specific physical findings as well as by a review of the maternal and obstetric histories. In this regard, certain laboratory investigations should be considered an integral part of the proper evaluation and management of the asphyxiated infant (Table 7-5). Other studies are performed when causes other than perinatal hypoxia-ischemia are suspected.

Medical management of the asphyxiated newborn infant is directed toward maintaining systemic homeostasis as well as optimal central nervous system function (Table 7-6). Specific treatment modalities to reverse or minimize the lingering effects of cerebral hypoxia-ischemia are based on both experimental investigations in animals and human infant responses to various therapeutic interventions. Control of physiologic blood oxygen, acid-base balance, and caloric balance are of utmost impor-

---

Table 7-6 Management of the Asphyxiated Infant

General Principles
    Ensure physiologic oxygen and acid-base balance
    Maintain environmental temperature and humidity
    Correct caloric, fluid, and electrolyte disturbances
    Maintain blood volume and hemostasis
    Treat infection
    Minimize hyperbilirubinemia

Specific Therapy for Postasphyxial Encephalopathy
    Treat seizures
        Phenobarbital: 20–60 mg/kg IV or IM initially, 5–8 mg/kg/day thereafter
        Diphenylhydantoin: 20 mg/kg IV or IM initially, 5–8 mg/kg/day thereafter
        Diazepam: 0.1–0.2 mg/kg IV for status epilepticus
        Paraldehyde: 0.1 mg/kg diluted 1:10 in 0.25 N saline PR or IV for status epilepticus
    Maintain blood glucose concentrations between 60 and 200 mg/dl
    Diagnose and treat brain edema
        Restrict fluids to minimal maintenance requirements
        Controlled hyperventilation ($Paco_2$ = 20–25 torr)
        Osmotic diuretics
            Furosmide 1 mg/kg IV
            Mannitol 1 g/kg IV

---

tance to prevent further neurologic damage in an already compromised infant. Hypovolemia must be corrected by whole blood transfusion. Body temperature is monitored closely and maintained by appropriate adjustments of environmental temperature and humidity.

Blood Glucose Concentrations

The maintenance of adequate blood glucose concentrations during and following perinatal asphyxia is important to prevent the adverse effects of superimposed hypoglycemia on the immature brain.[24,100,230,232] In the past, investigators suggested that "supranormal" levels of blood glucose might benefit the asphyxiated infant by providing greater supplies of organic fuel to the hypoxic brain for energy production via anaerobic glycolysis.[24,100,102] More recent studies have indicated that glucose supplementation of juvenile and adult experimental animals actually accentuates hypoxic-ischemic brain damage.[108,155,181] However, Voorhies et al.[240] have demonstrated in the immature rat that, unlike in adults, glucose supplementation and its associated hyperglycemia do not increase the severity of brain injury induced by hypoxia-ischemia. Age-specific differences in the rates of glucose uptake and metabolism by brain account for the age-related differences in the tissue damaging influence of glucose during hypoxic-ischemic stress.[233]

Certain clinical implications are inherent in the experimental studies described above. The data suggest that obstetricians and neonatologists need not restrict or curtail glucose administration to an acutely asphyxiated fetus or newborn infant for fear of accentuating brain damage. On the contrary, maternal glucose supplementation during labor and delivery may prolong central respiratory drive and reduce cardiovascular depression with its associated systemic hypotension and secondary cerebral ischemia.[24,100,102,240] The relative preservation of respiratory and cardiovascular function, in turn, should reduce the need for extensive resuscitation at birth and afford a more favorable neurologic outcome. A controlled clinical trial of glucose supplementation for mothers at risk for delivering an asphyxiated infant would clarify the beneficial—or deleterious—role of glucose in perinatal cerebral hypoxia-ischemia.

Barbiturates

Experimental animal studies suggest that barbiturates might protect the fetus and newborn infant against asphyxia, both by prolonging survival and by preventing or reducing the subsequent development of hypoxic-ischemic brain damage.[32,40,89] The mechanism of this protective effect is unknown, but barbiturates are known to reduce energy demands in the brain,[135] inhibit synaptic transmission,[10,146] and preserve an optimal cerebral energy balance during perinatal hypoxia.[235] In all experimental instances in which barbiturates have been found to influence favorably the outcome of perinatal asphyxia, the anesthetic was administered prior to the onset of the metabolic stress. Controlled clinical trials are required to clarify the protective influence of barbiturate *pretreatment* on asphyxia in the fetal and newborn human infant.

High-dose barbiturates have been administered to newborn infants sustaining cerebral hypoxia-ischemia before or at birth.[68,88] In a controlled clinical study, Goldberg et al.[88] randomized 32 full-term severely asphyxiated newborn infants to barbiturate-treated and control groups. All infants exhibited evidence of postasphyxial encephalopathy and required mechanical ventilation. Thiopental was begun at a mean postnatal age of 2 hr and was given as an infusion over 24 hr. Despite barbiturate therapy, no significant difference in the frequency of seizures or in intracranial pressure was noted between the two groups. Furthermore, early treatment with barbiturate did not favorably influence neonatal mortality and long-term neurologic morbidity. Of additional importance was the fact that systemic hypotension occurred significantly more often in the treated group (88% vs. 60%), requiring vasopressor support in these infants. The authors concluded that barbiturate therapy offers little benefit to the previously asphyxiated newborn infant and may actually perpetuate systemic cardiovascular derangements (see also ref. 68).

Cerebral Edema

The role of cerebral edema in aggravating postasphyxial encephalopathy of newborn infants is unresolved. Published reports indicate that edema is a prominent feature of human perinatal cerebral hypoxia-ischemia[5,75,119,179] and that it is associated with hypoxic-ischemic brain damage in experimental animals.[18,191] However, the critical question remains whether cerebral edema itself causes or contributes to brain tissue injury. Investigations in adult animals suggest that edema does accentuate tissue necrosis,[106,185,208] but parallel studies in perinatal animals have not been accomplished. Furthermore, there have been no clinical trials to indicate that the use of therapeutic agents known to reduce cerebral edema in any way ameliorates the extent of ultimate brain damage in asphyxiated newborn infants.

The existence of cerebral edema is ascertained clinically by the presence of bulging fontanelles, splayed sutures, and rapidly increasing head size in a previously asphyxiated newborn infant. The presence and extent of edema can then be determined by the presence of focal or widespread hypodensities with slitlike ventricles on CT or US scan. If cerebral edema is suspected by examination and documented radiographically, and if the infant is deteriorating clinically, then procedures to reduce the edema should be instituted (see Table 7-5). Oral and intravenous fluids are restricted to minimal maintenance requirements. If the situation is critical, controlled hyperventilation ($Paco_2$ = 20–25 torr) and/or hyperosmolar and diuretic agents (mannitol, glycerol, and/or furosemide) are used to reduce cerebral blood volume and dehydrate the brain. Although these procedures might be successful in preventing brain herniation and its attendant mortality, there is no information that they reduce the extent of brain damage.

Given the current dilemmas in the brain-oriented therapy of newborn infants sustaining cerebral hypoxia-ischemia, it is not surprising that management practices vary widely among neonatal intensive care units.[61] Thus there is presently no uniform standard of care, and it remains for future research to uncover new and effective modes of therapy for the neurologically compromised infant. Prevention or at least optimal management of prepartum and intrapartum asphyxia remains the best available means of reducing the incidence and severity of perinatal hypoxic-ischemic brain damage.

Seizures

Treatment of neonatal seizures arising from postasphyxial encephalopathy is directed toward the correction of any underlying systemic metabolic derangement or structural lesion of the brain, if present, and toward the early control of convulsive activity with anti-epileptic medications. Seizures of metabolic origin are treated by replacement of the deficient agent. Hypoglycemia is corrected by the intravenous injection of 2 to 3 mL/kg 25% glucose followed by an infusion of 15% glucose at a rate of 4 to 5 mL/kg/hr to maintain blood glucose levels well above 40 mg/dL. Hypocalcemia is corrected by the slow intravenous administration of 2 mL/kg 5% calcium gluconate, repeated as necessary to maintain serum calcium concentrations above 7 to 8 mg/dL depending upon the gestational age of the infant. Hypomagnesemia (less than 1 mEq/L) is corrected with 2 mL/kg 2% to 3% magnesium sulfate injected intravenously.

Once it has been established that a metabolic derangement is not contributing to seizure activity in an asphyxiated newborn infant, an anticonvulsant medication is employed in an attempt to control repetitive or continuous seizure activity (see Table 7-6). If convulsions are fragmentary and of short duration, phenobarbital and/or hydantoin (Dilantin)

(20 mg/kg) should be given intravenously followed by 3 to 5 mg/kg/day, with frequent monitoring of blood anticonvulsant levels.[71,129,169] Higher loading doses of phenobarbital are frequently required, as posthypoxic seizures are often refractory to therapy.[79] Status epilepticus, defined as continuous tonic or clonic convulsive activity lasting more than 30 min or frequent intermittent convulsive activity lasting more than 1 hr, is treated with short-acting anticonvulsant medications, specifically diazepam or paraldehyde. Maintenance therapy with phenobarbital and/or hydantoin then is instituted.[116,167]

PROGNOSIS

As mentioned previously, perinatal cerebral hypoxia-ischemia contributes substantially to perinatal mortality and morbidity. The outcome of infants sustaining cerebral hypoxia-ischemia is influenced by several factors, including the duration and severity of the insult; gestational age; presence of seizures; and associated infectious, metabolic, and traumatic derangements. Because of these many variables, a prognosis for any single infant is difficult to formulate. However, certain clinical and laboratory abnormalities in the setting of perinatal cerebral hypoxia-ischemia are associated with a high incidence of neurologic disability (Table 7-7).

The degree of maturity at birth is an important predictor of mortality in infants asphyxiated at birth.[137] Scott[203] investigated a group of infants who were either stillborn or without spontaneous, sustained respirations for a minimum of 20 min. Thirty-two percent of the premature infants and 70% of the full-term infants survived; however, the long-term morbidity of the survivors was 11% and 36%, respectively. Nelson and Ellenberg[159] also reported an appreciably higher death rate in premature

---

Table 7-7 Predictors of Mortality and Neurologic Morbidity

Fetal assessment
   Presence of meconium
   Heart rate monitoring
   Blood acid-base analysis
Extended Apgar score
Onset of respirations
Neonatal neurologic examination
US and/or CT scan
EEG

---

infants but an increased risk for cerebral palsy in the full-term survivors. The low morbidity among the premature infants was related in part to the small number of survivors in this group.

Abnormalities of fetal heart rate monitoring and acid-base status during labor are associated with less than optimal long-term neurologic outcome.[132,134,168] Painter et al.[168] studied the postnatal maturation of 50 high-risk full-term infants who had undergone intrauterine electronic monitoring and found a significant positive correlation between severe variable and late decelerations during labor and poor scores on developmental testing at one year of age. Low et al.[132] demonstrated a similar positive correlation between poor outcome and the severity and duration of fetal hypoxia as determined by scalp and umbilical artery acid-base analysis during labor and at delivery. These and other studies also provide evidence for the accuracy of abnormal fetal heart rate patterns and acid-base balance in predicting fetuses likely to exhibit low Apgar scores and develop postasphyxial encephalopathy.[38,110,117,166]

Despite its simplicity, the Apgar score provides prognostic information for the potential of ultimate brain damage. The 1-min Apgar score was initially used to predict neonatal mortality.[8] Drage and Berendes[57] later suggested that the 5-min Apgar score was a better predictor of ultimate neurologic impairment than the 1-min score. Dweck et al.[66] found that 2 of 9 term infants whose 1-min Apgar scores were 3 or less were abnormal at 2 or 3 years of age. Thomson et al.[220] found that of 25 full-term infants with Apgar scores of 0 at 1 min or less than 4 at 5 min, only 1 exhibited severe neurologic handicap at a five- to ten-year follow-up. These studies indicate the inaccuracy of the 1- and 5-min Apgar scores in predicting long-term neurologic outcome. However, Nelson and Ellenberg[158] evaluated 39 full-term infants whose 20-min Apgar scores were 3 or less; 8 of the 14 survivors had cerebral palsy when examined at age 7. Thus the extended Apgar score remains a reliable predictor of ultimate neurologic morbidity, especially when very low scores are obtained at 20 min.

The time from birth until onset of spontaneous, sustained respirations also has been correlated with long-term neurologic function. Mulligan et al.[151] reported a 19% immediate mortality and an 18% morbidity among 39 surviving full-term infants in whom spontaneous respirations did not take place for more than 1 minute following birth. D'Souza et al.[58] followed for up to five years 15 full-term infants who had previously survived apnea for 10 or more minutes at birth. Of this group, 2 exhibited severe neurologic deficit, and 5 had delayed language development. Full-term infants who were apneic for 30 or more minutes were universally and severely damaged.[213] These data suggest that prolonged delay in the initiation of spontaneous respirations is an indicator of irreversible brain damage.

Neurologic examination in the immediate neonatal period provides a useful index for predicting later developmental outcome, especially in the full-term infant.[2,4,27,59,70,128,159,200] Sarnat and Sarnat,[200] using their staging criteria for perinatal postasphyxial encephalopathy (see Table 7-4), showed that Stage I newborn infants invariably recover without neurologic deficit. Infants in Stage II later develop normally if clinical and EEG abnormalities are fully reversed within 5 days of birth. Stage III encephalopathy is associated with high mortality (50%) and universal morbidity among the survivors. Similar outcome data have been provided by Finer et al.[70] when applied to a larger population of asphyxiated full-term infants using the Sarnat staging system.

The data pertaining to long-term follow-up of low birth weight infants are much more complex than those of full-term neonates because of the multiple medical problems that follow premature birth. Respiratory distress syndrome, intermittent apnea and bradycardia, anemia, sepsis, meningitis, and undernutrition occur with such frequency that correlations between acute perinatal asphyxia and ultimate neurologic deficits are difficult, although not impossible.[14,62,170] All of these conditions can damage the brain through cerebral hypoxia-ischemia. In addition, periventricular and intraventricular hemorrhage frequently accompanies prematurity, hemorrhage itself contributing substantially to neonatal mortality and long-term morbidity (see Chapter 8). Finally, mortality, especially in the very low birthweight groups, is high, thereby excluding those infants most likely to be permanently brain damaged.[14,41,67,105,137,158,203] With these limitations in mind, outcome data suggest an incidence of neurodevelopmental deficits ranging from 15% to 40% of infants weighing less than 1,500 g at birth.[41,62,113,196,198,214] As in full-term infants sustaining hypoxia-ischemia, the major long-term deficits in premature infants include cerebral palsy, mental retardation, learning disability, and partial or complete blindness or deafness.

The contribution of neonatal convulsive activity to mortality and ultimate neurologic morbidity is not entirely clear. The absence or presence of seizures in an asphyxiated newborn infant is believed by some investigators to be a strong discriminator between later normal and abnormal development.[151,157,193] Conversely, Finer et al.[70] found no relationship between the presence of postasphyxial seizures and ultimate outcome. However, seizures occurring within the first 24 hr following birth did correlate with a significantly increased incidence of neurologic handicap at follow-up when these infants were compared with infants whose seizures occurred later. Prolonged seizures refractory to anticonvulsant medication as well as tonic or myoclonic seizures also appear to portend a poor outcome.[15,26,144] Thus the long-term prognosis of infants sustaining seizures in the newborn period appears to reflect more the severity of the underlying insult to brain than the convulsive activity itself.

Neurodiagnostic procedures are also helpful in delineating abnormalities in brain that predict the presence of permanent damage and a high likelihood of long-term neurologic handicap. The presence of hypodensities on CT scan, at least in full-term infants, correlates with less than optimal motor and mental development.[73,128,147,202] In this regard, Lipper et al.[128] found a close correlation between the extent of hypodensities on CT with neurodevelopmental abnormalities at 1 year. Echogenic abnormalities on US also have predictive value, especially the presence of large, intracerebral lesions presumed to represent areas of hemorrhagic infarction.[31,55,90,93,142,214] Finally, in those few medical centers where CBF has been measured in newborn asphyxiated infants, a persistently low flow state is associated with poor developmental outcome.[131,239] It remains to be determined to what extent MR imaging and spectrometry will predict with even greater sophistication the ultimate outcome of infants sustaining perinatal cerebral hypoxia-ischemia.

REFERENCES

1. Ahdab-Barmada M, Moossy J, Painter M: Pontosubicular necrosis and hyperoxemia. *Pediatrics* 1980;66:840–847.

2. Amiel-Tison C: Cerebral damage in full term newborn infants: Etiologic factors, neonatal status and continuous term follow-up. *Biol Neonate* 1969;40:234–238.

3. Amiel-Tison C: Neurological evaluation of the maturity of newborn infants. *Arch Dis Child* 1968;43:87–97.

4. Amiel-Tison C, Ellison P: Birth asphyxia in the fullterm newborn: Early assessment and outcome. *Dev Med Child Neurol* 1986;28:671–682.

5. Anderson JM, Belton NR: Water and electrolyte abnormalities in the human brain after severe intrapartum asphyxia. *J Neurol Neurosurg Psychiatry* 1974;37:514–520.

6. Antoine C, Silverman F, Young BK: Current status of continuous fetal pH monitoring, in Petrie RH (ed): *Clinics in Perinatology*. Philadelphia, WB Saunders, 1982, pp 409–422.

7. Apgar V: A proposal for a new method of evaluation of the newborn infant. *Curr Res Anesth Analg* 1953;32:260–265.

8. Apgar V, James LS: Further observations on the newborn scoring system. *Am J Dis Child* 1962;104:419–428.

9. Ashwal S, Dale PS, Longo LD: Regional cerebral blood flow: Studies in the fetal lamb during hypoxia, hypercapnia, acidosis and hypotension. *Pediatr Res* 1984;18:1309–1316.

10. Astrup J, Moller Sorenson P, Rahbek Sorenson H: Inhibition of cerebral oxygen and glucose consumption in the dog by hypothermia, pentobarbital and lidocaine. *Anesthesiology* 1981;55:263–268.

11. Banker BW, Larroche JC: Periventricular leukomalacia of infancy. *Arch Neurol* 1962;7:386–410.

12. Barmada MA, Moossy J, Shuman RM: Cerebral infarcts with arterial occlusion in neonates. *Ann Neurol* 1979;6:495–502.

13. Baxi LV: Current status of fetal oxygen monitoring, in Petrie RH (ed): *Clinics in Perinatology.* Philadelphia, WB Saunders, 1982, pp 423–432.

14. Bennett FC, Robinson NM, Sells CJ: Growth and development of infants weighing less than 800 grams at birth. *Pediatrics* 1983;71:319–323.

15. Bergman I, Painter MJ, Hirsch RP, Crumrine PK, David R: Outcome in neonates with convulsions treated in an intensive care unit. *Ann Neurol* 1983;14:642–647.

16. Borit A, Herndon RM: The fine structure of plaques fibromyeliniques in ulegyria and status marmoratus. *Acta Neuropathol* 1970;14:304–308.

17. Brand MM, Durbridge TC, Rosan RC, Northway WH: Neuropathological lesions in respiratory distress syndrome: Acute and chronic changes during hypoxia and oxygen therapy. *J Reprod Med* 1972;8:267–279.

18. Brann AW, Myers RE: Central nervous system findings in the newborn monkey following severe *in utero* partial asphyxia. *Neurology* 1975;25:327–338.

19. Brazelton TB: Neonatal behavioral assessment scale, in *Clinics in Developmental Medicine.* Philadelphia, LB Lippincott, 1973.

20. Brierley JB: The influence of brain swelling, age and hypotension upon the pattern of cerebral damage in hypoxia, in *Proceedings of the Fifth Conference of Neuropathology.* New York, Excerpta Medica, 1966.

21. Brierley JB, Brown AW, Excell BJ: Brain damage in the rhesus monkey resulting from profound arterial hypotension. Its nature, distribution and general physiological correlates. *Brain Res* 1969;13:68–74.

22. Brierley JB, Graham DI: Hypoxia and vascular disorders of the central nervous system, in Adams JH, Corsellis JAN, Duchen LW (eds): *Greenfield's Neuropathology IV.* New York, John Wiley and Sons, 1984, pp 125–207.

23. Brierley JB, Meldrum BS, Brown AW: The threshold and neuropathology of cerebral "anoxic-ischemic" cell change. *Arch Neurol* 1973;29:367–374.

24. Britton SW, Kline RF: Age, sex, carbohydrate, adrenal cortex and other factors in anoxia. *Am J Physiol* 1945–46;145:190–202.

25. Brown JD, Vannucci RC: Cerebral oxidative metabolism during intrauterine growth retardation. *Biol Neonate* 1978;34:170–173.

26. Brown JK, Cockburn F, Forfar JO: Clinical and chemical correlates in convulsions of the newborn. *Lancet* 1972;1:135–139.

27. Brown JK, Purvis RJ, Forfar JO, Cockburn F: Neurological aspects of perinatal asphyxia. *Dev Med Child Neurol* 1974;16:567–580.

28. Brown RM, Kehr W, Carlsson A: Functional and biochemical aspects of catecholamine metabolism in brain under hypoxia. *Brain Res* 1975;85:491–509.

29. Cabel LA, Devaskar U, Siassi B, Hodgman JE, Emmanouilides G: Cardiogenic shock associated with perinatal asphyxia in preterm infants. *J Pediatr* 1980;96:705–710.

30. Cady EB, Dawson MJ, Hope PL, Tofts PS, Costello AM, Delpy DT, Reynolds EOR, Wilke DR: Non-invasive investigation of cerebral metabolism in newborn infants by phosphorus nuclear magnetic resonance spectroscopy. *Lancet* 1983;1:1059–1062.

31. Calvert SA, Hoskins EM, Fong KW, Forsyth SC: Periventricular leukomalacia: Ultrasonic diagnosis and neurological outcome. *Acta Pediatr Scand* 1986;75:489–496.

32. Campbell AGM, Milligan JB, Talner NS: The effect of pretreatment with pentobarbital, meperidine, or hyperbaric oxygen on the response to anoxia and resuscitation in newborn rabbits. *J Pediatr* 1968;72:518–527.

33. Cassady G: The small-for-date infant, in Avery GB (ed): *Neonatology: Pathophysiology and Management of the Newborn.* Philadelphia, JB Lippincott, 1981, pp 262–286.

34. Cavazzuti M, Duffy TE: Regulation of local cerebral blood flow in normal and hypoxic newborn dogs. *Ann Neurol* 1983;11:247–257.

35. Chanez C, Tordet-Cardiroit C, Roux JM: Studies and experimental hypotrophy in the rat. *Biol Neonate* 1971;18:56–65.

36. Chase HP, Welsh NN, Dabiere CS, Vasan NS, Butterfield LJ: Alterations in human brain biochemistry following intrauterine growth retardation. *Pediatrics* 1972;50:403–411.

37. Christensen E, Melchior J: Cerebral palsy—a clinical and neurolopathological study, in *Clinics in Developmental Medicine 25.* London, Spastics Society, 1967.

38. Cibils LA: Clinical significance of fetal heart rate patterns during labor: V. Variable decelerations. *Am J Obstet Gynecol* 1978;132:791–803.

39. Clifford SH: The effects of asphyxia on the newborn infant. *J Pediatr* 1941;18:567–578.

40. Cockburn F, Daniel SS, Dawes GS, James LS, Myers RE, Niemann W, Rodriquez de Curet H, Ross BB: The effect of pentobarbital anesthesia on resuscitation and brain damage in fetal rhesus monkeys asphyxiated on delivery. *J Pediatr* 1969;75:281–291.

41. Cohen RS, Stevenson DK, Malachowski N, Ariagno RL, Kimble KJ, Hopper AO, Johnson JD, Veland K, Sunshine P: Favorable results of neonatal intensive care for very low-birth-weight infants. *Pediatrics* 1982;69:621–625.

42. Comline RS, Silver M: The composition of foetal and maternal blood during parturition in the ewe. *J Physiol* 1972;222:233–256.

43. Commey JOO, Fitzhardinge PM: Handicap in the preterm small-for-gestational age infant. *J Pediatr* 1979;94:779–786.

44. Courville CB: *Birth and Brain Damage.* Pasadena, CA, Courville Publishers, 1971.

45. Coyle JT, Molliver ME: Major innervation of newborn rat cortex by monoaminergic neurons. *Science* 1977;196:444–447.

46. Crockard A, Iannotti F, Hunstack AT, Smith RD, Harris RJ, Symon L: Cerebral blood flow and edema following carotid occlusion in the gerbil. *Stroke* 1980;11:494–498.

47. Dahlquist G, Persson B: Effect of intrauterine growth retardation on the postnatal development of D-β-hydroxybutyrate dehydrogenase activity in rat brain. *Biol Neonate* 1976;28:353–364.

48. Dauber IM, Krauss AN, Symchych PS, Auld PAM: Renal failure following perinatal anoxia. *J Pediatr* 1976;88:851–855.

49. Davis JN, Carlsson A: The effect of hypoxia on monoamine synthesis levels and metabolism in rat brain. *J Neurochem* 1973;21:783–790.

50. Davis JN, Carlsson A, MacMillan V, Seisjö B: Brain tryptophan hydroxylation: Dependence on arterial oxygen tension. *Science* 1973;182:72–74.

51. Dawes GS, Jacobson HM, Mott JC, Shelley HJ: Some observations on foetal and newborn rhesus monkeys. *J Physiol* 1960;152:271–298.

52. Dawes GS, Mott JC, Shelley HJ: The importance of cardiac glycogen for the maintenance of life in foetal lambs and newborn animals during anoxia. *J Physiol* 1959;146:516–538.

53. De Reuck J: The human periventricular arterial blood supply and the anatomy of cerebral infarctions. *Eur Neurol* 1971;5:321–334.

54. De Reuck J, Chattha AS, Richardson EP: Pathogenesis and evolution of periventricular leukomalacia in infancy. *Arch Neurol* 1972;27:229–236.

55. DeVries LS, Dubowitz V, Lary S, Whitelaw A, Dubowitz LMS, Kaiser A, Silverman M, Wigglesworth JS: Predictive value of cranial ultrasound in the newborn baby: A reappraisal. *Lancet* 1985;2:137–140.

56. Doyle LW, Nahmias C, Firnau G, Kenyon DB, Garnett ES, Sinclair JC: Regional cerebral glucose metabolism of newborn infants measured by positron emission tomography. *Dev Med Child Neurol* 1983;25:143–151.

57. Drage JS, Berendes H: Apgar scores and outcome of the newborn. *Pediatr Clin North Am* 1966;13:637–643.

58. D'Souza SW, McCartney E, Nolan M, Taylor IG: Hearing, speech and language in survivors of severe perinatal asphyxia. *Arch Dis Child* 1981;56:245–252.

59. D'Souza SW, Richards B: Neurological sequelae in newborn babies after perinatal asphyxia. *Arch Dis Child* 1978;53:564–569.

60. Donn SM, Bowerman RA: Neonatal posthemorrhagic porencephaly: Ultrasonographic features. *Am J Dis Child* 1982;136:707–709.

61. Donn SM, Goldstein GW, Schork A: Asphyxia neonatorum: A national survey of management practices. *Pediatr Res* 1986;20:461A.

62. Driscoll JM, Driscoll YT, Steir ME, Stark RI, Dangman BC, Perez A, Wung J, Kritz P: Mortality and morbidity in infants less than 1,001 grams birth weight. *Pediatrics* 1982;69:21–26.

63. Dubowitz LMS, Dubowitz V, Goldberg C: Clinical assessment of gestational age in the newborn infant. *J Pediatr* 1970;77:1–10.

64. Duffy TE, Kohle SJ, Vannucci RC: Carbohydrate and energy metabolism in perinatal rat brain: Relation to survival in anoxia. *J Neurochem* 1975;24:271–276.

65. Dunnihuo DR, Quilligan EJ: Carotid blood flow distribution in the *in utero* sheep fetus. *Am J Obstet Gynecol* 1973;116:648–656.

66. Dweck HS, Huggins W, Dorman LP, Saxon SA, Benton JW, Cassady G: Developmental sequelae in infants having suffered severe perinatal asphyxia. *Am J Obstet Gynecol* 1974;119:811–815.

67. Ergander U, Eriksson M, Zetterström R: Severe neonatal asphyxia. *Acta Paediatr Scand* 1983;72:321–325.

68. Eyre JA, Wilkinson AR: Thiopentone induced coma after severe birth asphyxia. *Arch Dis Child* 1986;61:1084–1089.

69. Fazekas JF, Alexander AD, Himwich HE: Tolerance of the newborn to anoxia. *Am J Physiol* 1941;134:281–287.

70. Finer NN, Robertson CM, Richards RT, Pinnell LE, Petters KL: Hypoxic-ischemic encephalopathy in term neonates: Perinatal factors and outcome. *J Pediatr* 1981;98:112–117.

71. Fischer JH, Lockman LA, Zaske D, Kriel R: Phenobarbital maintenance dose requirements in treating neonatal seizures. *Neurology* 1981;31:1042–1044.

72. Fishman R: Brain edema. *N Engl J Med* 1975;293:706–711.

73. Fitzhardinge PM, Flodmark O, Fitz CR, Ashby S: The prognostic value of computed tomography as an adjunct to assessment of the term infant with postasphyxial encephalopathy. *J Pediatr* 1981;99:777–781.

74. Fitzhardinge PM, Steven EM: The small-for-date infant. Neurological and intellectual sequelae. *Pediatrics* 1972;50:50–57.

75. Flodmark O, Becker LE, Harwood-Nash DC, Fitzhardinge PM, Fitz CR, Chuang SH: Correlation between computed tomography and autopsy in premature and full-term neonates that have suffered perinatal asphyxia. *Neuroradiology* 1980;137:93–103.

76. Freeman RK: Contraction stress testing for primary fetal surveillance in patients at high risk for uteroplacental insufficiency, in Petrie RH (ed): *Clinics in Perinatology.* Philadelphia, WB Saunders, 1982, pp 265–270.

77. Friede RL: *Developmental Neuropathology.* New York, Springer-Verlag, 1975.

78. Friede RL: Pontosubicular lesions in perinatal anoxia. *Arch Pathol* 1972;94:343–346.

79. Gal P, Toback J, Boer H, Erkan N, Wells T: Efficacy of phenobarbital monotherapy in treatment of neonatal seizures: Relationships to blood levels. *Neurology* 1982;32:1401–1404.

80. Gibson GE, Blass JP: Impaired synthesis of acetycholine in brain accompanying mild hypoxia and hypoglycemia. *J Neurochem* 1976;27:37–42.

81. Gibson GE, Duffy TE: Impaired synthesis of acetylcholine by mild hypoxic hypoxia or nitrous oxide. *J Neurochem* 1981;36:28–33.

82. Gibson GE, Peterson C, Sansone J: Decreases in amino acid and acetycholine metabolism during hypoxia. *J Neurochem* 1981;37:192–201.

83. Gibson GE, Shimada M, Blass JP: Alterations in acetycholine synthesis and cyclic nucleotides in mild cerebral hypoxia. *J Neurochem* 1978;31:757–760.

84. Gilles FH, Murphy SF: Perinatal telencephalic leucoencephalopathy. *J Neurol Neurosurg Psychiatry* 1969;32:404–413.

85. Gimovsky ML, Caritis SN: Diagnosis and management of hypoxic fetal heart rate patterns, in Petrie RH (ed): *Clinics in Perinatology.* Philadelphia, WB Saunders, 1982, pp 313–324.

86. Glass HG, Synder FF, Webster E: The rate of decline in resistance to anoxia of rabbits, dogs and guinea pigs from the onset of viability to adult life. *Am J Physiol* 1944;140:609–615.

87. Goldberg RN, Cabal LA, Sinatra FR, Plajstek CE, Hodgman JE: Hyperammonemia associated with perinatal asphyxia. *Pediatrics* 1979;64:336–341.

88. Goldberg RN, Moscoso P, Bauer CR, Bloom FL, Curless RG, Burke B, Boncalari E: Use of barbiturate therapy in severe perinatal asphyxia: A randomized controlled trial. *J Pediatr* 1986;109:851–856.

89. Goodlin RC, Lloyd D: Use of drugs to protect against fetal asphyxia. *Am J Obstet Gynecol* 1970;107:227–231.

90. Graziani LJ, Pasto M, Stanley C, Pidcock F, Desai H, Desai S, Branca P, Goldberg B: Neonatal neurosonographic correlates of cerebral palsy in preterm infants. *Pediatrics* 1986;78:88–95.

91. Grunnet ML: Periventricular leukomalacia complex. *Arch Neurol* 1979;103:6–10.

92. Gutberlet RL, Cornblath N: Neonatal hypoglycemia revisited. *Pediatrics* 1976;58:10–17.

93. Guzzetta F, Shackelford GD, Volpe S, Perlman JM, Volpe JJ: Periventricular intraparenchymal echodensities in the premature newborn: Critical determinant of neurologic outcome. *Pediatrics* 1986;78:995–1006.

94. Hamilton PA, Cady EB, Wyatt JS, Hope PL, Delpy DT, Reynolds EOR: Impaired energy metabolism in brains of newborn infants with increased cerebral echodensities. *Lancet* 1986;1:1242–1246.

95. Hedner T: Central monoamine metabolism and neonatal oxygen deprivation. *Acta Physiol Scand* 1978;460(Suppl):1–34.

96. Hedner T, Lundborg P, Engel J: Effect of hypoxia on monoamine synthesis in brains of developing rats. *Biol Neonate* 1977;31:122–126.

97. Hernandez MJ, Brennan RW, Bowman GS: Autoregulation of cerebral blood flow in the newborn dog. *Brain Res* 1980;184:199–202.

98. Hernandez MJ, Brennan RW, Vannucci RC, Bowman GS: Cerebral blood flow and oxygen consumption in the newborn dog. *Am J Physiol* 1978;234:R209–R215.

99. Hill A, Melson GL, Clark HB, Volpe JJ: Hemorrhagic periventricular leukomalacia: Diagnosis by real time ultrasound and correlation with autopsy findings. *Pediatrics* 1982;69:282–284.

100. Himwich HE, Bernstein AO, Herrlich H, Chesler A, Fazekas JF: Mechanism for the maintenance of life in the newborn during anoxia. *Am J Physiol* 1942;135:387–391.

101. Hobel CJ: Intrapartum assessment of fetal distress. *Am J Obstet Gynecol* 1971; 110:336–342.

102. Holowach-Thurston J, Haubart RE, Jones EM: Anoxia in mice: Reduced glucose in brain with normal or elevated glucose in plasma and increased survival after glucose treatment. *Pediatr Res* 1974;8:238–243.

103. Hon EH, Koh SK: Management of labor and delivery, in Avery GB (ed): *Neonatology: Pathophysiology and Management of the Newborn.* Philadelphia, JB Lippincott, 1981, pp 120–131.

104. Hope PL, Cady EB, Tofts PS, Hamilton PA, Costello AM, Delpy DT, Chu A, Reynolds EOR, Wilke DR: Cerebral energy metabolism studied with phosphorus NMR spectroscopy in normal and birth-asphyxiated infants. *Lancet* 1984;2:366–369.

105. Horwood SP, Boyle MH, Torrance GW, Sinclair JC: Mortality and morbidity of 500- to 1499-gram birth weight infants live-born to residents of a defined geographic region before and after neonatal intensive care. *Pediatrics* 1982;69:613–620.

106. Hossman KA: Treatment of experimental cerebral ischemia. *J Cereb Blood Flow Metabol* 1982;2:275–297.

107. James LS, Weisbrot IM, Prince CE, Holaday DA, Apgar V: The acid-base status of human infants in relation to birth asphyxia and onset of respiration. *J Pediatr* 1958; 52:379–394.

108. Kalimo H, Rehncrona S, Söderfeldt B, Olsson Y, Siesjö BK: Brain lactic acidosis and ischemic cell damage: 2. Histopathology. *J Cereb Blood Flow Metabol* 1981;1:313–327.

109. Kaplan SL, Feigin RD: Inappropriate secretion of antidiuretic hormone complicating neonatal hypoxic-ischemic encephalopathy. *J Pediatr* 1978;92:431–432.

110. Keegan KA, Waffarn F, Quilligan EJ: Obstetric characteristics and fetal heart rate patterns of infants who convulse during the newborn period. *Am J Obstet Gynecol* 1985;153:732–737.

111. Kellaway P, Hrachovy RA: Status epilepticus in newborns: A perspective on neonatal seizures. *Adv Neurol* 1983;34:93–101.

112. Kirschbaum TH, DeHaven JC, Shapiro N, Assali NS: Oxyhemoglobin dissociation characteristics of human and sheep maternal and fetal blood. *Am J Obstet Gynecol* 1966;96:741–757.

113. Kitchen WH, Ford GW, Rickards AL, Lissenden JV, Ryan MM: Children of birth weight <1000 g: Changing outcome between ages 2 and 5 years. *J Pediatr* 1987;110:283–288.

114. Knobloch H, Sotos JF, Sherand ED: Prognostic and etiologic factors in hypoglycemia. *J Pediatr* 1967;70:876–884.

115. Kohle SJ, Vannucci RC: Glycogen metabolism in fetal and neonatal rat brain: Influence of birth. *J Neurochem* 1977;28:441–443.

116. Koren G, Butt W, Rajchgot P, Mayer J, Whyte H, Pape K, MacLeod SM: Intravenous paraldehyde for seizure control in newborn infants. *Neurology* 1986;36:108–111.

117. Krebs HE, Petres RE, Dunn LJ: Intrapartum fetal heart rate monitoring: VIII. Atypical variable decelerations. *Am J Obstet Gynecol* 1983;145:297–305.

118. Kreusser KL, Schmidt RE, Shackelford GD, Volpe JJ: Value of ultrasound for identification of acute hemorrhagic necrosis of thalamus and basal ganglia in an asphyxiated term infant. *Ann Neurol* 1984;16:361–363.

119. Larroche JCL: in *Developmental Pathology of the Neonate*. Amsterdam, Elsevier/North Holland, 1977.

120. Larroche JC: Fetal encephalopathies of circulatory origin. *Biol Neonate* 1986;50:61–74.

121. Leech RW, Alvord EC: Anoxic-ischemic encephalopathy in the human neonatal period: The significance of brain stem involvement. *Arch Neurol* 1977;34:109–113.

122. Leech RW, Olson MI, Alvord EC: Neuropathologic features of idiopathic respiratory distress syndrome. *Arch Pathol Lab Med* 1979;103:341–343.

123. Leonard JC, Younkin DP, Chance B, Subramanian YH, Leigh JS, Alavi A, Kressel HY, Zimmerman R, Delivoria-Papadopoulos M: Nuclear magnetic resonance: An overview of its spectroscopic and imaging applications in pediatric patients. *J Pediatr* 1985;106:757–761.

124. Levene MI, Wigglesworth JS, Dubowitz V: Hemorrhagic periventricular leukomalacia in the neonate: A real-time ultrasound study. *Pediatrics* 1983;71:794–797.

125. Leviton A, Gilles FH: Acquired perinatal leukoencephalopathy. *Ann Neurol* 1984;16:1–8.

126. Levitsky LL, Speck SM, Skulman R: Metabolic response to fasting in experimental intrauterine growth retardation. *Biol Neonate* 1976;30:11–16.

127. Linde L, Rasof B, Dunn O: Mental development in congenital heart disease. *Am J Dis Child* 1967;71:198–203.

128. Lipper EG, Voorhies TM, Ross G, Vannucci RC, Auld PAM: Early predictors of one-year outcome for infants asphyxiated at birth. *Dev Med Child Neurol* 1986;28:303–309.

129. Lockman LA, Kriel R, Zaske D, Thompson T, Virnig N: Phenobarbital dosage for control of neonatal seizures. *Neurology* 1979;29:1445–1449.

130. Lou HC, Lassen NA, Friis-Hanson B: Impaired autoregulation of cerebral blood flow in the distressed newborn infant. *J Pediatr* 1979;94:170–173.

131. Lou HC, Skov H, Pedersen H: Low cerebral blood flow: A risk factor in the neonate. *J Pediatr* 1979;95:606–609.

132. Low JA, Galbraith RS, Muir DW, Killen HL, Pater EA, Karchmar EJ: Factors associated with motor and cognitive deficits in children after intrapartum fetal hypoxia. *Am J Obstet Gynecol* 1984;148:533–539.

133. Low JA, Galbraith RS, Muir D, Killen H, Worthington D, Karchmar J, Campbell D: Intrauterine growth retardation: A preliminary report on long term morbidity. *Am J Obstet Gynecol* 1978;130:534–545.

134. Low JA, Pancham SR, Piercy WN, Worthington D, Karchmar J: Intrapartum fetal asphyxia: Clinical characteristics, diagnosis and significance in relation to pattern of development. *Am J Obstet Gynecol* 1977;129:857–872.

135. Lowry OH, Passoneau JV, Hasselberger FX, Schulz DW: Effect of ischemia on known substrates and cofactors of the glycolytic pathway in brain. *J Biol Chem* 1964;239:18–30.

136. Lucas W, Kirschbaum T, Assali NS: Cephalic circulation and oxygen consumption before and after birth. *Am J Physiol* 1966;210:287–292.

137. MacDonald HM, Mulligan JC, Allen AC, Taylor PM: Neonatal asphyxia. I. Relationship of obstetric and neonatal complications to neonatal mortality in 38,405 consecutive deliveries. *J Pediatr* 1980;96:898–902.

138. Malamud N: Status marmoratus: A form of cerebral palsy following either birth injury or inflammation of the central nervous system. *J Pediatr* 1960;37:610–619.

139. Malamud N, Itabashi HH, Caster J, Messinger HB: An etiologic and diagnostic study of cerebral palsy. *J Pediatr* 1964;65:270–293.

140. Manning FA, Morrison I, Lange IR, Harman C: Antepartum determination of fetal health: Composite biophysical profile scoring, in Petrie RH (ed): *Clinics in Perinatology*. Philadelphia, WB Saunders, 1982, pp 285–296.

141. McBride MC, Kemper TL: Pathogenesis of four-layered microgyric cortex in man. *Acta Neuropathol* 1982;57:93–98.

142. McMenamin JB, Shackelford GD, Volpe JJ: Outcome of neonatal intraventricular hemorrhage with periventricular echodense lesions. *Ann Neurol* 1984;15:285–290.

143. Meis PJ, Hall M, Marshall JR, Nobel CJ: Meconium passage: A new classification for risk assessment during labor. *Am J Obstet Gynecol* 1978;131:509–513.

144. Mellitis ED, Holden KR, Freeman JM: Neonatal seizures. II. A multivariate analysis of factors associated with outcome. *Pediatrics* 1982;70:177–185.

145. Ment LR, Duncan CC, Ehrenkranz RA: Perinatal cerebral infarction. *Ann Neurol* 1984;16:559–568.

146. Michenfelder JD: The interdependency of cerebral function and metabolic effects following massive doses of thiopental in the dog. *Anesthesiology* 1974;41:231–236.

147. Miligner AD, Wertheimer IS: Preliminary results of a computed tomography study of neonatal brain hypoxia-ischemia. *J Comput Assist Tomogr* 1980;4:457–463.

148. Miller FC: Prediction of acid-base values from intrapartum fetal heart rate data and their correlation with scalp and funic values, in Petrie RH (ed): *Clinics in Perinatology*. Philadelphia, WB Saunders, 1982, pp 353–362.

149. Mott JC: The ability of young mammals to withstand total oxygen lack. *Br Med Bull* 1961;17:144–148.

150. Mujsce DJ, Boyer MA, Vannucci RC: CBF and brain edema in perinatal cerebral hypoxia-ischemia. *Pediatr Res* 1987;21:494A.

151. Mulligan JC, Painter MJ, O'Donoughue PA, MacDonald HM, Allen AC, Taylor PM: Neonatal asphyxia. II. Neonatal mortality and long-term sequelae. *J Pediatr* 1980;96:903–907.

152. Myers RE: Experimental models of perinatal brain damage: Relevance to human pathology, in Gluck L (ed): *Intrauterine Asphyxia and the Developing Fetal Brain*. Chicago, Year Book Medical Publishers, 1977, pp 37–97.

153. Myers RE, Beard R, Adamsons K: Brain swelling in the newborn rhesus monkey following partial asphyxia. *Neurology* 1969;19:1021–1018.

154. Myers RE, Hill DE, Holt AB, Scott RE, Mellitis ED, Cheek DB: Fetal growth retardation produced by experimental placental insufficiency in the rhesus monkey. *Biol Neonate* 1971;18:379–394.

155. Myers RE, Yamaguchi S: Nervous system effects of cardiac arrest in monkeys. Preservation of vision. *Arch Neurol* 1977;34:65–74.

156. Naulty JS: Obstetric anesthesia, in Avery GB (ed): *Neonatology: Pathophysiology and Management of the Newborn.* Philadelphia, JB Lippincott, 1981, pp 132–144.

157. Nelson KB, Broman S: Perinatal risk factors in children with severe motor and mental handicaps. *Ann Neurol* 1977;2:371–377.

158. Nelson KB, Ellenberg JH: Apgar scores as predictors of chronic neurologic disability. *Pediatrics* 1981;68:36–44.

159. Nelson KB, Ellenberg JH: Neonatal signs as predictors of cerebral palsy. *Pediatrics* 1979;64:225–232.

160. Nelson NM: Respiration and circulation before birth; Respiration and circulation after birth, in Smith CC, Nelson NM (eds): *The Physiology of the Newborn Infant.* Springfield, IL, Charles C Thomas, 1976, pp 15–263.

161. Norman MG: On the morphogenesis of ulegyria. *Acta Neuropathol* 1981;53:331–332.

162. Norman MG: Unilateral encephalomalacia in cranial nerve nuclei in neonates: Report of two cases. *Neurology* 1974;24:424–427.

163. Nwaesei CG, Pape KE, Martin DJ, Becker LE, Fitz CR: Periventricular infarction diagnosed by ultrasound: A postmortem correlation. *J Pediatr* 1984;105:106–110.

164. O'Dougherty M, Wright FS, Loewenson RB, Torres F: Cerebral dysfunction after chronic hypoxia in children. *Neurology* 1985;35:42–46.

165. Ohno K, Ito U, Inaba Y: Regional cerebral blood flow and stroke index after left carotid artery ligation in the conscious gerbil. *Brain Res* 1984;297:151–157.

166. Page FO, Martin JN, Palmer SM, Martin RW, Lucas JA, Meeks GR, Bucovaz ET, Morrison JC: Correlation of neonatal acid-base status with Apgar scores and fetal heart rate tracings. *Am J Obstet Gynecol* 1986;154:1306–1311.

167. Painter MJ, Bergman I, Crumrine P: Neonatal seizures. *Pediatr Clin North Am* 1986;33:91–109.

168. Painter MJ, Depp R, O'Donoghue PD: Fetal heart rate patterns and development in the first year of life. *Am J Obstet Gynecol* 1978;132:271–277.

169. Painter MJ, Pippenger C, MacDonald H, Pitlick W: Phenobarbital and diphenylhydantoin levels in neonates with seizures. *J Pediatr* 1978;92:315–319.

170. Paneth N, Stark RI: Cerebral palsy and mental retardation in relation to indicators of perinatal asphyxia. *Am J Obstet Gynecol* 1983;147:960–966.

171. Papile L, Rudolph A, Heymann MA: Autoregulation of cerebral blood flow in the preterm fetal lamb. *Pediatr Res* 1985;19:159–161.

172. Parisi JE, Collins GH, Kim RC, Crosley CJ: Prenatal symmetrical thalamic degeneration with flexion spasticity at birth. *Ann Neurol* 1983;13:94–97.

173. Paul RH: The evaluation of antepartum fetal well-being using the nonstress test, in Petrie RH (ed): *Clinics in Perinatology.* Philadelphia, WB Saunders, 1982, pp 253–264.

174. Paul RH, Yonekura ML, Contrell CJ, Turkey S, Pavlova Z, Sipos L: Fetal injury prior to labor: Does it happen? *Am J Obstet Gynecol* 1986;154:1187–1193.

175. Perelman RH, Farrell PM: Analysis of causes of neonatal death in the United States with specific emphasis on fetal hyaline membrane disease. *Pediatrics* 1982;70:570–575.

176. Picard L, Claudon M, Roland J, Jeanjean E, André M, Plenat P, Vert P: Cerebral computed tomography in premature infants, with an attempt at staging developmental features. *J Comput Assist Tomogr* 1980;4:435–444.

177. Platt LD, Eglinton GS, Sipos L, Broussard PM, Paul RH: Further experience with the fetal biophysical profile. *Obstet Gynecol* 1983;61:480–485.

178. Poland RL and others: Use and abuse of the Apgar score. *Pediatrics* 1986; 78:1148–1149.

179. Pryse-Davis J, Beard RW: A necropsy study of brain swelling in the newborn with special reference to cerebellar herniation. *J Pathol* 1972;109:51–56.

180. Pulsinelli WA, Levy DE, Duffy TE: Regional cerebral blood flow and glucose metabolism following transient forebrain ischemia. *Ann Neurol* 1982;11:499–509.

181. Pulsinelli WA, Waldman S, Rawlinson D, Plum F: Hyperglycemia converts neuronal damage into brain infarction. *Neurology* 1982;32:1239–1246.

182. Purves MJ: in *The Physiology of the Cerebral Circulation*. Cambridge, Massachusetts, Cambridge University Press, 1972.

183. Purves MJ, James IM: Observations on the control of cerebral blood flow in the sheep fetus and newborn lamb. *Circ Res* 1969;25:651–667.

184. Quencer RM, Parker JC, Hinkle DK: Maturation of normal primate cerebral tissue: Preliminary results of a computed tomographic-anatomic correlation. *J Comput Assist Tomogr* 1980;4:464–465.

185. Raichle ME: The pathophysiology of brain ischemia. *Ann Neurol* 1983;13:2–10.

186. Ranck JB, Windle WF: Brain damage in the monkey, *Macaca mulatta*, by asphyxia neonatorum. *Exp Neurol* 1959;1:130–154.

187. Rayburn WF: Antepartum fetal assessment, in Petrie RH (ed): *Clinics in Perinatology*. Philadelphia, WB Saunders, 1982, pp 231–252.

188. Reddy GD, Gootman N, Buckley NM, Gootman PM, Crane L: Regional blood flow changes in neonatal pigs in response to hypercapnia, hemorrhage and sciatic nerve stimulation. *Biol Neonate* 1984;25:249–262.

189. Reivich M, Brann AW, Shapiro H: Reactivity of cerebral vessels to CO_2 in the newborn rhesus monkey. *Eur Neurol* 1971;6:132–136.

190. Reivich M, Brann AW, Shapiro H, Myers RE: Regional cerebral blood flow during prolonged partial asphyxia, in Myer JS, Reivich M, Lechner H (eds): *Research on the Cerebral Circulation*. Springfield, IL, Charles C Thomas, 1972, pp 216–227.

191. Rice JE, Vannucci RC, Brierley JB: The influence of immaturity on hypoxic-ischemic brain damage in the rat. *Ann Neurol* 1981;9:131–141.

192. Rorke LB: *Pathology of Perinatal Brain Injury*. New York, Raven Press, 1982, pp 4–12.

193. Rose RL, Lombroso CT: Neonatal seizure states. *Pediatrics* 1970;45:404–425.

194. Rosen MG, Scibetta JJ, Chik L, Borgstedt AD: An approach to the study of brain damage: The principles of fetal electroencephalography. *Am J Obstet Gynecol* 1973;115:37–43.

195. Rosenberg AA, Jones MD, Traystman RJ, Simmons MA, Molteni RA: Response of cerebral blood flow to changes in PCO_2 in fetal, newborn and adult sheep. *Am J Physiol* 1982;242:H862–866.

196. Rothberg AD, Maisels MJ, Bagnato S, Murphy J, Gifford K, McKinley K: Infants weighing 1,000 grams or less at birth: Developmental outcome for ventilated and non-ventilated infants. *Pediatrics* 1983;71:599–602.

197. Roux JM, Tordet-Caridroit C, Chanez C: Studies on experimental hypotrophy in the rat. *Biol Neonate* 1970;15:342–347.

198. Saigal S, Rosenbaum P, Stoskopf B, Sinclair JC: Outcome in infants 501 to 1000 gm birthweight delivered to residents of the McMaster Health Region. *J Pediatr* 1984; 105:969–976.

199. Saint-Anne Dargassies S: Neurological maturation of the premature infant of 28 to 41 weeks gestational age, in Falkner F (ed): *Human Development*. Philadelphia, WB Saunders, 1966, pp 306–325.

200. Sarnat HB, Sarnat MS: Neonatal encephalopathy following fetal distress—A clinical and electroencephalographic study. *Arch Neurol* 1976;33:695–706.

201. Schneider H, Balowitz L, Schachinger H, Hanefeld F, Dröszus JU: Anoxic encephalopathy with predominant involvement of basal ganglia, brain stem and spinal cord in the perinatal period. *Acta Neuropathol* 1975;32:287–298.

202. Schrumpf JD, Sehring S, Killpack S, Brady JP, Hirata T, Mednick JP: Correlation of early neurologic outcome and CT findings in neonatal brain hypoxia and injury. *J Comput Assist Tomogr* 1980;4:445–450.

203. Scott H: Outcome of very severe birth asphyxia. *Arch Dis Child* 1976;51:712–716.

204. Seltzer ME, Myers RE, Holstein SF: Prolonged partial asphyxia: Effects of fetal brain water and electrolytes. *Neurology* 1972;22:732–737.

205. Shapiro HM, Greenberg JH, Naughton KVH, Reivich M: Heterogeneity of local cerebral blood flow-PACO$_2$ sensitivity in neonatal dogs. *J Appl Physiol* 1980;49:113–118.

206. Shen EY, Huang CC, Chyou SC, Hung HY, Hsu CH, Huang FY: Sonographic findings of the bright thalamus. *Arch Dis Child* 1986;61:1096–1099.

207. Shuman RM, Selednik LJ: Periventricular leukomalacia: A one-year autopsy study. *Arch Neurol* 1980;37:231–235.

208. Siesjö BK: Cell damage in the brain: A speculative synthesis. *J Cereb Blood Flow Metab* 1981;1:155–185.

209. Silbert A, Wolff PH, Stickler GB, Weidman WH: Children with congenital heart disease. *Pediatrics* 1969;43:192–200.

210. Slotkin TA, Cowdery TS, Orband L, Pachman S, Whitmore WL: Effects of neonatal hypoxia on brain development in the rat: Immediate and long-term biochemical alterations in discrete areas. *Brain Res* 1986;374:63–74.

211. Sokol RJ, Rosen MG, Chik L: Fetal electroencephalographic monitoring related to infant outcome. *Am J Obstet Gynecol* 1977;127:329–333.

212. Stafford A, Weatherall JAC: The survival of young rats in nitrogen. *J Physiol* 1960;153:457–472.

213. Steiner H, Neligau G: Perinatal cardiac arrest. *Arch Dis Child* 1975;50:692–702.

214. Stewart AL, Thorburn RJ, Hope PL, Goldsmith M, Lipscomb AP, Reynolds EOR: Ultrasound appearance of the brain in very preterm infants and neuro-developmental outcome at 18 months of age. *Arch Dis Child* 1983;58:598–604.

215. Szymonowicz W, Preston H, Yu VYH: The surviving monozygotic twin. *Arch Dis Child* 1986;61:454–458.

216. Szymonowicz W, Schafler K, Cussen LJ, Yu VYH: Ultrasound and necropsy study of periventricular hemorrhage in preterm infants. *Arch Dis Child* 1984;59:637–642.

217. Takashima S, Ando Y, Takeshita K: Hypoxic-ischemic brain damage and cerebral blood flow changes in young rabbits. *Brain Dev* 1986;8:274–277.

218. Takashima S, Taraka K: Development of cerebrovascular architecture and its relationship to periventricular leukomalacia. *Arch Neurol* 1978;35:11–16.

219. Thakkar N, O'Neil W, Duvally J, Liu C, Ambler M: Möbius syndrome due to brainstem tegmental necrosis. *Arch Neurol* 1977;34:124–126.

220. Thomson AJ, Searle M, Russell G: Quality of survival after severe birth asphyxia. *Arch Dis Child* 1977;52:620–626.

221. Thurston JH, McDougal DB: Effect of ischemia on metabolism of the brain of the newborn mouse. *Am J Physiol* 1969;216:348–352.

222. Ting P, Yamaguchi S, Bacher JD, Killens RH, Myers RE: Hypoxic-ischemic cerebral necrosis in midgestational sheep fetuses: Physiopathologic correlations. *Exp Neurol* 1983;80:227–245.

223. Towbin A: Central nervous system damage in the human fetus and newborn infant. *Am J Dis Child* 1970;119:529–542.

224. Vannucci RC: Pathogenesis of perinatal hypoxic-ischemic brain damage, in Thompson RA, Green JR, Johnsen SD (eds): *Perinatal Neurology and Neurosurgery*. New York, Spectrum Publications, 1985, pp 17–39.

225. Vannucci RC, Duffy TE: Cerebral metabolism in newborn dogs during reversible asphyxia. *Ann Neurol* 1977;1:528–534.

226. Vannucci RC, Duffy TE: Cerebral oxidative and energy metabolism of fetal and neonatal rats during anoxia and recovery. *Am J Physiol* 1976;230:1269–1275.

227. Vannucci RC, Duffy TE: The influence of birth on carbohydrate and energy metabolism in rat brain. *Am J Physiol* 1974;226:933–940.

228. Vannucci RC, Hernandez MJ: Perinatal cerebral blood flow, in Sinclair JC, Warshaw JB, Bloom RS (eds): *Perinatal Brain Insult*. Mead Johnson Symposium on Perinatal and Developmental Medicine 17, 1981, pp 17–29.

229. Vannucci RC, Lyons DT, Vasta F: Regional cerebral blood flow during hypoxia-ischemia in the immature rat. *Stroke* 1988;19:245–250.

230. Vannucci RC, Nardis EE, Vannucci SJ: Cerebral metabolism during hypoglycemia and asphyxia in newborn dogs. *Biol Neonate* 1980;38:276–286.

231. Vannucci RC, Plum F: Pathophysiology of perinatal hypoxic-ischemic brain damage, in Gaull GE (ed): *Biology of Brain Dysfunction*. New York, Plenum, 1975, vol 3, pp 1–45.

232. Vannucci RC, Vannucci SJ: Cerebral carbohydrate metabolism during hypoglycemia and anoxia in newborn rats. *Ann Neurol* 1978;4:173–179.

233. Vannucci RC, Vasta F, Vannucci SJ: Cerebral metabolic responses of hyperglycemia immature rats to hypoxia-ischemia. *Pediatr Res* 1987;21:524–529.

234. Vannucci RC, Voorhies TM: Perinatal cerebral hypoxia-ischemia: Pathogenesis and neuropathology, in Sarnat HB (ed): *Topics in Neonatal Neurology*. Orlando, FL, Grune & Stratton, 1984, pp 27–60.

235. Vannucci RC, Wolff JW: Oxidative metabolism in fetal rat brain during maternal anesthesia. *Anesthesiology* 1978;48:238–244.

236. Vasan NS, Chase HP: Brain glycosaminoglycans (mucopolysaccharides) following intrauterine growth retardation. *Biol Neonate* 1976;28:196–206.

237. Vohr BR, Oh W, Rosenfield AG, Cowett RM, Berstein J: The preterm small-for-gestational age infant: A two-year follow-up study. *Am J Obstet Gynecol* 1979;133:425–431.

238. Volpe JJ: in *Neurology of the Newborn*, II. Philadelphia, WB Saunders, 1987.

239. Volpe JJ, Hercovitch P, Pearlman J, Kreusser KL, Raichle ME: Positron emission tomography in the asphyxiated term newborn: Parasagittal impairment of cerebral blood flow. *Ann Neurol* 1985;17:287–296.

240. Voorhies TM, Rawlinson D, Vannucci RC: Glucose and perinatal hypoxic-ischemic brain damage in the rat. *Neurology* 1986;36:1115–1118.

241. Wagner KR, Ting P, Westfall MV, Yamaguchi S, Bacher, Myers RE: Brain metabolic correlates of hypoxic-ischemic cerebral necrosis in mid-gestational sheep fetuses: Significance of hypotension. *J Cereb Blood Flow Metab* 1986;6:425–434.

242. Weisbrot IM, James LS, Prince CE, Holaday DA, Apgar V: The acid-base homeostasis of the newborn infant during the first 24 hours of life. *J Pediatr* 1958;52:395–406.

243. Welsh FA, Vannucci RC, Brierley JB: Columnar alterations of NADH fluorescence during hypoxia-ischemia in immature rat brain. *J Cereb Blood Flow Metab* 1982;2:221–228.

244. Westwood M, Kramer MS, Munz D, Lovett JM, Walters GV: Growth and development of full-term nonasphyxiated small-for-gestational-age newborns: Follow-up through adolescence. *Pediatrics* 1983;71:376–382.

245. Wigglesworth JS: Experimental growth retardation in the foetal rat. *J Pathol Bacteriol* 1964;88:1–16.

246. Wilson ER, Mirra SS, Schwartz JF: Congenital diencephalic and brain stem damage: Neuropathologic study of three cases. *Acta Neuropathol* 1982;57:70–74.

247. Windle WF: *Physiology of the Fetus.* Springfield, IL, Charles C Thomas, 1971.

248. Windle WF: Brain damage at birth: Functional and structural modification with time. *JAMA* 1968;206:1967–1972.

249. Winick M: *Malnutrition and Brain Development.* New York, Oxford University Press, 1976.

250. Yoshioka H, Kadomoto Y, Mino M, Morikawa Y, Kasubuchi Y, Kusunoki T: Multicystic encephalomalacia in liveborn twin with a stillborn macerated co-twin. *J Pediatr* 1979;95:798–800.

251. Young RSK, Hernandez MJ, Yagel SK: Selective reduction of blood flow to white matter during hypotension in newborn dogs: A possible mechanism of periventricular leukomalacia. *Ann Neurol* 1982;12:445–448.

252. Younkin DP, Delivoria-Papadopoulos M, Leonard JC, Subramanian VH, Eleff S, Leigh JS, Chance B: Unique aspects of human newborn cerebral metabolism evaluated with phosphorus nuclear magnetic resonance spectroscopy. *Ann Neurol* 1984;16:581–586.

253. Younkin D, Reivich M, Jaggi J, Obrist W, Delivoria-Papadopoulos M: Noninvasive method of estimating human newborn regional cerebral blood flow. *J Cereb Blood Flow Metab* 1982;2:415–420.

254. Zuspan FP, Quillidan EJ, Iams JD, van Geijn HP: NICHD consensus development task force report: Predictors of intrapartum fetal distress—The role of electronic fetal monitoring. *J Pediatr* 1979;95:1026–1030.

8

Acute Perinatal Brain Injury: Intracranial Hemorrhage

Robert C. Vannucci

PERIVENTRICULAR/INTRAVENTRICULAR HEMORRHAGE

Periventricular (PVH) and intraventricular hemorrhage (IVH) together comprise the most commonly encountered acute perinatal brain insults and are major causes of death and disability, especially in low birth weight infants.[33,56,128,159] Hemorrhage is associated with respiratory distress syndrome in 50% to 95% of cases, and is the most common neuropathologic finding in infants dying with this pulmonary disorder.[81] It has been estimated that PVH/IVH occurs in 35% to 60% of premature infants with birth weight less than 1,800 g; the more immature the infant at birth, the greater the likelihood that hemorrhage will occur.[11,13,114,120,136] Improvement in the obstetric and neonatal management of the complex problems faced by the premature neonate has led to the survival of many infants who have sustained IVH. Although the long-term outcome of these infants is still understood incompletely, there is evidence that those with the most severe hemorrhages have a high incidence of subsequent neurodevelopmental handicap.[36,68,70,90,111,143,145] While an understanding of the pathogenesis of IVH and thereby its prevention are appropriate long-range goals, the accurate diagnosis, identification of adverse risk factors, and management of posthemorrhagic complications are of immediate importance in the care of the high-risk newborn infant.

This work was supported by Grants 09109 and 15738 from the National Institute of Child Health and Human Development, and Grant 19190 from the National Heart and Lung Institute.

PATHOGENESIS OF PVH/IVH

Neuroanatomic Factors

Many etiologic factors are related to the occurrence of IVH, but prematurity itself is the most consistent finding. The association of PVH/IVH with prematurity is based in large part on the neuroanatomic features of the periventricular region of the fetal and newborn brain at 5 to 8 months gestational age (Table 8-1). The germinal matrix (GM) (Figure 8-1) develops laterally and inferiorly to the lateral ventricles of the cerebral hemispheres and immediately beneath the ependymal lining. The GM is the site of origin of primitive neuroblasts (precursors of neurons) and of spongioblasts (precursors of astrocytes and oligodendrocytes) that migrate from the subependymal zone into the evolving cerebral cortex and midline gray matter structures (basal ganglia, thalamus, and hypothalamus). Prior to the 26th week, the GM extends along the entire length of the lateral ventricles, including the anterior horns, bodies, posterior, and temporal horns. With increasing age and the continued migration of primitive cells (predominantly or exclusively spongioblasts), the GM slowly involutes so that by 32 to 34 weeks it is represented by a narrow zone of cells between the lateral ventricle and the head of the caudate nucleus at the level of the foramen of Monro.[22,55,134,161] The GM is identified rarely in the term infant.

Neuropathologic investigations have demonstrated that the sites of origin of PVH differ among premature infants of varying gestational age. In the extremely premature infant, PVH occurs typically in the GM along the body of the lateral ventricle and caudate nucleus. In infants older than 28 weeks gestational age, hemorrhage is more likely to occur adjacent to the anterior horn of the lateral ventricle at the head of the caudate

---

Table 8-1 Pathophysiology of Perinatal PVH/IVH

Neuroanatomic Features of the Germinal Matrix
   Primitive cellular architecture
   Immature vascular bed

Extrinsic Factors That Promote Hemorrhage
   Altered cerebral blood flow (increased or decreased)
   Increased cerebral blood volume
   Change in vascular:parenchymal (transmural) pressure gradient
   Prior vascular and/or parenchymal injury

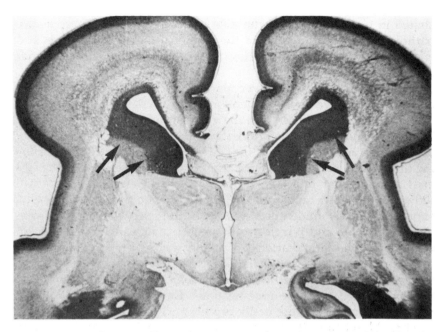

Figure 8-1 Coronal section of brain of a premature infant at 24 weeks gestation. Note the well-developed darkly stained germinal matrix (arrows) adjacent to the lateral ventricle of each cerebral hemisphere.

nucleus.[55,80] Thus, PVH is focused on those regions of GM characterized by the presence of clusters of closely packed cells separated by acellular areas of low structural resistance.

Vascular Factors

The predilection for hemorrhage to occur in the GM relates to features of the vascular anatomy and blood supply intrinsic to this primitive region of brain. In the past, investigators emphasized the peculiar structure of the deep venous system of the brain as a causal factor in GM hemorrhage. The terminal, choroidal, and thalamostriate veins drain the subependymal areas of the immature brain; these vessels converge anteriorly to form the internal cerebral vein. The direction of blood flow changes at this juncture as the internal cerebral vein makes an acute bend to course posteriorly to join the great vein of Galen. Thrombosis and venous occlusion within this deep venous system have been demonstrated in newborn infants who died with IVH.[74,130,147] These neuro-pathologic observations led to the proposal that venous stasis and engorgement result in extravasation of blood into the GM and surrounding areas of brain.[74,75,147]

In contrast to the theory of a venous origin for PVH/IVH, Wigglesworth and colleagues have directed attention to the arterial side of the cerebral vasculature.[48,113,161] Studies on the vascular anatomy of the immature brain have shown that the arteries supplying blood to the developing basal ganglia and, presumably, the GM are large relative to those perfusing the cerebral cortex.[55,160] Furthermore, blood vessels within the GM exist as a vascular rete (i.e., a primitive arteriovenous anastomosis), rather than a mature capillary bed.[113] The rete is composed of thin-walled sinusoidal vessels unidentifiable as either arterioles, capillaries, or venules. Hambleton and Wigglesworth[55] injected a colored barium-gelatin solution into the carotid arteries of infants who had died with IVH and found prominent leaks within the GM. No such leaks occurred when the jugular veins were injected with the same material at the same infusion pressure. Based on these investigations, they proposed that cerebral vessels within the GM are easily ruptured when exposed to increased cerebral blood flow (CBF) or increased cerebral perfusion pressure brought about by systemic stresses known to alter CBF.

Pathophysiologic Factors

The neuroanatomic features of the GM and its vascular bed provide the structural framework (or lack thereof) for hemorrhage to occur, whereas systemic physiologic disturbances most likely account for production of the hemorrhage itself (see Table 8-1). Whether the precipitating factor is an alteration in blood flow within the GM or a change in perfusion pressure is unknown; but the two variables are intimately related. Blood flow is related directly to perfusion pressure and inversely to vascular resistance. Perfusion pressure is influenced primarily by arterial blood pressure. Vascular resistance is regulated by the interstitial pressure within the surrounding brain tissue itself, measured as intracranial pressure (ICP), and by the elasticity of the blood vessel wall (intramural pressure). Under physiologic conditions in mature cerebral arteries (arterioles), perfusion pressure and vascular resistance are finely tuned to maintain CBF constant, that is, CBF is autoregulated. When autoregulation is disrupted by hypoxia or respiratory acidosis, cerebral capillaries become exposed to the direct driving force of systemic blood pressure; the vessels then may rupture and bleed. Cerebral vascular autoregulation is impaired in premature infants asphyxiated at birth, during which CBF becomes pressure-passive to alterations in systemic blood pressure.[88] It is also possible, although not documented in human infants, that the immature blood vessels of the GM do not autoregulate even under physiologic conditions. Then any increase in systemic blood pressure would result in an elevation of cerebral perfusion pressure.

The physiologic events that accompany the transition from fetal to postnatal life may contribute to IVH, especially in the premature infant. During the first few days following birth, the newborn loses body fluid. The brain appears to participate in this process, as indicated by an early postnatal shrinkage in head size.[162] A decline in ICP parallels the decrease in brain volume.[121,157] The lowering of ICP or increasing systemic blood pressure increases the pressure gradient from blood vessel to interstitial space and, therefore, might increase cerebral perfusion pressure to the extent that the immature vascular channels of the GM rupture and cause hemorrhage.[22] Any factor that accentuates brain shrinkage, for example, plasma hyperosmolality, might contribute to this tendency to hemorrhage.

There appears to be a baseline incidence of PVH/IVH in premature infants that relates to the anatomic vulnerability of the GM. When hemodynamic alterations are superimposed on this susceptible structure, the predisposition to hemorrhage is increased.[30] In particular, mechanical ventilation, pneumothorax, volume expansion, and bicarbonate administration have been implicated as postnatal factors exacerbating the bleeding tendency.[30,39,86,137,153]

Animal Studies

Investigations in experimental animals have contributed to our understanding of the pathogenesis of human perinatal PVH/IVH.[123] The brain of the fetal monkey at term, like the human fetus, is relatively mature and no longer possesses a prominent GM. This lack of a GM explains why Myers and colleagues have been unable to produce IVH in the monkey despite the presence of experimentally induced hypoxic-ischemic brain damage.[11,104,105] An alternative explanation is that PVH/IVH is not causally associated with the tissue necrosis (infarction) that arises from cerebral hypoxia-ischemia. However, both PVH/IVH and periventricular hemorrhagic infarction certainly coexist in premature human infants, although their etiologies differ.

Reynolds et al.[122] have been successful in producing IVH in midgestation fetal sheep. Asphyxia alone was not associated with an increased frequency of IVH,[146] whereas asphyxia combined with raised arterial (maternal transfusion) and/or venous (superior vena cava obstruction) blood pressures did cause hemorrhage. Furthermore, arterial hypertension, induced by blood transfusion and norepinephrine infusion without asphyxia, also resulted in an increased incidence of IVH. The study indicates that hypoxia-acidosis is not a prerequisite for IVH, but that its presence increases the likelihood of hemorrhage in the midst of fluctuations in cerebral perfusion pressure.

The newborn dog provides an excellent model of IVH, since its size allows for systemic physiologic monitoring as well as for studies of regional CBF and metabolism.[16,29,99,150] PVH/IVH occurs with increased frequency in newborn dogs subjected to either acute hypoxemia, respiratory acidosis, or arterial hypertension. Goddard et al.[41] produced IVH in two of five normoxic puppies by the rapid induction of severe hypercapnic acidosis. Such extremes of respiratory acidosis would be expected to dilate maximally those cerebral blood vessels known to be sensitive to the vasoactive effect of carbon dioxide, even in these young animals.[16,60,133] Whether or not the primitive blood vessels of the GM exhibit carbon dioxide sensitivity is not known.

In further studies, Goddard et al.[42] produced intracranial hemorrhage in newborn dogs by phenylephrine-induced arterial hypertension. Both GM hemorrhages and IVH were observed. PVH/IVH also occurred when pups were subjected to rapidly induced hypovolemic hypotension (partial exsanguination) followed by rapid volume expansion by reinfusion of blood to produce normotension.[43,98] Paradoxically, this procedure led to elevations in CBF (131%–142% of control), greatest in hindbrain structures, even during the period of systemic hypotension, with further increases in flow during volume reexpansion.[44] The investigators hypothesized that the changes in CBF reflected peripheral vasoconstriction concurrent with cerebral vasodilation in response to partial exsanguination, which was accentuated during systemic reperfusion. The rapidity of the changes in blood flow might also have contributed to the increased incidence of IVH.

In a recent investigation, Ment et al.[99] subjected newborn dogs to normotensive hypoxemia and produced PVH/IVH. Regional CBF, measured during the hypoxic insult, was increased significantly in the GM. This study indicates that the immature blood vessels of the GM respond appropriately to systemic hypoxia, but it remains to be determined whether or not they respond similarly to elevations in blood carbon dioxide tensions.

To determine the presence and extent to which GM blood vessels autoregulate,[59] Pasternak and Groothuis[117] subjected newborn dogs to phenylephrine-induced systemic hypertension during which CBF of the GM and other brain regions was determined. The results showed that over the blood pressure range 35 to 70 torr, blood flow within the GM did not change, whereas flows increased progressively to twice the normal value (50 mL/100 g/min) at blood pressures in the range of 75 to 105 torr. The findings indicate that CBF autoregulation of the GM is confined to a narrow range and that blood flow becomes pressure passive at even modestly elevated systemic blood pressures. As discussed previously, a pressure-passive state exposes the GM capillaries to the direct driving force of systemic blood pressure, thereby increasing perfusion pressure and the potential for vascular rupture.

The above-described experimental investigations are helpful in clarifying the contributions of hypoxia, acidosis, and alterations in systemic blood pressure to the pathogenesis of PVH/IVH. Hypoxemia is not an absolute prerequisite for IVH, since arterial or venous hypertension and possibly hypercapnia alone can lead to intracranial hemorrhage. However, hypoxemia or asphyxia, especially when combined with elevations in arterial or cephalic venous pressure, does increase the likelihood of PVH/IVH. Therefore, it is probable that the cerebral vasodilatation resulting from systemic hypoxia or hypercapnia initiates the pathophysiologic events that culminate in PVH/IVH.

It is unlikely that hypoxic-ischemic brain damage plays any major role in the genesis of IVH, since hemorrhage occurs during the course of, rather than following, the systemic stress, long before pathologic alterations in brain tissue are apparent histologically. That hypoxic-ischemic brain damage need not precede intracranial hemorrhage is supported by the absence of ischemic infarction in many cases of IVH in human newborn infants.[50,80,107,134]

NEUROPATHOLOGY OF PVH/IVH

Neuropathologic alterations observed in perinatal PVH/IVH reflect the extent of the hemorrhage as well as the interval of infant survival following the vascular insult to the brain. Pathologic alterations in brains of infants dying acutely or subacutely are characterized by: (a) one or more areas of hemorrhage originating in the GM and/or adjacent structures and extending into the periventricular and subcortical white matter; (b) disruption of the ependyma; and (c) casts of blood partially or completely filling and often distending the ventricular system and spreading into the subarachnoid space[26,80,128] (Figures 8-2 to 8-4). Smaller hemorrhages may be confined to the GM or limited to one lateral ventricle.

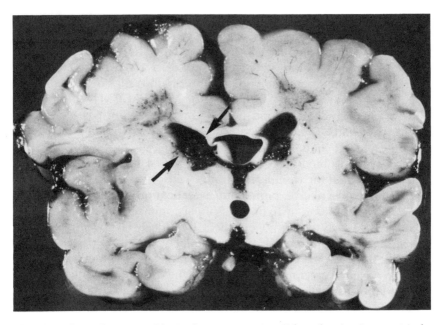

Figure 8-2 Coronal section of brain from a premature infant showing intraventricular hemorrhage. Blood clot is present primarily in the slightly expanded left lateral ventricle (arrows) and in the third ventricle. A germinal matrix hemorrhage is present on the right.

The chronic neuropathologic changes seen following PVH/IVH include: (a) one or more areas of cavitation within the periventricular white matter which may communicate with the ventricular system (porencephaly); (b) hydrocephalus, resulting either from meningeal fibrosis (communicating) or periventricular gliosis (obstructive); (c) cystic degeneration and sclerosis of periventricular white matter (periventricular leukomalacia); and (d) atrophy of the cerebral and cerebellar gray matter.[26,76,107] Whether these white and gray matter lesions in brains are primarily of hypoxic-ischemic origin or the direct consequence of IVH is unknown. In an analysis of the pathology of 170 infants who died with respiratory distress syndrome, Leech et al.[81] noted a conspicuous temporal dichotomy between hemorrhagic and nonhemorrhagic lesions in brain. GM and IVH were associated with short survival; death occurred usually within 4 days of birth. In contrast, periventricular leukomalacia was most prominent in the brains of infants dying after 4 days of age. These and other pathologic observations suggest that although hypoxic-ischemic brain damage and IVH may coexist, they have separate pathogenic mechanisms.[50]

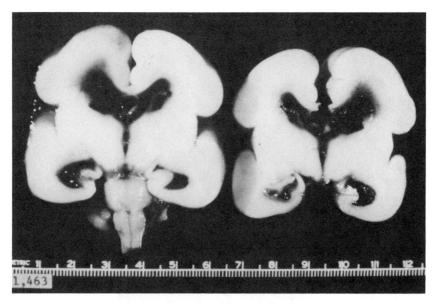

Figure 8-3 Coronal section of brain from a premature infant showing intraventricular hemorrhage. Blood clot is seen in both lateral and third ventricles, all of which are mildly expanded.

It is possible that IVH itself leads to ischemic necrosis (infarction) of vulnerable regions within the immature brain. Major hemorrhage from the GM into the lateral ventricles acutely increases ICP, which, if high enough, may disrupt drainage of blood through the deep venous system. Venous engorgement occurs with ultimate hemorrhagic necrosis of periventricular white matter. In this regard, Guzzetta et al.[52] have shown that periventricular hemorrhagic infarcts associated with IVH often are asymmetric and situated ipsilaterally to the lateral ventricles containing a large blood clot. Furthermore, Volpe et al.[154] measured regional CBF in newborn infants sustaining IVH and showed large areas of parenchymal ischemia well beyond the confines of the primary intraventricular and intracerebral hemorrhage.[96,97] It must be emphasized that periventricular hemorrhagic infarcts also occur in the absence of IVH;[52,81] in this instance, the pathogenic mechanism most likely is severe perinatal asphyxia.[149]

Hydrocephalus is a major complication of perinatal IVH. The pathologic hallmark of hydrocephalus is ventricular enlargement combined with evidence of disrupted cerebrospinal fluid (CSF) pathways.[74,75,107] Sites of obstruction include the aqueduct of Sylvius and the outlet foramina of Luschka and Magendie (obstructive hydrocephalus). Oblitera-

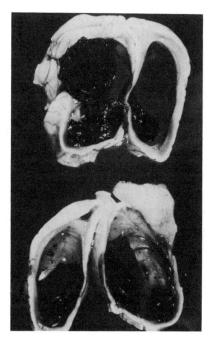

Figure 8-4 Coronal sections of the brain from a premature infant showing massive intraventricular hemorrhage with severe ventricular dilatation.

tion of the subarachnoid pathways results in communicating hydrocephalus. Both forms of hydrocephalus may occur acutely when blood clots are large enough to impede flow of CSF, while subacute and chronic forms are the consequence of periaqueductal gliosis and adhesive arachnoiditis. There also is evidence in experimental animals and humans that untreated communicating hydrocephalus may lead to the obstructive variety by a mechanism that distorts and ultimately constricts the aqueduct of Sylvius to the point of CSF obstruction.[10,108] Combined forms of hydrocephalus following perinatal IVH have been visualized by air and metrizamide ventriculography.[57]

RISK FACTORS

Numerous risk factors, of which prematurity is by far the most important, predispose the fetus and newborn infant to PVH/IVH (Figure 8-5). As mentioned previously, neuropathologic studies have demonstrated an inverse relationship between birth weight or gestational age and the incidence of hemorrhage.[26,33,160] More recent studies utilizing cranial

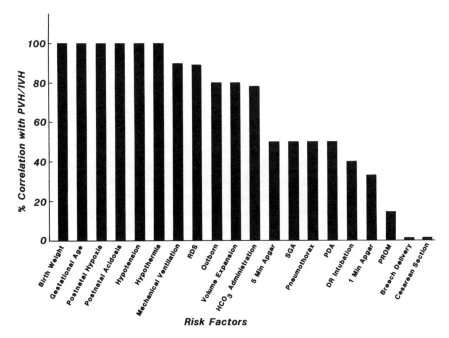

Figure 8-5 Risk factors associated with PVH/IVH in premature infants. Explanation of specific variables: low birth weight; low gestational age; presence of postnatal hypoxia, mechanical ventilation; occurrence of respiratory distress syndrome (RDS); need for volume expansion and/or bicarbonate administration; low 1- or 5-min Apgar score; small for gestational age (SGA); occurrence of pneumothorax; presence of patent ductus arteriosus (PDA); need for intubation in the delivery room (DR); premature rupture of membranes (PROM); breech delivery or cesarean section.

ultrasound (US) have confirmed the histologic observation that the more immature the infant at birth, the more likely the hemorrhage will occur.[83,94,120,140] Furthermore, increasing prematurity is associated with the most severe hemorrhages.[109]

Numerous investigations have focused on risk factors other than prematurity.[5,18,19,30,83,89,94,138,144,148] Of major importance is the fact that none of a variety of maternal complications of pregnancy, other than premature labor, have been demonstrated to be significantly related to the occurrence of PVH/IVH in the newborn infant. Negative correlations have been found for all major maternal conditions, including diabetes, hypertension, preeclampsia, heart disease, maternal age, and gravidity. Obstetric complications also do not appear to predispose the infant to PVH/IVH; this has been shown for placenta previa, abruptio placentae, premature rupture of membranes, prolonged labor, fetal distress, and multiple pregnancy. Similarly, obstetric intervention in the form of instrumental vaginal delivery or cesarean section poses no increased risk to the fetus over that of spontaneous vaginal delivery.[85,142] Vaginal breech presentation is no more deleterious than vertex presentation, despite its inherent risk of intrapartum asphyxia and mechanical trauma. In a single study, severe bruising at birth was a significant antecedent of hemorrhage.[138] Thus, complications of pregnancy, labor, and delivery contribute little to the overall incidence of PVH/IVH beyond that of prematurity itself.

In contrast to the absence of correlations between prepartum and intrapartum adverse events and PVH/IVH, numerous neonatal complications substantially increase the likelihood of hemorrhage in premature infants (Figure 8-5). Of these, immediate postpartum asphyxia and respiratory distress syndrome with their attendant hypoxia-acidosis, systemic hypotension, and hypothermia are strongly associated with hemorrhage.[40,59] Other significant risk factors include those therapeutic interventions required to reverse or minimize hypoxia-acidosis; especially major resuscitation at birth with intubation, mechanical ventilation, volume expansion, and bicarbonate administration.[46,137,138] To the extent that obstetric problems predispose to these adverse neonatal events, complications of pregnancy may contribute to the risk of PVH/IVH.

Pneumothorax, usually a complication of respirator therapy, also is considered a risk factor for PVH/IVH.[62,86] Pneumothorax leads to major alterations in systemic blood pressure, particularly arterial hypertension, which, in turn, influences cerebral hemodynamics adversely.[45,58] Even without pneumothorax, systemic hypertension—either continuous or episodic—is common among premature infants and contributes to the risk of PVH/IVH by increasing perfusion pressure within the GM vascular bed.[12,103,163]

Thus, both multivariate and univariate analyses of multiple risk factors for the occurrence of PVH/IVH in humans support the findings of experimental studies in animals that hypoxia, acidosis, and alterations in systemic blood pressure are the antecedent events that culminate in hemorrhage in susceptible newborns. Furthermore, these risk factors operate almost exclusively in the newborn period rather than prior to or during labor and delivery, which undoubtedly accounts for the low incidence of intracranial hemorrhage in stillborn fetuses.[161] The very fact that adverse events during pregnancy, labor, and delivery contribute so little to the risk of PVH/IVH suggests that birth itself and the infant's physiologic adjustment to extrauterine life is a prerequisite for hemorrhage to occur. Indeed, for the extremely small premature infant, few, if any, risk factors exist other than the process of being born.[159]

CLINICAL MANIFESTATIONS

The clinical spectrum of perinatal PVH/IVH ranges from an acute, catastrophic deterioration leading occasionally to death, to no symptoms or signs at all and no detectable sequelae.[57,77,153,156] The former clinical picture is characterized by an abrupt decrease in muscle tone and spontaneous activity, systemic hypotension, full fontanelles with splayed sutures, focal and major motor seizures, and abnormal eye movements. The most consistent nonradiographic laboratory findings include an abrupt fall in hematocrit or failure of the hematocrit to rise with blood transfusion and metabolic acidosis. Less dramatic presentations consist of subtle changes in tone and/or activity, brief multifocal seizures, and transient apnea and bradycardia. The ability to diagnose PVH/IVH clinically is related to the severity of hemorrhage visualized on US or CT (see below). Lazzara et al.[77] were able to predict PVH/IVH clinically in 81% of cases in which subsequent computed tomography (CT) scans demonstrated blood clot occupying more than one-half of the lateral ventricular volume. The ability to diagnose lesser degrees of hemorrhage was far less accurate and ranged from 22% to 35% of CT scan–proven cases.[77,114]

ALTERATIONS IN CEREBROSPINAL FLUID

Prior to the advent of US and CT scanning, the only way to diagnose perinatal IVH was by lumbar or ventricular puncture and analysis of CSF. Although lumbar puncture is not 100% reliable in diagnosing IVH,[77,136] it does provide valuable information regarding the presence or absence of subarachnoid hemorrhage or IVH. Hellmann and Vannucci[57,58] studied 19 premature infants who underwent at least two lumbar punctures, the first performed prior to any clinical evidence of IVH and the second upon clinical suspicion of hemorrhage later confirmed by CT scan or autopsy. Seven of the 19 initial CSF samples contained fewer than 30 red blood cells (RBC)/mL and 13 specimens contained fewer than 500 RBC/mL. Repeat CSF analysis upon suspicion of IVH revealed a 100-fold increase in the mean red cell count. Furthermore, there was no overlap of the ranges, as the red cell count increased in every infant.

Other abnormalities in CSF also occurred coincident with or following IVH. The mean leukocyte (white blood cell [WBC]) count of CSF prior to onset of IVH was low, as has been shown for apparently healthy newborn infants.[32,53,109,125] The increases in the WBC count of the posthemorrhage CSF were proportional to the increases in RBC counts. Protein concentrations of prehemorrhagic CSF were within the range of previously reported values;[32,53,125] but following IVH were greater than 200 mg/dL in all specimens. CSF glucose concentrations were within the normal range prior to any indication of IVH. Concentrations of glucose were unchanged immediately posthemorrhage but ultimately declined to very low levels in the majority of infants.

Thus, CSF analysis of the premature infant diagnoses IVH reliably when the fluid is deeply xanthrochromic, and contains greater than 40,000 RBC/mL and has greater than 200 mg/dL protein content. Hypoglycorrhachia (low CSF glucose) adds further support for the prior occurrence of IVH.

Hypoglycorrhachia is prominent following perinatal IVH.[25,57,93,106] The origin of the low CSF glucose has not been clarified entirely; but studies from our laboratory have demonstrated that elevated CSF lactate and lactate/pyruvate ratios are associated with low CSF glucose concentrations for up to 2 weeks posthemorrhage.[58] Also, erythrocytes and leukocytes in CSF metabolize glucose to lactic acid anaerobically, accounting, at least in part, for the observed metabolic alterations. Disrupted brain oxidative metabolism resulting from PVH/IVH may also contribute to the lingering abnormalities in CSF glucose and lactate homeostasis.[58,152]

RADIOGRAPHIC ABNORMALITIES

Computed Tomography

Computed tomographic scanning revolutionized our ability to diagnose PVH/IVH in the living newborn infant.[2,13,69,114] CT scan surveys documented an overall incidence of hemorrhage in between 40% and 45% of infants less than 1,500 g birth weight and less than 35 weeks gestational age.[2,13,114] CT enabled the clinician to determine not only the site and extent of hemorrhage but also the degree of acute or subacute ventricular enlargement and any neuropathologic sequelae. The correlation of CT with autopsy evidence of IVH has been extremely accurate, although not absolute.[2,37]

Several grading systems have been used to quantify the extent of PVH/IVH visualized on CT scan. The most widely utilized method was reported originally by Papile, Burstein, and colleagues[13,114] and consisted of four specific grades of hemorrhage: grade I, subependymal (GM) hemorrhage only; grade II, IVH without ventricular enlargement; grade III, IVH with acute ventricular enlargement; and grade IV, IVH also with extensive intracerebral hemorrhage (Figure 8-6). It must be emphasized that parenchymal hemorrhage distant from the GM with or without IVH or acute ventricular dilatation most likely represents hemorrhagic infarction arising from a pathogenic mechanism distinct from that

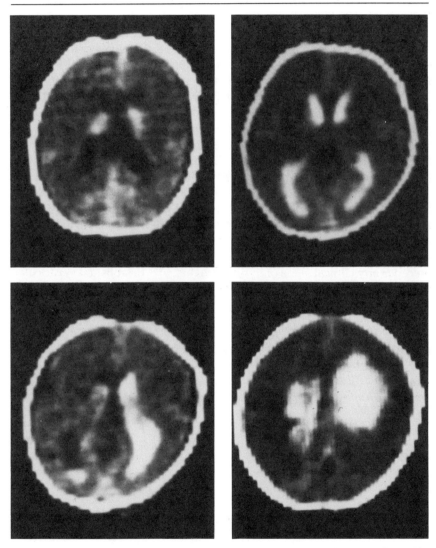

Figure 8-6 Representative CT scans of germinal matrix/intraventricular hemorrhage. The four scans depict increasing severity of PVH/IVH. Grade I (upper left), germinal matrix hemorrhage only; grade II (upper right), IVH without ventricular dilatation; grade III (lower left), IVH with ventricular dilatation; grade IV (lower right), IVH with parenchymal hemorrhage.

producing PVH/IVH.[52,61] Interpretation of the CT scan must take into account the interval between the presumed hemorrhage and the radiographic procedure, since retraction of the blood clot may lead to an underestimation of the extent of hemorrhage,[38] and dissolution of the clot may result in the absence of hemorrhagic densities on the scan after 10 to 15 days.[3,79,136]

The incidence and severity of PVH/IVH in premature infants as determined by CT scanning are readily discernible. In 100 consecutively studied infants with birth weights less than 1,500 g, Burstein et al.[13] found 44 exhibited hemorrhage within the first week of postnatal life (Table 8-2). The severity of hemorrhage was relatively equally distributed among the four grades described above. In a larger population of infants less than 35 weeks gestational age, Ahmann et al.[2] found 77 (40%) who had sustained PVH/IVH within 24 to 96 hr of birth (Table 8-3). Unlike the study of Burstein et al.,[13] moderate to severe hemorrhage predominated in the group, as did mortality and neurologic morbidity.

The subacute and chronic neuropathologic sequelae of PVH/IVH can be visualized radiographically by sequential CT scanning.[3,78,79,129] Progressive ventricular dilatation following IVH often occurs, particularly in those infants that sustained larger hemorrhages.[2,13,78,79] Dilatation can be observed immediately or up to 3 weeks posthemorrhage[3] and often precedes any clinical signs of hydrocephalus.[2,155] Established ventricular enlargement implies either hydrocephalus or cerebral atrophy. The distinction between these two pathologic entities may be difficult and

Table 8-2 Incidence of Severity of PVH/IVH in 100 CT Scanned Premature Infants Weighing < 1,500 g

Grade of Hemorrhage	No. Infants	Progressive Hydrocephalus	Deaths
None	56	0	13
I	10	0	3
II	10	0	4
III	14	5	8
IV	10	3	7
Total	44	8	22

Grade I = subependymal (GM) hemorrhage only; grade II = IVH without ventricular enlargement; grade III = IVH with ventricular enlargement; grade IV = IVH with extensive intracerebral hemorrhage.

Source: Reprinted with permission from "Intraventricular Hemorrhage and Hydrocephalus in Premature Newborns: A Prospective Study with CT" by J Burstein, LA Papile, and R Burstein in *American Journal of Roentgenology* (1979;132:631–635), Copyright © 1979, American Roentgen Ray Society.

Table 8-3 Incidence and Severity of PVH/IVH in 191 CT Scanned Premature Infants < 35 Weeks Gestational Age

Grade of Hemorrhage	No. Infants	Progressive Hydrocephalus	Deaths
None	114 (60%)	0	8
SEH	6 (4%)	0	0
Mild IVH	16 (8%)	0	2
Moderate IVH	20 (10%)	4	3
Severe IVH	35 (18%)	8	17
Total	77 (40%)	12	22

Mild IVH = blood filling < one-fourth of lateral ventricles; moderate IVH = blood filling < one-half of lateral ventricles; SEH = subependymal (GM) hemorrhage only; severe IVH = blood filling > one-half of lateral ventricles.

Source: Reprinted with permission from *Annals of Neurology* (1980;7:118–124), Copyright © 1980, Little, Brown & Company.

requires additional clinical and laboratory information, including serial measurements of head size, direct or indirect measurements of ICP, and the presence or absence of associated abnormalities on CT. Expansion of the subarachnoid spaces over the convexities of the cerebral hemispheres suggests cerebral atrophy. Dilatation of the lateral, third, and fourth ventricles suggests communicating hydrocephalus or ventricular obstruction at the level of the outlet foramina of Luschka and Magendie. Lateral and third ventricular enlargement with a normal size or small fourth ventricle connotes obstruction along the aqueduct of Sylvius.

Sequential CT scanning also reveals chronic alterations in periventricular white matter and the development of porencephalic cysts.[3,38,79,118,129] Cystic lesions presumably arise as a consequence of liquefaction of necrotic brain parenchyma destroyed previously by tissue hemorrhage. As anticipated, contralateral motor deficits (hemiparesis) often are an associated clinical finding.[118]

Cranial Ultrasonography

Imaging of the brain by ultrasonography (US) has proved a useful and accurate substitute for CT scanning.[47,126,136] The brain can be visualized in the coronal and sagittal plane using the anterior fontanelle as the acoustic window. Excellent visualization of the lateral, third, and fourth ventricles as well as the GM, periventricular white matter, caudate nucleus, and thalamus is possible. Hemorrhages appear as echogenic, castlike structures adjacent to or within the ventricular system (Figure 8-7).

The sensitivity and specificity of ultrasonographic diagnosis of PVH/IVH compared with CT has been demonstrated repeatedly.[47,126,136] However, neither method of brain imaging is 100% accurate in detecting intracranial hemorrhage when compared to postmortem examination.[37,112] In view of its accuracy, portability and the absence of ionizing radiation, US has become the standard diagnostic tool for the study of the presence and evolution of PVH/IVH and its complications.

Sequential US scanning has provided important information regarding the time of occurrence and early evolution of PVH/IVH in the newborn period. Szymonowicz and Yu[138] studied 30 premature infants weighing less than 1,250 g at birth and found that GM hemorrhage temporally preceded IVH, which, in turn, preceded the development of intracerebral

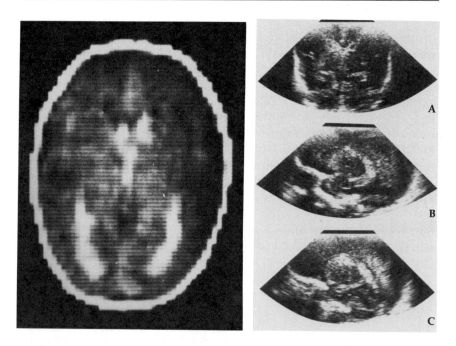

Figure 8-7 Germinal matrix and intraventricular hemorrhage in a 2-day-old premature infant: correlation of CT scan with ultrasound. The CT scan shows blood in the periventricular region and in both lateral ventricles. Ultrasound scans in coronal view **(A)** and in left **(B)** and right **(C)** sagittal views show blood in the germinal matrix, body, trigone, and temporal horn of both lateral ventricles.

hemorrhage. The hemorrhagic diathesis was essentially complete by 4 postnatal days. In a more detailed sequential US study, de Crespigny et al.[24] determined that of 47 infants weighing less than 1,500 g at birth, 10 (21%) had already suffered PVH/IVH by 1 hr of postnatal life and 32 (68%) by 24 hr. These and other data[7,120] indicate that PVH/IVH begins typically within 24 hr following birth and evolves to its maximum extent over the ensuing 48 to 72 hr. Therapeutic strategies focused on prevention of PVH/IVH must take into account the early initiation of the hemorrhage (see below).

Like CT scanning, the early and late evolution of neuropathologic sequelae of PVH/IVH are definable readily on US. Thus, sequential scanning allows the clinician to ascertain the presence and extent of ventricular dilatation following hemorrhage, as well as the development of porencephaly[48,84,120,126,132,140] (Figures 8-8 and 8-9).

POSTHEMORRHAGIC HYDROCEPHALUS

Sequential CT or US scanning has demonstrated that 50% or more of the premature newborn infants who sustain IVH develop posthemorrhagic hydrocephalus.[3,4,64,65,116,132] Not unexpectedly, the incidence of hydrocephalus is greatest in those infants with the most severe hemorrhage, although the condition may occur following mild PVH/IVH.[35]

Hydrocephalus may be asymptomatic in the newborn period, because the lateral ventricles of the cerebral hemispheres can enlarge before the classic signs of increased ICP (increasing head size, bulging fontanelles, separated cranial sutures) develop.[2,155] Ventricular dilatation without a concurrent increase in head size presumably relates to decreased tensile strength of the cerebral white matter in the immature brain, owing to a paucity of myelin and a relatively high water content. Apparently, less pressure is required to compress the immature periventricular white matter than to overcome the restrictive forces of the dura mater and skull vault.

Posthemorrhagic hydrocephalus results from blockage of CSF flow either within the ventricular system of the brain (obstructive) and/or within the basal cisterns along the subarachnoid pathways surrounding the brain (communicating). Approximately 50% of infants with posthemorrhagic hydrocephalus exhibit rapidly progressive ventricular enlargement in association with increased ICP.[64] It is likely that obstructive hydrocephalus is present in most if not all of these infants. Often a shunting procedure will be required as definitive therapy. The remaining infants with hydrocephalus exhibit gradual ventricular dilatation over

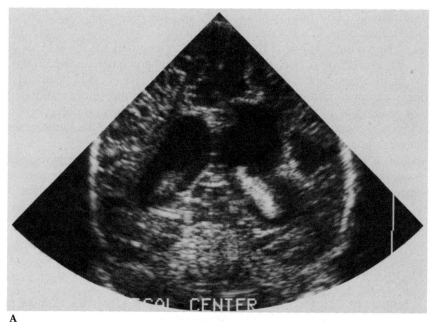

A

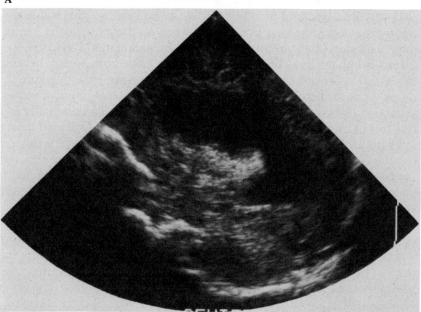

B

Figure 8-8 Coronal **(A)** and right sagittal **(B)** ultrasound scans of a premature infant showing posthemorrhagic hydrocephalus. Residual blood clot is seen in both lateral ventricles.

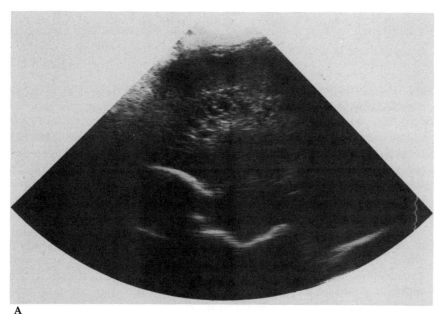

A

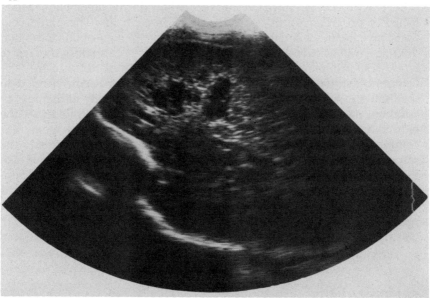

B

Figure 8-9 Sequential right sagittal ultrasound scans of a premature infant showing the evolution of periventricular leukomalacia with cyst formation. Scans **A** and **B** were performed at 2 and 4 weeks, respectively, following the occurrence of periventricular hemorrhagic infarction.

3 or more weeks in the absence of substantial elevations of ICP, that is, normal pressure communicating hydrocephalus.[4,64] Ventricular enlargement in these latter infants either stabilizes or reverts toward normal size or becomes progressive, ultimately requiring surgical intervention.[4,48,64]

MANAGEMENT

The immediate management of the newborn infant with PVH/IVH is focused on both the systemic and central nervous system derangements that result from brain parenchymal hemorrhage and rupture of blood into the ventricular system. Apnea, bradycardia, and hypotension are treated with cardiorespiratory support and blood is replaced as required. Seizures are treated with the appropriate anticonvulsant medication, usually phenobarbital. Blood within the ventricular system will ultimately dissipate even without therapeutic intervention. In a controlled study in which daily lumbar punctures were performed in an attempt to prevent hydrocephalus, no effect on the development of posthemorrhagic hydrocephalus could be demonstrated even though blood and protein were removed and ICP was lowered.[91]

Several procedures have been advocated for the management of established or progressive posthemorrhagic hydrocephalus. These interventions have included serial lumbar punctures,[17,66,116] external ventricular drainage,[63,64] ventriculoperitoneal shunting,[4,6,48,63] and drug therapy to retard CSF production and/or reduce intracranial hypertension.[63,135,141] Differences in the reported rates of success of these procedures relate to the timing of initiation and the duration of each modality of therapy. In addition, sequential CT and US scanning have demonstrated that the natural history of untreated posthemorrhagic ventricular enlargement is commonly one of spontaneous resolution.[3,4,65,84] Furthermore, the response to therapy also depends upon whether the hydrocephalus is of the obstructive or communicating variety.[63] That hydrocephalus unresponsive to serial lumbar punctures is probably obstructive in nature is supported by our own investigations in infants with progressive posthemorrhagic ventricular dilatation in whom sequential removal of CSF was unsuccessful and obstructive hydrocephalus was demonstrated by ventriculography.[57]

PREVENTION

It is possible that continued improvements in obstetric and neonatal management of premature infants will reduce the incidence and severity of PVH/IVH. However, there is likely a minimal incidence of hemorrhage that cannot be eliminated, except perhaps by the prevention of preterm birth.

Stringent guidelines for the current management of the sick premature newborn should help diminish the incidence of PVH/IVH. In this regard, Szymonowicz et al.[139] altered neonatal practice to include early intubation of distressed infants in the delivery room, prevention of hypothermia, rapid correction of hypoxia-acidosis and hypotension with ventilation and pharmacologic agents, and early recognition and treatment of pneumothorax. Muscular paralysis was accomplished if the activity of the infant led to respiratory instability. These therapeutic maneuvers were associated with PVH/IVH in only 36% of infants compared to a previously reported incidence of 60%. Thus, meticulous neonatal care to avoid or minimize the metabolic stresses of hypoxia-acidosis as well as fluctuations in systemic blood pressure appear to reduce the likelihood of hemorrhage in the high-risk premature newborn infant.

Pharmacologic intervention directed at ameliorating alterations in cerebral vascular reactivity and metabolism might provide protection from perinatal PVH/IVH. Several medications have been administered to premature infants in the early hours following birth in an attempt to prevent or minimize intracranial hemorrhage. These drugs have included phenobarbital, a CNS depressant;[28,72,102] ethamsylate, a hemostatic agent;[8,21,101] and indomethacin, a prostaglandin inhibitor.[95] Clinical traits of all three drugs have yielded contradictory results, thereby dampening early enthusiasm for a neonatal pharmacologic approach to the prevention of PVH/IVH.[27,31,67] Clinical investigations to confirm or deny the efficacy of these medications are still in progress.

Of obstetric importance is a recently published study on the use of maternally administered phenobarbital to prevent early neonatal PVH/IVH. Morales and Koerten[100] randomized 150 pregnant women in premature labor (less than 32 weeks) to phenobarbital treated and control groups. The prematurely delivered newborn infants were subjected to US examination to assess the presence and extent of intracranial hemorrhage. PVH/IVH occurred significantly less often in the treated infants, with a reduction in the incidence of hemorrhage from 47% to 21%. Furthermore, the incidence of severe hemorrhage was significantly less in the experimental group (5% vs. 20%). This investigation provides the impetus for further clinical trials of phenobarbital therapy in mothers suffering premature labor.

OUTCOME

The acute mortality of newborn infants with PVH/IVH is substantial and is dependent upon several factors, including the size of the hemorrhage, the maturity of the infant at birth, and associated disorders, especially the requirement for mechanical ventilation.[36,38,69,145,153] In general, the more immature the infant and the more extensive the hemorrhage, the greater the risk of death in the neonatal period. An intangible factor that also affects mortality is the philosophy prevailing in any particular neonatal intensive care unit regarding the aggressiveness of supportive measures for an infant with documented IVH or other serious ailments.

The long-term neurologic morbidity of survivors of PVH/IVH is related largely to the size of the hemorrhage.[15,49,70,90,111,143,153] Infants with grade I (GM) hemorrhage with few or no acute symptoms show no or only mild neurologic abnormalities on follow-up examination. Hemorrhages of grades II and III severity (IVH with or without ventricular enlargement) also may produce no residua but are associated with mild to moderate abnormalities in as many as 40% of infants. Severe IVH with extensive parenchymal hemorrhage is associated with major motor deficits, psychomotor retardation, hearing loss, and blindness in the vast majority of infants. Furthermore, posthemorrhagic hydrocephalus complicating IVH appears to increase ultimate neurologic morbidity over that of IVH alone.[20,49,90,111]

The long-term neurologic outcome of infants who have sustained PVH/IVH continues to be examined in medical centers throughout the world. Such investigations may, we hope, provide objective information upon which to base accurate prognostic assessments and therapeutic interventions.

INTRACRANIAL HEMORRHAGE OTHER THAN PVH/IVH

This chapter would not be complete without some discussion of intracranial hemorrhage distinct from PVH/IVH. As mentioned in Chapter 7, hemorrhage accompanies severe perinatal hypoxia-ischemia frequently, usually in the form of hemorrhagic infarction. Occasionally, the brains of asphyxiated infants also exhibit isolated primary hemorrhage in sites remote from the cerebral hemispheres, including the choroid plexus (with or without IVH), brain stem, and cerebellum.[14,26,34,51,73,92,110,119,127,153,161] Presumably, such hemorrhages arise as a consequence of hypoxic-ischemic tissue injury or of major hemodynamic fluctuations that occur during or after the asphyxial process.

In addition to perinatal hypoxia-ischemia, the single most frequently encountered event associated with intracranial hemorrhage is "cerebral birth trauma." Other etiologies are far less common (Table 8-4).

Subarachnoid Hemorrhage

Bleeding into the subarachnoid space is often the consequence of hemorrhage into the parenchyma of the brain, into the subdural space, or into the ventricular system.[34,153] Isolated or primary subarachnoid hemorrhage is also a frequent occurrence that can accompany even an uncomplicated vaginal delivery. Many infants probably sustain at least a minor subarachnoid hemorrhage at birth, with bleeding arising from easily disrupted veins that bridge the pia and arachnoid membranes. Nearly all of these infants are asymptomatic following birth, and the bleeding would never have been discovered were it not for the performance of a lumbar puncture. In a few of the infants, symptoms of "cerebral irritation" occur in the form of seizures usually on the second or third postnatal day. The infants appear entirely well between the seizures, which resolve spontaneously within hours to days. Long-term prognosis of infants with primary subarachnoid hemorrhage is excellent.

Table 8-4 Etiologies of Intracranial Hemorrhage Other Than PVH/IVH in Premature and Term Infants

---

Hypoxia-Ischemia (Asphyxia)
Physical Birth Trauma
Coagulation Defects
   Thrombocytopenia
   Deficiency of coagulation factors
Congenital Vascular Anomalies
   Aneurysm
   Arteriovenous malformation
   Coarctation of the aorta
Neoplasms
   Glioma
   Medulloblastoma
   Choroid plexus papilloma
   Miscellaneous
Unknown

Subdural Hemorrhage

Hemorrhage into the subdural space is usually the consequence of birth trauma. Recall that the major venous sinuses that drain blood from the brain are sheathed in dura mater and fixed firmly within the falx cerebri or tentorium cerebelli or to the inner surface of the skull. Any bleeding from the sinuses or their tributaries extravasates into the subdural space between the dura and arachnoid membranes.

Volpe[153] has suggested that four major varieties of subdural hemorrhage occur in newborn infants in accordance with the rupture of specific veins or venous sinuses. The location of the evolving hematoma will, in turn, determine the type and extent of neurologic dysfunction exhibited by the infant in the early postpartum period, and will also influence ultimate prognosis. Such lesions are usually of traumatic origin; on occasion, the physical injury may have been minor when superimposed upon a preexisting hemorrhagic diathesis (see Table 8-4).

Traumatic laceration of the tentorium cerebelli leads to bleeding into the subdural space of the posterior fossa.[9,23,54,131] The venous channels most frequently affected include the vein of Galen, straight sinus, and/or transverse or sigmoid sinuses. With clot formation, compression of the cerebellum and adjacent brain stem occurs, leading, in turn, to major fluctuations in systemic blood pressure, heart rate, and respiratory pattern. Death of the infant ensues if the hematoma is not evacuated promptly. Infratentorial subdural hemorrhage, even if smaller in amount, is associated with seizures, signs of brain stem dysfunction (cranial nerve palsies), and occasionally hydrocephalus. These symptoms and signs are often delayed for hours to days following birth as a reflection of the slowly enlarging blood clot. Surgical removal of the hematoma is indicated whenever the infant exhibits major neurologic manifestations.

Occipital osteodiastasis is a lesion in which a traumatic delivery (usually breech) causes separation of the cartilaginous joint between the squamous and lateral portions of the occipital bones.[113,158] The underlying dura mater and transverse sinus are ruptured, leading to massive bleeding into the subdural space of the posterior fossa. Laceration of the underlying cerebellum is a frequent accompaniment. The condition is often rapidly fatal.

Laceration of the falx cerebri, which separates the two cerebral hemispheres, is less common than trauma to the tentorium cerebelli. Tearing of the inferior leaf of the falx will include the inferior sagittal sinus, leading to hemorrhage into the inferior longitudinal fissure located above the corpus callosum. The relatively large size of the fissure prevents cerebral or brain stem compression unless a large hematoma evolves. Therefore, surgical evacuation usually is not required, as the clot will ultimately resolve spontaneously.

The most common location in which subdural hematomas arise is in the area that surrounds the convexity of the cerebral hemispheres. This hemorrhage arises from disruption of bridging, superficial veins or, rarely, from laceration of the superior sagittal sinus.[34,113,153] Unlike older infants (e.g., the battered child), the hematoma typically is unilateral and confined to the lateral aspect of the convexity of the skull vault. An overlying cephalohematoma is often present. Symptoms and signs in the affected infant range from none at all to focal neurologic deficits (hemiparesis, focal seizures, ipsilateral third cranial nerve dysfunction). Signs of brain stem compression evolve only if the hemorrhage has been massive, leading to brain herniation. Treatment is usually supportive, and surgical evacuation only required occasionally.

Traumatic subdural hematomas are sometimes accompanied by bleeding into the substance of the brain. Parenchymal hemorrhage reflects the occurrence of brain contusion with associated disruption of blood vessels within the area of tissue injury. The location of the hemorrhage is dependent upon the site and nature of the external forces causing the trauma, the two most common sites being the cerebral and cerebellar hemispheres. Brain stem hemorrhage occurs only if the injury has been catastrophic.

Subdural hemorrhage in the newborn infant is usually the consequence of a traumatic delivery. Factors that predispose both the premature and term infant to subdural hemorrhage are referable to the mother, the infant, the nature of the labor process, and the manner of delivery (Table 8-5).[153] Of these factors, the inappropriate use and application of forceps (particularly midforceps operations) and the vaginal delivery of a breech infant with a hyperextended head are probably the most important mechanisms by which traumatic hemorrhage occurs. These maneuvers produce compressive forces to the skull and intracranial contents. If these forces are excessive, they result in fracture or displacement of bones, stretching and laceration of dural structures, including veins and sinuses, and shearing of brain tissue (contusion).

Diagnostic Procedures

Diagnostic procedures to ascertain the presence, location, and extent of intracranial hemorrhage include skull and spine radiographs, CT, and/or US scanning. Radiographs may reveal a linear or comminuted skull

Table 8-5 Risk Factors in Neonatal Subdural Hemorrhage

At Risk	Predisposing Factor
Mother	Primiparous
	Older multiparous
	Small pelvis
Infant	Large full-term
	Premature
Labor	Precipitate
	Prolonged
Delivery	Breech extraction
	Foot, face, or brow presentation
	Difficult forceps extraction
	Difficult rotation

Source: Adapted with permission from *Pediatrics* (1983;72:589–601), Copyright © 1983, American Academy of Pediatrics.

fracture, occipital osteodiastasis, or a dislocation of one or more cervical vertebrae. CT scanning accurately localizes a subdural hematoma and/or any underlying hemorrhage into the brain substance with or without associated contusion (Figure 8-10). CT scanning will also help determine the presence or absence of subarachnoid hemorrhage. Until recently, US scanning has been useful only in the delineation of parenchymal hemorrhage, although the recent introduction of the 10-MHz probe has allowed visualization of the subdural and subarachnoid compartments. Presently, all newborn infants suspected of having intracranial hemorrhage should undergo CT scanning with or without US correlation.

Management

As previously mentioned, management strategies regarding intracranial hemorrhage are dependent primarily on the presence and extent of neurologic compromise exhibited by the infant in the immediate newborn period. First, the cause of the hemorrhage must be ascertained, for not all lesions are of traumatic or hypoxic-ischemic origin. Coagulation defects must be reversed promptly with replacement of the deficient agent. Blood transfusion may be required if the hemorrhage has been

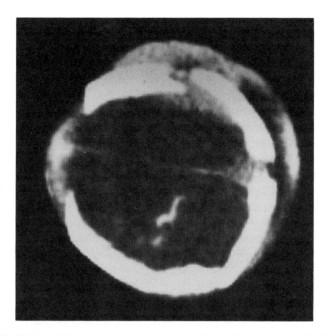

Figure 8-10 CT scan showing a right convexity subdural hematoma and a left cerebral hemispheric hemorrhagic contusion. Also apparent is a cephalohematoma overlying the skull on the right.

extensive enough to produce systemic oligemia. Surgical intervention is warranted to remove a congenital malformation of blood vessels or tumor producing hemorrhage. Lastly, surgical evacuation of the hematoma itself must be contemplated if the infant shows signs of clinical deterioration, that might lead to an early death or permanent neurologic deficit.

Prognosis

The long-term prognosis of newborn infants who survive intracranial hemorrhage depends primarily on the extent of concurrent injury to the brain itself. Thus, the majority of infants who sustain uncomplicated convexity subdural or subarachnoid hemorrhage exhibit no long-term neuropsychologic sequelae. Even infants who have sustained posterior fossa subdural hemorrhage can do well, especially those who have undergone prompt neurosurgical intervention.[153] Infants with primary parenchymal hemorrhage and/or contusion often are left with permanent deficits, usually in the form of spastic hemiparesis, ataxia, or cognitive delay. Fortunately, modern-day obstetric practice with emphasis on prompt diagnosis and treatment of dysfunctional labor and avoidance of potentially traumatic instrumental delivery has greatly reduced the incidence of traumatic lesions to the immature brain, thereby minimizing the need for acute neonatal intervention and long-term follow-up.

REFERENCES

1. Abroms IF, Mclennan JE, Mandell F: Acute neonatal subdural hematoma following breech delivery. *Am J Dis Child* 1977;131:192–194.

2. Ahmann PA, Lazzara A, Dykes FD, Brann AW, Schwartz JF: Intracranial hemorrhage in the high-risk preterm infant: Incidence and Outcome. *Ann Neurol* 1980;7:118–124.

3. Albright L, Fellows R: Sequential CT scanning after neonatal intracerebral hemorrhage. *AJNR* 1981;2:133–137.

4. Allan WC, Holt PJ, Sawyer LR, Tito AM, Meade SK: Ventricular dilation after neonatal periventricular intraventricular hemorrhage: Natural history and therapeutic implications. *Am J Dis Child* 1982;136:589–593.

5. Bada HS, Korones SB, Anderson GD, Magill HL, Wong SP: Obstetric factors and relative risk of neonatal germinal layer/intraventricular hemorrhage. *Am J Obstet Gynecol* 1984;148:798–804.

6. Bada HS, Salmon JH, Pearson DH: Early surgical intervention in posthemorrhagic hydrocephalus. *Child's Brain* 1979;5:109–115.

7. Bejar R, Curbelo V, Coen RW, Leopold G, James H, Gluck L: Diagnosis and follow-up of intraventricular hemorrhages by ultrasound studies of infant's brain through the fontanelles and sutures. *Pediatrics* 1980;66:661–673.

8. Benson JWT, Drayton MR, Hayward C, Murphy JF, Osborne JP, Rennie JM, Schulte JF, Speidel BD, Cooke RWI: Multicentre trial of ethamsylate for prevention of periventricular haemorrhage in very low birthweight infants. *Lancet* 1986;2:1297–1300.

9. Blank NK, Strand R, Gilles FH, Palakshappa A: Posterior fossa subdural hematomas in neonates. *Arch Neurol* 1978;35:108–111.

10. Bovit A, Sidman RL: New mutant mouse with communicating hydrocephalus and secondary aqueductal stenosis. *Acta Neuropathol* 1972;21:316–331.

11. Brann AW, Myers RE: Central nervous system findings in the newborn monkey following severe *in utero* parital asphyxia. *Neurology* 1975;25:327–338.

12. Brazy JE, Lewis DV: Changes in cerebral blood volume and cytochrome aa$_3$ during hypertensive peaks in preterm infants. *J Pediatr* 1986;108:983–987.

13. Burstein J, Papile LA, Burstein R: Intraventricular hemorrhage and hydrocephalus in premature newborns: A prospective study with CT. *Am J Roentgenol* 1979;132:631–635.

14. Cartwright GW, Culbertson K, Schreiner RL, Gang BP: Changes in clinical presentation of term infants with intracranial hemorrhage. *Dev Med Child Neurol* 1979;21:730–737.

15. Catto-Smith AG, Yu VYH, Bajuk B, Orgill AA, Astbury J: Effect of neonatal periventricular haemorrhage on neurodevelopmental outcome. *Arch Dis Child* 1985;60:8–11.

16. Cavazzuti M, Duffy TE: Regulation of local cerebral blood flow in normal and hypoxic newborn dogs. *Ann Neurol* 1982;11:247–257.

17. Chaplin ER, Goldstein GW, Myerberg DZ, Hunt JV, Tooley WH: Posthemorrhagic hydrocephalus in the preterm infant. *Pediatrics* 1980;65:901–909.

18. Clark CE, Clyman RI, Roth RS, Sniderman SH, Lane B, Ballard RA: Risk factor analysis of intraventricular hemorrhage in low-birth-weight infants. *J Pediatr* 1981; 99:625–628.

19. Cooke RWI: Factors associated with periventricular haemorrhage in very low birth-weight infants. *Arch Dis Child* 1981;56:425–431.

20. Cooke RWI: Early prognosis of low birthweight infants treated for progressive posthaemorrhagic hydrocephalus. *Arch Dis Child* 1983;58:410–414.

21. Cooke RWI, Morgan MEI: Prophylactic ethamsylate for periventricular haemorrhage. *Arch Dis Child* 1984;59:82–83.

22. de Courten GM, Rabinowicz T: Intraventricular hemorrhage in premature infants: Re-appraisal and new hypothesis. *Dev Med Child Neurol* 1981;23:389–403.

23. Craig WS: Intracranial haemorrhage in the newborn. *Arch Dis Child* 1938;13:39–43.

24. de Crespigny LC, Mackay R, Murton LJ, Roy RND, Robinson PH: Timing of neonatal cerebroventricular haemorrhage with ultrasound. *Arch Dis Child* 1982;57:231–233.

25. Deonna T, Calame A, Van Melle G, Prodham LS: Hypoglycorrhachia in neonatal intracranial hemorrhage: Relationship to post-hemorrhagic hydrocephalus. *Helv Paediatr Acta* 1977;32:351–361.

26. Donat JF, Okazaki H, Kleinberg F: Intraventricular hemorrhages in full-term and premature infants. *Mayo Clin Proc* 1978;53:437–441.

27. Donn SM, Goldstein GW, Roloff DW: Prevention of intraventricular hemorrhage with phenobarbital therapy: Now what? *Pediatrics* 1986;77:779–780.

28. Donn SM, Roloff DW, Goldstein GW: Prevention of intraventricular hemorrhage in preterm infants by phenobarbital. *Lancet* 1981;2:215–217.

29. Duffy TE, Cavazzuti M, Cruz NF, Sokoloff L: Local cerebral glucose metabolism in newborn dogs: Effects of hypoxia and halothane anesthesia. *Ann Neurol* 1982;11:233–246.

30. Dykes FD, Lazzara A, Ahmann P, Blumenstein B, Schwartz J, Brann AW: Intraventricular hemorrhage: A prospective evaluation of etiopathogenesis. *Pediatrics* 1980; 66:42–49.

31. Epstein MF: Three hot topics in neonatology. *Pediatr Alert* 1986;11:17–18.

32. Escobedo M, Barton LL, Volpe J: Cerebrospinal fluid studies in an intensive care nursery. *J Perinat Med* 1975;3:204–210.

33. Fedrick J, Butler NR: Certain causes of neonatal death. II. Intraventricular hemorrhage. *Biol Neonate* 1970;15:257–290.

34. Fenichel GM, Webster DL, Wong WKT: Intracranial hemorrhage in the term newborn. *Arch Neurol* 1984;41:30–34.

35. Fishman MA, Dutton RV, Okumura S: Progressive ventriculomegaly following minor intracranial hemorrhage in premature infants. *Dev Med Child Neurol* 1984;26:725–731.

36. Fitzhardinge PM, Pape K, Arstikaitis M, Boyle M, Ashby S, Rowley A, Netley C, Sawyer PR: Mechanical ventilation of infants less than 1,501 gm birth weight: Health, growth and neurologic sequelae. *J Pediatr* 1976;88:531–541.

37. Flodmark O, Becker LE, Harwood-Nash DC, Fitzhardinge PM, Fitz CR: Correlation between computerized tomography and autopsy in premature and full-term neonates that have suffered perinatal asphyxia. *Radiology* 1980;119:111–114.

38. Flodmark O, Fitz CR, Harwood-Nash DC: CT diagnosis and short-term prognosis of intracranial hemorrhage and hypoxic-ischemic brain damage in neonates. *J Comput Assist Tomogr* 1980;4:775–787.

39. Fujimura M, Salisburg DM, Robinson RO, Howat P, Emerson PM, Keeling JW, Tizard JPM: Clinical events relating to intraventricular haemorrhage in the newborn. *Arch Dis Child* 1979;54:409–414.

40. Garcia-Prats JA, Procianoy RS, Adams JM, Rudolph AJ: The hyaline membrane disease—intraventricular hemorrhage relationship in the very low birth weight infant: Perinatal aspects. *Acta Paediatr Scand* 1982;71:79–84.

41. Goddard J, Lewis RM, Alcala H, Zeller RS: Intraventricular hemorrhage—an animal model. *Biol Neonate* 1980;37:39–52.

42. Goddard J, Lewis R, Armstrong DL, Zeller RS: Moderate, rapidly induced hypertension as a cause of intraventricular hemorrhage in the newborn beagle model. *J Pediatr* 1980; 96:1057–1060.

43. Goddard-Finegold J, Armstrong D, Zeller RS: Intraventricular hemorrhage following volume expansion after hypovolemic hypotension in the newborn beagle. *J Pediatr* 1982; 100:796–799.

44. Goddard-Finegold J, Michael LH: Cerebral blood flow and experimental intraventricular hemorrhage. *Pediatr Res* 1984;18:7–11.

45. Goldberg RN: Sustained arterial blood pressure elevation associated with pneumothoraces: Early detection via continuous monitoring. *Pediatrics* 1981;68:775–777.

46. Goldberg RN, Chung D, Goldman SL, Bancalari E: The association of rapid volume expansion and intraventricular hemorrhage in the preterm infant. *J Pediatr* 1980; 96:1060–1063.

47. Grant EG, Borts FT, Schellinger D, McCullough DC, Sivasubramanian KN, Smith Y: Real-time ultrasonography of neonatal intracranial hemorrhage and comparison with computed tomography. *Radiology* 1981;139:687–691.

48. Graziani L, Dave R, Desai H, Branca P, Waldnoup L, Goldberg B: Ultrasound studies in preterm infants with hydrocephalus. *J Pediatr* 1980;97:624–630.

49. Greisen G, Petersen MB, Pedersen SA, Baekgaard P: Status at two years in 121 very low birth weight survivors related to neonatal intraventricular and mode of delivery. *Acta Paediatr Scand* 1986;75:24–30.

50. Grunnet ML: Periventricular leukomalacia complex. *Arch Pathol Lab Med* 1979; 103:6–10.

51. Grunnet ML, Shields WD: Cerebellar hemorrhage in the premature infant. *J Pediatr* 1976;88:605–608.

52. Guzzetta F, Shackelford GD, Volpe S, Pearlman JM, Volpe JJ: Periventricular intraparenchymal echodensities in the premature infant: Critical determinants of neurologic outcome. *Pediatrics* 1986;995–1006.

53. Gyllensward A, Malmstrom S: The cerebrospinal fluid in immature infants. *Acta Pediatr Scand* 1962;135(Suppl):54–62.

54. Haller ES, Nesbitt RE, Anderson GW: Clinical and pathologic concepts of gross intracranial hemorrhage in perinatal mortality. *Obstet Gynecol Surv* 1956;11:179–182.

55. Hambleton G, Wigglesworth JS: Origin of intraventricular hemorrhage in the preterm infant. *Arch Dis Child* 1976;51:651–659.

56. Harcke HT, Naeye RL, Storch A, Blanc WA: Perinatal cerebral intraventricular hemorrhage. *J Pediatr* 1972;80:37–42.

57. Hellmann J, Vannucci RC: Intraventricular hemorrhage in premature infants. *Semin Perinatol* 1982;6:42–53.

58. Hellmann J, Vannucci RC: Perinatal intraventricular hemorrhage, in Wood JH (ed): *Neurobiology of Cerebrospinal Fluid.* New York, Plenum, 1983, pp 497–515.

59. Hernandez MJ, Brennan RW, Bowman GS: Autoregulation of cerebral blood flow in the newborn dog. *Brain Res* 1980;184:199–202.

60. Hernandez MJ, Brennan RW, Vannucci RC, Bowman GS: Cerebral blood flow and oxygen consumption in the newborn dog. *Am J Physiol* 1978;234:R209–R215.

61. Hill A, Melson GL, Clark HB, Volpe JJ: Hemorrhagic periventricular leukomalacia: Diagnosis by real time ultrasound and correlation with autopsy findings. *Pediatrics* 1982; 69:282–284.

62. Hill A, Perlman JM, Volpe JJ: Relationship of pneumothorax to occurrence of intraventricular hemorrhage in the premature newborn. *Pediatrics* 1982;69:144–149.

63. Hill A, Taylor DA, Volpe JJ: Treatment of post-hemorrhagic hydrocephalus by serial lumbar puncture: Factors that account for success or failure. *Ann Neurol* 1981;10:284.

64. Hill A, Volpe JJ: Normal pressure hydrocephalus in the newborn. *Pediatrics* 1981; 68:623–629.

65. Holt PJ, Allan WC: The natural history of ventricular dilatation in neonatal intraventricular hemorrhage and their therapeutic implications. *Ann Neurol* 1981;10:293–294.

66. Horbar JD, Walters CL, Philip AGS, Lucey JF: Ultrasound detection of changing ventricular size in post-hemorrhagic hydrocephalus. *Pediatrics* 1980;66:674–678.

67. Kauffman RE: Therapeutic interventions to prevent intracerebral hemorrhage in preterm infants. *J Pediatr* 1986;108:323–325.

68. Korobkin R: The prognosis for survivors of perinatal intraventricular hemorrhage, in Korobkin R, Guilleminault C (eds): *Advances in Perinatal Neurology.* New York, SP Medical and Scientific Books, vol 1, 1979, pp 141–151.

69. Krishnamoorthy KS, Fernandez RA, Momose KJ, DeLong GR, Moylan FMB, Todres ID, Shannon DC: Evaluation of neonatal intracranial hemorrhage by computerized tomography. *Pediatrics* 1977;59:165–172.

70. Krishnamoorthy KS, Kuehnle KJ, Todres ID, DeLong GR: Neurodevelopmental outcome of survivors with posthemorrhagic hydrocephalus following grade II neonatal intraventricular hemorrhage. *Ann Neurol* 1984;15:201–204.

71. Krishnamoorthy KS, Shannon DC, DeLong GR, Todres ID, Davis KR: Neurologic sequelae in the survivors of neonatal intraventricular hemorrhage. *Pediatrics* 1979; 64:233–237.

72. Kuban KCK, Leviton A, Krishnamoorthy KS, Brown ER, Teele RL, Baglivo JA, Sullivan KF, Huff KR, White S, Cleveland RH, Allred EN, Spritzer KL, Skouteli HN, Cayea P, Epstein MF: Neonatal intracranial hemorrhage and phenobarbital. *Pediatrics* 1986; 77:443–450.

73. Lacey DL, Terplan K: Intraventricular hemorrhage in full-term neonates. *Dev Med Child Neurol* 1982;24:332–337.

74. Larroche JCL: Hemorrhagies cerebrales intraventricularis chez le premature. I. Anatomie and physiopathologie. *Biol Neonate* 1964;7:26–56.

75. Larroche JCL: Post-hemorrhagic hydrocephalus in infancy. Anatomical study. *Biol Neonate* 1972;20:287–299.

76. Larroche JCL: *Developmental Pathology of the Neonate.* Amsterdam, Elsevier/North Holland, 1977.

77. Lazzara A, Ahmann P, Dykes F, Brann AW, Schwartz J: Clinical predictability of intraventricular hemorrhage in preterm infants. *Pediatrics* 1980;65:30–34.

78. Le Blanc R, O'Gorman AM: Neonatal intracranial hemorrhage: A clinical and serial computerized tomographic study. *J Neurosurg* 1980;53:642–651.

79. Lee BCP, Grassi AE, Schecher S, Auld PAM: Neonatal intraventricular hemorrhage: A serial computed tomograhic study. *J Comput Assist Tomogr* 1979;3:483–490.

80. Leech RW, Kohnen P: Subependymal and intraventricular hemorrhages in the newborn. *Am J Pathol* 1974;77:465–476.

81. Leech RW, Olsson MI, Alvord EC: Neuropathologic features of idiopathic respiratory distress syndrome. *Arch Pathol Lab Med* 1979;103:341–343.

82. Levene MI, De Vries L: Extension of neonatal intraventricular hemorrhage. *Arch Dis Child* 1984;59:631–636.

83. Levene MI, Fawer C-L, Lamont RF: Risk factors in the development of intraventricular haemorrhage in the preterm neonate. *Arch Dis Child* 1982;57:410–417.

84. Levene MI, Starte DR: A longitudinal study of post-haemorrhagic ventricular dilatation in the newborn. *Arch Dis Child* 1981;56:905–910.

85. Leviton A, Gilles F, Stassfeld R: The influence of route of delivery and hyaline membrane disease on the risk of neonatal intracranial hemorrhages. *Ann Neurol* 1977;2:451–454.

86. Lipscomb AP, Thorburn RJ, Reynolds EOR, Stewart AL, Blackwell RJ, Cosick G, Whitehead MD: Pneumothorax and cerebral hemorrhage in preterm infants. *Lancet* 1981;1:414–416.

87. Lorenzo AV, Welch K, Conner S: Spontaneous germinal matrix and intraventricular hemorrhage in prematurely born rabbits. *J Neurosurg* 1982;56:404–410.

88. Lou HC, Lassen NA, Friis-Hanson B: Impaired autoregulation of cerebral blood flow in the distressed newborn infant. *J Pediatr* 1979;94:170–173.

89. Low JA, Galbraith RS, Saverbrei EE, Muir DW, Killen HL, Pater EA, Karchmar EJ: Maternal, fetal and newborn complications associated with newborn intracranial hemorrhage. *Am J Obstet Gynecol* 1986;154:345–351.

90. Low JA, Galbraith RS, Saverbrei EE, Muir DW, Killen HL, Pater E, Karchmar EJ: Motor and cognitive development of infants with intraventricular hemorrhage, ventriculomegaly, or periventricular parenchymal lesions. *Am J Obstet Gynecol* 1986;155:750–756.

91. Mantovani JF, Pasternak JF, Matthew OF, Allan WC, Mills MT, Casper J, Volpe JJ: Failure of daily lumbar puncture to prevent the development of hydrocephalus following intraventricular hemorrhage. *J Pediatr* 1980;97:278–281.

92. Martin R, Roessmann D, Fanaroff A: Massive intracellular hemorrhage in low birthweight infants. *J Pediatr* 1976;89:290–293.

93. Mathew OP, Bland HE, Pickens JM, James E: Hypoglycorrhachia in the survivors of neonatal intracranial hemorrhage. *Pediatrics* 1979;63:851–854.

94. Meidell RM, Marinelli P, Pettett G: Perinatal factors associated with early-onset intracranial hemorrhage in premature infants: A prospective study. *Am J Dis Child* 1985;139:160–163.

95. Ment LR, Duncan CC, Ehrenkranz RA, Kleinman CS, Pitt BR, Taylor KJW, Scott DT, Stewart WB, Gettner P: Randomized indomethacin trial for prevention of intraventricular hemorrhage in very low birth weight infants. *J Pediatr* 1985;107:937–943.

96. Ment LR, Duncan CC, Ehrenkranz RA, Lange RC, Taylor KJ, Kleinman CS, Scott DT, Sivo J, Gettner P: Intraventricular hemorrhage in the preterm neonate: Timing and cerebral blood flow changes. *J Pediatr* 1984;104:419–425.

97. Ment LR, Ehrenkranz RA, Lange RC, Rothstein PT, Duncan CC: Alterations in cerebral blood flow in preterm infants with intraventricular hemorrhage. *Pediatrics* 1981; 68:763–769.

98. Ment LR, Stewart WB, Duncan CC, Pitt BR: Beagle puppy model of intraventricular hemorrhage. *J Neurosurg* 1982;57:219–222.

99. Ment LR, Stewart WB, Duncan CC, Pitt BR: Beagle puppy model of perinatal cerebral insults: Cerebral blood flow changes and intraventricular hemorrhage evoked by hypoxemia. *J Neurosurg* 1986;65:847–850.

100. Morales WJ, Koerten J: Prevention of intraventricular hemorrhage in very low birth weight infants by maternally administered phenobarbital. *Obstet Gynecol* 1986;68:295–299.

101. Morgan MEI, Benson JWT, Cooke RWI: Ethamsylate reduces the incidence of periventricular haemorrhage in very low birthweight babies. *Lancet* 1981;2:830–831.

102. Morgan MEI, Massey RF, Cooke RWI: Does phenobarbitone prevent periventricular hemorrhage in very low-birth-weight babies? A controlled trial. *Pediatrics* 1982;70:186–189.

103. Moscoso P, Goldberg RN, Jamieson J, Bancalari E: Spontaneous elevation in arterial blood pressure during the first hours of life in the very-low-birth-weight infant. *J Pediatr* 1983;103:114–117.

104. Myers RE: Two patterns of perinatal brain damage and their conditions of occurrence. *Am J Obstet Gynecol* 1972;112:246–276.

105. Myers RE: Fetal asphyxia due to umbilical cord compression. *Biol Neonate* 1975; 26:21–43.

106. Nelson RM, Bucciarelli RL, Nagel JW, Beale EF, Eitzman DV: Hypoglycorrhachia associated with intracranial hemorrhage in newborn infants. *J Pediatr* 1979;94:800–803.

107. Norman MG: Perinatal brain damage. *Perspect Pediatr Pathol* 1978;4:41–92.

108. Nugent GR, Al-Mefty O, Chou S: Communicating hydrocephalus as a cause of aqueductal stenosis. *J Neurosurg* 1979;51:812–818.

109. Otilia E: Studies on the cerebrospinal fluid in premature infants. *Acta Paediatr Scand* 1948;35(Suppl 8):9–100.

110. Palma PA, Miner ME, Morris FH, Adcock EW, Denson SE: Intraventricular hemorrhage in the neonate born at term. *Am J Dis Child* 1979;133:941–944.

111. Palmer P, Dubowitz LMS, Levene MI, Dubowitz V: Developmental and neurological process of preterm infants with intraventricular haemorrhage and ventricular dilatation. *Arch Dis Child* 1982;57:748–753.

112. Pape K, Bennett-Britton S, Szymonowicz E: Diagnostic accuracy of neonatal brain imaging: A post mortem correlation. *Pediatr Res* 1981;15:709.

113. Pape KE, Wigglesworth JS: *Haemorrhage, Ischemia and the Perinatal Brain.* Philadelphia, Spastic International Medical Publications, 1979.

114. Papile LA, Burstein J, Burstein R, Koffler H: Incidence and evolution of subependymal and intraventricular hemorrhage: A study of infants with birth weights less than 1,500 gm. *J Pediatr* 1978;92:529–534.

115. Papile L, Burstein J, Burstein R, Koffler H, Koops B: Relationship of intravenous sodium bicarbonate infusions and cerebral intraventricular hemorrhage. *J Pediatr* 1978; 93:834–836.

116. Papile L, Burstein J, Burstein R, Koffler H, Koops BL, Johnson JD: Posthemorrhagic hydrocephalus in low-birth-weight infants: Treatment of serial lumbar punctures. *J Pediatr* 1980;97:273–277.

117. Pasternak JF, Groothuis DR: Autoregulation of cerebral blood flow in the newborn beagle puppy. *Biol Neonate* 1985;48:100–109.

118. Pasternak JF, Mantovani JF, Volpe JJ: Porencephaly from periventricular intracerebral hemorrhage in a premature infant. *Am J Dis Child* 1980;134:673–675.

119. Pearlman JM, Nelson JS, McAlister WH, Volpe JJ: Intracerebellar hemorrhage in a premature newborn: Diagnosis by real-time ultrasound and correlation with autopsy findings. *Pediatrics* 1983;71:159–162.

120. Pearlman JM, Volpe JJ: Intraventricular hemorrhage in extremely small premature infants. *Am J Dis Child* 1986;140:1122–1124.

121. Philip AGS, Long JG, Donn SM: Intracranial pressure: Sequential measurements in full-term and premature infants. *Am J Dis Child* 1981;135:521–524.

122. Reynolds ML, Evans CAN, Reynolds EOR, Saunders NR, Durbin GM, Wigglesworth JS: Intracranial hemorrhage in the preterm sheep fetus. *Early Hum Dev* 1979; 3:163–186.

123. Rice JE, Vannucci RC, Brierley JB: The influence of immaturity on hypoxic-ischemic brain damage in the rat. *Ann Neurol* 1981;9:131–141.

124. Ross JJ, Dimette RW: Subependymal cerebral hemorrhage in infancy. *Am J Dis Child* 1965;110:531–542.

125. Sarff LD, Platt LH, McGracken GH: Cerebrospinal fluid evaluation in neonates: Comparison of high-risk infants with and without meningitis. *J Pediatr* 1976;88:473–477.

126. Saverbrei EE, Digney M, Harrison PB, Cooperberg PL: Ultrasonic evaluation of neonatal intracranial hemorrhage and its complications. *Radiology* 1980;139:677–685.

127. Scher MS, Wright FS, Lockman LA, Thompson TR: Intraventricular hemorrhage in the full-term neonate. *Arch Neurol* 1982;39:769–772.

128. Schoenberg BS, Mellinger JF, Schoenberg DG: Perinatal intracranial hemorrhage: Incidence and clinical features. *Arch Neurol* 1977;34:570–573.

129. Schrumpf JD, Sehring S, Killpack S, Brady JP, Hirata T, Mednick JP: Correlation of early neurologic outcome and CT findings in neonatal brain hypoxia and injury. *J Comp Assist Tomogr* 1980;4:445–450.

130. Schwartz P: *Birth Injuries of the Newborn.* New York, S Karger, 1961.

131. Serfontein GL, Rom S, Stein S: Posterior fossa subdural hemorrhage in the newborn. *Pediatrics* 1980;65:40–43.

132. Shankaran S, Slovis TL, Bedard MP, Poland RL: Sonographic classification of intracranial hemorrhage. A prognostic indicator of mortality, morbidity, and short-term neurologic outcome. *J Pediatr* 1982;100:469–475.

133. Shapiro HM, Greenberg JH, Haughton KVH, Reivich M: Heterogeneity of local cerebral blood flow—$PaCO_2$ sensitivity in neonatal dogs. *J Appl Physiol* 1980;49:113–118.

134. Sherwood A, Hopp A, Smith JF: Cellular reactions to subependymal plate haemorrhage in the human neonate. *Neuropathol Appl Neurobiol* 1978;4:245–261.

135. Shinnar S, Grammon K, Bergman EW, Epstein M, Freeman JM: Management of hydrocephalus in infancy: Use of acetazolamide and furosemide to avoid cerebrospinal fluid shunts. *J Pediatr* 1985;107:31–36.

136. Silverboard G, Horder MH, Ahmann PA: Reliability of ultrasound in diagnosis of intracerebral hemorrhage and post-hemorrhagic hydrocephalus: Comparison with computed tomography. *Pediatrics* 1980;66:507–514.

137. Simmons MA, Adcock EW, Bard H, Battaglia FC: Hypernatremia and intracranial hemorrhage in neonates. *N Engl J Med* 1974;291:6–10.

138. Szymonowicz W, Yu VYH: Timing and evolution of periventricular hemorrhage in infants weighing 1250 g or less at birth. *Arch Dis Child* 1984;59:7–12.

139. Szymonowicz W, Yu VYH, Walker A, Wilson F: Reduction in periventricular hemorrhage in preterm infants. *Arch Dis Child* 1986;61:661–665.

140. Szymonowicz W, Yu VYH, Wilson FE: Antecedents of periventricular haemorrhage in infants weighing 1250 g or less at birth. *Arch Dis Child* 1984;59:13–17.

141. Taylor DA, Fishman MA, Volpe JJ: Treatment of post-hemorrhagic hydrocephalus with glycerol. *Ann Neurol* 1981;10:297.

142. Tejani N, Verma U, Hameed C, Chayen B: Method and route of delivery in the low birth weight vertex presentation correlated with early periventricular/intraventricular hemorrhage. *Obstet Gynecol* 1987;69:1–4.

143. Tekolste KA, Bennett FC, Mack LA: Follow-up of infants receiving cranial ultrasound for intracranial hemorrhage. *Am J Dis Child* 1985;139:299–303.

144. Thorburn RJ, Lipscomb AP, Stewart AL, Reynolds EOR, Hope PL: Timing and antecedents of periventricular haemorrhage and of cerebral atrophy in very preterm infants. *Early Hum Dev* 1982;7:221–238.

145. Thorburn RJ, Stewart AL, Hope PL, Lipscomb AP, Reynolds EOR, Pape KE: Prediction of death and major handicap in very preterm infants by brain ultrasound. *Lancet* 1981; 1:1119–1121.

146. Ting P, Yamaguchi S, Bacher JD, Killems RH, Myers RE: Failure to produce germinal matrix or intraventricular hemorrhage by hypoxia, hypo-, or hypervolemia. *Exp Neurol* 1984; 83:449–460.

147. Towbin A: Cerebral intraventricular hemorrhage and subependymal matrix infarction in the fetus and premature newborn. *Am J Pathol* 1968;52:121–139.

148. Van De Bor M, Van Bel F, Lineman R, Ruys JH: Perinatal factors and periventricular-intraventricular hemorrhage in preterm infants. *Am J Dis Child* 1986;140:1125–1130.

149. Vannucci RC, Duffy TE: Cerebral oxidative and energy metabolism of fetal and neonatal rats during anoxia and recovery. *Am J Physiol* 1976;230:1269–1275.

150. Vannucci RC, Duffy TE: Cerebral metabolism in newborn dogs during reversible asphyxia. *Ann Neurol* 1977;1:528–534.

151. Vannucci RC, Hellmann J, Dubynsky O, Page RB, Maisels MJ: Cerebral oxidative metabolism in perinatal post-hemorrhagic hydrocephalus. *Dev Med Child Neurol* 1980; 22:308–316.

152. Vert P, Andre M, Sibout M: Continuous positive airway pressure and hydrocephalus. *Lancet* 1973;2:319.

153. Volpe JJ: *Neurology of the Newborn*. Philadelphia, WB Saunders, 1987.

154. Volpe JJ, Herscovitch P, Pearlman JM, Raichle ME: Positron emission tomography in the newborn: Extensive impairment of regional cerebral blood flow with intraventricular hemorrhage and hemorrhagic intracerebral involvement. *Pediatrics* 1983;72:589–601.

155. Volpe JJ, Pasternak JF, Allan WC: Ventricular dilatation preceding rapid head growth following neonatal intracranial hemorrhage. *Am J Dis Child* 1977;131:1212–1215.

156. Voorhies TM, Vannucci RC: Perinatal neurology, in Boyd R, Battaglia FC (eds): *Perinatal Medicine*. Boston, Buttersworth, 1983, pp 70–111.

157. Welch K: The intracranial pressure in infants. *J Neurosurg* 1980;52:693–699.

158. Wigglesworth JS, Husemeyer RP: Intracranial birth trauma in vaginal breech delivery: The continued importance of injury to the occipital bone. *Br J Obstet Gynaecol* 1977; 84:684–690.

159. Wigglesworth JS, Keith IH, Girling DJ, Slade SA: Hyaline membrane disease, alkali, and intraventricular haemorrhage. *Arch Dis Child* 1976;51:755–762.

160. Wigglesworth JS, Pape KE: An integrated model for haemorrhagic and ischemic lesions in the newborn brain. *Early Hum Dev* 1978;2:179–199.

161. Wiggleworth JS, Pape KE: Pathophysiology of intracranial haemorrhage in the newborn. *J Perinat Med* 1980;8:119–133.

162. Williams J, Chir B, Hirsch NJ, Corbet AJS, Rudolph AJ: Postnatal head shrinkage in small infants. *Pediatrics* 1977;59:619–622.

163. Wimberly PD, Lou HC, Pedersen H, Hejl M, Lassen NA, Friis-Hansen B: Hypertensive peaks in the pathogenesis of intraventricular hemorrhage in the newborn. Abolition by phenobarbitone sedation. *Acta Paediatr Scand* 1982;71:537–542.

9

Clinical Management of Fetal Hypoxemia

Wayne R. Cohen and Barry S. Schifrin

Electronic fetal monitoring systems provide continuous precise information about fetal heart rate. Changes in the pattern of heart rate yield indirect evidence relating to the state of fetal oxygenation. Skillful use of these data permits clinical judgments to be made about the quality of fetal oxygen supply. To utilize fetal monitoring most effectively, the clinician must have a general understanding of the mechanisms of fetal oxygenation. In this regard, a thorough review of the physiology of placental oxygen transfer and of the mechanisms by which the fetus adapts to reduced oxygen availability is presented in Chapter 5. The potential neuropathologic consequences of fetal asphyxia have been discussed in Chapters 6 to 8. Although it may be concluded that a minority of cases of permanent brain damage are a consequence of intrapartum fetal oxygen deprivation, the number of such cases is not insubstantial; moreover, they represent an important clinical entity because brain damage that occurs under these circumstances is potentially preventable.

The fetus has important physiologic mechanisms that enable it to maintain cardiovascular and metabolic homeostasis during periods of diminished oxygen availability. When very severe asphyxial stress occurs, oxygenation of vital organs is diminished, and the likelihood of both immediate and long-term complications increases. Currently available monitoring techniques are capable of identifying early signs of fetal hypoxemia; timely intervention can reduce the risk of perinatal death, and probably of neurologic disability. Of greater importance, these techniques can identify the normally oxygenated fetus with almost complete accuracy. This is information of paramount importance to determine the need for various obstetric interventions and the most appropriate timing of delivery.

FETAL HEART RATE MONITORING

Baseline Heart Rate

The control of myocardial excitability in the fetus is quite complex, and is based upon an interplay of factors controlling intrinsic rhythmicity as well as neurologic or humoral extrinsic influences. Of primary importance is the autonomic nervous system. This is the common pathway for many higher brain inputs that influence heart rate.

Beat-to-beat changes in the instantaneous heart rate are determined primarily by alterations in parasympathetic tone. More broad changes in rate that occur over a period of several beats are influenced to a greater degree by changes in sympathetic nerve activity. Because the autonomic nervous system is not completely developed in many species until very late in fetal or even neonatal life, other cardioactive systems probably play important roles in control of heart rate. For example, circulating catecholamines of adrenal medullary origin influence fetal heart rate and blood pressure, and probably are critical components in the fetal cardiovascular adaptive responses to hypoxemia (see Chapter 5).

An interplay of these intrinsic and extrinsic influences produces a fetal heart rate normally between 110 and 160 beats/min at term that displays irregular, apparently random oscillations, termed *variability*. Autonomic influences on the heart fluctuate rapidly in response to afferent signals that result from changes in venous return or metabolic demands, and in turn result in the continuous small variations in heart rate that constitute variability.[35,96,98] The beat-to-beat interval changes that are observed with each successive heart beat, and which, as noted, are primarily under vagal control, are referred to as short-term variability. This is the most important facet of variability for the clinical assessment of fetal oxygenation. Fluctuations in short-term variability are generally accompanied by similar trends in long-term variability, but they may on occasion be altered separately.[98]

It must be emphasized that the interpretation of heart rate variability is a pivotal aspect of fetal monitoring. To employ the system of heart rate pattern interpretation described in this chapter, a cardiotachometer capable of determining heart rate on a beat-to-beat basis must be used. Some monitoring techniques involve tachometric methods that average the heart rate, thus obscuring important information concerning variability.

Mean fetal heart rate decreases modestly during pregnancy,[49] probably in response to maturation and increasing predominance of the parasympathetic portion of the autonomic nervous system.[12,83] For the same reason, beat-to-beat variability in the heart rate tends to increase somewhat as term approaches.

Assessment of heart rate variability should be made by inspecting the pattern visually, and classifying the variability as increased, average, decreased, or absent (Figure 9-1). Although several sophisticated measures for electronic quantitation of heart rate variability have been proposed[47,61] their clinical utility has not been established. In fact, there is not always a good correlation between visual and electronically derived estimates of variability.[28]

Of great clinical pertinence, there seems to be a relationship between heart rate variability and the state of fetal oxygenation. Although acute hypoxemia may cause a temporary increase in heart rate variability,[91] more long-standing and clinically significant oxygen deprivation is almost always associated with marked diminution in variability.[78] Even if other heart rate pattern abnormalities were present, it is uncommon to deliver a hypoxemic newborn when the heart rate variability prior to delivery was normal.

Although fetal asphyxia results in decreased variability, other important clinical situations may produce the same effect (Table 9-1). For example, most analgesic drugs as well as sedative or hypnotic agents may

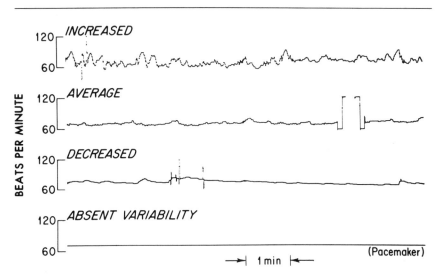

Figure 9-1 Heart rate variability patterns. Visual discrimination of increased, average, decreased, or absent variability is necessary for fetal heart rate pattern interpretation. The electronically produced pacemaker signal is an example of the complete absence of variability. *Source:* Reprinted from *Perinatal Medicine*, ed 2 (pp 223–243) by RJ Bolognese, RH Schwarz, and J Schneider (Eds) with permission of Williams & Wilkins Company, © 1982.

Table 9-1 Diminished Variability—Clinical Associations

Hypoxemia
Drugs
  Narcotics
  Barbiturates
  Tranquilizers
  Anesthetics
Physiologic
  Prematurity
  State
Anomalies
Arrhythmias

---

reduce variability. In addition, normally oxygenated premature babies may have less variability than their term counterparts. Of most importance, normal cyclic changes in fetal arousal levels (state) may sometimes be accompanied by diminished variability.[36,69] The heart rate pattern of the fetus in a normal state of diminished activity will usually manifest a transient increase in variability and/or a baseline acceleration if the fetus is stimulated by examination or sound. These responses, most obvious during antepartum monitoring, are also seen occasionally during labor.

Oxygen deprivation may increase or decrease the fetal heart rate, depending on the nature of the asphyxial event, and the milieu in which it occurs. Acute profound asphyxia always causes a fetal bradycardia. However, persistently low fetal heart rates may occur under other circumstances (Table 9-2).

In the absence of contractions, slowly developing asphyxia may produce a fetal tachycardia. Before ascribing increased fetal heart rates to hypoxia, however, one must exclude other etiologies (Table 9-3).[70,88] Maternal fever, with or without fetal infection, is the most common cause of

---

Table 9-2 Persistent Bradycardia—Clinical Associations

Hypoxia
Idiopathic
Drugs (e.g., propranolol)
Bradyarrhythmia
Hypoglycemia
Fetal hypopituitarism
Hypothermia

Table 9-3 Persistent Tachycardia—Clinical Associations

Hypoxia
Maternal fever
Fetal infection
Drugs (e.g., beta-mimetics)
Physiologic
   Prematurity
   Idiopathic
Tachyarrhythmia
Thyrotoxicosis

persistent fetal tachycardia. In the presence of contractions, the development of tachycardia between contractions often signifies worsening hypoxemia.

Occasionally, sinusoidal oscillations in the baseline fetal heart rate occur (Figure 9-2).[66] The pathophysiology and complete significance of this pattern are still undetermined. It has been observed during antepartum monitoring in several situations associated with fetal compromise, especially in severely anemic fetuses with erythroblastosis.[80] Reported cases of poor outcome accompanying this pattern have been described in various conditions[34,100] including postmaturity, diabetes mellitus, amnionitis, and preeclampsia. Certain structural cardiac and central nervous system anomalies and narcotic analgesics can also cause sinusoidal patterns.[27] Confusion exists in the literature concerning these patterns, largely because of the lack of uniform definition.[54,100] Because persistent sinusoidal patterns are sometimes manifestations of fetal compromise, fetal blood sampling should be performed when possible to

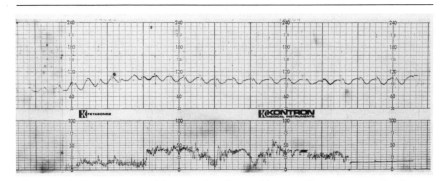

Figure 9-2 Persistent sinusoidal pattern in a fetus with severe intrapartum asphyxia.

ensure that fetal hypoxemia is not present. This is especially true when these patterns are observed in conjunction with any of the risk factors noted above. In particular, fetal anemia is a common denominator of many reported cases, and should be considered in appropriate clinical circumstances. Determination of fetal hematocrit from a scalp blood sample may be helpful.

Heart Rate Decelerations

Although many schemes for the classification of periodic heart rate decelerations have been proposed, the one most useful and widely applied is a modification of that of Hon and Quilligan.[44] Decelerations are categorized based upon their configuration and timing in relation to the uterine contraction. The use of this interpretation system requires fetal monitor paper speeds of 3 cm/min and a vertical scaling of 30 beats/min/ cm. The use of monitors with other scaling factors makes interpretation more difficult. In the 20 years that have elapsed since the introduction of this system, our knowledge of fetal monitoring and fetal physiology has grown dramatically, and allowed amplification and clarification of many of the original concepts.

Recurrent symmetric decelerations that begin and end at the same time as the contraction, and have their nadir at the peak of uterine pressure are called *early decelerations*. The associated change in heart rate is rarely more than 20 beats/min below the baseline. The presence of these decelerations, most common in the second stage of labor, does not require intervention unless they are accompanied by other fetal heart rate abnormalities. Most evidence suggests that there is no increased risk of hypoxemia or its consequences associated with early decelerations.[59,99]

Late decelerations are observed most commonly in association with acute or chronic uteroplacental vascular insufficiency.[15] They are the result of acute decrements in fetal oxygenation that result from reduction in intervillous blood flow during uterine contractions. When the reduction in oxygen delivery that accompanies this decrease in flow is of sufficient magnitude to exceed the fetal oxygen reserve, a late deceleration is produced as a result of central nervous system asphyxia and sometimes direct myocardial depression.[37] Although all late decelerations are manifestations of fetal hypoxemia and therefore warrant prompt attention, they are not always associated with fetal acidosis or adverse outcomes. Their potential impact must be assessed in relation to the clinical situation in which they occur, and according to other characteristics of the accompanying heart rate pattern. Experimental studies of late decelerations in animals have shown that they are accompanied by decreased oxygen consumption and arterial oxygen content.[77] As noted, the bradycardia may be influenced by cerebral and/or myocardial factors. Fetal hypoxemia probably causes stimulation of fetal chemoreceptors—and perhaps baroreceptors—and a vagally mediated deceleration in heart rate. This mechanism, because it requires an intact parasympathetic nervous system, manifests baseline variability in the heart rate between decelerations. Late decelerations with normal baseline variability occur most commonly as a consequence of acute fetal hypoxemia in a previously well-oxygenated fetus (Figure 9-3). But when the fetus is compromised by more long-standing or severe hypoxemia or acidosis, oxygen content may be low enough to cause a late deceleration based largely on direct myocardial depression (Figure 9-4).[52] Autonomic influences on heart rate are blunted, presumably as a consequence of central nervous system hypoxia. Therefore, these decelerations will be accompanied by diminished baseline variability because of reduced vagal stimulation.[43]

Late decelerations are recognized by four characteristics: (1) their shape is always relatively uniform, (2) they are repetitive in response to contractions of equal magnitude, (3) a lag time of at least 20 s exists between the onset of the contraction and that of the deceleration, and (4) the duration and amplitude of the deceleration is proportional to that of the accompanying contraction (Figure 9-5). The latter applies because these characteristics of the contraction govern the degree of diminution in uteroplacental blood flow that is produced.

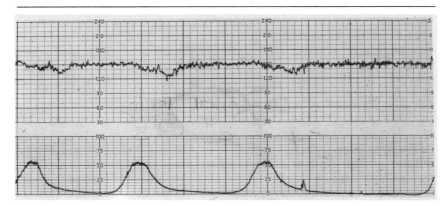

Figure 9-3 Late decelerations. The accompanying normal baseline rate and variability suggest that although the fetus is intermittently hypoxemic, its compensatory cardiovascular mechanisms are probably sufficient to maintain homeostasis at this time. Attempts at intrauterine resuscitation should be made, and fetal condition followed closely by further heart rate monitoring and serial pH measurements.

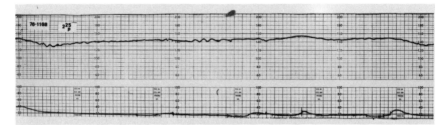

Figure 9-4 Late decelerations with mild contractions in a fetus with severe intrauterine growth retardation. The absence of heart rate variability and the adverse response to minimal stress characterize this as an ominous pattern.

The presence of late decelerations indicates that hypoxemia is present. Baseline heart rate changes that accompany the decelerations yield the most useful information concerning the degree of accompanying impairment. Of utmost importance in this regard is the heart rate variability. Paul et al.[78] showed that fetal acidosis accompanying late decelerations with diminished baseline variability is generally more severe than if the variability is normal. Similarly, the combination of baseline tachycardia and decreased variability between late decelerations is virtually always a sign of severe compromise.[4,15] This implies neither that hypoxemia is always absent with good variability nor that decreased variability is always accompanied by bad outcome; rather, accurate interpretation of

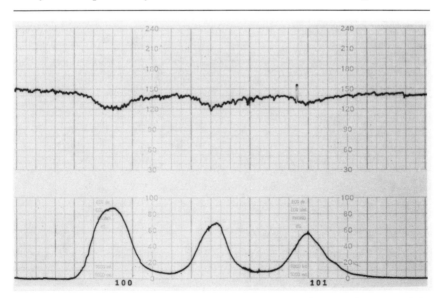

Figure 9-5 Late decelerations: The relation between the size of the deceleration and the magnitude of the contraction is demonstrated.

these features allows the obstetrician to make reasonable judgments regarding the probability of oxygen deprivation.

Variable decelerations are caused most often by compression of the umbilical cord during contractions.[16,42,43,90] They are possibly produced under certain circumstances by head compression or other factors, and can be recognized by the fact that there is usually considerable variation in their configuration and timing with relation to the contraction cycle (Figure 9-6).

The degree of fetal asphyxia that accompanies variable decelerations depends on the frequency, duration, and completeness of cord occlusion. There is a general correlation between the magnitude of the bradycardia in a variable deceleration and the severity of the acidosis that accompanies it.[59,62] However, the reliability of this criterion in clinical situations may be questioned because it does not take baseline heart rate changes into account. In fact, baseline tachycardia and/or diminished variability accompanying variable decelerations seem to be more useful indicators of severity than the size of the decelerations.

When fetal asphyxia is severe and baseline variability is absent, variable decelerations may be accompanied by a brief acceleration ("overshoot") that occurs before the heart rate pattern returns to baseline (Figure 9-7). In contrast, accelerations that precede or follow variable decelerations in the presence of good beat-to-beat variability are not ominous signs (see Figure 9-6).

Variable decelerations are occasionally observed in which the return to baseline is considerably more gradual than the drop in heart rate at the onset of the deceleration. The mechanism for the production of this configuration is unknown. Some evidence links this type of variable deceleration with more severe acidosis than those in which the return to

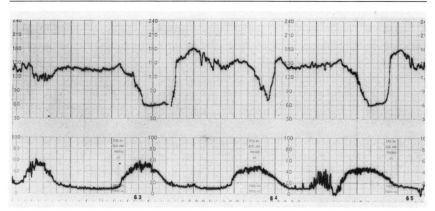

Figure 9-6 Recurrent variable decelerations with normal baseline rate and variability.

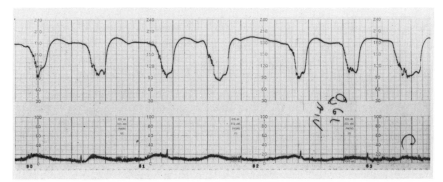

Figure 9-7 Variable decelerations. This is an ominous pattern because of the tachycardia and absent baseline variability that accompany the decelerations. In contrast to Figure 9-6, severe hypoxemia and acidosis were present in this case.

---

baseline is more abrupt, but baseline rate and variability have not generally been taken into consideration in these studies.[57] In the authors' experience, the variable decelerations that are associated with the most severe compromise are accompanied by absence of beat-to-beat variability and rather abrupt ascending and descending limbs. We do not consider delayed return to baseline or other atypical features to be clinically useful manifestations of severity.

The importance of assessing baseline heart rate changes between decelerations was emphasized by Gaziano.[32] He studied Apgar scores among groups of babies with normal fetal heart rate patterns, variable decelerations with normal baseline rate and variability, and similar decelerations with accompanying abnormal baseline characteristics. Significantly decreased Apgar scores were encountered only in the group in which variable decelerations were accompanied by abnormal baseline rate or diminished variability.

Prolonged decelerations are most commonly associated with preceding variable decelerations, and occasionally accompany manipulations of the fetus for vaginal examination or fetal blood sampling. Conditions that produce acute and relatively prolonged hypoxemia such as uterine hypertonus, tetanic contraction, maternal seizures, paracervical block anesthesia, or acute fetal blood loss may also result in prolonged decelerations. When they are manifestations of very severe or acute oxygen deprivation, they are generally associated with diminished variability. However, most prolonged decelerations, particularly those associated with good beat-to-beat variability, are not associated with adverse outcome. If the fetal heart rate pattern was normal prior to the deceleration, and an identifiable and correctable etiology exists, good outcome is the

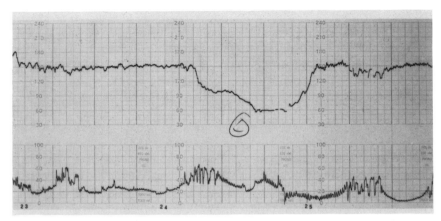

Figure 9-8 Prolonged deceleration. Although these patterns can be serious, those that occur in a fetus with a previously normal fetal heart rate pattern and in association with a demonstrable etiology generally resolve without serious sequelae.

rule[6,7,92] (Figures 9-8 to 9-10). Those fetuses that have manifested evidence of persistent hypoxemia prior to a prolonged deceleration are those most likely to suffer serious consequences.[55]

Iatrogenic Fetal Distress

The potential of many commonplace techniques to impair fetal oxygenation is now well known. The implications of these risks have been reviewed in detail elsewhere,[85] but certain issues are worthy of emphasis.

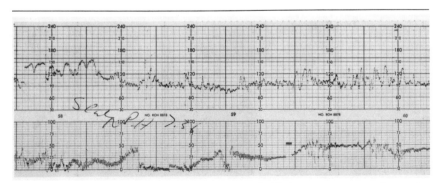

Figure 9-9 Prolonged fetal heart rate deceleration probably is response to excessive uterine activity. Maintenance of variability and normal scalp pH (7.36) indicate urgent intervention is not necessary. Pattern resolved after contractility diminished, and the baby was in good condition.

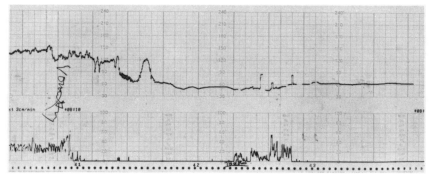

Figure 9-10 Prolonged fetal heart rate deceleration with absent variability and no apparent cause. Baby was born 15 min later and had evidence of acute severe asphyxia.

The deleterious effect of the supine position on uterine blood flow in a term gravida is well documented. Although a minority of women develop demonstrable hypotension when they are supine,[46] diminished cardiac output and uterine blood flow probably occur in many pregnant women when they assume the supine position. The importance of this fact with regard to the management of labor is evident. It has been documented that fetal oxygenation is better when babies are delivered vaginally or by cesarean section in the lateral rather than the supine position.[48,94]

The relationship between the magnitude of a uterine contraction and the degree of accompanying decrease in intervillous blood flow has been alluded to previously. It is therefore not surprising that the frequency of late decelerations increases when ecbolic agents are employed (Figure 9-11). These drugs should always be used with complete cognizance of their potential risks. These may be minimized by using a controlled intravenous infusion pump for administration of oxytocin, and careful

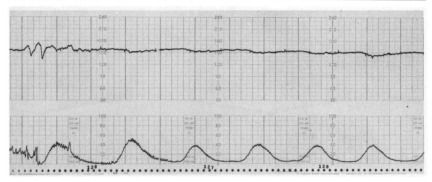

Figure 9-11 Small late decelerations associated with oxytocin-induced uterine tachysystole. Pattern returned to normal after oxytocin was discontinued and contractility normalized.

monitoring of uterine activity. The use of an internal uterine pressure catheter has advantages in this regard. Uterotonic agents must be used only when there is a clear indication, and the benefits of these drugs are perceived to outweigh the risks.

Of further importance with regard to possible iatrogenic fetal distress is the use of conduction anesthesia. Continuous peridural anesthesia is used frequently. It provides excellent pain relief with minimal side effects when used appropriately. However, the incidence of late decelerations in the presence of conduction anesthesia is potentially high.[84] This relates to the decrease in venous return and cardiac output that are the consequences of the sympathetic blockade induced by the use of anesthetic blocks. Late decelerations are even more frequent when oxytocin administration is combined with conduction anesthesia.[84] However, the potential hazards of anesthetic block techniques with regard to their effect on uterine blood flow can be minimized by keeping patients well hydrated and in the lateral position during epidural anesthesia.[17] In fact, with proper prehydration and subsequent management, epidural anesthesia has the potential to increase placental blood flow.[40] Continuous fetal heart rate monitoring will provide early warning if placental blood flow is compromised (Figure 9-12).

TREATMENT OF FETAL DISTRESS

As knowledge of perinatal physiology and mechanisms of abnormal fetal heart rate patterns has developed, simple methods for treating fetal

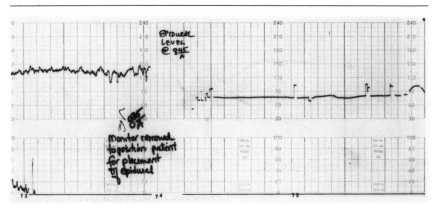

Figure 9-12 Continuous monitoring is mandatory when potentially harmful interventions are employed. The monitor was removed and an epidural level was given to a woman whose fetus had a normal heart rate pattern. A scalp electrode was applied 40 min later. Severe hypoxemia and acidosis accompanied this prolonged bradycardia. Had the monitor been recording continuously, fetal hypoxemia could have been recognized and treated earlier.

distress in utero have evolved. Although obstetric intervention in the presence of fetal oxygen deprivation may occasionally be urgent, there is usually time to invoke these methods of intrauterine resuscitation. In fact, delivery for fetal distress is rarely indicated until these potentially salutary avenues of correction have been tried and found fruitless.

In the vast majority of clinical situations, fetal hypoxemia is related primarily to a deficit in uterine or umbilical blood flow. Therefore, in the presence of late decelerations, all attempts should be made to maximize uterine blood flow. When recurrent variable decelerations suggest that cord compression is the source of asphyxia, techniques to relieve cord compression should be used in addition to those directed at uterine blood flow.

The importance of the lateral position has been emphasized previously. The maintenance of adequate intravascular volume is also crucial. Considerable volume deficits may occur in young women without demonstrable postural alterations in pulse or blood pressure. Under these circumstances, a redistribution of cardiac output occurs that favors flow to vital organs at the expense of the uterus. Therefore, an intravenous infusion of Ringer's lactate or similar crystalloid solution is vital whenever the diagnosis of fetal distress is entertained. When late decelerations have occurred purely as a result of depleted intravascular volume, this simple maneuver can be curative. The maintenance of hydration is of special importance if conduction anesthesia is employed.

Providing the mother with near-100% inspired oxygen by mask may also be beneficial,[3,56,72] and this maneuver may increase fetal oxygen content considerably under some circumstances (see Chapter 5). Nevertheless, because the transplacental exchange of oxygen is largely a flow-dependent process, the administration of oxygen is of secondary importance to the maneuvers mentioned above that enhance uterine blood flow.

The use of energy substrates including glucose has not been shown to be of value in the treatment of fetal distress during labor,[65] although hypoglycemia can perhaps potentiate fetal ischemic brain injury. The use of atropine to abolish fetal bradycardias has been suggested. The reasons this drug is probably not of benefit (and may be potentially harmful) have been described in Chapter 5.

Two other methods of in utero treatment of fetal heart rate pattern abnormalities have been described recently. Both remain experimental, but may ultimately achieve acceptance as clinical tools. In a randomized trial, Miyazaki and Nevarez[71] demonstrated the effectiveness of intrauterine infusion of saline to relieve recurrent variable decelerations that failed to respond to standard position changes or maternal oxygen therapy. Expanding the intrauterine volume with fluid in this manner probably reduces the risk or degree of cord compression during uterine contractions and may thus modify or eliminate variable decelerations. The role of this procedure in management of fetal distress is yet unclear. Whether amnioinfusion can ameliorate variable decelerations that would otherwise require operative delivery (i.e., generally those with abnormal baseline characteristics) is uncertain and requires clarification. Moreover, questions relating to possible risks (infection, increased intrauterine pressure, amniotic fluid embolus) remain unanswered.

Since uterine contractions frequently provoke fetal hypoxemia during labor, the use of a bolus of a beta-sympathomimetic drug has been recommended for treating fetal distress, and success has been reported.[51] These agents decrease uterine activity promptly, and may also have a beneficial effect on uterine blood flow. The real efficacy of this technique is not yet certain. It may prove useful as a temporizing measure in urgent situations when operative delivery cannot be accomplished promptly. Whether this maneuver would be useful and safe in the presence of a progressing etiology for fetal distress, such as abruptio placentae, is uncertain.

In summary, the management of late decelerations should include a careful examination of the mother and treatment of any correctable factors such as hypotension that might adversely affect uterine blood flow. The mother should be placed in the lateral position and acutely hydrated (assuming there is no cardiopulmonary contraindication to this). Oxytocin, if in use, should be discontinued immediately. A high inspired oxygen concentration should be provided. The initiation of conduction anesthesia in these situations should generally be proscribed.

The management of severe recurrent variable decelerations should include the above measures to maximize uteroplacental blood flow. In addition, altering the mother's position may sometimes be efficacious in relieving cord entrapment. To this end, changing the mother from one side to the other, to the knee-chest position, or to the Trendelenburg position may be helpful. When progressively severe variable decelerations are observed that do not respond to these maneuvers, a vaginal examination should be performed to rule out prolapse of the umbilical cord.[19] If an overt prolapse is discovered, and the fetal head is elevated out of the pelvis, the urgency of intervention can be determined by observing the fetal heart rate pattern. If a normal pattern or recovery from an abnormal one is observed, cesarean section can be carried out in a safe and unhurried fashion.

Occasionally, an occult prolapse of the cord will be manifested by recurrent variable decelerations. If the standard maneuvers of resuscitation prove fruitless, and the cord is not palpated vaginally, the patient should be prepared for cesarean section. With the mother in steep Trendelenburg position, the presenting part may be elevated.[22] Immediate delivery is indicated if this maneuver does not provoke an improvement in the heart rate pattern. If resolution of the abnormal pattern is observed, one should await complete recovery. At that time the fetus should be allowed to descend into the pelvis once again. If an ominous heart rate pattern occurs, elevation should be reinstituted and operative delivery performed after the fetus recovers. If the heart rate pattern appears to have improved considerably and remains stable, labor may be allowed to progress under close surveillance. Resolution of an occult cord prolapse has presumably occurred in these situations.

FETAL BLOOD SAMPLING

The development of a technique for fetal capillary blood sampling in the early 1960s by Erich Saling was a momentous landmark in the history of fetal evaluation.[82] Although no longer used as a primary screening tool, fetal blood sampling is an important corollary technique to fetal heart rate monitoring. Indeed, the two surveillance methods should be used in a complementary fashion to obtain the most useful and predictive information about fetal condition during labor.

Under conditions of oxygen deprivation, the fetus is unable to utilize pathways of aerobic intermediary metabolism. Therefore, glucose, the major fetal energy substrate, is metabolized primarily to the fixed organic acids lactate and pyruvate. The accumulation of these acids and the accompanying fall in fetal blood pH is a reflection of the magnitude and duration of oxygen lack. For this reason, measurement of fetal capillary pH is a way to estimate the state of fetal oxygenation. In addition to the progressive acidosis that accompanies anaerobic glycolysis, this is a much more inefficient means of energy production than its aerobic counterpart.

Volatile acids also accumulate during fetal oxygen deprivation. When placental perfusion is decreased as a result of impaired uterine or umbilical blood flow, the immediate result is an accumulation of carbon dioxide in the fetus. This increase in carbon dioxide partial pressure (Pco_2) is generally accompanied by a modest fall in pH, a respiratory acidosis. More prolonged hypoxemia results in a combined respiratory and metabolic acidosis. The latter may not resolve for a considerable time even after the hypoxic insult has abated.

Technique

The technique of fetal blood sampling is relatively easy, and experienced personnel can obtain adequate samples in at least 85% of cases with a measurement error of 0.03 to 0.05 pH units. The patient should be placed in the lateral position with her back at the edge of the bed. Lithotomy position should be avoided because it may interfere with maternal cardiac output and uterine blood flow. The assistant should stand in front of the mother to support the upper leg and thigh, which should be externally rotated. One should avoid having all personnel standing behind the mother, as isolation from visual contact with her caregivers can sometimes be frightening. The obstetrician, positioned behind the patient, prepares the perineum with antiseptic solution and inserts the amnioscope gently into the vagina until the presenting part is visualized. In vertex presentations, the sampling site should be over one of the parietal bones. Areas of obvious scalp edema and sutures or fontanels must be avoided. (In breech presentations the buttocks are the preferred site, with special care taken to avoid genital injury). Excess pressure with the amnioscope is counterproductive because it can produce local vascular stasis and acidosis within the circumscribed sampling area. After drying the scalp, a thin layer of silicone lubricant should be applied with a sterile swab. Using firm pressure the standard 2-mm guarded lancet is used to make a single horizontal puncture in the skin. Vertical incisions are less desirable because blood will not form droplets of the necessary size as readily. Several seconds usually pass before blood appears on the skin surface. When the drop reaches approximately 3 mm in diameter, its surface should be touched with the end of a heparinized glass capillary tube. The blood is collected by gravity. The capillary tube should be rotated between the fingers as the blood is collected in order to ensure rapid mixing with the heparin. After an adequate sample has been obtained, the tube should be handed to an assistant, and taken for immediate analysis. Under direct vision pressure should then be applied to the lancet incision with a sterile swab. The incision must be observed through at least one contraction after hemostasis has apparently been achieved.

Interpretation of Blood pH Values

The capillary fetal pH during labor normally ranges from 7.40 to 7.25 in the first stage.[50,53,64] Values less than 7.20 are generally considered abnormal and suggestive of significant asphyxia. Those between 7.20 and 7.24 are equivocal and require further evaluation.[10,64,82] A gradual decline in the fetal pH may occur during normal labor; most investigators find this is accelerated in the second stage. Second stage progression in acidosis, which is probably the result of a combination of increased uterine contractility and expulsive efforts of the mother, may be avoided or blunted when women labor and deliver in the lateral position, presumably because this posture maximizes uterine blood flow.[48] The validity of scalp pH measurements as an index of fetal oxygenation is supported by the generally good agreement between scalp capillary pH, cord blood pH and Apgar scores.[10,45,97] Pertinent information from experimental studies in pregnant monkeys revealed a very high correlation between the pH of blood in the fetal carotid artery and jugular vein and simultaneous samples from the fetal scalp.[1]

The predictive value of fetal pH samples in the clinical management of fetal distress has been evaluated extensively.[5,9,24,45,97] When using pH alone to predict Apgar scores, about 8% to 10% of values are spuriously low, and 6% to 10% are falsely normal.[4,9] Low Apgar scores accompanying normal capillary pH values may occur for several reasons. Poor respiratory effort or tone could be related to sedative or anesthetic drugs, infection, or birth trauma with normal pH. Premature babies often have low Apgar scores despite apparently adequate oxygenation because low birth weight babies normally have diminished tone and reflex responsivity in comparison to their term counterparts. Improper timing of the pH sample probably accounts for most false-normal values. Presumably, this relates to the fact that hypoxemic episodes may occur between the time of the blood sample and delivery.

Erroneously low pH values may be the result of local factors such as excessive caput succedaneum formation. Often these misleadingly low values occur because the fetus has recovered from an episode of acidosis between the sampling period and delivery.

Because lactate and carbon dioxide cross the placenta, severe maternal acidosis may produce a low fetal pH despite adequate oxygen transfer.[81] Maternal acidemia may itself be potentially harmful because passive fetal acidemia may adversely affect placental blood flow, deactivate fetal enzyme systems, alter the oxygen carrying capacity of fetal blood, and deplete buffer-base reserves. Comparison of the pH in maternal and fetal blood samples has been advocated as a means for differentiating acidosis due to fetal asphyxia from that which is related to maternal acidosis. Indeed, if the fetus is significantly acidotic and maternal pH and blood gases are normal, the fetal acidosis is almost certainly primary. Transplacental passage of bicarbonate ions from a mother who is hyperventilating could artificially obscure a fetal metabolic acidosis.

It has been suggested that if the difference in fetal and maternal pH is more than 0.1 unit, fetal asphyxia is likely.[58] Although this is a useful generalization, subtraction of these two values does not always provide accurate information about fetal condition. More complex methods to evaluate these differences have been developed, but they lack clinical applicability.

Spurious pH values may also result from technical problems that beset the collection of fetal scalp blood and the measuring system. Careful attention to the details of blood sample collection and prompt transportation to the laboratory are critically important. Calibration of the measuring devices should be done regularly, and the operator should be familiar with the technical requirements of the equipment.

The obstetrician will profit most from fetal blood sampling information when it is used to follow trends in the fetal acid base status in the presence of heart rate pattern abnormalities. Indications for fetal blood sampling are: uncertain diagnosis of fetal heart rate pattern; recurrent decelerations with good variability; persistent tachycardia or decreased variability without previously normal patterns.

The greatest virtue of the technique is that knowledge of a normal pH may permit one to allow progression of labor when the fetal heart rate pattern suggests a possible abnormality.[101] A clear understanding of the relationship between fetal heart rate patterns and pH values is therefore of great importance.[41]

Fetal acidosis is found rarely in association with persistent tachycardia or bradycardia unless these baseline abnormalities are associated with diminished variability or recurrent decelerations.[63] The presence of a persistent beat-to-beat arrhythmia or a sinusoidal pattern should be an indication for blood sampling. Although neither of these abnormalities is necessarily associated with acidosis, they preclude the use of usual criteria for the assessment of fetal oxygenation from monitoring data.

As noted previously, the impact of a variable deceleration is better judged by the accompanying baseline heart rate abnormalities than by the duration and depth of the bradycardia. Some studies have not found a correlation between the magnitude of variable or late decelerations and the severity of fetal acidosis.[102] When a blood sample is obtained in the presence of variable decelerations, it is vital that it be timed just prior to a contraction. In this way it will serve as a measure of fetal reserve and the ability to recover from the stress of the previous contraction. Moreover, umbilical cord compression results in rapid reduction in carbon dioxide transfer across the placenta, and in a fetal respiratory acidosis. Scalp blood samples obtained at the nadir of a large variable deceleration commonly show acidosis. This is often respiratory in nature and resolves rapidly after the contraction. Acidosis that persists until the onset of the next contraction more likely has a metabolic component, and places the fetus in greater jeopardy.

Late decelerations are always accompanied by fetal hypoxemia.[15,77] As noted, however, because of certain compensatory cardiovascular mechanisms, not all heart rate patterns with late decelerations are accompanied by acidosis. In general, intervention should not be considered unless there is evidence of progressive oxygen deprivation. It is reassuring that experiments in monkeys have shown that late decelerations appear prior to neuropathologic evidence of brain damage.[2] In fact, during labor they are probably an early sign of hypoxemia, and generally occur before loss of acceleration and variability.[73] Late decelerations that are associated with baseline tachycardia or diminished variability are much more likely to be associated with significant asphyxia than those with a normal baseline.[15,68,78,102] When a prolonged deceleration occurs in a fetus with good reserve and normal oxygenation, significant acidosis is unlikely in the first several minutes. If the bradycardia is persistent, and the etiology is not readily discernible or remediable, serial scalp sampling may help guide judgments concerning intervention. Prompt delivery is indicated if the bradycardia is not responsive to resuscitative maneuvers described above and if the pH is falling or variability is absent for several minutes.

It has been emphasized that although diminished variability may be a consequence of asphyxia, it has numerous other causes. In fact, decreased variability unaccompanied by other heart rate changes is generally not associated with measurable acidosis or reduced fetal oxygen tension.[4] Variability almost always diminishes considerably when hypoxemia becomes persistent. Although experimental studies have shown that the initial response to hypoxemia may be an increase in variability, persistence of distress eventually causes variability to diminish in human fetuses.

Based on our current understanding of the pathophysiology of fetal heart rate abnormalities and their accompanying acid-base aberrations, we have chosen to consider baseline heart rate and variability as indices of fetal reserve. The nature of the deceleration waveform is used to gain insight into the mechanism of the hypoxic insult. Therefore, we do not emphasize the magnitude of heart rate decelerations per se in determining severity, but rather find it more useful to determine the impact of a deceleration by assessing the changes that accompany it in baseline rate and variability.[18,20,21] The principle underlying this approach is based on the idea that loss of central nervous system (primarily parasympathetic) control of heart rate will occur when fetal compensatory cardiovascular mechanisms are no longer able to sustain normal brain flow and oxygenation. The resulting decrease in variability and/or development of tachycardia foreshadows the potential for hypoxic tissue damage.

COMPLICATIONS OF FETAL MONITORING

Maternal Infection

Several investigators have demonstrated an increase in maternal infection risk after vaginal delivery among women whose babies were monitored during labor, but other retrospective studies have not confirmed this association.[31,95] In most studies, confounding variables that might have influenced the occurrence of postpartum infection such as social class, duration of labor and ruptured membranes, and route of delivery were not considered thoroughly. In a careful analysis that attempted to address such factors, Gibbs et al.[33] were unable to demonstrate any influence of electronic fetal monitoring on infection rates. Other studies reached similar conclusions.[26,31,38] Despite this encouraging evidence that has failed to confirm suspicions about the infectious potential of fetal monitoring, the fact that internal monitoring involves invasion of the uterus with foreign materials (scalp electrode and pressure catheter) suggests that a risk might be present. Reasonable care to provide asepsis should be used when monitors are applied. It is likely that restricting the use of intrauterine pressure catheters to specific indications (oxytocin infusion, abnormal heart rate pattern) may also serve to diminish the risk.

Neonatal Complications

Local scalp erythema, cellulitis, or abscess formation in association with scalp electrodes have been described.[25,75] Most of these respond to conservative local therapy and do not produce serious sequelae. However, antibiotic treatment is sometimes necessary, and rare instances of serious, even lethal infections have been described. The use of scalp electrodes should be avoided or considered carefully in certain situations likely to be associated with an increased risk of infection. This is true of prolonged rupture of the membranes, prolonged labor, or suspected amnionitis. The potential benefits of internal monitoring must be weighed against risks in these situations. The use of the scalp electrode should be contraindicated in the presence of maternal genital infections such as herpes simplex.

Excessive trauma from the scalp electrode may occasionally occur, but this can be minimized by observing the proper techniques of application and removal. The electrode should be inserted with the protective sheath covering the electrode tip, thus minimizing contamination from the vagina or cervix. Application should take place over one of the skull bones. Introduction of the electrode into the relatively thin scalp of the premature infant has been reported to result in cerebrospinal fluid leaks.[93] Obviously, when malpositions or malpresentations are present, extreme care must be taken to apply the electrode away from the face, eyelids, or genitalia. Removal of the electrode should be accomplished only by grasping it at its base and rotating it counterclockwise without traction. Traction on the wires or the electrode may cause local scalp lacerations and increased infection risk. Proper technique must also be observed during placement of the intrauterine catheter in order to minimize risks of infection or trauma. The sheath surrounding the flexible catheter should be held between the fingers and not allowed to extend beyond the fingertips. The introducer should be placed just inside the cervix and fixed there as the internal catheter is advanced past the fetus. Forceful insertion of the catheter or inappropriate advancement of the external sheath may cause laceration of placental vessels or uterine perforation.[13,29]

The fetal blood sampling incision is also an area where infection may begin. Appropriate precautions must be used to minimize the introduction of bacteria to this site. The use of multiple scalp incisions or X-shaped incisions is not necessary, and may increase the potential for local complications. Of greater consequence is the fact that in rare instances scalp blood sampling can result in serious or even fatal hemorrhage. This has been reported only among fetuses with coagulation disorders, or after vacuum extractor application over a sampling site;[79] but one should always be aware of the potential for this complication. For this reason it is mandatory that the scalp puncture site be observed for several minutes even after hemostasis appears to have occurred.

Obstetric Complications

Concerns have been raised about indirect complications that may result from fetal monitoring techniques. The influence of fetal monitoring on cesarean section rates and the excess morbidity necessarily associated with that mode of delivery has been evaluated. Although some studies have shown an increase in the likelihood of cesarean section among monitored patients, others do not support this notion.[8,74]

It seems that monitoring techniques themselves cannot be indicted as causes of the increase in cesarean section rate noted by some investigators. It is more likely that inappropriate interpretation of monitoring information has resulted in over-zealous intervention. Clearly, the ability to make the most appropriate decisions in the presence of abnormal heart rate patterns requires considerable experience and insight. The application of definitions of fetal distress that were extant prior to the advent of electronic monitors is erroneous and will lead to unnecessary interventions. The use of modern methods of monitoring requires a commitment to learning new interpretive approaches.

CLINICAL CONSIDERATIONS

Application of the foregoing principles of fetal monitoring to clinical events requires the knowledge afforded by experience and study, coupled with a systematic approach to the problem (Figure 9-13). Fetal heart rate patterns have been categorized into four groups, based upon the likelihood of accompanying asphyxia[20,21,87] (Table 9-4). This scheme can guide evaluation and intervention; however, it must be used with the understanding that it consists of generalizations and many clinical problems breach boundaries between categories.

Suspicious signs (tachycardia, bradycardia, decreased variability) are infrequently associated with hypoxia. They assume graver significance when they accompany variable or late decelerations.[100] On rare occasions a fetus with severe, preterminal asphyxia will present with an abnormal baseline and no other heart rate pattern abnormalities. When suspicious patterns are diagnosed, the patient should be evaluated thoroughly to ensure that any correctable factors that could contribute to fetal hypoxia (e.g., hypotension, supine position) are treated promptly. Oxytocin stimulation, regional anesthesia, or other potentially compromising techniques should be withheld until it is established that fetal oxygenation is adequate.

Threatening heart rate patterns (recurrent variable or late decelerations with normal baseline rate and variability) are somewhat more worrisome. A prompt evaluation of fetal condition and search for treatable causes of hypoxia should be made. Maneuvers of intrauterine resuscitation designed to enhance uterine blood flow—and to reduce cord compression if variable decelerations are present—should be undertaken. Fetal blood

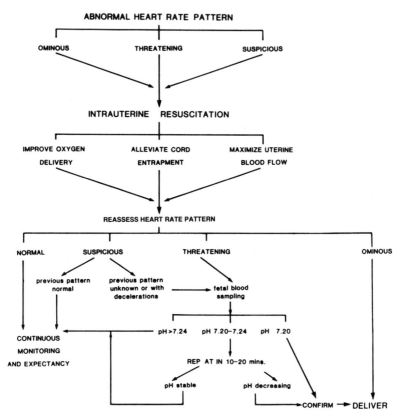

Figure 9-13 Logic diagram indicating a method for managing abnormal heart rate patterns. *Source:* Adapted by permission from "Fetal Distress" by W Cohen in *Obstetrical Decision Making* (p 139) by EA Friedman (Ed), BC Decker Inc, Toronto, © 1982.

sampling may be helpful in these situations and careful attention must be directed to the condition of the baseline heart rate between decelerations. Intervention is generally not necessary if the baseline rate is stable, and the variability is normal. Delivery should be considered in the presence of a rising baseline rate, loss of variability, or decreasing pH (Figure 9-14).

Prolonged decelerations deserve the same resuscitative efforts described for variable decelerations. If no improvement in the fetal heart rate occurs, and variability is absent, delivery should be expedited promptly. However, when variability is normal, a good outcome is the rule even when the bradycardia persists for extended periods of time. Serial scalp blood samples may be helpful in this situation to verify that

Table 9-4 Classification of Fetal Heart Rate Patterns

Classification	Baseline features	Periodic features
Reassuring	Stable rate Average variability	None Uniform accelerations Early decelerations
Suspicious	Decreased variability Tachycardia Bradycardia	No decelerations
Threatening	Stable rate Average variability	Late decelerations Variable decelerations
Ominous	Absent variability Tachycardia Bradycardia	Late decelerations Variable decelerations

Sources: Seminars in Perinatology (1978;2:155–167), Copyright © 1978, Grune & Stratton Inc; Perinatal Medicine, ed 2 (pp 223–243) by RJ Bolognese, RH Schwarz, and J Schneider (Eds), Williams & Wilkins Company, © 1982.

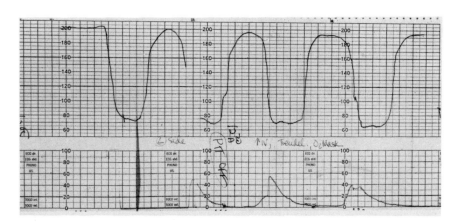

Figure 9-14 Large, variable decelerations in a 26-week-gestation fetus who died within minutes of delivery. Tachycardia and absence of variability mark this as a very ominous pattern.

the fetal adaptive cardiovascular mechanisms are maintaining acid-base homeostasis.

Ominous fetal heart rate patterns (concurrence of recurrent decelerations and abnormal baseline heart rate or variability) demand swift evaluation and attempts at improvement because they are so often a manifestation of severe fetal asphyxia. Preparation for immediate cesarean section should be made, and delivery carried out if conservative measures do not result in prompt, demonstrable improvement in the heart rate pattern.

Recently, a variant of the ominous pattern has been described[89] in which absent variability accompanies small variable decelerations with overshoot (Figure 9-15). Late decelerations are absent. The baseline rate is stable and is normal or slightly elevated. Sometimes the fetal pH may be normal and accelerations present. Some of the babies are terminally ill from asphyxia, and others will survive with residual neurologic handicap. The precise significance of this pattern is not yet clear. It may be that in many cases intervention will prove to be of little benefit.

The presence of meconium in the amniotic fluid may sometimes result from intrauterine asphyxia; however, severe asphyxia neither leads invariably to nor is a prerequisite for meconium passage or aspiration. In fact, most fetuses who pass meconium are not compromised in utero. Therefore, the presence of meconium should be an indication for fetal heart rate monitoring to determine whether hypoxemia exists. Intervention for fetal distress should not be undertaken solely because meconium is present, but should be based also on information from the accompanying fetal heart rate pattern and, if appropriate, fetal blood pH. Aspiration

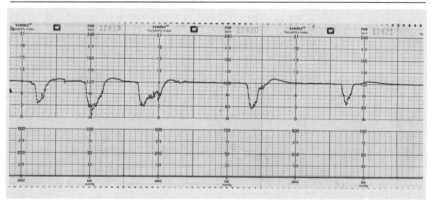

Figure 9-15 Small variable decelerations with terminal overshoot and absence of baseline variability in a 41-week-fetus with oligohydramnios and postmaturity syndrome. This is an ominous pattern that probably represents long-standing oxygen deprivation.

of meconium can occur in utero during severe asphyxial episodes;[11] it is therefore especially vital to avoid fetal asphyxia when this threat to the airway exists. Consequently, when abnormal fetal heart rate patterns are present, the threshold for intervention should be lower when meconium is present than when the amniotic fluid is clear. Because of the considerable risks of aspiration at delivery, personnel and equipment for immediate suctioning of the newborn's airway must be available.

Assessment of uterine activity is an important aspect of heart rate pattern interpretation. Uterine blood flow decreases in proportion to the duration, amplitude and frequency of contractions; therefore, uterotonic drugs must not be used if compromised fetal oxygenation is suspected. As indicated above, some advocate that the mother be given a uterine relaxant drug when severe fetal distress is diagnosed. By abolishing contractions and enhancing uterine blood flow, the fetal condition may be improved while preparations for operative delivery are undertaken. Even if this were to become an approved technique, it would likely be applicable in only a minority of situations.

It should be emphasized that the decision to expedite delivery in the presence of fetal distress should be made only after all appropriate attempts at intrauterine resuscitation have proved futile. The success of these attempts may be judged by following the trends in fetal pH and heart rate patterns. In general, if a cause of a hypoxic event can be removed, the fetus will fare better if allowed to recover in utero than if delivered in a hypoxic condition requiring vigorous delivery room resuscitation. Even if intrauterine treatment of hypoxia provides just transient improvement, it may permit the careful delivery of a well-oxygenated fetus rather than the hasty and potentially traumatic delivery of a hypoxic one.

The timing of delivery should be determined by the likelihood of recovery, and a judgment based on all available information must be made in each case. When emergency delivery requires a choice between a midforceps operation and cesarean section, the latter is generally preferred. There is convincing evidence that midforceps delivery carries a high frequency of trauma and some suggestion that this risk may be potentiated in the presence of asphyxia.[14,30]

SUMMARY

The introduction of various methods of fetal monitoring has opened new horizons for obstetrics. Nevertheless, important questions concerning the efficacy of these techniques remain unanswered.[86] Of particular importance in this regard is how to determine what populations benefit most from monitoring. Intrapartum asphyxia is more common among high-risk patients, and they should receive priority when monitoring resources are limited. Whether the economic costs and medical risks of monitoring make it appropriate for low-risk patients is still uncertain. Occasional instances of significant asphyxia certainly occur in this group and detection and treatment of these cases is gratifying.

The controversy concerning the use of electronic monitoring is ongoing.[21,39,76] Although most retrospective analyses have concluded that monitoring is beneficial, several randomized clinical trials have failed to document improvement in short or long-term outcome attributable to the technique. Existing studies are clearly inadequate to provide definitive answers and more research is required. Despite the lingering uncertainty in the obstetric literature, monitoring of high risk pregnancies is prevalent in most institutions, and advocates of universal monitoring abound. Presumably, this paradox is rooted in the conviction of individual practitioners that information obtained from this technology is useful.

The most disturbing aspect of the evaluation of monitoring risks is the observation that unnecessary intervention may result from improper interpretation of fetal monitoring information. In this regard, it is important to emphasize that fetal heart rate monitoring and scalp blood sampling are sophisticated techniques. In order to obtain a benefit from them, and to avoid inherent risks, the obstetrician must make a commitment to understanding the nuances and pitfalls of this technology.

REFERENCES

1. Adamsons K, Beard RW, Meyers RE: Comparison of the composition of arterial, venous and capillary blood of the fetal monkey during labor. *Am J Obstet Gynecol* 1970;107: 435–440.

2. Adamsons K, Meyers RE: Late decelerations and brain tolerance of the fetal monkey to intrapartum asphyxia. *Am J Obstet Gynecol* 1977;128:893–900.

3. Althabe O Jr, Schwarcz RL, Pose SV, Escarena L, Caldeyro-Barcia R: Effects on fetal heart rate and fetal PO_2 of oxygen administration to the mother. *Am J Obstet Gynecol* 1967; 98:858–870.

4. Beard RW, Filshie GM, Knight CA, Roberts GM: The significance of the changes in the continuous fetal heart rate in the first stage of labor. *J Obstet Gynaecol Br Commonw* 1971; 78:865–881.

5. Beard RW, Morris ED, Clayton SG: pH of foetal capillary blood as an indicator of the condition of the fetus. *J Obstet Gynaecol Br Commonw* 1967;74:812–822.

6. Boehm F, Growdon J: The effect of eclamptic convulsions on the fetal heart rate. *Am J Obstet Gynecol* 1974;120:851–852.

7. Boehm FH: Prolonged end stage fetal heart rate deceleration. *Obstet Gynecol* 1975;45: 579–582.

8. Boehm FH, Davidson KK, Barrett JM: The effect of electronic fetal monitoring on the incidence of cesarean section. *Am J Obstet Gynecol* 1981;140:295–298.

9. Bowe ET: Fetal blood sampling in labor. *Bull Sloane Hosp Women* 1969;15:103–106.

10. Bretscher J, Saling E: pH values in the human fetus during labor. *Am J Obstet Gynecol* 1967;97:906–911.

11. Brown BL, Gleicher N: Intrauterine meconium aspiration. *Obstet Gynecol* 1981; 57:26–29.

12. Caldeyro-Barcia R, Mendez-Bauer C, Poseiro JJ, Escarcena LA, Pose SV, Arnt IV, Gulin L, Althabe O, Bieniarz J: Control of the human fetal heart rate during labor, in Cassels DE (ed): *The Heart and Circulation in the Newborn Infant.* New York, Grune & Stratton, 1966.

13. Chan WH, Paul RH, Toews J: Intrapartum fetal monitoring. Maternal and fetal morbidity and perinatal mortality. *Obstet Gynecol* 1973;41:7–13.

14. Chiswick ML, James DK: Kielland's forceps: Association with neonatal morbidity and mortality. *Br Med J* 1979;1:7–9.

15. Cibils L: Clinical significance of fetal heart rate patterns during labor. II. Late decelerations. *Am J Obstet Gynecol* 1975;123:473–494.

16. Cibils LA: Clinical significance of fetal heart rate patterns during labor. Variable decelerations. *Am J Obstet Gynecol* 1975;132:791–805.

17. Clark RB: Prevention of spinal hypotension associated with cesarean section. *Anesthesiol* 1976;45:670–674.

18. Cohen WR: Invasive electronic and biochemical fetal monitoring, in Iffy L, Charles D (eds): *Operative Perinatology.* New York, NY, Macmillan, 1984, pp 489–514.

19. Cohen WR: Umbilical cord prolapse, in Nelson NM (ed): *Current Therapy in Neonatal-Perinatal Medicine.* Toronto, BC Decker, 1985, pp 69–70.

20. Cohen WR, Schifrin BS: Diagnosis and management of fetal distress during labor. *Semin Perinatol* 1978;2:155–167.

21. Cohen WR, Schifrin BS: Diagnosis and treatment of fetal distress, in Bolognese RJ, Schwarz RH, Schneider J (eds): *Perinatal Medicine,* ed 4. Baltimore, Williams & Wilkins, 1982, pp 223–243.

22. Cohen WR, Schifrin BS, Doctor G: Elevation of the fetal presenting part, a method of intrauterine resuscitation. *Am J Obstet Gynecol* 1975;123:646–649.

23. Cohen WR, Yeh S-Y: The abnormal fetal heart rate baseline. *Clin Obstet Gynecol* 1986; 29:73–82.

24. Coltart TM, Trickey NRA, Beard RW: Fetal blood sampling: Practical approach to management of fetal distress. *Br Med J* 1969;1:342–346.

25. Cordero L Jr, Hon EG: Scalp abscess: A rare complication of fetal monitoring. *J Pediatr* 1971;78:533–536.

26. D'Angelo LJ, Sokol RJ: Time-related peripartum determinants of postpartum morbidity. *Obstet Gynecol* 1980;55:319–323.

27. Epstein H, Waxman A, Gleicher N, Laverson NH: Meperidine-induced sinusoidal fetal heart rate pattern and reversal with naloxone. *Obstet Gynecol* 1982;59:225–255.

28. Escarcena L, McKinney RD, Depp R: Fetal baseline heart rate variability estimation. I. Comparison of clinical and stochastic quantification techniques. *Am J Obstet Gynecol* 1979; 135:615–621.

29. Fernandez-Rocha L, Oulette R: Fetal bleeding: An unusual complication of fetal monitoring. *Am J Obstet Gynecol* 1976;125:1153–1155.

30. Friedman EA, Sachtleben MR, Bresky PA: Dysfunctional labor. XII. Long term effects on infant. *Am J Obstet Gynecol* 1977;127:779–783.

31. Gassner CB, Ledger WJ: The relationship of hospital-acquired maternal infection to invasive intrapartum monitoring techniques. *Am J Obstet Gynecol* 1976;126:33–37.

32. Gaziano EP: A study of variable decelerations in association with other heart rate patterns during monitored labor. *Am J Obstet Gynecol* 1979;135:360–363.

33. Gibbs RS, Jones PM, Wilder CJY: Internal fetal monitoring and maternal infection following cesarean section. A prospective study. *Obstet Gynecol* 1978;52:193–197.

34. Gleicher N, Runowicz CD, Brown BL: Sinusoidal fetal heart rate pattern in association with amnionitis. *Obstet Gynecol* 1980;56:109–111.

35. Glick G, Braunwald E: Relative roles of the sympathetic and parasympathetic nervous systems in the reflex control of heart rate. *Circ Res* 1965;16:363–375.

36. Griffin RL, Caron FJM, VanGeijn HP: Behavioral states in the human fetus during labor. *Am J Obstet Gynecol* 1985;152:828–833.

37. Harris JL, Krueger TR, Parer JT: Mechanisms of late decelerations of the fetal heart rate during hypoxia. *Am J Obstet Gynecol* 1982;144:491–496.

38. Hawrylyshyan PA, Bernstein P, Papsin FR: Risk factors associated with infection following cesarean section. *Am J Obstet Gynecol* 1981;139:294–298.

39. Hobbins JC, Freeman R, Queenan JT: The fetal monitoring debate. *Obstet Gynecol* 1979;54:103–109.

40. Hollmen AI, Jouppila R, Jouppila P, Koivula A, Vierola H: Effect of extradural analgesia using bupivacaine and 2-chloroprocaine on intervillous blood flow during normal labour. *Br J Anaesth* 1982;54:837–842.

41. Hon E: Electronic evaluation of the fetal heart rate. VI. Fetal distress—a working hypothesis. *Am J Obstet Gynecol* 1962;83:333–353.

42. Hon E: Additional observations on "pathologic" bradycardia. *Am J Obstet Gynecol* 1974;118:428–441.

43. Hon EH, Bradfield AN, Hess OW: The electronic evaluation of the fetal heart rate. V. The vagal factor in fetal bradycardia. *Am J Obstet Gynecol* 1961;82:291–300.

44. Hon EH, Quilligan EJ: The classification of fetal heart rate. II. A revised working classification. *Conn Med* 1967;31:779–784.

45. Hon EH, Yeh S: Electronic evaluation of the fetal heart rate. X. The fetal arrhythmia index. *Med Res Eng* 1969;8:14–19.

46. Howard BK, Goodson JH, Mengert WF: Supine hypotensive syndrome in late pregnancy. *Obstet Gynecol* 1953;1:371–377.

47. Huey JR, Jr, Paul RH, Hadjiev AA, Jilek J, Hon EH: Fetal heart rate variability: An approach to automated assessment. *Am J Obstet Gynecol* 1979;134:691–695.

48. Humphrey MD, Chang A, Wood EC, Morgan S, Hounslow D: A decrease in fetal pH during the second stage of labor when conducted in the dorsal position. *J Obstet Gynaecol Br Commonw* 1974;81:600–602.

49. Ibarra-Polo AA, Guiloff FE, Gomez-Rogers C: Fetal heart rate throughout pregnancy. *Am J Obstet Gynecol* 1972;113:814–818.

50. Ingemarsson I, Arulkumaran S: Fetal acid-base balance in low-risk patients in labor. *Am J Obstet Gynecol* 1986;155:66–69.

51. Ingemarsson I, Arulkumaran S, Ratnam SS: Single injection of terbutaline in term labor. I. Effect on fetal pH in cases with prolonged bradycardia. *Am J Obstet Gynecol* 1985; 859–865.

52. Itskovitz J, Goetzman BW, Rudolph AM: The mechanism of late deceleration of the heart rate and its relationship to oxygenation in normoxemic and chronically hypoxemic fetal lambs. *Am J Obstet Gynecol* 1982;142:66–73.

53. Jacobson L, Rooth G: Interpretative aspects of the acid base composition and its variation in fetal scalp blood and maternal blood during labor. *J Obstet Gynaecol Br Commonw* 1971;78:971–980.

54. Johnson TRB, Compton AA, Rotmensch J, Work BA, Johnson JWC: Significance of sinusoidal fetal heart rate pattern. *Am J Obstet Gynecol* 1981;139:446–453.

55. Katz M, Naftali S, Meizner I, Insler V: Is end-stage deceleration of the fetal heart ominous? *Br J Obstet Gynaecol* 1982;89:186–189.

56. Khazin AF, Hon EH, Hehre FW: Effects of maternal hyperoxia on the fetus. *Am J Obstet Gynecol* 1971;109:628–637.

57. Krebs H-B, Petres RE, Dunn LJ: Intrapartum fetal heart rate monitoring. VIII. Atypical variable decelerations. *Am J Obstet Gynecol* 1983;145:297–305.

58. Kubli F: Current understanding of the relationship of fetal heart rate patterns to fetal blood gas measurements, in Lauersen NH, Hochberg HM (eds): *Clinical Perinatal Biochemical Monitoring*. Baltimore, Williams & Wilkins, 1981, pp 49–65.

59. Kubli FW, Hon EH, Khazin AF, Takemura H: Observations on heart rate and pH in the human fetus during labor. *Am J Obstet Gynecol* 1969;104:1190–1206.

60. Langer O, Cohen WR: Persistent fetal bradycardia during maternal hypoglycemia. *Am J Obstet Gynecol* 1984;149:688–690.

61. Laros RK, Wong WS, Heilbron DC, Parer JT, Shnider SM, Naylor H, Butler J: A comparison of methods for quantitating fetal heart rate variability. *Am J Obstet Gynecol* 1977; 128:381–392.

62. Low JA, Boston RW, Pancham SR: The role of the fetal heart rate pattern in the recognition of fetal asphyxia with metabolic acidosis. *Am J Obstet Gynecol* 1971;109:992–999.

63. Low JA, Cox MJ, Karchmar EJ, McGrath MJ, Pancham SR, Piercy WN: The prediction of intrapartum fetal metabolic acidosis by fetal heart rate monitoring. *Am J Obstet Gynecol* 1981;139:299–305.

64. Lumley J, McKinnon L, Wood C: Lack of agreement on normal values for fetal scalp blood. *J Obstet Gynaecol Br Commonw* 1971;78:13–21.

65. Mann LI, Prichard JW, Symmes D: The effect of glucose loading on the fetal response to hypoxia. *Am J Obstet Gynecol* 1970;107:610–618.

66. Manseau P, Vaquier J, Chavinine J, Sureau C: Le rythme cardiaque foetal "sinusoidal." *J Gynecol Obstet Biol Rep* 1972;1:343–352.

67. Marsh TD, Lagrew DC, Cook LN, Lavery JP: Unexplained fetal baseline bradycardia in congenital panhypopituitarism. *Am J Obstet Gynecol* 1987;156:977–979.

68. Martin CB: Regulation of the fetal heart rate and genesis of FHR patterns. *Semin Perinatol* 1978;2:131–146.

69. Martin CB: Behavioral states in the human fetus. *J Reprod Med* 1981;26:425–432.

70. Maxwell KD, Kearney KK, Johnson JWC, Eagan JW, Tyson JE: Fetal tachycardia associated with intrauterine fetal thyrotoxicosis. *Obstet Gynecol* 1980;55:185–225.

71. Miyazaki FS, Nevarez F: Saline amnioinfusion for relief of repetitive variable decelerations: A prospective randomized study. *Am J Obstet Gynecol* 1985;153:301–306.

72. Morishima H, Daniel S, Richards R, James LS: The effect of increased maternal PaO_2 upon the fetus during labor. *Am J Obstet Gynecol* 1975;123:257–264.

73. Murata Y, Martin CB, Ikenowe T, Hashimoto T, Taira S, Sakata H: Fetal heart accelerations and late decelerations during the course of intrauterine death in chronically catheterized rhesus monkeys. *Am J Obstet Gynecol* 1982;144:218–223.

74. Neutra RR, Greenland S, Friedman EA: Effect of fetal monitoring on cesarean section rates. *Obstet Gynecol* 1980;55:175–180.

75. Okada DM, Chow AW: Neonatal scalp abscess following intrapartum fetal monitoring: Prospective comparison of two spiral electrodes. *Am J Obstet Gynecol* 1977;127:875–878.

76. Parer JT: FHR monitoring: Answering the critics. *Contemp Ob/Gyn* 1981;17:163–174.

77. Parer JT, Krueger TR, Harris JL: Fetal oxygen consumption and mechanisms of heart rate response during artificially produced late decelerations of fetal heart rate in sheep. *Am J Obstet Gynecol* 1980;136:478–482.

78. Paul RH, Suidan AK, Yeh S, Schifrin BS, Hon EH: Clinical fetal monitoring. VII. The evaluation and significance of intrapartum baseline FHR variability. *Am J Obstet Gynecol* 1975;123:206–210.

79. Roberts IF, Stone M: Fetal hemorrhage: Complication of vacuum extractor after fetal blood sampling. *Am J Obstet Gynecol* 1978;132:109.

80. Rochard F, Schifrin BS, Goupil F, Legrand H, Blottiere J, Sureau C: Nonstressed fetal heart rate monitoring in the antepartum period. *Am J Obstet Gynecol* 1976;126:699–706.

81. Roversi GD, Cannussio V, Spennacchio M: Recognition and significance of materno-genic fetal acidosis during intensive monitoring of labor. *J Perinatol Med* 1975;3:53–63.

82. Saling E: *Foetal and Neonatal Hypoxia in Relation to Clinical Obstetric Practice.* Baltimore, Williams & Wilkins, 1968.

83. Schifferli PY, Caldeyro-Barcia R: Effects of atropine and beta-autonomic drugs on the heart rate of the human fetus, in Boreus L (ed): *Fetal Pharmacology.* New York, Raven Press, 1973.

84. Schifrin BS: Fetal heart rate patterns following epidural anesthesia and oxytocin infusion during labour. *J Obstet Gynaecol Br Commonw* 1972;79:332–339.

85. Schifrin BS: Iatrogenic fetal distress. *Int Anesthesiol Clin* 1973;11:119–140.

86. Schifrin BS: Polemics in perinatology: The future of fetal monitoring. *J Perinatol* 1987; 6:331–332.

87. Schifrin BS, Dame L: Fetal heart rate patterns. Prediction of Apgar scores. *JAMA* 1972;219:1322–1325.

88. Shenker L: Fetal cardiac arrhythmias. *Obstet Gynecol Surv* 1979;34:561–572.

89. Shields JR, Schifrin BS: Perinatal antecedents of cerebral palsy. *Obstet Gynecol* 1988;71:899–905.

90. Siassi B, Blanco C, Martin CB: Baroreceptor and chemoreceptor responses to umbilical cord occlusion in fetal lambs. *Biol Neonate* 1979;35:66–73.

91. Stange L, Rosen KG, Hokegard K-H, Karlsson K, Rochlitzer F, Kjellmer I, Joellson I: Quantification of fetal heart rate variability in relation to oxygenation in the sheep fetus. *Acta Obstet Gynecol Scand* 1977;56:205–209.

92. Tejani N, Mann L, Bhakthavathsalan A: Prolonged fetal bradycardia with recovery: Its significance and outcome. *Am J Obstet Gynecol* 1975;122:975.

93. Turbeville DF, McCaffree MA: Fetal scalp electrode complications: Cerebrospinal fluid leak. *Obstet Gynecol* 1979;54:469–470.

94. Waldron LW, Wood C: Cesarean section in the lateral position. *Obstet Gynecol* 1971; 37:706–710.

95. Wiechetek WJ, Horiguchi T, Dillon TF: Puerperal morbidity and internal fetal monitoring. *Am J Obstet Gynecol* 1974;119:230–233.

96. Wolf S: Central autonomic influences on cardiac rate and rhythm. *Mod Concepts Cardiovasc Dis* 1969;38:29–34.

97. Wood C, Lumley J, Renou P: A clinical assessment of fetal diagnostic methods. *J Obstet Gynaecol Br Commonw* 1967;74:823–825.

98. Yeh S, Forsythe A, Hon E: Quantification of beat-to-beat interval differences. *Obstet Gynecol* 1973;41:355–363.

99. Young BK, Katz M, Klein SA, Silverman F: Fetal blood and tissue pH with moderate bradycardia. *Am J Obstet Gynecol* 1979;135:45–47.

100. Young BK, Katz M, Wilson SJ: Sinusoidal fetal heart rate. I. Clinical significance. *Am J Obstet Gynecol* 1980;136:587–593.

101. Zalar RW, Quilligan EJ: The influence of scalp sampling on the cesarean section rate for fetal distress. *Am J Obstet Gynecol* 1979;135:239–246.

102. Zanini B, Paul RH, Huey JR: Intrapartum fetal heart rate: Correlation with scalp pH in the preterm fetus. *Am J Obstet Gynecol* 1980;136:43–47.

10

Resuscitation of the Newborn

Michael F. Epstein

Perinatal mortality in the United States has declined in the last two decades at least in part because of improved assessment of the physiologic and biochemical status of the fetus during its transition to newborn life.[28] The actual practices of delivery room care and resuscitation of the newborn have undergone few important revisions from the suggested practices of 30 years ago.[25] What has changed is the expectation that every woman admitted in labor with a live fetus in the third trimester will be delivered of a live newborn who will reach the nursery with the potential for normal survival.

That expectation has led to changes in the monitoring and management of labor and also to an appropriate emphasis on the assessment and immediate care of the newly born infant. Both the American College of Obstetricians and Gynecologists and the American Academy of Pediatrics have stated that there must be availability to the delivery suite of someone with primary responsibility for and the required skills in infant resuscitation at all times.[3] This has little practical effect on the obstetrician practicing in a medical center where the delivery room is frequently crowded with anesthesiologists, pediatric residents, and neonatologists; however, for the physician delivering babies in smaller, less heavily staffed hospitals, it may mean that the obstetrician's "two-patient" approach must continue beyond the delivery, through the safe arrival of the infant into the nursery. Attempts to identify in advance those deliveries that will require the presence of a pediatrician are bound to fail since even the uncomplicated, spontaneous vaginal delivery at term may result in a depressed baby.[22]

Newborn resuscitation has frequently been viewed with mystery and foreboding by the inexperienced. This is partly because of the small size of the patient and partly the result of an inappropriate focus placed on the mechanics of intubation, umbilical vein catheterization and administration of unfamiliar drugs in unusually small amounts. In fact, these procedures are not inherently difficult, especially for one with surgical skills. They are perceived as difficult because most obstetricians are called upon to use them so infrequently. Fewer than 2% of newborns need to be intubated, and fewer than 0.5% need administration of drugs via an umbilical catheter. Moreover, the need for these procedures can be minimized by prompt, proper attention to earlier steps in assessment and treatment of the mildly to moderately asphyxiated infant.

This chapter's goals are to provide the obstetrician with two important tools: 1) a simple and rapid system for continuous assessment of the newborn in the first 5 min of life, and 2) a simple and rapid plan to provide appropriate support determined by that moment-to-moment assessment of the baby's needs. Attainment of these goals depends on understanding the basic adaptive tasks that the transition from fetal to newborn physiology demands. There have been many reviews of resuscitation of the newborn directed at pediatricians, neonatologists, and anesthesiologists.[8,11] This chapter will try to make those same concepts relevant and useful for the physician who has just delivered the baby.

PHYSIOLOGY

The immediate adaptation from fetal to newborn at delivery involves fundamental changes in respiratory and circulatory functions.[24,26] During fetal life, cardiorespiratory function is directed at supporting the placenta's primary role in gas exchange. In contrast, at birth that role is transferred to the newborn's lungs by a series of alterations in lung inflation and perfusion.

The fetus is characterized by two major cardiorespiratory differences from the newborn. First, the lungs are fluid-filled and do not function as organs of gas exchange. Second, the circulation is arranged so that most blood avoids the purposeless trip through these nonventilated lungs, passing more directly to and from the placenta to ensure maximum efficiency of gas exchange and delivery to the tissues. This decreased pulmonary blood flow is accomplished via two right-to-left shunts, one at the ductus arteriosus and the other at the foramen ovale. For the newborn to survive, these two characteristics of fetal cardiorespiratory physiology (lungs that are fluid-filled and minimally perfused) must be altered abruptly at the time of delivery.

Lung Fluid

The fetal lungs should not be thought of as balloons, growing passively through gestation in preparation for postdelivery inflation. Rather, the lungs are active metabolic and secretory organs with complicated patterns of parenchymal and mesenchymal interaction combined with coordinated vascular development. This results at term in the development of thousands of alveolar sacs lined with surface active material in close apposition to a rich capillary bed, that is, an organ adapted for large-volume gas exchange.[14] However, the lungs at delivery are also full of pulmonary fluid. This fluid is not amniotic fluid aspirated by the breathing fetus. Rather, it is a combination of filtered plasma and phospholipids, proteins, and other compounds, secreted actively by lung parenchyma. This liquid fills the lungs to a volume that approximates the resting newborn infant's residual lung capacity achieved after several hours of air breathing, that is, approximately 30 mL/kg body weight. Therefore, the term baby has 100 to 120 mL of fluid in the lungs before delivery.

This fluid must either be expelled out through the nose or mouth by the pressure on the fetal thorax during expulsion through the birth canal at delivery or forced down the trachea, bronchi, and alveoli and into the pulmonary interstitium by the baby's first several breaths. The lung liquid is absorbed from the interstitium into lymphatics and the pulmonary capillary bed and into the circulation.[20] Karlberg et al. have shown that the force needed to move the air-liquid meniscus down the tracheobronchial tree with the first breath may well reach pressures greater than 30 to 50 cm H_2O, compared to the 3 to 5 cm H_2O with which the resting newborn breathes after several hours.[17]

The clearance of the lung liquid is followed quickly by achievement in the lung of a functional residual volume that allows efficient and effective breathing. This process depends on stabilization of the alveoli at the end of each expiratory phase of the respiratory cycle by surfactant. This group of compounds (primarily saturated phosphatidylcholine, or lecithin, phosphatidylglycerol, and a lung-specific protein) reduces the surface tension at the air/tissue interface and allows for maintenance of alveolar patency throughout the respiratory cycle. A deficiency of surfactant results in hyaline membrane disease or respiratory distress syndrome of the premature.

This orderly process of replacement of lung liquid with air, establishment of a residual lung capacity, and the maintenance of efficient and effective breathing can be disrupted by many fetal and neonatal conditions that range from physical blockage of the airway (e.g., meconium aspiration) to inadequate respiratory effort (e.g., neuromuscular disease or extreme prematurity). Although the precise mechanisms underlying it are uncertain, replacement of lung fluid with air is clearly an absolute requirement for adjustment to extrauterine life. Without effective inflation of the lungs and continued ventilation, fetal to neonatal transition will fail.

Pulmonary Blood Flow

The second important adaptation at delivery is the conversion of the circulatory system. In the fetus, blood is routed through the ductus arteriosus and the foramen ovale from right to left by passing the lungs so as to provide the blood most enriched with oxygen directly from the placenta to vital organs, avoiding a useless passage through the lungs. At delivery, respiratory function switches from the placenta to the lungs, and blood flow must change similarly to match perfusion with ventilation.

The basic determinant of the direction of blood flow in and around the heart and great vessels is the relationship between pulmonary (PVR) and systemic (SVR) vascular resistance. The fetal and neonatal pulmonary arterial bed is rich in muscle and these resistance vessels are responsive to hypoxia and acidosis. Rudolph and Yuan described the marked increase in PVR in newborn calves in response to a lowering of the partial pressure of oxygen Po_2 and/or pH.[23] The fetus, with its baseline Po_2 of 25 to 28 torr, maintains its pulmonary resistance vessels in a state of tonic vasoconstriction, resulting in a high PVR. At the same time, with 40% of the fetal cardiac output flowing to the low-resistance placental bed, the SVR in the fetus is quite low. The gradient between high PVR and low SVR leads to shunting of nearly all the right ventricular output to the aorta via the ductus arteriosus. The small amount of blood that does reach the pulmonary circulation (less than 5% of cardiac output) and returns to the left atrium exerts far less pressure than is measured in the right atrium, which receives the venous return from the superior vena cava as well as the umbilical venous return. This imbalance in right and left atrial return leads to an opening of the flap valve on the foramen ovale located in the atrial septum. The consequent right-to-left shunt at the foramen ovale completes the fetal circulation.

At delivery, with the first effective breath and the constriction of the umbilical arteries (either spontaneously or via cord clamping), the circulation begins to change. Inflation of the lung with air decreases the physical compression of the pulmonary vessels and local diffusion of oxygen begins to relieve the vasoconstriction. While the PVR begins to decrease, the removal of the placenta from the systemic circulation and the cooling of the skin capillary bed results in an increase in SVR. These combined alterations in resistance lead to a diminution and ultimate cessation of the right-to-left shunt through the ductus arteriosus. Right ventricular output goes to the lungs, the blood is oxygenated there, and returns to the left atrium. Left and right atrial pressures are equalized and the foramen ovale closes, resulting in an intact atrial septum. The fetal shunts have closed and ongoing maintenance of oxygenation results in their continued state of closure. The neonatal circulation is established in a pattern which persists throughout life.

This transition is, however, reversible in its initial stages, and a compromise of oxygenation or severe respiratory or metabolic acidosis may result in a marked increase in pulmonary vascular resistance and a return to the pattern of fetal circulation. This condition, referred to as persistent fetal circulation (PFC) or persistent pulmonary hypertension of the newborn (PPHN), can be seen in the term or postterm baby with severe meconium aspiration pneumonia and/or perinatal asphyxia. PFC remains a most difficult and frustrating condition to treat and continues to be associated with a mortality rate of 25% to 50%. When the pulmonary arterial bed remains tightly constricted in the newborn, perfusion of the lungs is sometimes impossible to accomplish even if adequate ventilation is achieved.

Another situation in which right-to-left shunting may continue into the newborn period is one in which low systemic blood pressure exists due to blood loss, sepsis, or myocardial injury from asphyxia. This condition is less severe than pulmonary hypertension and easier to diagnose because systemic blood pressure is measured more readily than pulmonary pressure.

The success of the newborn's cardiorespiratory adaptations at delivery can be summarized most succinctly in a single phrase—adequate oxygenation. The establishment of a patent airway and the initiation and maintenance of adequate breathing result in adequate oxygenation, and the circulatory adjustments follow. Appreciation of the central role of initiation and continued maintenance of adequate breathing will provide the proper focus for the assessment and management of every baby in the delivery room.

ASSESSMENT OF THE NEWBORN

Nowhere in medicine should treatment precede assessment or diagnosis, and the delivery room is no exception. Most errors in resuscitation stem from inaccurate or inadequate assessment of the baby's condition, and encompass those of commission as well as omission. Both types of mistakes may result in a baby in worse condition than if correct assessment had led to a proper approach.

The great majority of babies need little if any help in order to accomplish the fetus-to-newborn transition successfully. Our longevity as a species supports the logic of that observation; however, when this transition is not proceeding well on its own, there is a pressing need for prompt and appropriate action. All obstetricians are accustomed to acting promptly. The challenge in newborn resuscitation is to choose expeditiously the response most appropriate to the baby's needs. Endotracheal intubation of the well infant who only needs lung liquid suctioned gently from the nares with a bulb syringe is as inappropriate as expectantly observing the apneic, bradycardic baby who is in severe difficulty. The choice of the appropriate action should be based on experience, thought, and a preset plan which matches assessment to action in a dynamic and specific fashion.

Assessment of the newborn in the delivery room is best accomplished by the Apgar score, first described over 30 years ago.[1] In a setting in which laboratory tests, x-rays, and observation over prolonged periods of time are impossible, the components of the Apgar score remain dependable diagnostic criteria. The work of Dawes in the asphyxiated newborn monkey has elegantly correlated the hypoxia, hypercarbia, and acidemia that accompany the failure to initiate respiration at delivery with the sequence of gasping, absent respiratory efforts and rapid fall in heart rate.[6] The correlation between cord blood pH and 1-min Apgar score has been demonstrated in human infants as well.[15]

The Apgar score system is perhaps most hampered by the ease with which it can be used and consequently, by the lack of rigor which has crept into its current application. Although most babies have scores of at least 8 at and beyond 1 min of age, there is value in accurately assigning an Apgar score to every baby even if it appears well. By so doing, one will develop proficiency in the observation and confidence in acting upon a lower score when a baby is not well. It is well worth the effort to develop good habits in regard to diagnostic skills in the delivery room because they are only as good as our care and attention in using them.

The Apgar score has been assigned routinely at 1 and 5 min after delivery. The 1-min score correlates closely with the pH of umbilical cord arterial blood, while the 5-min score has been correlated more closely with later neurologic outcome.[19] However, the Apgar score is most useful when used in a continuous manner, rather than only assigned at 1 and 5 min. By so doing, one can alter resuscitative measures continuously to adapt to the changing situation of an individual baby. The score consists of five diagnostic criteria which are assigned 0, 1, and 2 points depending on the baby's condition (Table 10-1). The Apgar score can be assigned easily by the delivery physician within 20 s of delivery in the following manner. Three of the five criteria are observable in the brief walk from the delivery bed to the warming table. Color, respiratory effort, and tone are all either in front of your eyes or in your hands. At the warming table, the right hand can use the bulb syringe to suction out the mouth and nose, either eliciting a reflex response or failing to do so. Simultaneously, the left hand can reach down to the umbilical cord stump and palpate the baby's heart rate. Thus, within 20 to 30 s after delivery, one can assign the first of a repetitive series of assessment scores to establish whether the baby is well or is mildly, moderately, or severely asphyxiated. It is that assessment that allows the obstetrician to decide on a further course of action with each baby.

One exception to these observations is the very low birth weight (VLBW) baby. Infants of less than 1,500 g birth weight may have low Apgar scores in the absence of acidosis.[10] These premature infants of 32 or fewer weeks may not be asphyxiated but may nonetheless have low scores simply on the basis of prematurity. Poor respiratory effort, poor color, poor tone, absent reflex responsiveness, and rapid onset of bradycardia are all characteristics consistent with prematurity alone and may not indicate asphyxia. This observation does not argue for a less aggressive approach to these babies. Rather, it should encourage a more rapid and vigorous resuscitative effort since these babies may not suffer from asphyxia and may be resuscitated easily with early attention to adequate ventilation. Some individuals have advocated routine endotracheal intubation of all VLBW infants at delivery.[7] This remains controversial. In addition, the presence of a low Apgar score in a VLBW baby should not discourage the aggressive management of these babies in the

Table 10-1 Apgar Scoring System

	0	1	2
Heart rate	0	<100 beats/min	>100 beats/min
Respiratory effort	Apnea	Irregular, shallow, or gasping respirations	Vigorous and crying
Color	Pale, blue	Pale or blue extremities	Pink
Muscle tone	Absent	Weak, passive tone	Active movement
Reflex irritability	Absent	Grimace	Active avoidance

neonatal intensive care unit. This management has resulted in greatly improved survival and outcome for this group of very small and immature babies[12] (Table 10-2).

TREATMENT

The delivery room treatment of the newborn infant is based on the physician's assessment of how successfully the baby is accomplishing the changeover from fetus to newborn. As stated previously, nearly 90% of babies accomplish this transition without difficulty and without assistance. The identification of the other 10% in need of specialized assistance is accomplished by careful, continuous observation within the framework of the Apgar score.

Table 10-3 provides a flow sheet describing a step-by-step approach to the newborn based on Apgar score, and Table 10-4 lists the equipment and medications that should be available in the delivery room.

A few additional points require emphasis. First, if a severely asphyxiated infant fails to respond to ventilation with 100% oxygen, the most likely remediable cause is displacement of the endotracheal tube from the trachea. A brief pause in cardiac massage is warranted every half-minute to ensure that chest motion (not that of the lower rib cage over the stomach) is adequate, with good breath sounds bilaterally. If in doubt over endotracheal tube placement, direct visualization of the tube passing through the cords is essential. Cardiac massage, umbilical venous catheters, and drugs are all for naught unless a secure airway and adequate ventilation with 100% oxygen are achieved first. This most funda-

---

Table 10-2 Birth Weight Specific Neonatal Mortality Statistics for Inborn Babies at Brigham and Women's and Beth Israel Hospitals, 1983[a]

Weight (g)	Live born	Discharged alive	Survival (%)
601–700	16	4	25
701–800	30	17	56
801–900	27	23	85
901–1,000	30	27	90
1,001–1,500	127	111	87

[a]Data from Brigham and Women's Hospital and Beth Israel Hospital, Boston, 1983.

Table 10-3 Apgar Score

8, 9, or 10—No Asphyxia

Pink, active, responsive, crying baby with rapid heart rate

1. Gently suction airway, including nares, with bulb syringe.
2. Dry baby thoroughly, including head.
3. Maintain body temperature.
4. Perform brief physical examination.
5. Assign 5-min Apgar score.
6. Unite baby with parents.

5, 6, 7—Mild Asphyxia

Slightly cyanotic baby, moving with decreased muscle tone, breathing slowly or periodically, heart rate >100 beats/min

1. Repeat steps 1, 2, and 3 in rapid succession.
2. Stimulate to breathe more frequently by gentle but forceful slapping of soles of feet or rubbing spine or sternum.
3. Provide enriched O_2 ambient atmosphere via 100% O_2 and anesthesia bag and mask held by baby's face.
4. If improving, complete steps 4, 5, and 6 as above when Apgar score reaches 8.
5. If heart rate falls to <100 beats/min, Apgar score is then ≤4.
6. Administer naloxone 0.01 mg/kg IM if mother has received a narcotic analgesic during labor.

3 or 4—Moderate Asphyxia

Cyanotic baby, poor tone, weak respiratory efforts, heart rate <100 beats/min

1. Repeat steps 1, 2, and 3 and call for additional personnel to continuously monitor heart rate, manage airway, provide cardiac massage, and so on. Resuscitation for the severely asphyxiated infant is a three- to four-person job.
2. Brief trial of stimulation plus O_2 mask. If no improvement by 1 min, perform steps 3 (and 4, if needed).
3. Ventilate with bag and mask, using 100% O_2 and pressure adequate to move the chest. Continue bagging until heart rate >100 beats/min, color pink, and spontaneous respirations have begun. If the chest cannot be adequately moved with bag and mask ventilation, intubate.
4. If heart rate <60 beats/min, perform external cardiac massage.

0, 1, or 2—Severe Asphyxia

Deeply cyanotic, no muscle tone, absent respiratory effort or periodic gasps, heart rate slow or absent

1. Proceed directly to intubation and bag ventilation with 100% O_2 at 40–60 breaths/min at pressures great enough to move the upper chest wall. Use inspiratory time of 0.5–1 s.
2. Cardiac massage at rate of two compressions/s, using fingers wrapped around back and thumbs over the sternum.[27]

continues

Table 10-3 continued

3. If heart rate is not >100 beats/min despite 1 min of adequate ventilation with 100% O_2, administer 0.1–1.0 mL of 1:10,000 epinephrine via the endotracheal tube and follow with an equal volume of 0.9% NaCl or sterile water.[18] Bag as indicated to disperse this medication to the absorptive alveolar surface and if the heart rate remains <100 beats/min proceed to insert umbilical venous catheter, filled with 0.9% NaCl and capped with a syringe. Insertion of the catheter is facilitated by cutting the cord at a point 1–2 cm from the abdominal wall. The catheter is most safely inserted 2–3 cm until blood return is achieved to avoid administering hypertonic solutions directly into a small hepatic vein. All solutions must be flushed through the catheter to ensure their reaching the central circulation.

Delivery room treatment is directed at improving myocardial contractility and rate by initially correcting metabolic acidosis (2–4 mEq $NaHCO_3$-dextrose solution can be infused over 3–5 min). Next, epinephrine (0.1–1.0 mL, 1:10,000) or atropine (0.1 mL/kg) can be injected to reverse bradycardia. Finally, a slow infusion of 1.0–2.0 mL/kg of calcium gluconate may provide for further enhancement of cardiac output. None of these drugs is effective unless adequate ventilation with O_2 has been achieved.

If the heart rate is >100 bpm and adequate ventilation is achieved, either spontaneously or via assisted ventilation, the use of drugs is not necessary in the delivery room and the baby should be moved to the nursery. In the nursery, the following are done: measurement of vital signs (including HR, RR, BP, and temperature), arterial or capillary blood gases (Pao_2, $Paco_2$, and pH), and a chest x-ray allow a rational basis for further care. The administration of hypertonic $NaHCO_3$, cardiotonic drugs, or volume expanders all carry risk. If adequate ventilation and heart rate >100 beats/min can be achieved in the delivery room, their use should be withheld pending specific documentation of their need by the above studies.

Abbreviations: BP, blood pressure; HR, heart rate; $Paco_2$, arterial carbon dioxide pressure; Pao_2, arterial oxygen pressure; RR, respiratory rate.

---

mental of all lessons is the one neglected most often by the individual who does neonatal resuscitation infrequently and is the one most in need of emphasis. "Airway + Breathing must precede Cardiac output + Drugs" is a lesson known to all laypeople who have graduated from cardiopulmonary resuscitation (CPR) workshops and courses and is a lesson that is just as critical in the delivery room.

Second, the oropharyngeal suctioning of all babies—except those with thick meconium (see below)—should be done with a bulb syringe and not a suction catheter. Cordero and Hon identified a 14% incidence of significant arrhythmia or apneic episodes in babies suctioned with a catheter immediately after delivery.[5] None of a second group of babies suctioned immediately with a bulb syringe or suctioned with a catheter 5 min after delivery developed these problems. This probably reflects the great reactivity of vagal nerve endings in the laryngeal area in the presence of the

Table 10-4 Equipment Needed for Newborn Resuscitation[a]

1. *Well-lit, flat, stable, and heated area for observation and management of the infant.* Modern radiant warming tables provide an ideal setting. Standard infant care bassinets are inadequate for access to the baby.
2. *Oxygen source with adjustable flowmeter.* Ideally this gas should be warmed and humidified.
3. *Suction.* Bulb syringe should be available for all babies. Wall suction with adjustable vacuum and no. 8–no. 12 catheters provide ideal means for clearing the oropharynx and nares of thick meconium.
4. *Flow-through anesthesia bag with adjustable pressure valve.* These bags can provide 100% O_2 and allow the resuscitator to vary inspiratory and expiratory pressure without adjusting the O_2 flow at the wall outlet or the mask's seal on the baby's face. Self-inflating bags are not ideal since they cannot deliver more than 40% O_2, provide continuous O_2 flow out of the mask, or produce pressures greater than the preset pop-off valve allows (usually 25–35 cm H_2O).
5. *Masks of assorted size and configuration*
6. *Laryngoscope with Miller 1 and Miller 0 blades.* The former are necessary only in the larger, term baby of >3.5 kg. The 0 blade allows visualization of the vocal cords in all smaller babies.
7. *Endotracheal tubes of 3.5, 3.0, and 2.5 mm diameter.* Both flanged (Cole) and unflanged tubes should be available. The former have the advantages of being stiffer and maintaining a curve similar to that of the posterior pharynx, allowing easier placement. Moreover, the flange makes it less likely that the tube will be placed too far down the trachea and into the right mainstem bronchus, a common error. The unflanged tube is sometimes easier to insert in the <1,000 g infant.
8. *Umbilical catheters of 3.5 and 5.0 French size* with umbilical tape for securing the stump
9. *Syringes and needles*
10. *Medications*
    $NaHCO_3$ (0.9 mEq/mL or 0.45 mEq/mL)
    Dextrose (10% and 50%)
    Epinephrine (1:10,000)
    Atropine (0.4 mg/0.5 mL)
    Calcium gluconate (10%)
    Naloxone (0.02 mg/mL) (neonatal solution)
    Albumin (5%)
    NaCl (0.9%)

[a]O-negative packed red blood cells should be readily available in the Blood Bank for emergency use.

relative asphyxia present in all babies immediately after delivery. This risk of inducing apnea or bradycardia in an otherwise healthy newborn can be avoided by using a bulb syringe, rather than a suction catheter, in the first several minutes of life. Emptying the stomach with a catheter placed through the nose and esophagus is not indicated routinely; however, when gastric aspirate is needed for diagnostic studies (e.g., foam stability shake test for lung maturity or Gram stain and culture when a question of infection has been raised), or when there has been thick meconium passed into the amniotic fluid, aspiration of gastric contents should be done only after achievement of adequate oxygenation as indicated by Apgar score of ≥ 8 five minutes after delivery.

A third point to be emphasized is that the routine administration of unwarmed oxygen blown onto the newborn's face at a high flow rate is not without risk. Several authors have described slowing of respiration and heart rate induced by this maneuver; nevertheless, when indicated by an Apgar score in the 5 to 7 range, careful administration of low-flow "blow-by" oxygen (especially if warmed and humidified) accompanied by stimulation represents the treatment of choice for the mildly depressed infant.

Fourth, resuscitation is not a solo performance. Although both the American College of Obstetricians and Gynecologists and the American Academy of Pediatrics place the responsibility for resuscitation of the newborn with an individual, the principles and processes of resuscitation must be understood by all personnel working in the labor and delivery room area. Treatment of the moderately to severely depressed newborn calls for a coordinated team approach. One member must be skilled in management of the airway and ventilation and is ordinarily the coordinator for the other members of the team. The latter may be nurses, anesthesiologists, or other physicians, but all must be skilled in assignment of Apgar score (especially monitoring of the heart rate by auscultation or palpation), positioning of the baby to facilitate intubation, closed cardiac massage, and administration of drugs via an umbilical venous catheter. Drug therapy is facilitated by posting a list of drugs and dosages in all delivery rooms in view of the participants in a resuscitation.

Practice in the actual resuscitative procedures of bag and mask ventilation, endotracheal intubation, and catheterization of the umbilical vein is an important program for all hospitals in which babies are delivered. Bag and mask ventilation is perhaps best learned by applying the technique to a resuscitation doll, several of which are available commercially. This allows the operator to achieve dexterity in the application of the mask to a baby's face while adjusting oxygen flow and pressure applied to the bag with the other hand. Facility in the intubation of the newborn can be aided by the use of kittens anesthetized with ketamine, a short-acting hypnotic drug.[16] The pharyngeal and laryngeal anatomy of the kitten is quite similar to that of the newborn human infant, and several practice sessions per year for the delivery room staff responsible for resuscitation serves to maintain otherwise infrequently used skills. The same applies to umbilical vein cannulation. Every placenta with its attached cord offers the opportunity for practicing cannulation of the umbilical vein, and this procedure should be practiced frequently by the relevant staff. Full-scale mock resuscitation in the delivery room with the actual use of the warming table, oxygen, equipment, drugs, and umbilical vein cannulation is a valuable exercise to pursue on all delivery services.

SPECIAL SITUATIONS

The above guidelines for assessment and treatment of the newborn in the delivery room apply to all babies; however, two special situations may arise that call for an alteration or addition to the standard approaches. These are meconium-stained amniotic fluid and the pale, shocky infant.

Approximately 9% to 15% of all fetuses pass meconium into the amniotic fluid before delivery.[2] This situation places the fetus and newborn at risk for aspiration of this thick, viscid material into the mouth, pharynx, trachea, and bronchi either before, during, or after labor and delivery. Many instances of meconium aspiration into the lungs occur in utero due to fetal gasping and cannot be prevented by delivery room care. Moreover, it now appears that many babies who die with meconium aspiration syndrome and persistent fetal circulation (PFC) have chronic pulmonary vascular changes that antedate their intrapartum asphyxia and aspiration.[13,21] Nevertheless, many babies who have passed meconium in utero can be assisted by several therapeutic maneuvers taken to minimize the risk of aspiration after delivery. Removing all or most of the meconium from the nasopharynx and from the trachea before the first breath is taken or before positive-pressure ventilation is initiated has the goal of minimizing the severe pneumonitis, atelectasis, and air-leak phenomena of meconium aspiration syndrome.

The combined obstetric and pediatric approach recommended by Carson et al. calls for the obstetrician to suction the mouth and nares thoroughly before the delivery of the shoulders and the thorax.[4] The original recommendation to use a DeLee suction catheter should be amended in view of the risk of contact with potentially infectious body fluids. The use of a bulb syringe or a suction catheter connected to low vacuum wall suction is preferable. Clearing the upper airway before delivering the thorax may be critical, because a net change of intrathoracic pressure of several cm H_2O occurs from decompression of the chest during vaginal delivery.[17]

After delivery, the cord should be clamped and cut expeditiously and the baby handed immediately to the resuscitator, who intubates the trachea. Direct suctioning of the trachea can be accomplished by using one of several new adaptors to connect the suction apparatus to endotracheal tube. Repeated suctioning of the trachea is indicated until no further meconium is obtained; do not persist if the newborn's heart rate slows to 40 beats/min. A concerted effort should be made to remove meconium from the trachea of large, term, or postterm babies with thick meconium and intrapartum asphyxia since these babies continue to have a 25% to 30% case-fatality rate from severe meconium aspiration syndrome.

Prevention is the best hope, and access to the trachea for suctioning ensures a ready route for ventilation once suctioning is completed. Use of this approach at the Brigham and Women's Hospital in Boston has reduced the incidence of meconium aspiration from 5/1,000 births in 1975 to 1.1/1,000 births in recent years; however, there are still 1 to 2 babies/year (in a total annual population of 9,500) who die from meconium aspiration syndrome and PFC.

The second group of infants with specialized needs consists of those with significant pre- or intrapartum hemorrhage. Some infants present with pallor and shock in the delivery room. Shock results from a significant intrapartum blood loss, which may be due to premature placental separation, fetal-placental or fetal-maternal hemorrhage, avulsion of the umbilical cord from the placenta, vasa, or placenta previa, incision through an anterior placenta at cesarean section, twin-twin transfusion, or rupture of an abdominal viscus (liver or spleen) during a difficult delivery. These infants will be tachycardic (over 180 beats/min), tachypneic, and hypotensive with poor capillary filling and weak pulse. After stabilization of respiration and heart rate, immediate transfusion with type O Rh-negative packed red blood cells and fresh frozen plasma may be necessary. A volume of 20 mL/kg can be given rapidly through an umbilical venous catheter. If clinical improvement is not seen, causes of further blood loss should be sought, and more vigorous blood and colloid replacement should be continued.

If blood is not immediately available in the hospital, autologous cord blood from the placenta may be used.[9] A 20-mL syringe rinsed with 50 U of heparin and filled from placenta or cord (the surface of which has been prepared with povidone-iodine) provides a suitably anticoagulated specimen. Although there is a small risk of bacterial contamination, the provision of such a blood transfusion may be life-saving in certain circumstances.

REFERENCES

1. Apgar V: A proposal for a new method of evaluation of the newborn infant. *Anesth Analg* 1953;32:260–267.

2. Bacsik RD: Meconium aspiration syndrome. *Pediatr Clin North Am* 1977;24:463–480.

3. Brann AW, Cefalo RC: Assessment and care of the neonate in the delivery room, in Brann AW, Cefalo RC (eds): *Guidelines for Perinatal Care*. Washington DC, American Academy of Pediatrics/The American College of Obstetricians and Gynecologists, 1983, pp 67–73.

4. Carson BS, Lasey BW, Bowes WA, Simmons MA: Combined obstetric and pediatric approach to prevent meconium aspiration syndrome. *Am J Obstet Gynecol* 1976;126:712–715.

5. Cordero L, Hon EH: Neonatal bradycardia following nasopharyngeal stimulation. *J Pediatr* 1971;78:441–447.

6. Dawes G: *Foetal and Neonatal Physiology*. Chicago, Year Book Medical Publishers, 1968.

7. Drew JH: Immediate intubation at birth of the very low birth weight infant. *Am J Dis Child* 1982;136:207–210.

8. Epstein MF: Resuscitation in the delivery room, in Cloherty J, Stark A (eds): *Manual of Neonatal Care*, ed 2. Boston, Little, Brown, 1985, pp 73–84.

9. Golden SM, O'Brien WF, Lissner C, Cefalo RC, Schumacher H, Stass S: Hematologic and bacteriologic assessment of autologous cord blood for neonatal transfusions. *J Pediatr* 1980;97:810–812.

10. Goldenberg RL, Huddleston JF, Nelson KG: Apgar scores and umbilical arterial pH in preterm newborn infants. *Am J Obstet Gynecol* 1984;149:651–654.

11. Gregory GA: Resuscitation of the Newborn. *Anesthesiology* 1973;43:225–237.

12. Hack M, Fanaroff AA: Changes in the delivery room care of the extremely small infant (<750 g). *N Engl J Med* 1986;314:660–664.

13. Haworth SG, Reid L: Persistent fetal circulation: Newly recognized structural features. *J Pediatr* 1976;88:614–620.

14. Inselman LS, Mellins RB: Growth and development of the lung. *J Pediatr* 1981;98:1–15.

15. James LS, Weisbrat IM, Prince CE, Holaday DA, Apgar V: Acid base studies of human infants in relation to birth asphyxia and onset of respiration. *J Pediatr* 1958;52:379–394.

16. Jennings PB, Alden ER, Brenz RW: A teaching model for pediatric intubation utilizing ketamine sedated kittens. *Pediatrics* 1974;53:283–284.

17. Karlberg P, Cherry RB, Escardo FE, Koch G: Pulmonary ventilation and mechanics of breathing in the first minutes of life, including onset of respiration. *Acta Paediatr* 1962;51:121–136.

18. Lindemann R: Endotracheal administration of epinephrine during cardiopulmonary resuscitation. *Am J Dis Child* 1982;136:753.

19. MacDonald HM, Mulligan JC, Allen AC, Taylor PM: Neonatal Asphyxia I: Relationship of obstetric and neonatal complications to neonatal mortality in 38,405 consecutive deliveries. *J Pediatr* 1980;96:898–902.

20. Milner AD, Vyas H: Lung expansion at birth. *J Pediatr* 1982;101:879–886.

21. Murphy JD, Rabinovitch M, Reid LM: Pulmonary vascular pathology in fatal neonatal meconium aspiration. *Pediatr Res* 1981;15:673.

22. Primhak RA, Herber SM, Whineup G, Milner RDG: Which deliveries require pediatricians in attendance. *Br Med J* 1984;289:16–18.

23. Rudolph AM, Yuan S: Response of the pulmonary vasculature to hypoxia and H+ ion concentration changes. *J Clin Invest* 1966;45:399–411.

24. Scarpelli E: *Pulmonary Physiology of the Fetus, Newborn and Child*. Philadelphia, Lea and Febiger, 1975.

25. Smith CA, McKay RJ: Care of the newborn infant, in Nelson W (ed): *Textbook of Pediatrics*, ed 6. Philadelphia, WB Saunders, 1959, pp 301–303.

26. Smith CA, Nelson NM: *Physiology of the Newborn Infant*. Springfield, IL, Charles C Thomas, 1976.

27. Todres ID, Rogers M: Methods of external cardiac massage in the newborn infant. *J Pediatr* 1975;86:781–782.

28. Wegman ME: Annual Summary of Vital Statistics 1985. *Pediatrics* 1986;78:983–994.

11

Preterm Labor

Wayne R. Cohen

Premature delivery is a public health problem of considerable magnitude, and is the major contributor to perinatal mortality and morbidity. Current guidelines recommended by the American Academy of Pediatrics[5] suggest that we use the word "term" for births from 38 to 41 weeks, and "preterm" for those less than 38 weeks' menstrual age. The term "low birth weight" applies to all infants weighing below 2,500 g at delivery, whether they be truly preterm, or term babies suffering from growth deficiency.[13,115]

Although premature births account for about 8% of all deliveries in the United States, they contribute disproportionately to at least 75% of the perinatal mortality.[32,91,112] Approximately 200,000 low birth weight babies are delivered annually in the United States; of these, about 15,000 die and, conservatively, at least 10% of the survivors develop mental or neurologic disorders.

The first half of this century witnessed a marked decrease in infant mortality in the United States, coincident with generally improved nutritional and economic standards, and coupled with cognizance of the need for specialized equipment and personnel to deal with premature infants. As mortality data have improved, concern over the long-term sequelae of prematurity has mounted.

Analyses of outcomes of babies born during the 1940s and 1950s are distressing. Dann et al.[35] observed a high incidence of serious visual defects (59%) in a group of 100 children born in 1940–1957 with birth weights between 660 and 1,325 g; this observation was significantly different from the findings in full-term siblings. Intelligence quotient distributions in the two groups were similar, although this was a selected sample because of its generally high socioeconomic status. Moreover, it was suggested that the outcome may have been bad among some of the children whose follow-up was not complete.

Similarly, Lubchenco et al.[84] reported a 68% incidence of central nervous system and visual handicaps in their series of low birth weight infants born between 1947 and 1950 and examined at 10 years of age. Many studies[38,83,84,113] suggested that although many premature babies do quite well, they tend to be smaller in height and weight during the first decade, have more disease during the first year of life, and have an increased risk of neurologic, intellectual, or sensory handicaps compared to term babies.

Recent data are somewhat more encouraging, particularly for the very low birth weight (VLBW) infant. Babies of 1,000 to 1,500 g birth weight treated in special care nurseries have an overall 85% survival. In a 1-year follow-up of 67 babies treated in an intensive care nursery, Fitzhardinge[47] found that their rates of growth from the projected full-term date of confinement to 1 year of age were the same as in term infants. Moreover, there was no difference in the distribution of intelligence quotients between the two groups. Marriage and Davies[89] examined 73 children who survived the neonatal period after mechanical ventilation, and found 15% with neurologic sequelae. Other studies show similar rates of long-term neurologic disability. Although not inconsequential, these rates are lower than anticipated; however, far more thorough and long-term analysis will be necessary before we fully understand the consequences of being born at very low weight.

Although demonstrable neurologic abnormality is an endpoint relatively easily defined, assessment of intelligence and behavior is more hazardous. Numerous racial, economic, environmental, and cultural differences influence intelligence quotients and behavior, and these confounding factors have not been considered in most studies. When they have been taken into consideration, it has been difficult to verify a role of low birth weight in retarded development.[32] The very factors of socioeconomic deprivation that are associated with low birth weight are also associated with a higher incidence of poor general health and lower scores on intellectual or developmental tests. Thus, in spite of a large volume of persuasive circumstantial evidence, no incontrovertible proof exists that links preterm birth per se with increased risks of long-term cognitive, behavioral, or functional handicap, at least with regard to babies weighing above 1,500 g at birth. But low birth weight is clearly a concomitant of these problems, and insofar as preterm delivery can be prevented, the prevalence of these handicaps in the population should diminish.

The recent increase in the survival of VLBW babies, especially those below 1,000 g, requires especially careful consideration. Some data suggest that the improved survival even in the 500 to 1000 g group has not been accompanied by higher rates of severe neurologic morbidity.[59] Nevertheless, the prevalence of cerebral palsy is quite high among VLBW babies. Kitchen et al.[79] reported a 12.5% incidence of cerebral palsy among 416 survivors. In another study, severe neurologic impairment was reported in 19% of babies born at 23 to 28 weeks' gestation.[141] In addition to obvious handicaps that can be diagnosed in the first year or two of life, many children born at very low birth weights have more subtle long-term neurologic abnormalities that may be manifest later in life as learning disabilities.[134] The contribution of persistent non-neurologic sequelae of newborn intensive care such as bronchopulmonary dysplasia to long-term morbidity is still unclear.

It is likely that an individual's global neurodevelopmental functioning is a consequence of numerous factors, including, but by no means limited to, perinatal events. Because of the complexity of the problem, it is difficult to implicate specific obstetric events, such as mode of delivery,[78] in poor outcome. There is, however, little doubt that the aggregate of perinatal practices that results in maximally appropriate prolongation of pregnancy when preterm birth threatens, and in delivery of small babies in optimal condition contributes to minimizing the chance of adverse outcome.

Mortality rates for low birth weight babies have diminished over the past decade. The advent of specialized neonatal intensive care nurseries has coincided with this decline, and it is tempting to ascribe causality to this relationship. Indeed, recognition of the fluid, electrolyte, and caloric requirements of premature babies, as well as understanding the importance of maintaining a neutral thermal environment, advances in the control of infections, and the introduction of sophisticated techniques of mechanical ventilation seem likely to have influenced mortality and morbidity. It has been argued that populations in special care nurseries represent a select and advantaged group in that they consist of babies having had sufficient vigor to be deemed salvageable and suitable for transfer to the intensive care unit. This may indeed bias some data, but even within individual neonatal intensive care units mortality has decreased as new advances have been incorporated into the standard of care.

Certain specific changes in pediatric care have clearly influenced morbidity statistics. A considerable proportion of long-term disabilities prior to neonatal intensive care consisted of retrolental fibroplasia and hearing loss. The prevalence of the former has been reduced considerably by ventilatory techniques that require less prolonged inspiration of high oxygen concentrations, and the latter by more conservative use of ototoxic aminoglycosides and more rigorous control of hyperbilirubinemia. It is unknown to what extent sensory deficits contributed to spuriously poor performance on cognitive or developmental evaluation reported for children born prematurely.

Whatever dynamics of cause and effect exist, it is clear that premature babies of very low birth weight are surviving today who could not have done so two decades ago. The fears that clinicians would be fruitlessly preserving the lives of severely handicapped individuals have, to an extent, proved false. As noted, normal outcome, even after delivery at extremely low birth weight is possible. Nevertheless, the frequency of handicap in survivors is considerable, and sufficient long-term data on surviving babies in the 500 to 750 g weight category are not yet available. In spite of this cautious new optimism, however, it should be stressed that preterm birth is still the major cause of mortality in the perinatal period and may contribute significantly to the prevalence of neurologic and cognitive disability in the population.

EPIDEMIOLOGY

Numerous factors have been found to be associated with spontaneous delivery of low birth weight or preterm infants.[1,45] Most are indeed simply associations, and little information is available that explores adequately whether these factors actually cause premature labor, or simply occur in conjunction with it, or perhaps are even caused by it. Considering the inherent pitfalls in the definition of prematurity, difficulties can be expected in interpreting the vast literature that deals with the epidemiology of preterm birth.

Most studies agree that delivery of low birth weight children commonly follows certain medical and obstetric conditions. Among most low birth weight populations, 30% to 50% have some antecedent maternal medical or obstetric abnormality.[21,92,130] These include hypertensive disorders, antepartum hemorrhage, multiple gestation, congenital anomaly, maternal infection, premature rupture of membranes, and iatrogenic causes related to indicated (or occasionally inappropriate) early induction of labor or cesarean section.[87]

OBSTETRIC HISTORY

Previous obstetric history predicts future reproductive performance. The British Perinatal Mortality Survey data showed that a previous premature delivery doubled the risks of perinatal death to subsequent infants if the prior baby was liveborn and increased it 2.6 times if stillborn. Data from the National Collaborative Perinatal Project suggested that in the United States when a previous delivery of a less-than-2,500 g baby has occurred, the rate of low birth weight of the subsequent pregnancy was 25% in whites and 33% in blacks, both considerably in excess of expectations.[51] In a study of 25,958 consecutive singleton deliveries, Funderburk et al. showed that perinatal mortality rates were directly proportional to the number of previous abortions and premature births.[51] For women who had three or more previous premature deliveries, the perinatal mortality rate was 18% for their next delivery.

The role of prior induced abortion in the etiology of premature delivery is not clear. In countries in which abortion has been used as a common means of birth control, prematurity rates appear to have risen dramatically.[104]

Some studies have shown a twofold increase in the risk of premature delivery for mothers who have had one or more previous induced or spontaneous abortions.[103] These studies do not discriminate between spontaneous and induced procedures, nor do they correct mortality rates for potentially confounding variables such as maternal age or nutrition. A comprehensive survey of the sequelae of induced abortion has demonstrated no subsequent risk of premature delivery.[34]

Schoenbaum et al.[116] found no increase in the risk of poor outcome after 27 weeks in pregnancies that followed one induced abortion. However, women who had a prior spontaneous abortion did have more complications, including premature delivery, in their subsequent pregnancy. Belsey[16] emphasized that data are insufficient to rule out an effect of previous induced abortion with certainty and suggested that abortion technique may be important in minimizing such effects. In this regard, during first trimester abortions, the operator should employ the minimum necessary gradual cervical dilatation and evacuate with suction, rather than sharp curettage. The use of laminaria or other devices that produce gradual dilatation prior to abortion is beneficial, particularly in second trimester procedures.

Spontaneous miscarriage seems to be associated with some increased risk of future premature delivery. However, it has not been demonstrated whether this results from the abortion itself, or from the dilatation and curettage that often accompany it; furthermore, it cannot be determined if the abortion merely identifies the population that is likely to deliver prematurely for some other reason, the same underlying factors perhaps giving rise to a spectrum of poor obstetric performance.

UTERINE FACTORS

Müllerian Anomalies

Maternal uterine abnormalities have been implicated as a cause of preterm birth.[52] Because these morphologic aberrations are uncommon, it is difficult to accumulate a meaningfully large series. The partially septate uterus appears to carry the most risk. In a group of 98 patients with bicornuate or septate uteri, approximately 30% had pregnancies with bad outcomes, more than half related to spontaneous abortion prior to viability.[71] Of pregnancies that reach the third trimester in an anomalous uterus, about 25% terminate in premature delivery. Operative repair of these defects seems to increase the likelihood of successful pregnancy in patients with uterine anomalies when other causes of reproductive failure have been excluded.[71]

The müllerian duct anomalies associated with in utero exposure to diethylstilbesterol have been implicated in various aspects of pregnancy wastage. Barnes et al.[10] found a 7.7% incidence of premature birth among a small number of women who had been exposed to diethylstilbesterol, but only 4.5% in a control population. This difference was, however, not statistically significant. Several cases of cervical incompetence have been described in exposed women,[53] but it is not known whether this is more common than in a control group. The delineation of an abnormality in the contour of the uterine cavity by radiography (T-shaped uterus) has also been implicated as a cause of pregnancy loss and preterm birth. Further work is necessary to delineate the role of estrogen-induced teratogenesis in the development of premature labor.

Incompetent Cervix

Occasionally, cervical incompetence may result in premature delivery. Typically, patients present in midpregnancy with asymptomatic cervical dilatation that eventually proceeds to abortion. The etiology of this disorder is unknown, as is its real incidence and contribution to perinatal mortality. Prior operative cervical trauma is documentable with an alarming frequency among patients with an incompetent cervix. Cone biopsy of the cervix was found associated with a 17% incidence of spontaneous preterm labors, compared with 3% in a control population in a case-control study by Jones et al.[72] There is not universal agreement about the role of cone biopsy in this regard, and if damage to the cervix or to the fibromuscular tissue in the distal lower segment is causative, this may be favorably modified by the more conservative conizations performed since the popularization of colposcopy and the availability of laser surgery.

The diagnosis of incompetent cervix is difficult and clinical criteria inconsistent.[7] Hysterosalpingography between pregnancies may be useful,[48] and measurement of the diameter of the cervical canal or of cervical compliance has been attempted; but no reliable means of diagnosis has yet been described.

Generally, the diagnosis is based upon careful obstetric history and serial cervical examinations during pregnancy to detect precocious cervical change. Ultrasonography can sometimes be helpful in this regard, and Jeanty et al. demonstrated that perineal scanning may be useful to delineate details of the cervical anatomic relationships during pregnancy.[69] Various suture techniques to occlude the cervical os mechanically and prevent further dilatation appear useful; mechanical support with a pessary is used by some individuals with success.[133]

The McDonald procedure, a simple purse-string suture to occlude the cervical os, is the most widely applied surgical approach.[93] It has the advantage of simplicity, ease of accomplishment, and minimal manipulation of the cervix; moreover, it can be applied even with a considerable degree of cervical effacement. Other approaches to especially difficult conditions have been described,[7] including an abdominal approach if the cervix is so distorted from previous surgery or trauma that traditional procedures are not feasible.

The author prefers a modification of the Shirodkar technique[117] when conditions permit. A 5 mm-wide band of woven Dacron or similar substance, is placed circumferentially in the portio vaginalis just below the bladder reflection. The suture is buried submucosally in the cervix. Although this may make retrieval at term difficult, an advantage is gained. Leaving a cerclage suture exposed provides a portal of entry to the cervix for bacteria, and may predispose to infection, a common reason for cerclage failure. In addition, many women complain of considerable vaginal discharge throughout pregnancy when exposed suture is present. This discharge is not only annoying to the patient, but may be difficult to distinguish from significant cervical or vaginal infection. Burial of the entire suture results in greater patient comfort, easier diagnosis and, perhaps, reduced risk of infection. This technique has the disadvantages of more difficult removal, and requirement for more surgical manipulation at the time of insertion and removal.

The use of interval cerclage is controversial. Most obstetricians prefer to place elective cerclage sutures during pregnancy at the end of the first trimester. This precludes potential risks of anesthetic or other drug use in the first trimester, and allows reasonable assurance that spontaneous miscarriage will not occur subsequently. The author's preference is to recommend cerclage between pregnancies for women in whom the diagnosis of cervical incompetence is reasonably certain. The possible risks of this approach are interference with fertility, and need for removal in case of early pregnancy loss. Both are exceedingly unlikely, and are outweighed by the advantage of not providing any anesthetic drugs or any surgical manipulation of the cervix during the pregnancy. Even if early miscarriage occurs, curettage can usually be performed with a flexible suction catheter without removing the cerclage. In cervical incompetence, spontaneous dilatation can occur with surprising suddenness, and examining the patient even several times weekly may not be sufficient to detect the first evidence of change. The use of interval cerclage prevents tragic losses or unnecessarily difficult procedures that may result if dilatation occurs sooner than expected.

Leiomyomata

The cervical factors mentioned above are associated with perhaps 1% to 3% of low birth weight deliveries. It has been suggested that uterine leiomyomata or intrauterine synechiae can result in premature labor. Although testimonials abound in this regard, data to substantiate these as predictable causes of prematurity are lacking. Gibbs[52] observed no such factors among 1,000 premature labors. The specific entity of degenerating leiomyomata during pregnancy has, in my experience, been a cause of premature labor.

INFECTION

Maternal Infection

Although it is commonly believed that severe infections (or indeed many severe acute or chronic disease states) increase the likelihood of premature delivery, appropriate population studies that take into account the influence of factors such as socioeconomic status and past reproductive history rarely have been accomplished to verify this contention. Experience from earlier in this century indicated that mothers with moderate to severe pulmonary tuberculosis are at increased risk for the delivery of low birth weight infants,[107] as might be those with hepatitis and other viral diseases. The hepatitis risk may apply primarily to underdeveloped countries. Similarly, although a report has suggested that mothers carrying the hepatitis B antigen, with or without clinical disease, are at increased risk for premature delivery, it remains to be confirmed.[120] Whether the carrier state is causative or merely a proxy for some other factor predisposing to early delivery is not certain.

Bacterial infection of the maternal urinary tract has been the focus of numerous studies. There is general agreement that the development of acute pyelonephritis confers an increased risk of preterm delivery. Moreover, patients with symptomatic bacteriuria during pregnancy are at risk to develop pyelonephritis.

Of great interest are the observations made by Kass, who suggested that patients with untreated asymptomatic bacteriuria were also at increased risk for preterm delivery.[1,74] He defined significant bacteriuria as two successive cultures of clean voided specimens having more than 100,000 colonies/mL of the same bacteria. Prematurity risks disappeared among patients whose bacteriuria responded to initial antibiotic treatment, but not among those who did not respond or who had a recurrence. Controversy exists regarding these observations. Some authors have suggested that no increased likelihood of prematurity exists,[109] whereas most have corroborated Kass' findings. Wren[140] documented a two- to threefold increase in the incidence of preterm labor in a group of untreated or unsuccessfully treated patients with asymptomatic bacteriuria compared to treated bacteriuric and nonbacteriuric control subjects. The weight of available evidence suggests that asymptomatic bacteriuria is a real and potentially curable cause of premature delivery.[1]

Fetoplacental Infection

Infections that arise in the fetoplacental unit or uterus may be associated with preterm birth. It is well known that overt chorioamnionitis is associated frequently with premature labor. A bacteriologic study found evidence of placental bacterial infection in 27% of premature deliveries, compared to 4.7% in term placentas,[114] and it has been suggested that as much as 25% of preterm delivery could be accounted for by histologic chorioamnionitis, much of which was subclinical.[58]

Bacteria are present in amniotic fluid in about 20% of preterm labor patients,[135] and in a small study, Iams et al.[66] identified bacterial metabolic products in the amniotic fluid in 5 of 6 women in preterm labor who had no evidence of bacteria in the fluid. These and related data are consistent with the idea that at least some cases of idiopathic preterm labor are in fact the result of clinically apparent or occult infections in the uteroplacental environment.

A mechanism to explain the role of infection in the onset of labor is now evolving. Bejar et al.[15] found phospholipase A_2 in bacteria that commonly cause amnionitis, neonatal sepsis, and urinary tract infection. This bacterial enzyme might stimulate the release of arachidonic acid from fetal membranes or decidua and thus stimulate prostaglandin synthesis and the initiation of labor.

If occult infection were an important cause of preterm labor, antibiotic therapy ought to be salutary. Indeed, several studies[94,129] suggest this is so. McGregor et al.[94] gave oral erythromycin or placebo in a randomized double-blind fashion to 58 women who were being treated for preterm labor, and who had evidence of cervical dilatation. The delay to delivery was significantly longer in the antibiotic-treated group. Elimination of group B streptococci from maternal urine with penicillin during prenatal care was also shown effective.[129] The frequency of preterm labor in the antibiotic group was 5%, compared with 38% in the placebo group. Perhaps urinary bacteria are also found frequently in the genital tract. If so, this might explain Kass' earlier findings on the benefits of treating asymptomatic bacteriuria.

An accumulating body of evidence supports the concept that asymptomatic bacterial infestation of the fetoplacental environs may cause or predispose to premature labor. These microorganisms may not be considered pathogenic under ordinary conditions; normal vaginal flora might, under certain circumstances, be sufficient to cause infection.[57] What cofactors are necessary to permit bacterial invasion and provocation of labor is unknown. Reports of benefits of antibiotic therapy to prevent or treat preterm labor are intriguing, but data are insufficient to recommend this as a clinical practice at this time.

Listeriosis seems to occur at higher than the expected rate in women with poor reproductive performance and its role in preterm birth has been observed.[11] Mycoplasma T-strains have been reported as possible causes of fetal infection in midtrimester abortion, but a prospective study has suggested that although maternal T-strain infestation is associated with lower birth weight, this was not related to true preterm delivery.[25] A similar association was reported with *Mycoplasma hominis*,[36] but other data have implicated genital mycoplasmas in preterm birth.[75]

Coitus

The role of sexual activity in promoting early labor has been suggested but not adequately investigated. The uterine contractions that normally accompany female orgasm and the systemic absorption of seminal prostaglandins are possible etiologies. Some women do experience uterine contractions that persist after orgasm during pregnancy.[55] Studies have suggested on the basis of retrospective information that orgasm during gestation may be more frequent in mothers of prematures.[56,106] However, these studies are subject to considerable bias. In interviews with 260 women, Solberg et al.[122] noted that none reported the immediate onset of labor after coitus or orgasm. Rayburn and Wilson[108] found no difference in the proportion of sexually active patients, or of coital or orgasmic frequency in 111 patients with premature labor compared to matched control subjects. Thus, although some would consider it prudent to interdict sexual activity for women demonstrated to be at high risk for premature delivery, no satisfactory data exist that establish a causal association between the two.

Iatrogenic Prematurity

Termination of pregnancy by induction of labor or cesarean section before term is occasionally mandated because of some complication that would place mother or fetus in jeopardy if the pregnancy were continued. Under such circumstances, all possible measures should be employed to reduce the risks of prematurity. In some instances, corticosteroid administration may be used to enhance fetal lung maturation. If local neonatal care is not adequate, preparations to transfer the neonate (or, preferably, the mother prior to delivery) to a suitable tertiary care setting should be made.

Of greatest concern are those cases of iatrogenic prematurity in which pregnancy is terminated electively, but inadvertently, prior to term. It has been estimated that there may be as many as 7,500 such cases in the United States each year[87] accounting for considerable unnecessary morbidity and even mortality. In this regard, it is obviously vital that an accurate estimation of fetal age or maturity be made prior to any elective termination of pregnancy. Amniocentesis and evaluation of amniotic fluid phospholipids is sometimes necessary. Frigoletto et al.[50] reported 1,497 elective repeat cesarean sections with a 0.13% incidence of iatrogenic prematurity. Their suggested management protocol includes estimation of gestational age by menstrual dates, early pregnancy pelvic examination, and a midtrimester ultrasonographic measurement of fetal biparietal diameter. They undertook amniocentesis only if these measurements did not all agree that the patient was at term. The two premature deliveries in their series were not managed according to this protocol.

Socioeconomic Factors

A number of medical and social conditions in addition to those already mentioned have been associated with an increased risk of the delivery of low birth weight infants.[1] Thus, women who are at the extremes of reproductive age, unmarried, anemic, of short stature, poorly nourished, or smokers, or have babies with congenital defects or occupy lower social strata, may be at risk.

The pervasive and undeniable association between low birth weight or preterm birth and low socioeconomic status is of most interest. As much as a 50% greater risk of preterm birth among women in lower socioeconomic strata has been documented.[1,21] Affluence has been demonstrated to be associated with a lower chance of prematurity in various nations and within racial groups.[1] In fact, this relationship holds regardless of how one measures social status.

Because most of the factors that seem to magnify risks of prematurity, such as young maternal age, poor pregnancy weight gain, short stature, toxemia, and inadequate prenatal care, are found more commonly among low socioeconomic populations, it is difficult to sort out whether they act independently or merely help identify the low socioeconomic group in which other factors operate to induce premature birth. More data are necessary to delineate the relative roles of socially determined variables and their effect on intrauterine growth retardation and preterm birth. A common denominator among many of these factors seems to be the poor nutritional status of those in lower social groups. Psychologic factors, including the kind of chronic environmental stress thought to prevail among lower social classes have also been implicated.

Because of the multiplicity of factors involved, and their complex interaction, controlled studies to sort out the most relevant variables are exceedingly difficult to design and execute. Moreover, the prevailing assumption that improving the social or medical care status of an individual will decrease the risk of premature delivery has not been proved.

TOCOLYSIS

A large number of methods have been utilized in attempts to arrest premature labor (Table 11-1). The available clinical information for a number of uterine relaxant drugs is described below. Emphasis is placed on the sympathomimetic compounds because they are the most widely used tocolytic agents, and their use has been sanctioned by the United States Food and Drug Administration.

Table 11-1 Methods To Arrest Preterm Labor

Bed rest
Hydration
Sedation
Ethanol
Beta-mimetic agents
Prostaglandin inhibitors
Magnesium sulfate
Diazoxide
Progestins

When interpreting data concerning tocolytic drugs, several principles of experimental design should be borne in mind. Designing a study to test the efficacy of a drug in inhibiting preterm labor should involve several considerations. True labor cannot be distinguished reliably from false labor except in retrospect, when entering active phase dilatation shows that delivery will occur. This is problematic because all methods of labor inhibition become less effective as labor advances, and the best results should be obtainable in the latent phase. Nevertheless, it would seem that if there is an attempt to validate the efficacy of any therapeutic regimen, the chances of treated patients being diagnosed incorrectly should be minimized. Thus, for study purposes, patients considered to be in labor should ideally manifest regular uterine contractions and progressive cervical effacement or, preferably, dilatation. The latter estimation has less inherent measurement error. Patients should be assigned randomly to experimental and placebo groups, and neither the investigators nor the subject should be aware of who is receiving the active drug. Groups should be large enough to allow sufficient statistical power in the study, and scrupulous care should be taken to demonstrate that the two groups are equivalent in all possible respects. The definition of successful therapy should be clearly and logically defined. Perhaps the best measure of success is not the duration of labor inhibition, but neonatal outcome.

These fundamental steps in research design have manifested themselves rarely. Literature concerning labor-inhibiting drugs is replete with data that are frequently overinterpreted. Almost all available studies lack control groups; some exceptions are indicated below. Clinicians may frequently conclude that a particular agent is quite capable of inhibiting uterine activity, but rarely can a judgment be made about its effectiveness in arresting labor.

Sympathomimetic Amines

The expectation that certain catecholamines and related compounds would inhibit uterine contractility was based on a firm historical experimental foundation. In 1927, Bourne and Burn[23] reported that uterine contractions diminished in two laboring women given intravenous epinephrine. The subsequent description of alpha- and beta-adrenergic receptors by Ahlquist[2] led to the observation that beta-adrenergic agonists inhibit uterine contractility, while it was enhanced by alpha-adrenergic drugs. Subsequently, Lands et al.[81] demonstrated the existence of two discrete populations of beta receptors: beta$_1$-receptor activity was associated with cardioaccelerator and lipolytic effects of catecholamines, whereas beta$_2$ stimulation involved smooth muscle relaxation. The uterus possesses beta$_2$-receptors.

The practical importance of these observations is considerable. Although many beta-adrenergic drugs clearly inhibit uterine activity, most are not useful clinically as uterine relaxants because of their considerable beta$_1$ activity. Thus, doses that result in uterine relaxation cause the undesirable side effects of peripheral vasodilatation and hypotension, as well as inotropic and chronotropic cardiac effects.

The recognition that adrenergic mechanisms produce uterine relaxation stimulated the search for clinically useful drugs with primarily beta$_2$ activity. The most promising have been relatives of naturally occurring catecholamines known as phenethanolamines. Their stereoconfiguration ensures that they have a relatively long duration of action and can be administered orally.

Isoxsuprine

Isoxsuprine was the first beta-mimetic drug used clinically for tocolysis in the United States. Preliminary reports were encouraging, and suggested that when given by intravenous infusion delivery could be delayed in a substantial number of cases. Although evidence of its effectiveness in inhibiting labor accumulated, isoxsuprine was found to cause maternal tachycardia frequently, and most studies reported a small incidence of palpitations, apprehension, nausea, or dizziness. Diastolic hypotension was common and occasionally severe, resulting in considerable maternal and fetal risks. Cardiovascular side effects as well as reported fetal and neonatal effects (hypoglycemia, hypocalcemia, ileus, transient renal failure, and hypotension) were recognized. This drug is now not used for tocolysis, in deference to ritodrine or terbutaline.

Ritodrine

Ritodrine is useful for labor inhibition because of its favorable ratio of uterine to cardiovascular effects. It is the only beta-agonist approved for use as a labor suppressant by the United States Food and Drug Administration. Barden[8] and Landesman et al.[80] demonstrated in 1971 that ritodrine given intravenously in doses of 50 to 100 μg/min could decrease uterine activity during term labor with only modest increases in maternal pulse pressure and heart rate and no significant fetal heart rate changes. Initial uncontrolled observations in premature labor appeared promising,[19] and a double-blind study was reported by Wesselius-de Casparis et al.[137] Their results showed that labor was inhibited successfully for more than 7 days in 80% of the ritodrine group and 48% of the placebo group. Both groups were treated with bed rest and sedation. The criteria for admission to the study were quite liberal, and insufficient information was provided to compare the distributions of dilatation prior to therapy in the two groups; in addition it is possible that many were not in labor.

Spellacy et al.[123] randomized 29 patients thought to be in premature labor to receive either ritodrine or placebo. They found no significant difference between the two groups in the degree of extension of pregnancy, birth weight, or neonatal mortality. Contrary results were obtained from a randomized multicenter trial involving 313 singleton pregnancies.[95] In this study the ritodrine group had a significant decrease in neonatal death rate and frequency of low birth weight and respiratory distress syndrome. In another study, Creasy et al.[33] treated 55 patients with oral ritodrine or placebo. All had just completed a successful course of tocolysis with parenteral ritodrine. If labor recurred, intravenous therapy was reinstituted. Although the number of days gained until delivery was the same in both groups, there were fewer relapses in the ritodrine treated group. The implied benefit would be a reduced need for hospitalization in patients treated with oral maintenance ritodrine after their initial episode of premature labor has been treated.

Ritodrine causes an increase in cardiac output, maternal heart rate, and pulse pressure, and is less likely to produce significant hypotension than isoxsuprine.[20,100] Its uterine and cardiovascular effects are blocked by propranolol, but not by phenoxybenzamine, suggesting that its mode of action is beta-receptor mediated.[118] No effect on uterine blood flow has been noted in normal pregnancies, but it may cause an increase in blood flow in pathologic pregnancies in which there is uteroplacental artery constriction.[28] However, in sheep, a dose-related but transient decrease in uterine blood flow was observed;[27,42] this was perhaps related to generalized vasodilatation in other vascular beds. No severe changes in the fetal acid-base milieu have been detected.

Because sympathomimetic amines activate glycogen phosphorylase, they may increase blood glucose and lactate. Maternal hyperglycemia is found commonly when these drugs are used as tocolytic agents, and blood glucose levels should be measured periodically during therapy. Although major changes in glucose tolerance do not seem to occur in normal mothers,[121] ritodrine and related drugs should be used with caution in women with diabetes mellitus. In fact, occasional cases of severe hyperglycemia or ketoacidosis have occurred in type I diabetics treated with these drugs.[97] Neonatal hypoglycemia may occur.[43]

Other maternal side effects include tremor (10%–15%) and anxiety or restlessness (5%–10%).[9] Decreases in serum potassium levels also occur.[77] This probably relates both to direct effects of beta agonists on membrane electrolyte pumps and to the movement of plasma potassium into cells as a consequence of hyperglycemia and concomitant insulin-mediated glucose transfer. Although the decrease in potassium is usually modest, it should be monitored closely; this is particularly true in women susceptible to cardiac arrhythmias.

Maternal pulmonary edema has been reported after the use of beta-mimetic drugs.[3] This complication occurs most frequently in association with multiple gestation, steroid therapy, and excessive hydration. When these factors, which may be associated with intravascular volume over-load, occur in conjunction with the cardiotonic and vasopressinlike effects of the sympathomimetic tocolytic drugs, pulmonary edema may result. Patients receiving these drugs must be monitored carefully for clinical signs of pulmonary congestion.

Other reported serious side effects include cerebral ischemia (in women with migraine),[11] cardiac arrhythmias, myocardial ischemia, and hypotension.[17] The presence of prominent cardiovascular effects should prompt a search for previously undetected cardiac disease.[110] In fact, prior to beginning ritodrine treatment the patient should have a careful cardiopulmonary examination and an electrocardiogram. Large decreases in maternal blood pressure are rare, and generally are limited to patients who are hypovolemic. When severe hypotension occurs during ritodrine administration in such patients, it is very difficult to reverse. For this reason, ritodrine (and related tocolytics) are contraindicated in the presence of vaginal bleeding when placenta previa or abruptio placentae (or any condition that may cause unexpected severe hemorrhage) is present.

The initial dose of ritodrine should generally be 50 to 100 μg/min IV. The infusion rate should be increased by 50 μg/min every 10 to 20 min until contractions stop, unacceptable side effects have occurred, or a maximum of 350 μg/min has been reached. Often the attained dose can be decreased by as much as 50% once tocolysis has been achieved without incurring further contractions. Although this approach is in common use, there is evidence that the use of a loading dose will result in more stable plasma levels.[128] It is generally recommended that the infusion be continued for at least 12 hr after contractions have ceased, and followed by oral doses of 40 to 80 mg/day in divided doses. The minimum effective dose should always be used in order to reduce the risks of side effects.

Terbutaline

Terbutaline has primarily beta$_2$-agonist properties. In asthmatic patients it has proved acceptable because of its generally mild cardiovascular side effects. Terbutaline effectively decreases the frequency and amplitude of myometrial contractions both in vivo and in vitro.[4,6,29,67,68]

The doses of terbutaline required to inhibit labor usually cause no change in diastolic blood pressure or in uterine blood flow and only a mild increment in maternal heart rate.[30] Because ritodrine may decrease uterine blood flow, terbutaline seems to be potentially advantageous with regard to fetal well-being; however, the two drugs have not been compared directly in this regard. Because of their identical mode of action, it is likely that they would have similar effects on uterine blood flow if given in comparable situations.

Maternal and fetal metabolic and cardiovascular alterations are qualitatively similar to those of ritodrine and related drugs.[60,68,121] The incidence of serious cardiovascular side effects is probably somewhat higher than with ritodrine when the drugs are given intravenously.[31]

Stubblefield and Heyl[125] reported their success with subcutaneous administration of terbutaline in the treatment of premature labor. Although this route has the disadvantage of not allowing immediate control over the drug, it has the virtues of ease of administration and minimum risks of overdosage. This technique has been used with success at the Beth Israel Hospital, Boston, for some time. The initial dosage is 0.25 to 0.50 mg subcutaneously every 1 to 2 hr until contractions cease, maternal pulse is 115 to 120 beats/min, or undesirable side effects occur. Oral maintenance dosages of 15 to 30 mg/day can then be instituted. Serious or intolerable side effects are quite uncommon with this regimen.

Certain precautions must be followed when using sympathomimetic drugs for labor inhibition. Because these agents may increase heart rate and cardiac output, they should not be employed in patients with heart disease, hypertension, or thyrotoxicosis. A constant infusion pump should be used for intravenous administration and blood pressure should be measured continuously or at frequent intervals. Patients must be well hydrated and maintained in the lateral position to minimize hypotension. Fetal heart rate monitoring is a necessity. Blood sugar and serum potassium should be measured periodically. These drugs should be used with great care in diabetics, whose insulin requirements may increase considerably during the infusion. Neonatal hypoglycemia is a possibility even in babies of nondiabetics, and should be anticipated. Maternal plasma potassium must be monitored (although replacement is rarely necessary unless signs or symptoms of hypokalemia occur), and scrupulous attention must be paid to the gravida's state of hydration and cardiopulmonary status.

An insufficient number of controlled studies are available to demonstrate with certainty whether any of the sympathomimetics (or any other labor-inhibiting drug) is efficacious.[26] More sophisticated comparisons of the cardiovascular effects of the available compounds must be made in the same experimental system in order to determine which drugs have the most favorable benefit/risk ratio. Very little information is available concerning the effect of these drugs on fetal cardiovascular dynamics;[119] it would be important to ascertain with clarity whether fetal or maternal effects differ in normal versus pathologic pregnancies.

Magnesium Sulfate

During the last several years, the use of magnesium sulfate ($MgSO_4$) to suppress preterm labor has become widespread.[124] The drug's use and side effects are quite familiar to obstetricians, who have long employed it in the treatment of preeclampsia. It compares favorably with ritodrine and terbutaline[14,64] in its efficacy, and because the serious side effects of $MgSO_4$ tend to be less common than those of sympathomimetics, $MgSO_4$ has been advocated as the first drug of choice for the treatment of preterm labor.[64] In monkeys, ritodrine seems to be capable of reducing placental perfusion, whereas $MgSO_4$ does not.[127] Although the clinical significance of this observation is not known, it has prompted some to avoid sympathomimetic drugs in favor of $MgSO_4$ if there is concern about fetal oxygenation.

When adrenergic agonists are unsuccessful in reducing contractility, benefit may sometimes be achieved by changing to $MgSO_4$.[14] Concomitant use of both agents should generally be avoided, as it considerably increases the frequency of side effects.[46,101]

Prostaglandin Inhibitors

Interest in the role of prostaglandins in the initiation of labor and in the production of uterine contractility for induction of labor or abortion engendered the idea that inhibitors of prostaglandin synthesis might suppress labor. Zuckerman et al.[143] showed that this indeed may be so. However, evidence showing that prostaglandin antagonists can result in closure of the fetal ductus arteriosus is of concern. Clinical reports of persistent fetal circulation, pulmonary hypertension, and congestive heart failure in the newborn and experimental evidence of decreased placental blood flow are disturbing.[88,96,107,139] Nevertheless, reported clinical experience with these drugs[99] has been generally favorable. The dose necessary to provide myometrial suppression may be insufficient to result in cardiovascular complications in most individuals and ductus closure may be unlikely to occur if the drug is given very early in gestation. Indomethacin should be used with extreme reluctance until more is known about the magnitude of the attendant risk.

Calcium Channel Blockers

Calcium channel blocking drugs are not widely used for treatment of premature labor, but derivatives of available agents hold great promise for the future. Existing drugs are potent myometrial relaxants in sheep[54] and rabbits[63] without severe cardiovascular side effects. However, evidence in experimental animals that calcium channel blockers may diminish uterine blood flow[82] and affect fetal oxygenation adversely are of concern. There is increasing experience with short-term use of verapamil for the treatment of supraventricular tachycardia in pregnant women, and no adverse fetal effects have been reported; but use of this class of drugs for the treatment of preterm labor is limited, and results are thus far not conclusive regarding efficacy or safety.[40,131] Widespread application must await proper clinical trials.

Effectiveness of Tocolysis

Now that beta-mimetic and other tocolytic drugs have been in widespread use for more than a decade, it is important to assess their impact on the problem of preterm delivery. Although there is no doubt that these drugs are effective myometrial relaxants, whether they are able to arrest advancing labor and to reduce the frequency or complications of preterm birth is less clear. In fact, there is some evidence that, although beta-mimetic drugs probably delay delivery somewhat, they have little demonstrable effect on reducing the frequency of low birth weight delivery, perinatal mortality, or respiratory complications in newborns.[128] There are probably several reasons for this. Many women in preterm labor have contraindications to tocolysis, and side effects that require discontinuation of the drugs are frequent. Furthermore, our ignorance regarding the early diagnosis of preterm labor, alluded to above, makes interpretation of existing data concerning efficacy very difficult. Finally, consideration must be given to the most appropriate endpoint to use in studies of the effects of tocolytic drugs. Attainment of long delays to delivery and birth weights above 2,500 g is desirable, but not necessarily the sole index of success. Delay of delivery for even 48 hr at very early gestational ages may allow time for significant further spontaneous or steroid-induced lung maturation. There is even the suggestion that some tocolytic drugs possess lung-maturing properties.[22] In addition, short delays in delivery may provide time for transfer of the pregnant mother to a hospital with neonatal intensive care facilities.

Therefore, the use of tocolytic drugs may in selected cases prolong pregnancy sufficiently to provide benefits. These drugs must always be used with a clear understanding of their benefits and risks, and with careful monitoring to ensure maximal patient safety.

COURSE OF LABOR

Friedman and Sachtleben[49] analyzed the labors of 1,000 mothers who gave birth to infants weighing between 1,000 and 2,500 g. When compared to term labors, nulliparous preterm labors showed shortening of latent and active phases, the phase of maximum slope, and the second stage. In multiparas, however, only the active phase duration was shortened, and its maximum slope increased. The degree of shortening of each aspect of labor was inversely proportional to birth weight.

The incidence of dysfunctional labor among nulliparas was 11.2%. Only the frequency of protracted active phase dilatation was significantly higher than in term labors (7.6% vs. 3.6%); but in multiparas, abnormal labors occurred with almost twelve times their frequency at term. There is thus a bimodal distribution of active phase duration in preterm labor, particularly obvious in multiparas. Many premature labors are quite short, and others prolonged. Dysfunctional labors are most common in the lowest birth weight groups. The explanation for these phenomena is unknown.

MANAGEMENT CONSIDERATIONS

Diagnosis

The first and most crucial decision to be made when faced with a patient experiencing uterine contractions prior to term is whether she is indeed in labor. Unfortunately, no criteria exist that enable this diagnosis to be confirmed with certainty, except by hindsight. In general, it should be required that regular uterine contractions be accompanied by objective changes in cervical dilatation or effacement. Confirmation requires serial examinations by the same individual, unless advanced dilatation is obvious. If the patient is deemed to be in labor, assessment of fetal weight and gestational age must be made by clinical examination, a review of obstetric milestones, and ultrasonography. The latter may provide the only reasonable estimate of gestational age or fetal weight, especially in women who have not had extensive prenatal care. Ultrasonography is of further value because women who labor prematurely are more likely to be carrying a fetus with a major anomaly or a malpresentation, or to have a multiple gestation or evidence of intrauterine growth retardation. Knowledge of such abnormalities could have a major bearing on decisions concerning the timing and route of delivery (Figure 11-1). In addition, ultrasound is vital if amniocentesis is to be used to assess fetal maturity or to search for evidence of amniotic fluid infection.

If the fetus appears to have completed 34 or more menstrual weeks of pregnancy, many authorities make no attempt, other than perhaps bed rest or intravenous hydration, to inhibit labor. This is because the mortality and morbidity among these babies is extremely low when cared for in major pediatric centers, and the risks of labor inhibition (coupled with risks inherent in the conditions leading to the premature initiation of the labor process) are not fully known and may exceed the risks of extrauterine life. The exception to this generalization would be situations in which fetal lung maturity is known to be incomplete despite advanced gestational age. Also, if sophisticated neonatal care is unavailable, attempts to inhibit labor should perhaps be more aggressive with a view toward transfer of the mother to a tertiary care unit prior to delivery. There is convincing evidence that delivery of low birth weight babies at other than tertiary centers may influence outcome adversely.[102]

Tocolysis

In the less-than-34 weeks fetus in labor, the next question relates to the advisability of arresting the labor. Various practical and ethical considera-

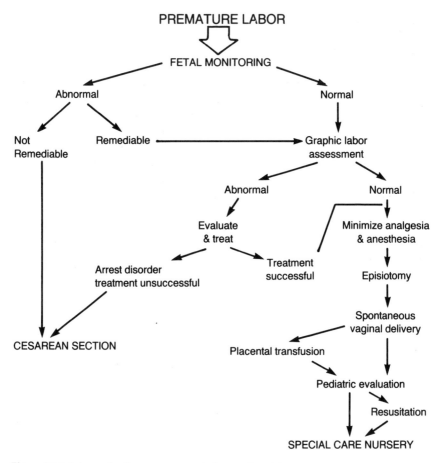

Figure 11-1 Schema for the management of premature labor.

tions are involved in this decision. Is the uterine milieu "hostile" in the sense of placing the fetus in special jeopardy? Does the maternal condition warrant continuing the pregnancy? Is the fetus so premature as to preclude any reasonable chance of extrauterine survival?

If evaluation of the mother and fetus reveals no conditions (e.g., preeclampsia, diabetes mellitus, sepsis) that mitigate against delaying delivery, an assessment of fetal condition must be made by continuous fetal heart rate monitoring.[24] In addition, a search for evidence of chorioamnionitis must be made, including cervical culture and Gram stain, maternal leucocyte count, and sometimes amniocentesis for evaluation of amniotic fluid. If the heart rate pattern is normal and there is no evidence of infection, tocolytic therapy may be considered, if indicated based on other considerations (see below). If evidence of fetal compromise is elicited, the most expedient and atraumatic means for immediate delivery should be contemplated. It would be unacceptable to impede the labor process and risk losing the fetus as a consequence.

Usually, during the initial evaluation of the patient with premature uterine contractions, she is placed on bed rest and given intravenous hydration. Some obstetricians add sedation to this regimen. Volume loading is presumed to inhibit oxytocin release. Although this is a harmless maneuver in women without cardiopulmonary disease, its effectiveness is unproven. Similarly, bed rest and sedation may have some effect in reducing uterine contractility. It is tempting to ascribe these benefits to alterations in sympathoadrenal activity, but this also has not been verified. Despite these uncertainties, there is evidence that about half of patients diagnosed with early preterm labor will have diminished uterine contractility when bed rest, hydration, and/or sedation are employed.[132] Although this might be interpreted to document our diagnostic inability to identify true preterm labor, there is evidence that even those women who respond to these simple measures are at increased risk of preterm birth.[130] Therefore, rest and hydration should be employed as soon as the diagnosis of preterm labor has been entertained, and contraindications to fluid loading have been ruled out.

A urinalysis should be performed and maternal urinary tract infection treated promptly. Specific conditions that would render labor inhibition potentially hazardous include amnionitis, rupture of the membranes, maternal disease (e.g., preeclampsia and cardiac disease), fetal disease (e.g., Rh isoimmunization, infection, and intrauterine death), or obstetric conditions such as suspected abruptio placentae. Moreover, when the cervix is dilated more than 4 cm, or especially if active phase dilatation can be documented, labor inhibition by any method is unlikely to succeed.

If the monitor pattern suggests that the immature fetus is in stable condition, and there are no fetal or maternal contraindications, consideration should be given to attempting to arrest labor. If bed rest, hydration, and perhaps sedation prove ineffective, pharmacologic intervention may be contemplated. Sympathomimetic drugs such as ritodrine or terbutaline should generally be the first choice. If specific contraindications to these agents exist, $MgSO_4$ is a reasonable alternative.

The idea that administration of corticosteroids to the mother can enhance lung maturation in premature fetuses is supported by considerable experimental and clinical evidence. However, there is a growing trend of skepticism concerning this therapeutic option, and answers concerning the efficacy and side effects of this therapy are not definitive.

Preliminary data do suggest safety, at least in mothers without medical complications. Pharmacologic delay of delivery for 1 or 2 days seems an attainable goal in many situations, and this would be enough time for the steroids to exert their effect. Even if the baby were born prematurely, the risk of it developing and succumbing to respiratory distress syndrome would be reduced considerably. However, although disorders of the pulmonary system represent the greatest threat to the small premature infant, other organ systems may also evoke morbidity and mortality by virtue of their immaturity.

When no correctable source of premature labor has been found, amnionitis, even in the presence of intact membranes, should be considered. If bacteria or white blood cells are observed in amniotic fluid, delivery should be expedited. Although the frequency of chorioamnionitis in asymptomatic patients is low,[41] amniocentesis should be considered when there are ruptured membranes when even a subtle suggestion of infection exists.

Labor and Delivery

When a preterm labor continues to progress, several guidelines should be adhered to. It is generally assumed that fetal distress is more common among premature than term babies, although proof for this does not exist. Nevertheless, fetal monitoring is exceedingly important if we are to optimize the chances of survival for premature babies. Monitoring is predictive of fetal condition in preterm fetuses as it is in term fetuses[138] and babies born after asphyxial heart rate patterns are more likely to be difficult to resuscitate, and to develop severe respiratory distress syndrome[37,90] than those with normal patterns. Although the characteristic heart rate patterns of very premature fetuses differ somewhat from those of fetuses at term, in general the same principles of management should apply (see Chapter 10).

The progress of labor should be followed using graphic techniques, and intervention considered only if the labor is abnormal. Premature fetuses are much more vulnerable to trauma and drug effects than are term babies. Thus, any potentially compromising technique should be avoided unless clearly indicated.

The dangers inherent in midforceps delivery and other extensive obstetric manipulations are now well known. Prohibition of these techniques in a vulnerable premature fetus is especially important, and prompt cesarean section is almost always preferable to midforceps operations when faced with fetal distress. This applies particularly to labors in which there has been an arrest of dilatation or descent that has not responded to oxytocin stimulation. When cesarean section is required, special attention to technique is important. The use of the Kroenig incision for cesarean section in prematures has been advocated.[44] It allows easy extension into the fundus when the need for a larger incision becomes apparent, and averts a transverse incision that will often prove too small if the lower uterine segment is not well developed. Jovanovic has cautioned against enlarging a lower segment incision bluntly, and advocates the use of scissors for this purpose to ensure adequate exposure.[73] Whatever incision is chosen, it should be large enough to deliver the fetal head with a minimum of exerted pressure. Carefully splinting the small baby's body with the forearm while protecting the head with the operator's upper hand is useful to avoid potentially traumatic manipulation and traction on the extremities.[39] The author has found that a lower segment incision extended cephalolaterally ("smiled up") if necessary often provides sufficient room, and may be preferable to a vertical incision in terms of risk of rupture in subsequent pregnancies.

Vaginal delivery should also progress with a minimum of interference. The concept that outlet forceps provide protection against cranial trauma has not been substantiated, and the author generally favors spontaneous delivery. The use of a large episiotomy to prevent excessive perineal pressure on the fetal skull is probably important.

Cesarean section can obviate some of the potential risks of trauma from vaginal delivery, and routine cesarean delivery has been advocated for all VLBW babies. The preponderance of existing evidence does not support this approach, and studies suggest that cesarean section per se provides no advantage over vaginal delivery in the VLBW baby with regard to survival[65] or morbidity.[12,18,79,126] Randomized clinical trials to help settle this controversy have been attempted. One enrolled only 40 subjects and had considerable methodologic difficulty;[136] another[85] was abandoned for lack of subjects, primarily because obstetricians were so convinced of the benefits of cesarean delivery they were reluctant to allow their patients to be entered into the study. Surely, this question deserves clear resolution. The fundamental desire is obviously to deliver preterm babies with the minimal amount of trauma and asphyxia compatible with good intrapartum care and safety. In the absence of fetal distress, neglected labor dysfunction, or instrumental delivery, it is likely that vaginal delivery is quite safe, and the superiority of cesarean section in this regard remains unproved.

Controversy exists over the need for placental transfusion after delivery. Immediate clamping of the cord could deprive the neonate of needed red blood cells and thus impair oxygen carrying capacity, and perhaps increase the risk of severe respiratory distress. On the other hand, excessive transfusion can result in hyperbilirubinemia, hypervolemia, and plethora. An empiric compromise that seems reasonable is to delay cord clamping for about 45 s. However, if the newborn does not initiate respiration promptly, it is much more important not to delay clamping the cord so as to expedite immediate resuscitative measures.

Of utmost importance is the fact that many prematures require urgent ventilatory assistance. Thus, whenever the delivery of a preterm infant is anticipated, all of the requisite equipment and skilled personnel should be available for immediate resuscitation. Furthermore, access to a specialized neonatal intensive care unit is mandatory.

Prevention

The recent trend of improved survival and decreased morbidity among premature babies is encouraging and probably relates to improvements in obstetric and pediatric medicine. Nevertheless, premature delivery is still common and remains a major contributor to perinatal death and later infirmity. Its economic burden to society and to the health care system is enormous. The financial and emotional impacts on involved families are incalculable.

The pharmacologic inhibition of premature labor is becoming more sophisticated, and new agents are likely to become available. However, because a relatively small proportion of patients who present with premature labor are suitable for tocolytic therapy,[142] it is clear that the greatest impact on preterm birth will be accomplished by its prevention. Physicians can play a direct role in this regard to a certain extent. Encouragement of adequate nutrition, preconceptional and prenatal education regarding the potential dangers of nicotine and other drugs, conservative management of placenta previa and other obstetric disorders, early detection and treatment of pregnancy bacteriuria, all seem to contribute to diminishing the risk of premature delivery. Bed rest in multiple gestations may also play a role. The establishment of regional referral centers capable of managing high-risk gravidas and neonates transferred to them is critically important to optimize the infant outcome in those situations that do result in delivery of low birth weight infants. The ability to predict reliably that a patient will enter labor prior to term would be of great benefit. Methods of preventing labor could be administered, developing early labor could be dealt with promptly, and appropriate plans made for the management of a premature infant if delivery were to occur.

Several investigators have proposed scoring systems based on known epidemiologic risk factors that identify women at risk for premature labor. Most systems have the drawback of a high false-positive rate. For example, Papiernik's method can identify 75% of patients destined to deliver prematurely. However, fully 35% of all patients must be considered at high risk and followed carefully in order to obtain this result.[104] The application of Papiernik's approach, however, has been associated with a considerable reduction in the frequency of preterm birth in France, and deserves further evaluation in other settings.

Creasy and others[62] have evolved similar programs, incorporating risk assignment, patient instruction in clinical signs of early premature labor, and frequent prenatal visits. Although this system was successful in reducing the frequency of preterm birth, the low-risk group still contributed 36% of the premature deliveries.[62] The applicability of such systems to a low socioeconomic population has been questioned.[86]

The observation that uterine activity seemed to be higher during pregnancy among women who delivered prematurely than those who did not prompted the development of ambulatory uterine contraction monitoring. When patients monitor their uterine activity at home, they may detect preterm labor and seek medical help sooner than if they depended on subjective evidence of labor.[76,98] This approach shows considerable promise, but large-scale prospective trials are necessary before routine use can be recommended.

Drug therapy for the prevention of premature labor has been attempted. Some studies have suggested that oral beta-mimetic drugs given after parenteral therapy for premature labor might reduce the likelihood of recurrence.[33] No effective oral sympathomimetic drug to prevent preterm labor has been found. Medroxyprogesterone acetate has no effect on length of gestation when given prophylactically. Although one group of investigators has suggested that the use of this drug might decrease the frequency of premature labor if it is administered early in gestation, this remains controversial.[70] This progestin did not seem to prolong gestation when given in the third trimester of twin pregnancy.[61] The role of bed rest in the prevention of prematurity is widely advocated, but the true efficacy of reductions in physical activity has not been tested. Similarly, preterm birth is more common among women who work at physically strenuous jobs. Whether ceasing work will reduce risk, or whether occupation is merely a proxy for other factors is uncertain. Many obstetricians recommend that women at high risk for premature labor cease or curtail vigorous physical activity during pregnancy. The virtue of this common approach remains to be proved.

Despite the potential benefits of accurate identification of women at risk for preterm birth, and the possible value of pharmacologic agents in the prevention of preterm labor, it is clear that socioeconomic variables, whether related to nutrition, wealth, geography, or stress, contribute most substantially to the burden of premature delivery. Thus, the greatest potential impact on reduction of this problem will come from major social, educational, and economic changes that will reduce the number of disadvantaged people in our society. Although such changes will require monumental efforts on the part of medicine and government, in them resides the strongest potential for reducing the serious consequences of premature birth. In the absence of such major social upheaval, the application of organized preterm birth prevention programs holds some promise. More importantly, the root biologic causes of preterm labor must be elucidated.

REFERENCES

1. Abramowicz M, Kass EA: Pathogenesis and prognosis of prematurity. *N Engl J Med* 1966;275:878–885.

2. Ahlquist RP: A study of adrenotropic receptors. *Am J Physiol* 1948;153:586–680.

3. Alper M, Cohen WR: Maternal pulmonary edema after ritodrine and dexamethasone treatment for threatened premature labor. *J Reprod Med* 1983;28:349–352.

4. Akerlund M, Andersson K-E: Effects of terbutaline on human myometrial activity and endometrial blood flow. *Obstet Gynecol* 1976;47:529–535.

5. American Academy of Pediatrics. Working party to discuss nomenclature based on gestational age and birth weight. *Arch Dis Child* 1970;45:730.

6. Andersson K-E, Bengtsson LP, Gustafson I, Ingemarsson I: The relaxing effect of terbutaline on the human uterus during term labor. *Am J Obstet Gynecol* 1975;121:602–609.

7. Ansari AH, Reynolds RH: Cervical incompetence. A review. *J Reprod Med* 1987;32:161–171.

8. Barden TP: Effect of ritodrine on human uterine motility and cardiovascular responses in term labor and the early postpartum state. *Am J Obstet Gynecol* 1972;112:645–652.

9. Barden TP, Peter JB, Merkatz IR: Ritodrine hydrochloride: A β-mimetic agent for use in preterm labor. I. Pharmacology, clinical history, administration, side effects and safety. *Obstet Gynecol* 1980;56:1–6.

10. Barnes AB, Colton T, Gundersen J, Noller KL, Tilley BC, Strama T, Townsend DE, O'Brien W: Fertility and outcome of pregnancy in women exposed in utero to diethylstilbesterol. *N Engl J Med* 1980;302:609–613.

11. Barresi JA: Listeria monocytogenes: A cause of premature labor and neonatal sepsis. *Am J Obstet Gynecol* 1980;136:410–411.

12. Barrett JM, Boehm FH, Vaughn WK: The effect of type of delivery on neonatal outcome in singleton infants of birth weight of 1000g or less. *JAMA* 1983;250:625–629.

13. Battaglia FC, Lubchenco LO: A practical classification of newborn infants by weight and gestational age. *J Pediatr* 1967;71:159–163.

14. Beall MH, Edgar BW, Paul RH: Smith-Wallace LVN: A comparison of ritodrine, terbutaline and magnesium sulfate for the suppression of preterm labor. *Am J Obstet Gynecol* 1985;53:854–859.

15. Bejar R, Curbelo V, Davis C, Gluck L: Premature labor. II. Bacterial sources of phospholipase. *Obstet Gynecol* 1981;57:479–482.

16. Belsey MA: Gestation, birth weight, and spontaneous abortion in pregnancy after induced abortion. *Lancet* 1979;1:142–145.

17. Benedetti TJ: Maternal complications of parenteral β-sympathomimetic therapy for premature labor. *Am J Obstet Gynecol* 1983;145:1–6.

18. Ben-Shlomo I, Zohar S, Marmor A, Blondheim DS, Sharir T: Myocardial ischemia during intravenous ritodrine treatment: Is it so rare? *Lancet* 1986;2:917–918 (letter).

19. Bieniarz J, Ivankovich A, Scommegna A: Cardiac output during ritodrine treatment in premature labor. *Am J Obstet Gynecol* 1974;118:910–920.

20. Bieniarz J, Motew M, Scommegna A: Uterine and cardiovascular effects of ritodrine in premature labor. *Obstet Gynecol* 1972;40:65–73.

21. Bloch H, Lippsett H, Redner B, Hirschl D: Reduction of mortality in the premature nursery. II. Incidence and causes of prematurity. Ethnic, socioeconomic, and obstetric factors. *J Pediatr* 1952;41:300–304.

22. Boog G, Ben Brahim M, Gandar R: β-mimetic drugs and possible prevention of respiratory distress syndrome. *Br J Obstet Gynaecol* 1975;82:285–288.

23. Bourne A, Burn JH: The dosage and action of pituitary extract and of the ergot alkaloids on the uterus in labour, with a note on the action of adrenalin. *J Obstet Gynaecol Br Emp* 1927;34:249–267.

24. Bowes WA, Gabbe SG, Bowes C: Fetal heart rate monitoring in premature infants weighing 1,500 grams or less. *Am J Obstet Gynecol* 1980;137:791–796.

25. Braun P, Lee Y, Klein JO, Marcy SM, Klein TA, Charles D, Levy P, Kass EH: Birth weight and genital mycoplasma in pregnancy. *N Engl J Med* 1971;284:167–171.

26. Breart G, Ringa V: Evaluation des traitements contre la prematurité, in Sureau C, Blot P, Gabrol D, Cavaille F, Germain G, (eds): *Control and Management of Parturition.* Paris/London, Colloques INSERM/John Libby Eurotext Ltd., 1986, pp 191–198.

27. Brennan SC, McLaughlin MK, Chez RA: Effects of prolonged infusion of β-adrenergic agonists on uterine and umbilical blood flow in pregnant sheep. *Am J Obstet Gynecol* 1977;128:709–715.

28. Brettes JP, Renaud R, Gandar R: A double-blind investigation into the effects of ritodrine on uterine blood flow during the third trimester of pregnancy. *Am J Obstet Gynecol* 1976;124:164–168.

29. Caritis SN, Morishima HO, Stark RI, Daniel SS, James LS: Effects of terbutaline on the pregnant baboon and fetus. *Obstet Gynecol* 1977;50:56–60.

30. Caritis SN, Mueller-Heubach E, Morishima HO, Edelstone DI: Effect of terbutaline on cardiovascular state and uterine blood flow in pregnant ewes. *Obstet Gynecol* 1977; 50:603–606.

31. Caritis SN, Toig G, Heddinger LA, Ashmead G: A double-blind study comparing ritodrine and terbutaline in the treatment of preterm labor. *Am J Obstet Gynecol* 1984; 150:7–14.

32. Clifford SH: High-risk pregnancy. I. Prevention of prematurity, *sine qua non* for reduction in mental retardation and other neurologic disorders. *N Engl J Med* 1964; 271:243–249.

33. Creasy RK, Golbus MS, Laros RK, Parer JT, Roberts JM: Oral ritodrine maintenance in the treatment of preterm labor. *Am J Obstet Gynecol* 1980;137:212–219.

34. Daling JR, Emanuel I: Induced abortion and subsequent outcome of pregnancy in a series of American women. *N Engl J Med* 1977;297:1241–1245.

35. Dann M, Levine SZ, New EV: Small premature infants. *Pediatrics* 1964;33:945–955.

36. DiMusto JC, Bohjalian O, Millar M: Mycoplasma hominis type I infection and pregnancy. *Obstet Gynecol* 1973;41:33–37.

37. Douvas SG, Meeks GR, Graves G, Walsh DA, Morrison JC: Intrapartum fetal heart rate monitoring as a predictor of fetal distress and immediate neonatal condition in low-birth weight ($\leq$1800 grams) infants. *Am J Obstet Gynecol* 1984;148:300–302.

38. Drillien CM: Growth and development in a group of children of very low birth weight. *Arch Dis Child* 1958;33:10–18.

39. Druzin M: Atraumatic delivery in cases of malpresentation of the very low birth weight fetus at cesarean section. *Am J Obstet Gynecol* 1986;154:941–942.

40. Dubecq JP, Gonnet JMT, Horvitz J: Place des anticalciques dans la tocolyse, in Sureau C, Blot P, Cabrol D, Cavaille F, German G (eds): *Control and Management of Parturition*. Paris/London, Colloques INSERM/John Libby Eurotex Ltd., 1986, pp 173–177.

41. Duff P, Kopelman JN: Subclinical intraamniotic infection in asymptomatic patients with refractory preterm labor. *Obstet Gynecol* 1987;69:756–759.

42. Ehrenkranz RA, Walker AM, Oakes GK, McLaughlin MK, Chez RA: Effect of ritodrine infusion on uterine and umbilical blood flow in pregnant sheep. *Am J Obstet Gynecol* 1976;126:343–349.

43. Epstein M, Nicholls E, Stubblefield P: Neonatal hypoglycemia after β-sympathomimetic tocolytic therapy. *J Pediatr* 1979;94:449–453.

44. Fanaroff AA, Merkatz IR: Modern obstetrical management of the low birth weight infant. *Clin Perinatol* 1977;4:215–237.

45. Fedrick J, Anderson ABM: Factors associated with spontaneous preterm birth. *Br J Obstet Gynaecol* 1976;83:342–350.

46. Ferguson JE, Hensleigh PA, Kredenster D: Adjunctive use of magnesium sulfate with ritodrine for preterm labor tocolysis. *Am J Obstet Gynecol* 1984;148:166–171.

47. Fitzhardinge PM: Early growth and development in low-birth weight infants following treatment in an intensive care nursery. *Pediatrics* 1975;56:162–172.

48. Fournil C, Hidden J, Lajoux P: Evaluation du calibre de l'isthme uterin en debut de grossesse. *Nouv Presse Med* 1977;6:523–533.

49. Friedman EA, Sachtleben MR: Preterm labor. *Am J Obstet Gynecol* 1969;104:1152–1158.

50. Frigoletto FD, Philippe M, Davies IJ, Ryan KJ: Avoiding iatrogenic prematurity with elective repeat cesarean section without the routine use of amniocentesis. *Am J Obstet Gynecol* 1980;137:521–524.

51. Funderburk SJ, Guthrie D, Meldrum D: Suboptimal pregnancy outcome among women with prior abortions and premature births. *Am J Obstet Gynecol* 1976;126:55–60.

52. Gibbs CE: Diagnosis and treatment of uterine conditions that may cause prematurity. *Clin Obstet Gynecol* 1973;16:159–170.

53. Goldstein DP: Incompetent cervix in offspring exposed to diethylstilbesterol in utero. *Obstet Gynecol* 1978;52:73s–75s.

54. Golichowski AM, Hathaway DR, Fineberg N, Peleg D: Tocolytic and hemodynamic effects of nifedipine in the ewe. *Am J Obstet Gynecol* 1985;151:1134–1140.

55. Goodlin RC: Orgasm and premature labor. *Lancet* 1969;2:646.

56. Goodlin RC, Keller DW, Raffin M: Orgasm during late pregnancy: Possible deleterious effects. *Obstet Gynecol* 1971;38:916–920.

57. Gravett MG, Hummel D, Eschenbach DA, Holmes KK: Preterm labor associated with subclinical amniotic fluid infection and with bacterial vaginosis. *Obstet Gynecol* 1986;67:229–237.

58. Guzick DS, Winn K: The association of chorioamnionitis with preterm delivery. *Obstet Gynecol* 1985;65:11–16.

59. Haas G, Buchwald-Saal, Leidig E, Mentzel H: Improved outcome in very low birth weight infants from 1977 to 1983. *Eur J Pediatr* 1986;145:337–340.

60. Hankins GDV, Hauth JC: A comparison of the relative toxicities of β-sympathomimetic tocolytic agents. *Am J Perinatol* 1985;2:338–345.

61. Hartikainen-Sorri A-L, Kauppila A, Tuimale R: Inefficacy of 17α-hydroxyprogesterone caproate in the prevention of prematurity in twin pregnancy. *Obstet Gynecol* 1980;56:692–695.

62. Herron MA, Katz M, Creasy RK: Evaluation of a preterm birth prevention program. *Obstet Gynecol* 1982;59:452–456.

63. Holbrook RH Jr, Lirette M, Katz M: Cardiovascular and tocolytic effects of nicardipine HCl in the pregnant rabbit: Comparison with ritodrine HCl. *Obstet Gynecol* 1987;69:83–87.

64. Hollander DI, Nagey DA, Pupkin MJ: Magnesium sulfate and ritodrine hydrochloride: A randomized comparison. *Am J Obstet Gynecol* 1987;156:631–637.

65. Hutson JM, Driscoll JM, Fox HE, Driscoll YT, Steir ME: The effect of obstetric management on neonatal mortality and morbidity for infants weighing 700–1000 grams. *Am J Perinatol* 1986;3:255–261.

66. Iams JD, Clapp DH, Contos DA, Whitehurst R, Ayers LW, O'Shaughnessy RW: Does extra-amniotic fluid infection cause preterm labor? Gas-liquid chromatography studies of amniotic fluid in amnionitis, preterm labor, and normal controls. *Obstet Gynecol* 1987;70:365–368.

67. Ingemarsson I: Effect of terbutaline on premature labor: A double-blind placebo-controlled study. *Am J Obstet Gynecol* 1976;125:520–524.

68. Ingemarsson I, Westgren M, Lindberg C, Ahren B, Lundquist I, Carlsson C: Single injection of terbutaline in term labor: Placental transfer and effects on maternal and fetal carbohydrate metabolism. *Am J Obstet Gynecol* 1981;139:697–701.

69. Jeanty P, d'Alton M, Romero R, Hobbins JC: Perineal scanning. *Am J Perinatol* 1986;3:289–295.

70. Johnson JWC, Austin KL, Jones GS, Davis GH, King TM: Efficacy of 17α-hydroxyprogesterone caproate in the prevention of premature labor. *N Engl J Med* 1975;293:676–680.

71. Jones HW, Wheeless CR: Salvage of the reproductive potential of women with anomalous development of the müllerian ducts: 1868–1968–2068. *Am J Obstet Gynecol* 1969;104:348–364.

72. Jones JM, Sweetnam P, Hibbard BM: The outcome of pregnancy after cone biopsy of the cervix: A case-control study. *Br J Obstet Gynaecol* 1979;86:913–916.

73. Jovanovic R: Incisions of the pregnant uterus and delivery of low-birth weight infants. *Am J Obstet Gynecol* 1985;152:971–974.

74. Kass EH: Pregnancy, pyelonephritis, and prematurity. *Clin Obstet Gynecol* 1970; 13:239–254.

75. Kass EH, McCormack WM, Lin JS, Rosner B, Munoz A: Genital mycoplasmas as a cause of excess premature delivery. *Trans Assoc Am Physicians* 1981;94:261–266.

76. Katz M, Gill PJ, Newman RB: Detection of preterm labor by ambulatory monitoring of uterine activity for the management of oral tocolysis. *Am J Obstet Gynecol* 1986; 154:1253–1256.

77. Kirkpatrick C, Quenon M, Desir D: Blood anions and electrolytes during ritodrine infusion in preterm labor. *Am J Obstet Gynecol* 1980;138:523–527.

78. Kitchen W, Ford GW, Doyle LW, Rickards AL, Lissenden JV, Pepperell RJ, Duke JE: Cesarean section or vaginal delivery at 24 to 28 weeks' gestation: Comparison of survival and two-year morbidity. *Obstet Gynecol* 1985;66:149–157.

79. Kitchen WH, Doyle LW, Ford GW, Rickards AL, Lissenden JV, Ryan MM: Cerebral palsy in very low birthweight infants surviving to 2 years with modern perinatal intensive care. *Am J Perinatol* 1987;4:29–35.

80. Landesman R, Wilson KH, Coutinho EM, Klima IM, Marcus RS: The relaxant action of ritodrine, a sympathomimetic amine, on the uterus during term labor. *Am J Obstet Gynecol* 1971;110:111–114.

81. Lands AM, Arnold A, McAuliff JP, Luduena FP, Brown TG: Differentiation of receptor systems activated by sympathomimetic amines. *Nature* 1967;214:597–598.

82. Lirette M, Holbrook RH, Katz M: Cardiovascular and uterine blood flow changes during nicardipine HCl tocolysis in the rabbit. *Obstet Gynecol* 1987;69:79–82.

83. Lubchenco LO, Bard H, Goldman AL, Coyer WE, McIntyre C, Smith DV: Newborn intensive care and long term prognosis. *Dev Med Child Neurol* 1974;16:421–431.

84. Lubchenco LO, Horner FA, Reed LH, Hix IE, Metcalf D, Cohig R, Elliot HC, Bourg M: Sequellae of premature birth. *Am J Dis Child* 1963;106:135–149.

85. Lumley J, Lester A, Renou P, Wood C: A failed RCT to determine the best method of delivery for very low birth weight infants. *Controlled Clin Trials* 1985;6:120–127.

86. Main DM, Richardson D, Gabbe SG, Strong S, Weller SC: Prospective evaluation of a risk scoring system for predicting preterm delivery in black inner city women. *Obstet Gynecol* 1987;69:61–66.

87. Maisels MJ, Rees R, Marks K, Friedman Z: Elective delivery of the term fetus: An obstetrical hazard. *JAMA* 1977;238:2036–2039.

88. Manchester D, Margolis HS, Sheldon RE: Possible association between maternal indomethacin therapy and primary pulmonary hypertension of the newborn. *Am J Obstet Gynecol* 1976;126:467–471.

89. Marriage KJ, Davies PA: Neurological sequelae in children surviving mechanical ventilation in the neonatal period. *Arch Dis Child* 1977;52:176–182.

90. Martin CB, Siassi B, Hon EH: Fetal heart rate patterns and neonatal death in low birthweight infants. *Obstet Gynecol* 1974;44:503–510.

91. McCormick MC: The contribution of low birth weight to infant mortality and childhood morbidity. *N Engl J Med* 1985;312:82–90.

92. McDonald AD: Congenital defects associated with prematurity. *Arch Dis Child* 1962;37:277–281.

93. McDonald IA: Suture of the cervix for inevitable miscarriage. *J Obstet Gynaecol Br Emp* 1957;64:346–350.

94. McGregor JA, French JI, Reller LB, Todd JK, Makowski E: Adjunctive erythromycin treatment for idiopathic preterm labor: Results of a randomized double blinded, placebo-controlled trial. *Am J Obstet Gynecol* 1986;154:98–103.

95. Merkatz IR, Peter JB, Barden TP: Ritodrine hydrochloride: A β-mimetic agent for use in preterm labor. II. Evidence of efficacy. *Obstet Gynecol* 1980;56:7–12.

96. Mogilner BM, Ashkenazy M, Borenstein R, Lancet M: Hydrops fetalis caused by maternal indomethacin treatment. *Acta Obstet Gynecol Scand* 1982;61:183–185.

97. Mordes D, Kreutner K, Metzger W, Colwell JA: Dangers of intravenous ritodrine in diabetic patients. *JAMA* 1982;248:973–975.

98. Morrison JC, Martin JN, Martin RW, Gookin KS, Wiser WL: Prevention of preterm birth by ambulatory assessment of uterine activity: A randomized study. *Am J Obstet Gynecol* 1987;156:536–543.

99. Niebyl JR, Witter FR: Neonatal outcome after indomethacin treatment for preterm labor. *Am J Obstet Gynecol* 1986;155:747–749.

100. Nochimson DJ, Riffel HD, Yeh SY, Kreitzer MS, Paul RH, Hon EH: The effects of ritodrine hydrochloride on uterine activity and the cardiovascular system. *Am J Obstet Gynecol* 1974;118:523–528.

101. Ogburn PL Jr, Hansen CA, Williams PP, Butler JC Jr, Joseph MS, Julian TM: Magnesium sulfate and β-mimetic tocolysis in preterm labor after single-agent failure. *J Reprod Med* 1985;30:583–587.

102. Paneth N, Kiely JL, Wallenstein S, Marcus M, Pakter J, Susser M: Newborn intensive care and neonatal mortality in low birth weight infants. *N Engl J Med* 1982;307:149–155.

103. Papaevangelou G, Vrettos AS, Papadatos C, Alexiou D: The effect of spontaneous and induced abortion on prematurity and birth weight. *J Obstet Gynaecol Br Commonw* 1973;80:418–422.

104. Papiernik E: L'accouchement prématuré et sa prevention. *Arch Fr Pediatr* 1977; 34:488–491.

105. Parsons MT, Owens CA, Spellacy WN: Thermic effects of tocolytic agents: Decreased temperature with magnesium sulfate. *Obstet Gynecol* 1987;69:88–90.

106. Pugh WE, Fernandez FL: Coitus in late pregnancy. *Obstet Gynecol* 1953;2:636–642.

107. Ratner B, Rostler AE, Salgado PS: Care, feeding and fate of premature and full term infants born of tuberculous mothers. *Am J Dis Child* 1951;81:471–491.

108. Rayburn WF, Wilson EA: Coital activity and premature delivery. *Am J Obstet Gynecol* 1980;137:972–974.

109. Robertson JG, Livingstone JRB, Isdale MH: The management and complications of asymptomatic bacteriuria in pregnancy. *J Obstet Gynaecol Br Commonw* 1960;75:59–65.

110. Ron-El R, Caspi E, Herman A, Schreyer P, Algom M, Schlezinger Z: Unexpected cardiac pathology in pregnant women treated with beta-adrenergic agents (ritodrine). *Obstet Gynecol* 1983;61:105–125.

111. Rosene KA, Featherstone HJ, Benedetti TJ: Cerebral ischemia associated with parenteral terbutaline use in pregnant migraine patients. *Am J Obstet Gynecol* 1982;405–407.

112. Rush RW, Keirse MJNC, Howat P, Baum JD, Anderson ABM, Turnbull AC: Contribution of preterm delivery to perinatal mortality. *Br Med J* 1976;2:965–968.

113. Saint-Anne Dargassies S: Long-term neurological follow-up of 286 truly premature infants. I. Neurological sequelae. *Dev Med Child Neurol* 1977;19:462–478.

114. Sarfati P, Pageaut G, Gauthier C: Le role de l'infection dans les avortements tardifs et les accouchements prématuré. *Cah Coll Med* 1968;13:1079–1092.

115. Schlesinger ER, Allaway NC: The combined effect of birth weight and length of gestation on neonatal mortality among single premature births. *Pediatrics* 1955;15:698–703.

116. Schoenbaum SC, Monson RR, Stubblefield PG, Darney PD, Ryan KJ: Outcome of the delivery following an induced or spontaneous abortion. *Am J Obstet Gynecol* 1980;136:19–24.

117. Shirodkar VN: A method of operative treatment for habitual abortion in the second trimester of pregnancy. *Antiseptic* 1955;52:299–305.

118. Siimes ASI, Creasy RK: Effect of ritodrine on uterine activity, heart rate, and blood pressure in the pregnant sheep: Combined use of α or β blockade. *Am J Obstet Gynecol* 1976;126:1003–1010.

119. Siimes ASI, Creasy RK, Heymann MA, Rudolph AM: Cardiac output and its distribution and organ blood flow in the fetal lamb during ritodrine administration. *Am J Obstet Gynecol* 1978;132:42–48.

120. Smithwick EM, Pascual E, Go SC: Hepatitis-associated antigen: A possible relationship to premature delivery. *J Pediatr* 1972;81:537–540.

121. Smythe AR, Sakakini J: Maternal metabolic alterations secondary to terbutaline therapy for premature labor. *Obstet Gynecol* 1981;57:566–570.

122. Solberg DA, Butler J, Wagner NN: Sexual behavior in pregnancy. *N Engl J Med* 1973;288:1098–1103.

123. Spellacy WN, Cruz AC, Birk SA, Buhi WC: Treatment of premature labor with ritodrine: A randomized controlled study. *Obstet Gynecol* 1979;54:220–223.

124. Spisso K, Harbert G, Thiagarajah S: The use of magnesium sulfate as the primary tocolytic agent to prevent premature delivery. *Am J Obstet Gynecol* 1982;142:840–845.

125. Stubblefield PG, Heyl PS: Treatment of premature labor with subcutaneous terbutaline. *Obstet Gynecol* 1982;59:457–462.

126. Tejani N, Verma U, Hameed C, Chayen B: Method and route of delivery in the low birth weight vertex presentation correlated with early periventricular/intraventricular hemorrhage. *Obstet Gynecol* 1987;69:1–4.

127. Thiagarajah S, Harbert GM, Bourgeois FJ: Magnesium sulfate and ritodrine hydrochloride: Systemic and uterine hemodynamic effects. *Am J Obstet Gynecol* 1985;153:66–74.

128. Thiery M: Betamimetics for the management of preterm labour, in Sureau C, Blot P, Cabrol D, Cavaille F, Germain G (eds): *Control and Management of Parturition.* Paris/London, Colloques INSERM/John Libby Eurotext Ltd., 1986, pp 151–162.

129. Thomsen AC, Morup L, Hansen KB: Antibiotic elimination of Group B streptococci in urine in prevention of preterm labour. *Lancet* 1987;1:591–593.

130. Tupper C: The problems of prematurity. *Can Med Assoc J* 1960;83:51–53.

131. Ulmsten U, Andersson KE, Wingerup L: Treatment of premature labor with the calcium antagonist nifedipine. *Arch Gynecol* 1980;229:1–5.

132. Valenzuela G, Cline S, Hayashi RH: Follow-up of hydration and sedation in the pretherapy of premature labor. *Am J Obstet Gynecol* 1983;147:396–398.

133. Vitsky M: Pessary treatment of the incompetent cervical os. *Obstet Gynecol* 1968;31:732–733.

134. Vohr BR, Goll CTG: Neurodevelopmental and school performance of very low birth weight infants: A seven-year longitudinal study. *Pediatrics* 1985;76:345–350.

135. Wahbeth CJ, Hill GB, Eden RD, Gall SA: Intra-amniotic bacterial colonization in premature labor. *Am J Obstet Gynecol* 1984;148:739–743.

136. Wallace RL, Schifrin BS, Paul RH: The delivery route for very-low-birth-weight infants. A preliminary report of a prospective randomized study. *J Reprod Med* 1984; 29:736–740.

137. Wesselius-de Casparis A, Thiery M, Yo Le Sian A, Baumgarten K, Brosena I, Garmisans O, Stolk JC, Vivier W: Results of a double-blind, multicentre study with ritodrine in premature labor. *Br Med J* 1971;3:144–147.

138. Westgren M, Hormquist P, Ingemarsson I, Svenningsen N: Intrapartum fetal acidosis in preterm infants: Fetal monitoring and long-term morbidity. *Obstet Gynecol* 1984;63:355–359.

139. Wilkinson AR, Aynsley-Green A, Mitchell MD: Persistent pulmonary hypertension and abnormal prostaglandin E levels in preterm infants after maternal treatment with naproxen. *Arch Dis Child* 1979;54:942–945.

140. Wren BG: Subclinical renal infection and prematurity. *Med J Aust* 1969;2:596–600.

141. Yu Vyh, Loke HL, Bajuk B, Szymonowicz W, Orgill AA, Astbury J: Prognosis for infants born at 23–28 weeks' gestation. *Br Med J* 1986;293:1200–1203.

142. Zlatnik FJ: The applicability of labor inhibition to the problem of prematurity. *Am J Obstet Gynecol* 1972;113:704–706.

143. Zuckerman H, Reiss U, Rubinstein I: Inhibition of human premature labor by indomethacin. *Obstet Gynecol* 1974;44:787–789.

12

Breech Presentation

Max Borten

Hazards associated with breech delivery have been recognized since antiquity, and have received considerable attention in the obstetric literature.[4,5,23,31,52,60,63,70] Contemporary suggestions that heavy reliance on cesarean section for breech presentation would lower the associated perinatal mortality and morbidity were made in the late 1940s and early 1950s by Goethels[40] and Hall and Kohl.[43] Wright[93] was first to advocate routine cesarean section for all breech presentations. He based his opinion on a 50% lower perinatal morbidity rate observed when the cesarean section rate for term breech presentations was 22%, twice the rate reported by others at that time.

Reports of unfavorable long-term outcome for breech infants delivered vaginally[1,32,51,74] further encouraged the liberal use of cesarean section as the primary mode of delivery.[59,82] However, legitimate questions have been raised concerning the appropriateness of such a pervasive policy.[76,86] For example, the excess morbidity and mortality associated with breech delivery varies with the type of breech presentation and infant birth weight.[22] Also, traumatic delivery, some of which may be preventable, contributes to the poor results.[44,84] Most importantly, breech deliveries occur frequently in conjunction with certain antepartum and intrapartum complications that cause morbidity and mortality themselves, such as multiple pregnancy, prematurity, placenta previa, and congenital malformations. Even if all complications associated with delivery per se could be eliminated, there would still remain some excess morbidity and mortality among breech presentations due to these associated risk factors. In the analysis of outcome in breech presentations, therefore, such concurrent relevant issues must be considered.

INCIDENCE

Breech presentation occurs in 3% to 4% of term pregnancies.[10] This rate increases in direct proportion to the degree of prematurity and inversely with fetal weight, reaching 40% in fetuses weighing less than 1,000 g. According to Hall and Kohl,[43] about 14% of multiparas with breech presentation had breech presentation in a previous pregnancy. This recurrence rate is accounted for by the fact that premature labor tends to recur in successive pregnancies; the more premature the fetus when labor begins, the greater the likelihood of presenting as a breech.

ETIOLOGY

Premature labor and all its predisposing conditions (premature rupture of membranes, multiple gestation, uterine anomaly, and so on) account for the majority of breech births. Ninety percent of the fetuses in breech presentation at 28 weeks of gestation will convert spontaneously if pregnancy continues to term and will deliver in cephalic presentation. Why up to 4% of term fetuses (10% of those that had been breech at 28 weeks) remain breech is unknown. Some obstetric factors—including placenta previa, contracted pelvis, and uterine anomaly—might mechanically prevent spontaneous version, and the presence of hydramnios may allow more fetal movement and increase the chance that the presentation will be breech.

Fianu and Vaclavinkova[33] studied 124 term breech pregnancies ultasonographically and found the placenta implanted in either the right or left cornual-fundal region in 72.6%; this contrasted with 4.8% in a control population of pregnancies with cephalic presentation. They concluded that cornual-fundal implantation reverses the usual polarity of the uterine ovoid so that the fetal head is encouraged to occupy the region in the fundus not occupied by the placenta. Luterkort et al.[58] followed 228 pregnancies in which breech presentation was diagnosed by ultrasound screening in the 33rd gestational week. Repeat ultrasound examinations were carried out in the 35th and 38th week to identify factors that might impede spontaneous conversion to a vertex presentation. No difference in the frequency of extended fetal legs and cornual-fundal placental implantation was found between the group of fetuses that remained in breech presentation and those that converted spontaneously to vertex presentation. An increased frequency of uterine and fetal malformations, oligohydramnios, and contracted pelvis was found in the group of fetuses that remained breech until birth.

In gestations with normal uterine volume and geometry, fetal factors may be involved in the genesis of breech presentation.[9] Neuromuscular and skeletal malformations as well as chromosomal anomalies have been found to be more common in infants delivered as breech. Although prematurity may play a role here, it has been suggested that a fetus unable to move its extremities normally may be unable to adopt the cephalic position.

CONGENITAL ABNORMALITIES

Congenital abnormalities are more frequent in breech (6.3%) than in cephalic (2.4%) presentations (Table 12-1). Braun et al.[9] considered breech presentation a potential marker for fetal abnormality. They found a higher incidence of malformation than expected on the basis of gestational age or birth weight and speculated that failure of the fetus to assume the cephalic presentation somehow resulted from dysfunction of the affected organs.

Many of the central nervous system anomalies common among breeches can be diagnosed by ultrasonography. Although most of these

---

Table 12-1 Congenital Abnormalities Most Commonly Associated with Breech Presentation

---

Central Nervous System
　Hydrocephalus
　Anencephaly
　Meningomyelocele
　Familial dysautonomia
Urinary System
　Potter's syndrome
Musculoskeletal System
　Congenital hip dislocation
　Myotonic dystrophy
Multiple Abnormalities
　Prader-Willi syndrome
　Werdnig-Hoffman syndrome
　Smith-Lemle-Opitz syndrome
　Fetal alcohol syndrome
　deLange syndrome
　Trisomy 13 syndrome
　Trisomy 18 syndrome
　Trisomy 21 syndrome

---

anomalies are not treatable, knowledge of their presence is of vital importance for counseling the patient and deciding on the most appropriate route of delivery.[8,57] Neilson[67] found that large infants (more than 8.5 lb) in breech presentation are as free from lethal congenital abnormalities as term pregnancies in general. Therefore, when considering a cesarean section for a labor abnormality associated with fetopelvic disproportion and breech presentation, the clinician should bear in mind that the probability of delivering an infant with a congenital anomaly is no greater than in comparable cephalic presentations.

Musculoskeletal abnormalities also seem to be more common among infants that present as breech. Congenital hip dysplasia is present in one-fifth of breech infants, and congenital dislocation of the hip is nine times more prevalent than with cephalic presentation. Torticollis, scoliosis, geniculate recurvation, and club foot are other deformations seen commonly in breech babies. These abnormalities are not true malformations, but are instead deformations resulting from intrauterine constraints of long-standing breech posture.

PREMATURITY

About one-third of all breech deliveries yield a premature infant. Cephalopelvic disproportion was once thought to be the principal cause of the complications of breech vaginal delivery; because disproportion is very uncommon in premature infants, the vaginal route was selected almost exclusively for delivery. The poor outcome of premature breech infants was mainly attributed to the inherent risks of prematurity. Recent evaluations reveal that the perinatal outcome for the premature breech is in fact worse than could be explained by prematurity alone. Indeed, the premature breech infant is exposed to definite risks based on complications quite different from its vertex counterpart.

Entrapment of the aftercoming head by an insufficiently dilated cervix is explained by the greater head/abdomen ratio in prematures relative to term babies. The fetal abdomen is delivered through a cervix that is not dilated enough to permit the greater cephalic diameters to negotiate readily. The damage inflicted by this condition may be compounded by the rapid descent of the aftercoming head, which affords little or no time for cranial molding.

Asphyxia and trauma, mainly to the central nervous system, also play important roles in the short- and long-term outcome results for premature breech infants. Another detrimental factor in the very premature breech baby relates to the risks of footling breech presentation. The smaller the breech, the less likely it is to be in frank breech presentation. While at least half the fetuses weighing 2,000 g or more in breech presentation are found in frank breech attitude, the proportion falls sharply for smaller fetuses. The frequency of cord accidents is inversely related to fetal weight. Moreover, footling breech fetuses are more likely to be delivered by potentially traumatic extractions that those in frank breech.

Ingemarsson et al.[50] evaluated the neurologic outcome at ages 1 and 5 years in 84 children who had presented as breech. Those delivered by cesarean section had considerably better outcome than those delivered vaginally. Tentorial rupture, subdural hematoma, and bleeding into the cerebrospinal fluid occurred significantly more often in the vaginally delivered group. In addition, there were more frequent transient neurologic abnormalities in the neonatal period and developmental or neurologic abnormalities at 1 and 5 years of age among those delivered vaginally. Critics of routine cesarean section for the premature breech in labor question the validity of such retrospective studies.[35,54,92]

Some investigators have attributed the recently improved outcome for low birth weight breech infants to the advanced perinatal care practices offered to all premature infants.[27] They point to the reduction of perinatal mortality in the very low birth weight vertex infants which was accomplished without a proportional increase in the rate of cesarean delivery for this group. Bodmer et al.[7] compared the condition at birth of preterm breech presentation in two time periods in which cesarean section as a delivery method increased from 8% to 89%. They found no reduction in the incidence of severe depression, birth trauma, and encephalopathy when cesarean section was utilized as the primary delivery mode in infants weighing over 1,000 g. Elimination of head entrapment by cesarean delivery of infants of less than 1,000 g was responsible for the improved outcome of breech infants 28 weeks of gestation or less.

There is clear need for carefully designed, prospective studies to be done comparing cesarean section and vaginal delivery. Such investigations should incorporate intensive intrapartum monitoring (which was not used in earlier studies). Until they are done and valid analytic results obtained, each case should be evaluated and managed on an individual basis.

TERM BREECH

Although prematurity accounts for a major portion of the perinatal morbidity and mortality associated with breech presentation, term breech delivery is also potentially hazardous. Contributing factors are prolapsed cord (less common as infant weight increases, but still a problem, primarily in footling breech), cord compression during the second stage of labor and during delivery, and mechanical problems at delivery. Some of the latter, such as the appearance of nuchal arms, which are often the result of an injudiciously rapid extraction of the fetal body, can be avoided.

Until recently, most of the concepts concerning the conduct of breech delivery were based on retrospective studies. Such studies compared the outcome of infants grouped according to various antepartum scoring systems and delivered by a variety of techniques.[62,81,87,91,95] No concrete data can be extracted concerning optimal mode of delivery (abdominal versus vaginal) because of the different composition of the populations studied and variations in their obstetric management. The increasingly common use of cesarean section in breech presentations has prompted prospective comparative evaluations of management plans.

Gimovsky et al.[38] evaluated breech births at 36 to 42 weeks' gestation and estimated fetal weight of 2,000 to 4,000 g. All index cases were managed by a preestablished protocol. They were matched with two control groups, one comprising breech cases not delivered according to the protocol and the other vertex vaginal deliveries. The protocol required adequate clinical as well as x-ray pelvimetric evaluation, strict adherence to Friedman's criteria for labor assessment,[34] and intrapartum biophysical and biochemical monitoring. Patients were subjected to cesarean section when any pelvic, labor, or fetal abnormality was encountered. When preselected in this manner, term breech fetuses could be safely delivered vaginally, irrespective of parity or type of breech presentation.

Collea et al.[13] randomized the delivery route (vaginal vs. cesarean section) in 208 women in labor at term with a singleton fetus in frank breech presentation. Of 93 women scheduled to undergo a cesarean section, 88 delivered according to protocol. (The remainder delivered vaginally before the surgery could be done.) Of the 115 in the vaginal delivery group, 112 had intrapartum roentgenographic pelvimetry; 52 required abdominal delivery because of one or more inadequate pelvic measurements. Eleven of the remaining 60 patients required cesarean section for labor problems, leaving 49 who delivered vaginally with no perinatal death. Acknowledging the lack of long-term follow-up, they concluded that it seemed reasonable to allow vaginal delivery in carefully selected cases of term frank breech presentation.

Gimovsky et al.[39] randomized the route of delivery in 105 women with nonfrank breech presentations at term in labor. All 35 women randomized to undergo a cesarean section were delivered according to protocol. Of the 70 women assigned to a trial of labor, 39 required a cesarean section. Twenty-three of them revealed inadequate pelvic dimensions on x-ray pelvimetry; the rest were deemed to have a failed trial of labor. The remaining 31 women delivered vaginally with no increase in neonatal morbidity but with significantly reduced maternal morbidity. It was concluded that, corrected for obstetric indications requiring cesarean section, women with a nonfrank breech presentation at term in labor can be expected to deliver vaginally with neonatal morbidity comparable to that seen in those delivered by cesarean section.

HYPEREXTENSION OF THE FETAL HEAD

In 1870, Parot[69] described the first well-documented case of spinal cord injury after breech delivery. Crothers and Putnam[17] reported in 1972 that 67% of a series of infants born with spinal cord injury had been delivered vaginally as breech. More recently, Bresnan and Abroms[11] found a 25% incidence of spinal cord transection among breech infants with hyperextended head who were delivered vaginally, but none in those delivered abdominally. Caterini et al.[12] reported the outcome of 108 deliveries in which hyperextended fetal head was diagnosed during labor. Of the 73 infants who were delivered vaginally, 10 died during the perinatal period; 5 of the survivors had signs of meningeal hemorrhage, and 15 showed medullary or vertebral lesions. Of the 35 infants delivered abdominally, all survived and there were only 2 with medullary or vertebral trauma.

The usual site of cord injury is the lower cervical region. Affected infants are sometimes stillborn; alternatively, they may survive for a short period of time in shock with respiratory depression and subsequent problems resembling the clinical picture of hyaline membrane disease. Those who survive generally suffer temporary or permanent paralysis and spasticity. The high incidence of spinal cord transection was once thought to be related directly to internal podalic version and breech extraction. However, recent reports confirm that spinal cord injury can occur in assisted or spontaneous breech deliveries, or even at cesarean section if the delivery technique is not gentle.

Hyperextension of the fetal head during labor is easily diagnosed radiographically by obtaining a flat film of the abdomen. Sometimes ultrasonography is sufficient. This information should be obtained before proceeding with x-ray cephalopelvimetry. If hyperextension of the fetal head is present, pelvimetry becomes superfluous because cesarean section is mandatory. Furthermore, the flat plate should not be obtained until the patient is in labor, because a hyperextended head may flex spontaneously after uterine contractions begin. If hyperextension is still present after labor is established, it cannot be expected to change subsequently. However, it should be borne in mind that with severe hyperextension of the fetal head, damage to the spinal cord may occur during labor prior to delivery. Therefore, the diagnosis should be made as early in labor as possible.

If hyperextension is diagnosed, a severe congenital abnormality must be ruled out. The incidence of Down syndrome among "star-gazing" fetuses is greater than expected in the general population.[20]

The etiology of hyperextension of the head or neck not associated with malformations is obscure. One proposed explanation is that it is secondary to hypertonicity of the extensor muscles of the neck. When contracture of these muscles is present at birth, it usually resolves spontaneously in 7 to 14 days, although it may persist for up to 2 months.[4]

Ballas and Toaff[2,3] have classified the degree of hyperextension of the fetal head and correlated it with perinatal outcome. They included only cases in which the angle between the head and the fetal spine could be measured on radiographs. Of 38 infants with a deflexion angle of less than 90 degrees, 25 were delivered vaginally and 13 by elective cesarean section; none sustained any cervical cord damage. Among the 20 mothers with a deflexion angle of more than 90 degrees, nine were delivered by cesarean section without trauma. The remaining 11 were delivered vaginally, and 8 babies sustained complete transection of the cervical cord.

In summary, all women with an infant in breech presentation should have a radiograph of the abdomen as soon as labor is diagnosed to rule out hyperextension of the fetal head. If the hyperextension is documented to be more than 90 degrees, the infant should be delivered by cesarean section. Any trial of labor under these circumstances is contraindicated because the spinal cord may be injured prior to or during delivery.

PROLAPSED CORD

Prolapse of the umbilical cord is a major factor contributing to the increased perinatal morbidity and mortality of breech presentation.[56] The incidence of cord prolapse is 0.24% to 0.5% in vertex presentations as contrasted with 2.3% to 6% among breeches,[10] a tenfold increase. It is apparently more common in multiparas than in nulliparas. Rupture of the membranes prior to labor doubles the incidence of cord prolapse.

The frequency of overt cord prolapse varies with the type of breech presentation; for example, it is increased threefold over vertex presentation in frank breech, 10 times in complete breech, and 20 times in footling. The more premature the fetus, the greater the likelihood of prolapse. Occult cord compression, diagnosed by continuous electronic monitoring of the fetal heart rate or by observation at delivery, is probably also more common among breeches.

Prolapse of the cord in breech presentation is not necessarily as dramatic an emergency as it is in cephalic presentation because the cord is less likely to be completely occluded by the softer, narrower, and more irregular presenting part. Nevertheless, immediate cesarean section is the most appropriate course of action under these circumstances. Because cord complications are so common, especially with complete and footling breech presentations, it is prudent to make all necessary preparations for cesarean section whenever allowing labor to evolve in the expectation of vaginal delivery. It follows that continuous electronic monitoring (and biochemical surveillance, when indicated) is imperative for all breech fetuses during labor.

PREMATURE RUPTURE OF MEMBRANES

Premature rupture of the membranes, defined as rupture 1 hr or more before the onset of labor, is encountered twice as often in breech as in cephalic presentations. This difference is most evident after 36 weeks of gestation. Except for footling breech, all breech cases with premature rupture of membranes can be managed in the same way as comparable cephalic presentations. Footling breech presentations are exceptions because of their frequent association with cord prolapse; as a consequence, they should be delivered as soon as fetal lung maturity is achieved.

ARREST OF THE AFTERCOMING HEAD

Entrapment of the fetal head is the most feared complication of breech delivery because it occurs at a stage of the delivery when a change in course is usually not feasible. The pathophysiology of this entity is probably different in the premature and term breech fetus.

In the premature, it is usually a soft tissue dystocia with entrapment of the head by an incompletely dilated cervix. In these situations, the cervix can sometimes be stretched with two or three right-angle retractors. Rarely it will prove necessary to cut the cervix using the incisions described by Dührssen.

After 36 weeks, when head size is equal to or smaller than abdominal size, arrest of the aftercoming head is more likely due to undiagnosed cephalopelvic disproportion. Transabdominal palpation to evaluate fetal head size or approximation of fetal head measurements from the estimated fetal weight are notoriously inaccurate. Many x-ray pelvimetric techniques, including computed tomography, although accurate for measuring the critical diameters of the maternal pelvis, do not evaluate fetal cephalic dimensions.

The Ball cephalopelvimetric technique (which the author utilizes) overcomes this drawback by comparing fetal cephalic and maternal pelvic volumes. The liberal use of x-ray cephalopelvimetry in breech presentation increases the accuracy of the diagnosis of disproportion considerably. In addition, it provides accurate information concerning the type of breech presentation. Ultrasonographic evaluation can sometimes be useful to estimate the fetal biparietal diameter[80] or to rule out major anomalies, and should be used as an adjunct to x-ray pelvimetry. Pelvic measurements adequate to accommodate the fetus suggest a safe passage for the aftercoming head but do not ensure it. A confounding factor, the effect of which cannot be measured prior to delivery, is the lack of cephalic molding associated with rapid head engagement, descent, and rotation.

It is generally felt to be good practice to apply Piper forceps to the aftercoming head if the head does not deliver quickly with application of gentle moderate suprapubic pressure and guidance to the fetal body. In a retrospective study, Milner[63] showed the benefit of using forceps to deliver the aftercoming head of infants weighing between 1,000 and 3,000 g. Unfortunately, the nonrandomized design of his study may have vitiated the conclusions. Also, this reported experience preceded recent major advances in neonatal care of low birth weight infants. Obviously the proper application of Piper forceps is vital to avoid iatrogenic damage. It should be done with the obstetrician kneeling to achieve the proper direction of blade application while the infant is suspended horizontally by an assistant using a towel to form a sling for the baby's trunk, abdomen, and limbs.

In both premature and term breech vaginal deliveries, attention should be directed to performing an ample episiotomy. It should preferably be cut in the midline to permit it to be extended, if necessary. The obstetrician should be prepared to retract the posterior vaginal wall with a Sims's or right-angle retractor to allow suctioning and clearing of the airway even before the head is delivered. Premature infants with arrest of the aftercoming head die mainly from asphyxia caused by occlusion of the airway by the mother's soft tissues. Appropriate intervention to expand the birth canal (i.e., to create a perineotomy) and to aspirate nasotracheal secretions may sometimes allow the infant to initiate respiration. The delivery of the head can then be accomplished slowly and atraumatically.

Another cause of arrest of the aftercoming head in breech presentation is extension of the fetal head. This can result in impingement of the chin against the pelvic inlet, especially if the fetal sacrum is directed posteriorly.[37] This obstruction can be relieved by recognizing the problem at once, promptly dislodging the chin, and rotating the face posteriorly. In prematures, because of the small cranial diameters, the obstetrician may be able to achieve good flexion instead; Piper forceps may be needed to effect delivery under these circumstances.

Myers[66] described a single-operator technique for flexing the aftercoming head that is useful for either vaginal or abdominal breech delivery. Its goal is to apply digital pressure to the occipital protuberance in order to splint the spinal column, and promote flexion. Avoid any form of traction to the body or shoulders that could exaggerate deflexion and risk injury to the fetal spinal column.

Entrapment of the aftercoming head seems to be most common in footling breeches. In a term frank breech presentation, the combined diameter of the thorax and the extended legs is generally equal to or greater than the diameter of the aftercoming head; therefore, normal descent of the fetal body makes cephalopelvic disproportion unlikely. This need not hold true in premature infants. The head dimensions of a smaller fetus are larger than those of the abdomen. Moreover, the soft tissues of the body are more compressible and thus able to negotiate an incompletely dilated cervix. Iffy et al.[49] reported a single case in which a cesarean section resulted in the successful rescue of a premature infant with an entrapped, deflexed head following delivery of the body and arms. Prompt action with appropriate anesthesia is required. Nonetheless, it must be stressed that this is not an innocuous procedure and ought not to be resorted to unless all other maneuvers to accomplish fetal extraction have failed.

TRAUMA

Trauma ranks high as a cause of perinatal mortality in breech presentation, together with prematurity and asphyxia.[91] The overall risk of traumatic injury to fetuses in breech presentation delivered vaginally is twice that of cephalic presentations. Injuries during breech delivery are most often the direct result of manipulations for extraction. Frequently injured areas are brain, abdominal viscera (liver, spleen, and adrenal glands), and musculoskeletal system.[84]

Traumatic intracranial hemorrhage occurs most commonly from rupture of the superior cerebral bridging veins. It results from excessive occipitofrontal pressure or oblique distortion of the head during labor and delivery. Posterior fossa bleeding may occur from extension of a tentorial tear into the lateral or straight sinuses. Subdural hemorrhage, once thought to occur only in term infants, has recently been found in premature babies as well. Occipital osteodiastasis, produced by excessive compressive forces, may be also associated with contusion and laceration of the underlying cerebellum. Probably as a result of both prematurity and intracranial trauma, cerebral palsy and epilepsy are seen three to four times more often than expected among children delivered as breech.

Liver and spleen lacerations may be the source of immediate post partum morbidity, but rupture of subcapsular hepatic hematomas may occur as late as 10 to 14 days postpartum. Adrenal glands in the newborn are one-third the size of the kidneys and are not so well protected as in the adult, where they are considerably smaller. A review of 12 cases of idiopathic adrenal calcification in children revealed that 10 of the children were delivered as breech.[84]

Trauma to skin and muscle tissue may be an important cause of neonatal morbidity and mortality. At autopsy of infants delivered as breech, Ralis[72] found the average hemorrhage within injured muscles to be equivalent to 20% to 75% of total blood volume. Furthermore, in six infants, there was histologic evidence to suggest that the cause of delayed death was renal crush injury syndrome.

PREDICTOR INDICES

The management of labor with breech presentation involves a sequence of decisions as new information becomes available. The use of static criteria systems should be abandoned in favor of a dynamic evaluation of all the factors potentially affecting outcome.[6,68,95] One such static system, the Zatuchni-Andros scoring index, has serious shortcomings. Briefly, it encourages vaginal delivery of a breech infant in certain patients, favoring multiparity over nulliparity, and early gestational age over term gestation. Lower estimated fetal weight and prior history of breech delivery are considered favorable signs. To the contrary, several recent reports suggest these criteria are not appropriate. Premature infants and those delivered by multiparas do not fare better than term infants or those delivered by nulliparas. In addition, this index does not take into consideration the dynamic evaluation of the progression of labor or electronic and biochemical fetal monitoring as important factors in the choice of delivery route.

LONG-TERM FOLLOW-UP

The concept that infants delivered as breech do not perform as well cognitively or neurologically as those delivered cephalically is entrenched in obstetric tradition. The literature concerning cerebral palsy and mental retardation makes frequent statements regarding the increased frequencies of these entities among breech infants.[25] Less severe psychoneurologic disabilities, including language difficulties, visual disturbances, and auditory impairment, may be associated with other factors, but their relationship to breech delivery was strongly suggested by Rauramo et al.[74] in 1961. Hyperkinetic syndrome (impulsivity, disorder of attention, and emotional lability) and learning disability (dyslexia and dyscalculia) are also more frequent in children who are products of breech delivery.[32]

Rosen et al.[75] compared the long-term neurologic development of 70 frank breech fetuses delivered vaginally with that of matched (birth weight and race) breech infants born by cesarean section, vertex infants born vaginally, and vertex infants born by cesarean section. All fetuses were alive at the onset of labor and without major congenital anomalies. No major neurologic abnormality was found to be attributable to the delivery route. Abdominal delivery did not appear to improve fetal mortality or morbidity when compared with those delivered vaginally when corrected for low birth weight infants and those with congenital anomalies.

The long-term follow-up of infants delivered as breech is an area of intensive current interest. Most of the previously reported studies are retrospective and suffer from serious methodologic shortcomings. The use of questionnaires mailed to parents of infants delivered as breech is heavily influenced by subjective interpretations; in general, it produces more optimistic results than does the use of medical records. The lack of good controls in various studies emphasizes the acute need for a well-planned prospective study comparing long-term outcome for breech and cephalic presentations by delivery method. The impact of the various labor and delivery management approaches deserves study as applied to the several types of breech presentation as well.

EXTERNAL CEPHALIC VERSION

External cephalic version is a technique for converting a breech or transverse presentation into a cephalic one by manual transabdominal manipulation of the fetus. Its value for reducing the incidence of breech presentation at term has been well documented.[73,83] Nonetheless, critics of version argue it is potentially hazardous as evidenced by reports of premature labor, premature rupture of membranes, cord entanglement or prolapse, abruptio placentae, uterine rupture, fetal death, and Rh isoimmunization.

Much of the criticism has been directed at the timing of the version. Spontaneous version to vertex presentation occurs in nearly 90% of breech cases diagnosed between 28 and 36 weeks of gestation, making unnecessary most version procedures done early in the third trimester. Spontaneous cephalic version of breech presentation in the last trimester is less likely to occur if associated with extended fetal legs, growth retardation, short umbilical cord, and nulliparity.[88] Similarly, persistent breech presentation can be seen in patients with oligohydramnios and those with cornual or lateral placental implantation.

Recent experience with the use of beta-adrenergic agonists as tocolytic agents suggests that external cephalic version can be performed successfully and safely in patients at term.[87] Terbutaline or ritodrine provide sufficient uterine relaxation to allow the external version to be accomplished atraumatically. Saling and Muller-Holve[77] and Fall and Nilsson[29] reported success rates near term of 60% to 70% with no return to breech after a successful version. Comparable results were reported by Morrison et al.,[64] Dyson et al.,[24] and Stine et al.[83] in larger samples of patients. The consensus is that the period between 37 and 40 weeks of gestation is most advantageous for performing version. There are several reasons for this: 1) the version is not difficult to perform with good uterine relaxation; 2) if labor, ruptured membranes, or fetal jeopardy is provoked, the fetal lungs are more likely to be mature; and 3) most of the spontaneous versions will have taken place by the 37th week, leaving primarily persistent breech presentations to be dealt with and thus minimizing the number of unnecessary procedures. Also, spontaneous return to a breech occurs infrequently in those converted successfully to cephalic presentations after 37 weeks of gestation.

Ferguson and Dyson[30] reported a similar success rate when intrapartum external cephalic version was attempted as an alternative to cesarean delivery. Women with ruptured membranes, multiple gestation, vaginal bleeding, or placenta previa were considered not to be candidates for this procedure. Although not recommended as a replacement for antepartum external cephalic version, it seems appropriate to attempt version in the patient who presents in labor with a previously undiagnosed breech presentation and has intact membranes.

For external cephalic version to be both successful and safe, proper selection of patients is of utmost importance. Contraindications, such as placenta previa, ruptured membranes, and bicornuate uterus should first be ruled out.

Constant monitoring of the mother and fetus by means of real-time ultrasonography and continuous electronic fetal heart rate monitoring is essential.[94] Hofmeyr and Sonnendecker[48] reported decreases in fetal movements and fetal heart rate variability and reactivity following external cephalic version; temporary baseline bradycardia was also seen in some cases. They attributed the changes in fetal response to a temporary decrease in uteroplacental flow during the procedure. Phelan et al.[71] found similar changes in addition to decelerations and occasional fetal tachycardia; temporarily decreased variability occurred significantly more often after the version was performed. Most of the observed fetal heart rate variations are transient and usually resolve shortly after cessation of manipulations. It is mandatory that there be adequate facilities available for immediate cesarean section in the event they do not. Rh-negative mothers should receive RhoGam after the procedure because of the risk of maternal-fetal hemorrhage and Rh isoimmunization.[61,65]

LABOR COURSE

Because fetopelvic relationships are difficult to assess clinically in the breech presentation, evaluation of labor progress is especially important in the decision making process for managing the delivery. Cesarean section is appropriate if pelvic inadequacy appears likely, as evidenced, for example, by disproportion on x-ray cephalopelvimetry, marked pelvic contraction, or an infant estimated to weigh more than 4,000 g.

Friedman[34] reported some degree of fetopelvic disproportion could be diagnosed in breech presentation by roentgenography in 15.5% of nulliparas and 5.8% of multiparas. The corresponding rates for vertex presentation were 7.8% and 1.5%, respectively. The incidence of disproportion among nulliparas would undoubtedly have been greater if those delivered electively by cesarean section had not been excluded.

When the course of labor was studied, nulliparous breech labor was found to be comparable to its vertex counterpart, with the exception of a significant shortening of the latent phase. In multiparas, the latent phases were comparable, but there was uniform lengthening of all other portions of labor with concomitant decreases in the maximum slopes of dilatation and descent. Labor curves in all types of breech presentation were nearly identical.

Patients whose membranes rupture spontaneously at or before the onset of labor have a shorter latent phase than those whose membranes rupture after labor has begun. As mentioned previously, the incidence of premature rupture of membranes in breech presentation is exceptionally high. When patients with premature rupture of the membranes were excluded, the latent phase duration in breech presentation was not different from that in the cephalic presentation.

Length of labor is also directly related to the station of the presenting part of the breech at the onset of labor. Progress of fetal descent in breech labor is different from that in vertex labors. Breech labor tends to begin with the presenting part at higher stations. It is generally accepted that the high fetal presenting part in breech labor is a serious problem and represents a condition in which the prognosis for vaginal delivery is guarded. Close analysis suggests this to be incorrect. Despite the initial high station, there is a rapid acceleration of descent, starting with the onset of the active phase of dilatation in most instances.

Dysfunctional labor patterns were encountered in significantly excess number in both nulliparas and multiparas with breech presentation. The overall incidence of labor abnormalities (primarily protraction disorders) was 29.7%. This rate was significantly greater than the 17.2% encountered in vertex presentations.

Fetal weight plays an important role in the appearance of these labor disorders, as it does in vertex presentations. Among labors associated with fetuses weighing more than 3,500 g, over 75% developed labor dysfunction. Most of the nulliparous breech labors associated with fetopelvic disproportion will develop a major labor aberration. Therefore, whenever a major labor abnormality appears, it should serve to alert the obstetrician to potentially serious and often previously unrecognized fetopelvic disproportion.

FETAL MONITORING

Most obstetricians feel that continuous fetal heart rate monitoring during breech labors is mandatory.[36] The high incidence of cord prolapse, prematurity, and abruptio placentae contribute to the increased risk of fetal compromise. Variable or late decelerations are seen in over half the breech presenting fetuses during labor. White and Cibils[90] reported a higher incidence of depressed neonates and neonatal deaths in this group of patients. They attributed this to the higher incidence of cord compression during the first and second stage of labor. Presence of fetal heart accelerations was associated with better outcomes (fewer depressed infants and neonatal deaths). The lowest fetal heart rates are consistently recorded at the time of delivery of the shoulders when maximum compression of the cord by maternal tissues is most likely to take place.[85,89] The drop in fetal heart rate during delivery of the head is comparable to that experienced during the delivery of the shoulders, and the recovery to normal heart rate is slower in breech than in cephalic presentation.

Eliot and Hill[28] and Hill et al.[47] reported routine fetal blood sampling during labor was helpful for early detection of fetal asphyxia. The largest drop in pH occurs during the interval of time between the breech reaching the perineum and the umbilicus appearing at the introitus. They found a close correlation between pH levels and the subsequent Apgar scores.[78]

Eilen et al.[26] found the type of acidosis is different in term breech fetuses with poor electronic fetal heart rate tracing as compared with fetuses showing mild abnormalities of their heart rate pattern. Fetuses with variable decelerations or tachycardia with reduced baseline variability had a metabolic acidosis associated with low Apgar scores. When acidosis was found in fetuses with normal heart tracings or those with sporadic variable decelerations, it was of the respiratory type, and corrected rapidly following birth. It is uncertain whether the pH of blood obtained from the buttocks or feet is representative of the perfusion of the vital centers and can be interpreted in the same way as scalp blood sample data.

ANESTHESIA

Controversy exists regarding the ideal mode of anesthesia for the conduct of labor and delivery of breech presentations. One school of thought holds that any procedure or medication that might interfere with the mother's spontaneous expulsive efforts during the second stage of labor could be deleterious because it might enhance the need for operative maneuvers such as breech extraction. It is also possible that attenuation or complete abolition of the mother's bearing-down efforts will reduce fetal intracerebral pressure changes during delivery and diminish the risk of intracranial hemorrhage. No data are available to confirm or refute these concepts.

Adherents to this notion of protection generally make use of parenteral narcotic analgesia during labor, and pudendal block for delivery. The pudendal block allows an adequate episiotomy to be cut while not disturbing abdominal muscular control, which, according to D'Esopo,[21] reduces fetal mortality and cranial trauma. Proponents of the Bracht maneuver (spontaneous breech delivery with support applied to counteract gravity forces only) consider the active participation of the woman in the expulsion process of vital importance; here, anesthesia is contraindicated.

Those who desire to diminish maternal control over the delivery utilize analgesia for labor and a saddle block anesthesia during the expulsive period, or epidural anesthesia for both labor and delivery.[19,79] Crawford et al.[15,16] reported the outcome of infants delivered as breech under epidural anesthesia. They found a reduced incidence of severe and prolonged neonatal depression in all birth weight categories. The incidence of breech extraction was not increased by the epidural anesthetic, although there was a significant prolongation of the second stage in this group. Confine et al.[14] found the first stage of labor to be similar in singleton breech labors conducted with and without extradural analgesia. They reported that, notwithstanding the prolongation of the second stage and lower 1-min Apgar score in those receiving extradural analgesia, the mean 5-min Apgar score and perinatal morbidity were similar in both groups.

Regardless of the anesthetic approach, the presence of a well-trained anesthesiologist during the delivery of a breech infant is vital. Immediate need for forceps application or other obstetric manipulations may arise unexpectedly. The potential requirement for rapid induction of general anesthesia always exists. In the case of an entrapped aftercoming head, use of Piper forceps, Dührssen incisions, or stretching of the cervix with right angle retractors obviously requires a well-anesthetized patient.

MANAGEMENT

Attitudes about the management of breech presentation have changed over the last 30 years. The more liberal use of cesarean section for the delivery of these infants has made breech presentation a factor in the increasing rate of cesarean section during the last two decades.[45] This trend evolved primarily from conclusions derived from retrospective evaluations of large numbers of breech deliveries. These showed an increased perinatal morbidity and mortality as well as an increase in subsequent psychoneurologic impairment in those infants delivered vaginally when compared with those delivered by cesarean section. However, most of these retrospective studies have the inherent problem of nonrandomized selection of patients as well as nonuniformity of indications for choosing delivery route. In addition to the unknown factors surrounding the decision to deliver an infant vaginally or by cesarean section, most retrospective studies cannot be controlled for differences between groups with regard to management of labor (e.g., use of labor graphs, electronic and biochemical monitoring, types of anesthesia, and forceps to the aftercoming head). The problem of extrapolating conclusions from retrospective studies is further compounded by the extraordinary recent advances achieved in the field of perinatal medicine that have improved the outcome for premature infants and refined the diagnosis and management of fetal asphyxia.

There should be no hesitation to perform a cesarean section if an abnormality of labor or evidence of fetal distress manifests itself. Nevertheless, careful evaluation of each case is imperative. The conduct of labor and delivery should be based on objective information concerning the progress of labor, pelvic architecture, and fetal condition. The management of a breech presentation should be overseen by the most experienced and skillful obstetrician available. If such help is not obtainable, cesarean section should be considered strongly.

Figure 12-1 illustrates the author's approach to breech presentation in labor. If the woman is not in labor or is in early labor and beyond 37 weeks of gestation, an external cephalic version using a uterine relaxant agent may be attempted under controlled and closely monitored conditions. This should be undertaken only if resources and personnel are at hand to perform immediate cesarean section.

If the patient is in labor, every effort should be made to establish gestational age, including careful history taking, clinical examination, and ultrasonography, if appropriate. Ultrasonographic evaluation to approximate fetal weight and to rule out the presence of a congenital malformation is especially indicated in the small fetus. In the presence of a lethal anomaly, there would be little to gain from cesarean section. Individual judgments must be made to determine an optimally sane route of delivery when nonlethal malformations are detected. Much data support the idea that a low birth weight breech infant without congenital malformations fares better when delivered by cesarean section,[18,28,41,53] although this is by no means a universally accepted opinion.

A flat plate film of the abdomen (or sometimes ultrasonograph) will disclose the degree of hyperextension of the fetal head. If hyperextension is not present, then x-ray cephalopelvimetry is indicated.[55] Hyperextension of more than 90 degrees or radiologically or clinically diagnosed cephalopelvic disproporton is an indication for cesarean section. In the absence of these complications, the woman is allowed to continue in labor

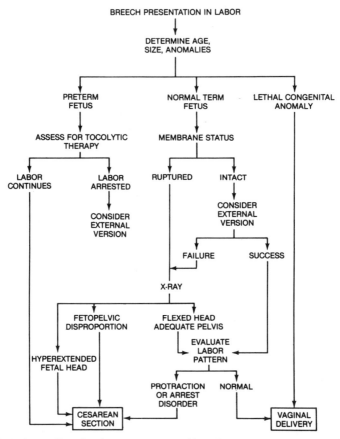

Figure 12-1 A paradigm for the management of breech presentation. *Source*: Adapted by permission from "Breech Presentation" by M Borten in *Obstetrical Decision Making*, ed 2 (p205) by EA Friedman, DB Acker, and BP Sachs (Eds), BC Decker Inc, Toronto, © 1987.

under constant electronic monitoring of the fetal heart rate and periodic biochemical evaluation of the fetal status, if indicated. The appearance of a labor abnormality or evidence of nonremediable fetal distress is an indication to expedite delivery by the abdominal route.

The facilities to perform an immediate cesarean section should be available at all times. The nature of the emergencies that may present during breech labor and delivery requires the continuous availability of an experienced anesthesiologist.

When performing a cesarean section in a breech presentation, the obstetrician should seek to accomplish delivery of the infant with the same caution and gentle dexterity used during a vaginal breech delivery.

Particular attention should be exercised to avoid traction on the infant's body. Correct flexion of the fetal head in utero is imperative. One exception to this is the hyperextended head which should be delivered through a large uterine incision with a minimum of manipulation.

CONCLUSIONS

The increase in the cesarean section rate for breech presentations has created a dilemma. Physicians in training now obtain relatively little experience in the nuances of the techniques involved in vaginal breech delivery. A self-fulfilling prophecy (to the effect that all breech fetuses will eventually be delivered abdominally) is thus in the process of being realized, because obstetricians with little training in this area are often reluctant (perhaps correctly) to attempt vaginal delivery even when it might otherwise seem to be a reasonable alternative.

It is sensible to consider breech presentation as a high-risk condition requiring the presence of a team of highly trained obstetricians, nurses, anesthesiologists, and perinatologists, who are in charge of the labor and delivery management. Unfortunately, many malpresentations are not diagnosed until labor is well established, at which time transfer to a regionalized high-risk center is not feasible. Nevertheless, a "breech team" in a medium-sized institution could provide the most advanced care. Benefits would be realized by both mother and infant due to the resulting standardization of care. This approach would also provide a forum for training physicians and offer an opportunity for collection of well-controlled, prospective data regarding the short- and long-term follow-up of the infants delivered in breech presentation. This information is essential if the continuing controversies concerning the safest mode of delivery are to be resolved.

REFERENCES

1. Alexopoulos KA: The importance of breech delivery in the pathogenesis of brain damage: End results of a long term follow-up. *Clin Pediatr* 1973;12:248–249.

2. Ballas S, Toaff R: Hyperextension of the fetal head in breech presentation: Radiological evaluation and significance. *Br J Obstet Gynaecol* 1976;83:201–204.

3. Ballas S, Toaff R, Jaffa AJ: Deflexion of the fetal head in breech presentation: Incidence, management and outcome. *Obstet Gynecol* 1978;52:653–655.

4. Behrman SJ: Fetal cervical hyperextension. *Clin Obstet Gynecol* 1962;5:1018–1030.

5. Benson WL, Boyce DC, Vaughn DL: Breech delivery in the primigravida. *Obstet Gynecol* 1972;40:417–428.

6. Bilodeau R, Marier R: Breech presentation at term. *Am J Obstet Gynecol* 1978;130:555–557.

7. Bodmer B, Benjamin A, McLean FH, Usher RH: Has use of cesarean section reduced the risks of delivery in the preterm breech presentation. *Am J Obstet Gynecol* 1986; 154:254–260.

8. Borno PR: Vaginal frank breech delivery of a hydrocephalic fetus after transabdominal encephalocentesis. *Am J Obstet Gynecol* 1978;132:336–338.

9. Braun FHT, Jones KL, Smith DW: Breech presentation as an indicator of fetal abnormality. *J Pediatr* 1975;86:419–421.

10. Brenner WE, Bruce RD, Hendricks CH: The characteristics and perils of breech presentation. *Am J Obstet Gynecol* 1974;118:700–712.

11. Bresnan MJ, Abroms IF: Neonatal spinal cord transection secondary to intrauterine hyperextension of the neck in breech presentation. *J Pediatr* 1974;84:734–737.

12. Caterini H, Langer A, Sama JC, Devanesan M, Pelosi MA: Fetal risk in hyperextension of the fetal head in breech presentation. *Am J Obstet Gynecol* 1975;123:632–636.

13. Collea JV, Chein C, Quilligan EJ: The randomized management of term frank breech presentation. *Am J Obstet Gynecol* 1975;123:632–636.

14. Confine E, Ismajovich B, Rudick V, David MP: Extradural analgesia in the management of singleton breech delivery. *Br J Anaesth* 1985;57:892–895.

15. Crawford JS: An appraisal of lumbar epidural blockade in patients with a singleton fetus presenting by the breech. *J Obstet Gynaecol Br Commonw* 1974;81:867–872.

16. Crawford JS, Davis P, Pearson JF: Significance of the individual components of the Apgar score. *Br J Anaesth* 1973;45:148–158.

17. Crothers B, Putnam MC: Obstetrical injuries of the spinal cord. *Medicine* 1927;6:41–44.

18. Cruikshank DP, Pitkin RM: Delivery of the premature breech. *Obstet Gynecol* 1977; 50:367–369.

19. Darby S, Thornton CA, Hunter DJ: Extradural analgesia in labor when the breech presents. *Br J Obstet Gynaecol* 1976;83:35–38.

20. Daw E: Management of the hyperextended fetal head. *Am J Obstet Gynecol* 1976; 124:113–115.

21. D'Esopo AD: Management of breech presentation. *Bull Sloane Hosp* 1956;2:90–93.

22. DeCrespigny LJC, Pepperell RJ: Perinatal mortality and morbidity in breech presentation. *Obstet Gynecol* 1979;53:141–150.

23. Duenhoelter JH, Wells CE, Reisch JS, Santos-Ramos R, Jiminez JM: A paired controlled study of vaginal and abdominal delivery of the low birth weight breech fetus. *Obstet Gynecol* 1979;54:310–313.

24. Dyson DC, Ferguson JE, Hensleigh P: Antepartum external cephalic version under tocolysis. *Obstet Gynecol* 1986;67:63–68.

25. Eastman NJ, deLeon M: The etiology of cerebral palsy. *Am J Obstet Gynecol* 1955; 69:950–961.

26. Eilen B, Fleisher A, Schulman H, Jagani N: Fetal acidosis and the abnormal fetal heart rate tracing: The term breech fetus. *Obstet Gynecol* 1984;63:233–236.

27. Effer SB, Saigal S, Rand C, Hunter DJS, Stoskoff B, Harper AC, Nimrod C, Milner R: Effect of delivery method on outcomes in the very low-birth weight breech infant: Is the improved survival related to cesarean section or other perinatal care maneuvers? *Am J Obstet Gynecol* 1983;145:123–128.

28. Eliot BW, Hill JG: Method of breech management incorporating use of fetal blood sampling. *Br Med J* 1972;4:703–715.

29. Fall O, Nilsson BA: External cephalic version in breech presentation under tocolysis. *Obstet Gynecol* 1979;53:712–715.

30. Ferguson JE, Dyson DC: Intrapartum external cephalic version. *Am J Obstet Gynecol* 1985;152:297–298.

31. Fianu S: Fetal mortality and morbidity following breech delivery. *Acta Obstet Gynaecol Scand* 1976;56S:5–77.

32. Fianu S, Joelsson I: Minimal brain dysfunction in children born in breech presentation. *Acta Obstet Gynaecol Scand* 1979;58:295–299.

33. Fianu S, Vaclavinkova V: Site of placental attachment as a factor in etiology of breech presentation. *Acta Obstet Gynaecol Scand* 1978;57:371–372.

34. Friedman EA: *Labor: Clinical Evaluation and Management,* ed 2. New York, Appleton-Century-Crofts, 1978.

35. Galloway WH, Bartholmew RA, Colvin ED, Grimes WH, Fish JS, Lester WM: Premature breech delivery. *Am J Obstet Gynecol* 1967;99:975–984.

36. Garite TJ, Linzey ME, Freeman RK, Dorchester W: Fetal heart rate patterns and fetal distress in fetuses with congenital anomalies. *Obstet Gynecol* 1979;53:716–720.

37. Gerber AH: Arrest of the after-coming head in breech birth caused by chin to pubic rotation. *Am J Obstet Gynecol* 1979;109:418–420.

38. Gimovsky ML, Petrie RH, Todd ND: Neonatal performance of the selected term vaginal breech delivery. *Obstet Gynecol* 1980;56:687–691.

39. Gimovsky ML, Wallace RL, Schifrin BS, Paul RH: Randomized management of the nonfrank breech presentation at term: A preliminary report. *Am J Obstet Gynecol* 1983;146:34–40.

40. Goethels TR: Cesarean section as method of choice in management of breech delivery. *Am J Obstet Gynecol* 1938;38:105–109.

41. Goldenberg RL, Nelson KG: The premature breech. *Am J Obstet Gynecol* 1977;127:240–244.

42. Greenhill JP, Friedman EA: *Biological Principles and Modern Practice of Obstetrics.* Philadelphia, WB Saunders, 1974.

43. Hall JE, Kohl S: Breech presentation. *Am J Obstet Gynecol* 1956;72:977–990.

44. Helfferich M, Favier J: Breech delivery. *Am J Obstet Gynecol* 1971;110:58–61.

45. Hibbard LT: Changing trends in cesarean section. *Am J Obstet Gynecol* 1976;125:798–804.

46. Hibbard LT, Schumann WR: Prophylactic external cephalic version in obstetric practice. *Am J Obstet Gynecol* 1973;116:511–518.

47. Hill JG, Eliot BW, Campbell AJ, Pickett-Hears AA: Intensive care of the fetus in breech labour. *Br J Obstet Gynaecol* 1976;83:217–275.

48. Hofmeyr GJ, Sonnendecker EWW: Cardiotocographic changes after external cephalic version. *Br J Obstet Gynaecol* 1983;90:914–918.

49. Iffy L, Apuzzio JJ, Cohen-Addad N, Zwolska-Demlzuk B, Francis-Lane M, Olenczak J: Abdominal rescue after entrapment of the aftercoming head. *Am J Obstet Gynecol* 1986;154:623–624.

50. Ingemarsson I, Westgren M, Svenningsen WW: Long-term follow-up of preterm infants in breech presentation delivered by cesarean section. A prospective study. *Lancet* 1978;2:172–175.

51. Johnson CE: Breech presentation at term. *Am J Obstet Gynecol* 1970;106:865–871.

52. Jurado L, Miller GL: Breech presentation. *Am J Obstet Gynecol* 1968;101:183–189.

53. Karp LE, Doney JR, McCarthy T, Meis PJ, Hall M: The premature breech: Trial of labor or cesarean section? *Obstet Gynecol* 1979;53:88–92.

54. Kaupplla O, Gronroos M, Aro P, Aittoniemi P, Kuoppala M: Management of low birth weight breech delivery: Should cesarean section be routine? *Obstet Gynecol* 1981;57:289–294.

55. Kopelman JN, Duff P, Karl RT, Schipull AH, Read JA: Computed tomographic pelvimetry in the evaluation of breech presentation. *Obstet Gynecol* 1986;68:455–458.

56. Lanka LD, Nelson HB: Breech presentation with low fetal mortality. A comparative study. *Am J Obstet Gynecol* 1969;104:879–882.

57. Lauderdale JM: Transabdominal decompression of the breech hydrocephalus. *Obstet Gynecol* 1964;23:938–939.

58. Luterkort M, Persson PH, Weldner BM: Maternal and fetal factors in breech presentation. *Obstet Gynecol* 1984;64:55–59.

59. Lyons DR, Papsin FR: Cesarean section in the management of breech presentation. *Am J Obstet Gynecol* 1978;130:558–561.

60. Manzke H: Morbidity among infants born in breech presentation. *J Perinat Med* 1978;6:127–140.

61. Marcus RG, Crewe-Brown H, Krawitz S: Fetomaternal haemorrhage following successful and unsuccessful attempts at external cephalic version. *Br J Obstet Gynaecol* 1975;82:578–580.

62. Mark C, Robert PHR: Breech scoring index. *Am J Obstet Gynecol* 1968;101:572–573.

63. Milner RDG: Neonatal mortality of breech deliveries with and without forceps to the aftercoming head. *Br J Obstet Gynaecol* 1975;82:783–785.

64. Morrison JC, Myatt RE, Martin JN, Meeks JR, Martin RW, Bucovaz ET, Wiser WL: External cephalic version of the breech presentation under tocolysis. *Am J Obstet Gynecol* 1986;154:900–903.

65. Murray J, Dewhurst CJ, Archer GD: External version in the rhesus negative woman. *J Obstet Gynaecol Br Commonw* 1974;81:873–874.

66. Myers SA: A new technique for flexion of the aftercoming head during breech delivery. *Am J Obstet Gynecol* 1986;155:33–34.

67. Neilson DR: Management of the large breech infant. *Am J Obstet Gynecol* 1970;107:345–348.

68. Ohlsen JH: Outcome of term breech delivery in primigravidae: A fetopelvic breech index. *Acta Obstet Gynecol Scand* 1975;54:141–151.

69. Parot J: Rupture of the spinal cord in the newborn. *L'Union Med* 1870;9:137–139.

70. Patterson SP, Mulliniks RC, Schreier PC: Breech presentation in the primigravida. *Am J Obstet Gynaecol* 1967;98:404–410.

71. Phelan JP, Stine LE, Mueller E, McCart D, Yeh S-Y: Observations of fetal heart rate characteristics related to external cephalic version and tocolysis. *Am J Obstet Gynecol* 1984;149:658–661.

72. Ralis ZA: Birth trauma to muscles in babies born in breech delivery and its possible fatal consequences. *Arch Dis Child* 1975;50:4–7.

73. Ranney R: The gentle art of external cephalic version. *Am J Obstet Gynecol* 1973;116:239–251.

74. Rauramo L, Gronroos M, Kivikoski A: A comparative study of the obstetrical history of pupils in schools for backward children and elementary school pupils. *Acta Obstet Gynaecol Scand* 1961;40:321–338.

75. Rosen MG, Debanne S, Thompson K, Bilenker RM: Long-term neurological morbidity in breech and vertex births. *Am J Obstet Gynecol* 1985;151:718–720.

76. Rovinsky JJ, Miller JA, Kaplan S: Management of breech presentation at term. *Am J Obstet Gynecol* 1973;115:497–515.

77. Saling E, Muller-Holve W: External cephalic version under tocolysis. *J Perinat Med* 1975;3:115–119.

78. Saling EZ: Oxygen-conserving adaptation of the foetal circulation, in Apley J (ed): *Modern Trends in Pediatrics*. London, Butterworths, 1970, p 51–68.

79. Salvatore CA, Cicivizzo E, Turatti S: Breech delivery with saddle block anesthesia. *Obstet Gynecol* 1965;26:261–264.

80. Scher E: Evaluation of cephalometry by ultrasound in breech presentation. *Am J Obstet Gynecol* 1969;103:1125–1130.

81. Sinder C, Wentsler NE: Breech presentation with follow-up. *Obstet Gynecol* 1965;25:322–328.

82. Smith RS, Oldham RR: Breech delivery. *Obstet Gynecol* 1970;36:151–161.

83. Stine LE, Phelan JP, Wallace R, Eglinton GS, Van Dorsten JP, Schifrin BS: Update on external cephalic version performed at term. *Obstet Gynecol* 1985;65:642–646.

84. Tank ES, Davis R, Holt JF, Morley GW: Mechanisms of trauma during breech delivery. *Obstet Gynecol* 1971;38:761–767.

85. Teteris NJ, Botschner AW, Ullery JC, Essig GF: Fetal heart rate during breech delivery. *Am J Obstet Gynecol* 1970;107:762–766.

86. U.S. Department of Health and Human Services, Public Health Service, and National Institutes of Health. Breech presentation, in *Cesarean Childbirth*. NIH Publication No. 82-2067, Bethesda, MD, 1981, pp 375–385.

87. Van Dorsten JP, Schifrin B, Wallace R: Randomized controlled trial of external cephalic version with tocolysis in late pregnancy. *Am J Obstet Gynecol* 1981;141:417–424.

88. Westgren M, Edvall H, Nordstrom L, Svalenius E: Spontaneous cephalic version of breech presentation in the last trimester. *Br J Obstet Gynaecol* 1985;92:19–22.

89. Wheeler T, Green K: Fetal heart rate monitoring during breech labor. *Br J Obstet Gynaecol* 1975;82:208–214.

90. White PC, Cibils LA: Clinical significance of fetal heart rate patterns during labor. VIII. Breech presentations. *J Reprod Med* 1984;29:45–51.

91. Wolter DF: Patterns of management with breech presentation. *Am J Obstet Gynecol* 1976;125:733–739.

92. Woods JR: Effects of low-birth-weight breech delivery on neonatal mortality. *Obstet Gynecol* 1979;53:735–740.

93. Wright RC: Reduction of perinatal mortality and morbidity in breech delivery through routine use of cesarean section. *Obstet Gynecol* 1959;14:758–763.

94. Ylikorkala O, Hartikanien-Sorri AL: Value of external version in fetal malpresentation in combination with use of ultrasound. *Acta Obstet Gynaecol Scand* 1977;56:63–67.

95. Zatuchni GI, Andros GJ: Prognostic index for vaginal delivery in breech presentation at term. Prospective study. *Am J Obstet Gynecol* 1967;98:854–857.

13

Cesarean Section

Benjamin P. Sachs and David B. Acker

HISTORICAL PERSPECTIVE

In the United States and Europe cesarean sections were rarely carried out until the end of the 19th century. The president of the American Gynecological Society, Thaddeus A. Reamy,[75] stated in 1886 that he had never performed a cesarean section over a 16-year period and 3,000 cases. However, by 1891 21 of 70 active fellows of the American Gynecological Society had performed a cesarean delivery.[45]

The first reported cesarean section in the United States was in 1822 in Nassau County, New York and was performed by a 14-year-old patient on herself in a snowbank.[32] The first documented operation by a physician was in 1827 by Dr. John Lambert Richmond.[66] Although it has been claimed that Dr. Jesse Bennett performed the first cesarean section in 1794, recent historical evidence finds this unlikely.[46] On the rare occasion in the 19th century when a cesarean section was performed, surgeons believed that the uterus should be left unsutured. Credit is largely due to American physicians for having shown that suture of the uterus improved maternal survival. Frank E. Polin of Springfield, Kentucky was the first accredited American physician to use sutures in a cesarean section.[75] The operation was performed in 1852 on a woman in labor for 40 hr with a hydrocephalic fetus. Dr. Polin used silver wire sutures and the patient was reported to have survived. Among 16 cases of cesarean section done soon after, in which the uterus was sutured, eight mothers survived, a remarkable figure for the time.[11] Brickell published in 1868 the first American report of the use of sutures.[11] In 1882, Max Sanger, an assistant of Credé from Leipzig, published a monograph strongly urging the use of uterine sutures.[72] The basis for this recommendation was the success of American physicians using this technique.

Further improvement in the safety of cesarean surgery was accomplished by enhancing its timeliness. In the 19th century it was considered that a patient should be fully dilated before a cesarean delivery was performed. Credit must go to Harris[31] and Sanger[72] for their demonstration that an earlier cesarean section could improve maternal survival. More progress came with a report by Harris in 1879 of an analysis of 100 cesarean sections performed in the United States.[33] It was recommended that instead of using chloroform, local anesthesia be sprayed on the incision line.

Most early cesarean sections were performed through an incision in the uterine fundus. Osiander (1805) was the first to recommend a vertical incision through the lower uterine segment.[20] Another German physician, Kehrer, of Heidelberg, described a low transverse incision in 1881; Kroenig furthered the work of Kehrer by recommending a uterovesical-peritoneal reflection for this procedure.[75]

By the 20th century the operation was in wide use in the United States. At a White House Conference on Child Health and Protection in 1933, the maternal loss from cesarean section was reported to range from 4.2% to 16.1%.[62] In New York at this same time, as reported by the State Maternal Mortality Committee, the incidence of cesarean section was 2.2% in the city's hospitals;[35] yet mothers who underwent a cesarean section represented almost one-fifth of all the maternal deaths.

THE OPERATION

Abdominal Incision

This can either be vertical or transverse. The former is simpler, quicker, and provides greater exposure than a Pfannensteil incision. However, a vertical incision has a greater risk for wound dehiscence and it is less cosmetic than the transverse incision. A transverse skin incision with transection of the rectus muscles (Maylard) can provide exposure equal to that of a midline incision. A repeat transverse incision is technically more difficult to perform than a midline incision, and there is a greater risk of bladder injury. To avoid this damage, it is important to enter the peritoneum as high as possible.

Uterine Incision

The uterus may be approached either transperitoneally or extra-peritoneally. The latter approach was popular in the era before antibiotics were available and may have reduced the risk of sepsis. However, it is rarely utilized currently. The low transverse uterine incision is the technique most favored, except in rare circumstances. The advantage of the lower uterine segment incision is in superior wound healing and thus less chance of dehiscence in future pregnancies. In addition, postoperative ileus and adhesion formation are less problematic than with incisions through the uterine corpus. If additional exposure is required a U-shaped uterine incision can be made with scissors. This form of incision allows for greater exposure and much less risk of extension. It is particularly useful in the delivery of macrosomic infants and for cases in which the lower uterine segment is not well developed.

The low vertical uterine incision (Kroenig) is widely used in France. However, it is less commonly utilized in the United States. It is advantageous when the lower uterine segment is poorly developed or there is a Bandl's ring of the uterus. Furthermore, this type of incision facilitates the atraumatic delivery of a premature fetus.

The classical cesarean section is defined by a vertical incision made into the anterior wall of the upper uterine segment. This incision is rarely needed in current obstetric practice. Examples of medical conditions that may warrant its use include placenta previa, carcinoma of the cervix, inaccessible lower uterine segment, or transverse lie (especially with the back down).

Incision of the Pregnant Uterus in the Delivery of a Low Birth Weight Infant

In many cases requiring a cesarean section for delivery of a low birth weight infant the lower uterine segment is poorly developed. An alternative to a low vertical or classical uterine incision is a U-type incision into the uterus.[39] This leaves a more durable scar in the uterus and obviates the need for a repeat cesarean section. It does provide in most instances sufficient exposure for the atraumatic delivery of the premature infant (see Chapter 11).

ANESTHESIA FOR CESAREAN SECTION

Preoperative Management

Premedication is usually omitted prior to cesarean section as most sedatives cross the placenta and may depress the infant. Prior to undertaking a cesarean section, either under general or regional anesthesia, it is important to give the patient a nonparticulate antacid (see Chapter 3). It has been shown that if aspiration occurs after having ingested antacids, serious consequences are less likely.[21] Patients should be placed in left lateral tilt position in order to prevent inferior vena caval and aortic compression.

There is a question as to whether routine cross-match of blood prior to cesarean section is justifiable because of the shortage of stored blood and the infrequent need for a transfusion. It is recommended that patients who are at high risk for hemorrhage, for example, those with uterine distension secondary to polyhydramnios or large uterine fibroids, or those with preexisting severe anemia, should have blood available prior to the surgery. As long as it is known that the patient has no unusual antibodies, blood need not be cross-matched prior to routine cesarean delivery. In an era when the safety of the blood supply has been questioned, it has been proposed that patients bank their own blood during pregnancy. Autologous donation is clearly the safest approach.

It is important that an intravenous line be established prior to carrying out a cesarean section. Ringer's lactate with 5% glucose is used commonly. However, there is a concern with the overutilization of glucose-containing solutions, particularly when there is fetal distress. Maintenance of maternal euglycemia should be the goal. Elevated maternal glucose may lead to secondary fetal hyperglycemia and hyperinsulinemia.[53,68]

Delivery Times

The induction-delivery time interval under general anesthesia is less important than the uterine incision-delivery time with respect to the risk of neonatal depression. If the fetus is not in distress and the mother is on her left side and adequately hydrated, an induction-delivery time of less than 20 min is not associated with an increased chance of neonatal depression.[17] Longer induction delivery intervals may result in mild neonatal depression attributable to the volatile maintenance agents.[16] A number of studies have shown that the interval between uterine incision and delivery is critical.[17,19] It is thought that once an incision is made into the uterus it leads to reflex uterine contractions and outpouring of catecholamines, both of which may lead to decreased uteroplacental perfusion. Under regional anesthesia that blocks the effects of sympathetic release, the uterine-delivery time appears to be less important.

PROPHYLACTIC CESAREAN SECTION AT TERM

Feldman and Freeman[27] asked whether prophylactic cesarean section in all pregnancies at approximately 38 weeks' gestation would improve perinatal outcome by preventing subsequent unpredictable events. If there is some proven adverse outcome for the fetus, how does this weigh against the additional risk for the mother? These authors were intrigued by this issue as a result of a malpractice case in which the plaintiff's attorney argued "would this baby be alive, healthy, and undamaged today if it had been delivered by cesarean section 1 week earlier?" Following a complicated statistical analysis, the authors came to the conclusion that patients should be given the opportunity to consider an elective prophylactic cesarean section. We would question the authors' findings for two reasons. First, their argument hinges very much on a precise estimate of the risk to a fetus in an uncomplicated pregnancy after 37 weeks' gestation. This study relied upon data collected prior to the widespread use of electronic fetal monitoring, and their risk estimates may thus be excessive. Second, it is extremely difficult to weigh the risks of cesarean delivery to the mother against the suggested improved outcome for the fetus. These judgments are based on numerous medical, ethical, and personal values difficult to quantify.

EPIDEMIOLOGY OF CESAREAN SECTION

Today in the United States almost one in four infants is delivered by cesarean section. Over the last 20 years the cesarean delivery rate has quadrupled. Prior to 1965 the reported rate was under 5%.[52] Today many regions of the country report rates of almost 25%.[74] This high cesarean delivery rate is controversial and has raised a number of important issues. Most revolve around the question of whether the rise in cesarean section rate improved the outcome for mothers and infants and, if so, has this improvement outweighed any increased maternal risk?

The reasons for the increase in the cesarean section rate between 1970 and 1978 were investigated by a National Institutes of Health (NIH) Task Force.[52] They reported that 30% of the rise was due to a diagnosis of dystocia, 25% to 30% to repeat cesarean section, 10% to 25% to cesarean delivery for breech presentation, and 10% to 15% to fetal distress (Table 13-1). At the time this Task Force presented its data, the national cesarean section rate was 17.9%. The further rise that has occurred since that time has been assumed to be due to a number of factors including: 1) virtual abandonment of vaginal breech deliveries in many places;

Table 13-1 Cesarean Section Rate 1970 to 1975: Major Indications

Indication	Cesarean sections for each indication (%)	Contribution to rise in rate (%)
Dystocia	31	30
Repeat cesarean	31	25–30
Breech presentation	22	10–25
Fetal distress	5	10–15

Source: Adapted with permission from *American Journal of Obstetrics and Gynecology* (1981;139: 902–909), Copyright © 1981, The CV Mosby Company.

2) concern about risks of midforceps deliveries; 3) increased cesarean delivery for the very low birth weight infant, and for multiple pregnancies; 5) techniques for fetal monitoring; and 6) the medicolegal environment. Although the last is very difficult to prove, it may be the most important factor to have influenced the recent increase in the number of cesarean sections. Failure to perform a timely cesarean section is often the "complaint" in malpractice suits (see Chapter 23).

Electronic Fetal Monitoring

Intrapartum electronic fetal monitoring has achieved widespread use in the United States, and in some centers is routine for almost all deliveries. This has occurred despite a number of recent reports that have failed to prove that routine fetal monitoring improves outcome in low-risk obstetric patients.[40,42] Although some institutions have reported that the use of electronic fetal monitoring did not influence the cesarean section rate,[50] it is likely that fetal monitoring has increased the cesarean section rate overall for a number of reasons: 1) in today's medicolegal environment, changes in the fetal heart rate pattern are more likely to lead to cesarean delivery even though they may not be pathologic in nature; 2) a minority of obstetric services in the country utilizes fetal scalp pH sampling; 3) the predictive value of abnormal fetal heart rate patterns is poor.[5,6,73]

A number of studies have evaluated the predictive value of fetal monitoring, using Apgar scores and in some cases a scalp pH less than 7.25 as endpoints.[16,73] Bissonnette et al. used a 1-min Apgar score less than 7 and a pH of less than 7.25 and reported a false-positive rate of 42.1%[8] and a false-negative rate of 19.1%. In another study of 355 cases by Bowe et al. using a 1-minute Apgar score less than 7 and a pH less than 7.20, a false-positive rate of 30.3% and a false-negative rate of 17.9% were found.[10] These findings are consistent with what we know about any screening test, that is, the predictive value is dependent on the incidence of the disease, which in this case is fetal hypoxia. Because the incidence of birth asphyxia is very small in low-risk populations, no screening test can be expected to have a good positive predictive value. The NIH consensus conference on cesarean sections reported that 5% of all cesarean sections in 1978 were for fetal distress.[52] Some pundits have argued that electronic fetal monitoring may also lead to an increase in the incidence of cesarean section for dystocia because monitored patients are generally confined to bed. This is an important question and one that has not been addressed adequately.

Demographic Factors Influencing the Cesarean Section Rate

There are a number of demographic factors that influence the cesarean section rate. These include:

Maternal Age

The cesarean section rate increases by a factor of 2 to 3 for women over the age of 30 years.[41,43,52,61] The explanation usually given for this observation is that older women have a higher incidence of dysfunctional labor[14] and also are more likely to have medical complications that influence the need for cesarean births. There is some evidence to support this contention although the precise contribution of these factors to the cesarean section rate is uncertain. Whatever the reason for the higher cesarean section rate among older patients, it is clear that as more women in the United States are delaying childbirth, the issue will become increasingly important.

Prenatal Care

It is controversial as to whether the absence of prenatal care is associated with a higher cesarean section rate.[52,58,59,81] Part of the problem may be that there are a number of potential confounding variables in such an analysis, including socioeconomic factors. However, it is of interest that Boston City Hospital reported a cesarean section rate of 17% in 1984[18] despite the fact that it provides care for the indigent population of the city among whom many receive little prenatal care. Similarly, the primary cesarean section rate at the Bronx Municipal Hospital Center, which cares for a similar population, has been 9% to 11% over the past 3 years. It is likely that the influence of many factors, including the general obstetric care philosophy, frequency of low birth weight, and fetal distress override the effects of poor prenatal care.

Maternal Demographics

These include marital status, maternal education, ethnicity, and whether the patient received care in an urban or rural setting. It is unclear from the literature whether these factors impact on the cesarean delivery rate.[59,80,81]

Hospital Teaching Status

A number of studies have shown that the cesarean delivery rate is higher in teaching hospitals compared to nonteaching hospitals.[41,52] However, most of these studies did not control for the differences in population. Teaching hospitals are often larger, are located in urban settings and serve high-risk populations. Also, many have special care nurseries and, therefore, attract patients who are at high risk for premature delivery. Williams and Hawes found no association between cesarean birth rates and teaching hospitals when they controlled for these risk factors.[81] Furthermore, in a report from teaching hospitals in California by Williams and Chen, there had been a lower cesarean section rate than expected over a 3-year period.[80]

Hospital Size and Neonatal Intensive Care Unit

Larger hospitals are generally located in urban settings, care for more indigent women, and thus have a high cesarean section rate. Furthermore, the presence of a neonatal intensive care unit should reflect the fact that more high-risk patients are delivered at that institution. Nevertheless, neither factor has been clearly associated with a high cesarean section rate.[80] The Department of Public Health of the Commonwealth of Massachusetts studied cesarean sections in 1981.[18] The cesarean delivery rate for first births at various hospitals ranged from 0 to 31.4% with an average of 18.5%. With the exception of one institution, none of the ten hospitals with a high cesarean section rate had a neonatal intensive care unit. These findings remained unchanged even when the delivery rates were calculated after controlling for birth weight.

Private or Clinic Care

In a recent review of 65,647 deliveries at four Brooklyn, New York hospitals between 1977 and 1982,[34] it was found that private physicians performed significantly more cesarean sections than house officers and attending physicians. Private patients were more likely to have been given the diagnosis of dystocia, malpresentation, or fetal distress. The perinatal mortality in this study was lower among private patients. However, infants of private patients had a significantly higher incidence of low Apgar scores and birth injuries than infants of clinic patients.

Hospital Ownership

Economic incentives have been cited as a reason for the high cesarean section rate.[43,52] If this is correct then one would predict that for-profit institutions would have higher cesarean section rates. In an analysis of data from hospitals in 1981, Placek et al. showed that the highest cesarean section rates were in proprietary hospitals followed by nonprofit hospitals and then government hospitals.[60] However, in New York City nonprofit and proprietary hospitals were found to have similar rates. Williams and Hawes found a positive correlation between cesarean section rates and nonprofit institutions but not proprietary hospitals.[81] Thus, there is no clear relationship between hospital ownership and cesarean delivery rates.

Insurance Coverage

The analysis of insurance status of patients and their cesarean section rate is confounded by a number of variables such as maternal age, socioeconomic factors, parity, race, and so on. The literature in this area is also confusing,[52,60] and it is difficult to draw concrete conclusions. However, it is of interest that two studies have shown that the primary cesarean section rate is lower for members of health maintenance organizations.

COMPARISONS OF NATIONAL CESAREAN SECTION RATES

A recent study of the cesarean section rates in 19 industrialized countries of North America, Europe, and the Pacific region showed that there was a marked difference in rates, with the highest occurring in the United States (Tables 13-2, 13-3).[78] The number of vaginal deliveries following a previous cesarean section was the lowest in the United States and the

Table 13-2 Cesarean Section Rates Per 100 Hospital Deliveries: 1970, 1975, 1980, and 1983

	1970	1975	1980	1983
United States	5.5	10.4	16.5	20.3
England and Wales	5.0	6.0	9.0	10.1
Denmark	5.7	7.5	—	12.8
Holland	5.3	5.9	8.9	11.4
(hospital deliveries)				

Source: Adapted with permission from *New England Journal of Medicine* (1987;316:386–387), Copyright © 1987, Massachusetts Medical Society.

Table 13-3 Cesarean Section Rates Per 100 Hospital Deliveries by Indication

Region, Year(s)	Multiple gestation	Breech presentation	Cephalo-pelvic disproportion	Fetal distress	Repeat cesarean
United States, 1983	43.6	75.8	97.9	68.7	95
Norway, 1980–1983	26.3	45.2	NA	NA	57
Denmark, 1983	42.5	75.4	70.5	21.6	NA
Canada, 1980–1981	20.1	54.2	88.8	23.0	96
England and Wales, 1980	NA	75.8	96.6	34.6	NA
Scotland, 1982	27.6	67.3	94.5	19.3	61

Abbreviations: NA, not available.

Source: Adapted with permission from *New England Journal of Medicine* (1987;316:386–387), Copyright © 1987, Massachusetts Medical Society.

highest in Norway. Despite those national differences, all countries reported a rise in their cesarean delivery rate over the past 15 years. A disturbing phenomenon is reports of high cesarean section rates in less-developed countries. For example, in northeastern Brazil it was 19%,[37] and 27% in Puerto Rico and metropolitan Mexico City.[78]

RISK OF CESAREAN SECTION

Maternal Mortality

The maternal mortality rate is the number of maternal deaths during pregnancy or within a set time postpartum per 100,000 terminated pregnancies (or livebirths). The American College of Obstetricians and Gynecologists (ACOG)[2] and the American Medical Association[3] define maternal mortality as the total number of maternal deaths during pregnancy or within 42 days of delivery per 100,000 terminated pregnancies. The National Center for Health Statistics[49] and the World Health Organization[82] define it as the number of maternal deaths (direct and indirect) during pregnancy or within 42 days of delivery per 100,000 livebirths.

Table 13-4 summarizes the findings of five American and two European studies that examined maternal mortality rates associated with cesarean section. The death rate for all cases in which a cesarean section was performed ranged from 0 to 105.3 per 100,000 cesarean sections. The lowest rate was reported by Frigoletto et al. from the Boston Hospital for Women[29] and the highest rate was for the state of Georgia.[69] The mean for these studies was 22.8 per 100,000 cesarean sections. For only those deaths directly related to the cesarean section, the mortality rate ranged from 0 to 60.7 per 100,000 cesarean sections (Table 13-5). The mean was 27 per 100,000 cesarean sections.

A problem arises in that these seven studies are not directly comparable. Two of them were hospital based, three were statewide reviews, and two dealt with national statistics. The strengths of a hospital-based study are that it has accurate data but may not include patients who die at home or in another institution. However, state or national population based studies rely upon vital statistics records, which are recognized to have problems with the reliability of reporting. The study by Rubin et al. from Georgia[69] identified deaths by linking birth and death certificates and then investigating each case. Thus, the difference in approach may account for the wide range of reported mortality rates. Nevertheless, the risk of cesarean section does appear to differ by country and region in the United States.

Table 13-4 Studies of Cesarean Section–Related Maternal Mortality

Study, Years	Population	No. deaths from C/S	Total No. C/S	Mortality per 100,000 C/S
Evrard and Gold[24], 1965–1975	Rhode Island	9	12,941	69.5
British study[64], 1973–1975	England and Wales	81	100,870	80.3
Frigoletto et al[29], 1968–1978	Boston Hospital for Women	0	10,231	0.0
Rubin et al.[69], 1975–1976	Georgia	16	15,188	105.3
Petitti et al.[58], 1975–1976	Hospitals in professional study	213	350,892	60.7
Moldin et al.[48], 1973–1979	Sweden	13	68,075	19.1
Sachs et al.[70], 1976–1984	Massachusetts	27	121,217	22.2
Total		359	679,414	52.8 (95% CL ± 46)

Abbreviations: CL, confidence limits; C/S, cesarean section.

A committee on maternal welfare was established in the Commonwealth of Massachusetts in 1941. Its principal objective was to improve the safety of childbirth using derivative information through investigation of every maternal death, to educate providers of health care and to institute public health policy. Under the stewardship of the late J.F. Jewett between 1953 and 1985, the committee was comprised of obstetricians from both teaching and community hospitals, pathologists, internists, anesthesiologists, and a representative from the Department of Public Health. In problem cases relevant specialists were consulted.

Between 1954 and 1985 there were 886 maternal deaths in the Commonwealth of Massachusetts.[70] The maternal mortality rate fell from 50 per 100,000 livebirths (1954–1957) to 10 per 100,000 livebirths (1982–1985).

The cesarean rate in Massachusetts rose from 13.9% in 1976 to 21.8% in 1984.[18] A total of 121,217 cesarean sections were performed during this time. Twenty-seven women died after a cesarean section, a mortality rate of 22.2 per 100,000 cesarean sections. However, only seven of these

Table 13-5 Studies of Maternal Death Due to a Cesarean Section

Study (years)	No. deaths related to C/S	Total No. C/S	Mortality rate[a] directly related to C/S
Evrard and Gold[24], 1965–1975	4	12,941	30.9
British study[64], 1973–1975	61	100,870	60.5
Frigoletto et al[29], 1968–1978	0	10,231	0.0
Rubin et al.[69], 1975–1976	9	15,188	59.3
Moldin et al.[48], 1973–1979	8	68,075	11.8
Sachs et al.[70], 1976–1984	7	121,217	5.8
Total	89	328,522	27 (95% CL ± 15.1)

Abbreviations: CL, confidence limits; C/S, cesarean section.

[a]Number maternal deaths due directly to complications of a cesarean section per 100,000 procedures.

deaths were directly related to the operative procedure, resulting in a corrected mortality rate of 5.8 per 100,000 cesarean sections.

The leading causes of cesarean section–related deaths were pulmonary embolus (22%) followed by anesthesia (17%), sepsis (15%), and hemorrhage (15%). In Massachusetts in the 1980s pulmonary embolus was the second leading cause of maternal death in the state.[70] Anesthesia-related mortality fell from 2.3 in 1954–1957 to 0.3/100,000 livebirths in 1982–1985.

A number of studies have attempted to examine the relative risk of cesarean versus vaginal delivery.[24,29,48,57,58,69] However, in those cases the comparison was made between all cesarean section–related deaths versus all other maternal deaths. This probably overestimates the risk of a cesarean section. A pure study would be to compare the maternal mortality directly due to the cesarean section–related complication in patients with no antecedent risk versus a vaginal delivery group including direct maternal deaths and excluding cases of ectopic pregnancies, abortions, and indirect deaths. However, most published studies do not meet these criteria.

In Massachusetts between 1976 and 1984, 27 patients died following cesarean section (Table 13-6). However, only seven of these deaths were due directly to the operative delivery, a corrected mortality rate of 5.8 per 100,000 procedures. In contrast, during the same time period there were 57 deaths associated with vaginal delivery, excluding ectopic pregnancies, septic abortions, and nonmaternal deaths. This calculates to a mortality rate of 10.8 per 100,000 vaginal deliveries. Thus, one can conclude that in Massachusetts during the time interval studied, a cesarean section was at least as safe as a vaginal delivery for the mother with respect to mortality.

Cesarean Section–Related Morbidity

Although a cesarean section is at least as safe as a vaginal delivery with respect to maternal mortality, maternal morbidity is significantly higher

Table 13-6 Relative Risk of a Cesarean Section versus a Vaginal Delivery in Massachusetts, 1976–1984

Year	No. cesarean deaths direct[a]	Total no. cesarean deaths[b] (preventable)[c]	No. vaginal deaths (preventable)[c]
1976	4(3)	4(3)	2(1)
1977	0	1(0)	4(1)
1978	0	3(2)	8(2)
1979	0	2(0)	6(4)
1980	0	4(0)	10(0)
1981	1(0)	3(0)	10(4)
1982	0	2(1)	7(5)
1983	2(2)	8(3)	9(5)
1984	0	0	1(0)
Total	7(5)	27(9)	57(22)
Total rate	5.8/100,000 cesarean sections	22.3/100,000 cesarean sections	10.8/100,000 vaginal deliveries

[a]Number of maternal deaths directly due to a cesarean section.
[b]All maternal deaths in which a cesarean section was performed.
[c]Deaths deemed by Massachusetts Maternal Mortality Committee to be preventable.

Source: Adapted with permission from *New England Journal of Medicine* (1987;316:667–672), Copyright © 1987, Massachusetts Medical Society.

in patients who undergo cesarean delivery. Table 13-7 shows the results of nine studies published since 1976 that reviewed cesarean section–related maternal morbidity.[4,26,30,38,47,51,56,63,65] These studies represented a total of 26,000 procedures. Six of the studies were from university centers and four from community hospitals.

Intraoperative Morbidity

In one study the incidence of major intraoperative complications was 0.4%.[38] This included four cases of bladder perforation, three of uterine bleeding requiring hysterectomy, two of broad ligament lacerations, and one of injury to the bowel. In another series, cesarean hysterectomy was required in 0.1% of patients.[77] Overall, in the four studies that examined the incidence of intraoperative morbidity, the incidence of major events ranged from 0.1% to 2.1%.

Table 13-7 Cesarean Section–Related Maternal Morbidity

Study, Years	Population	No. cesearean sections	Complication rate (%)
Jones[38], 1963–1975	Charlotte Memorial Hospital, Charlotte, North Carolina	2,563	33
Green and Sarubbi[30], 1975	North Carolina Memorial, Chapel Hill, North Carolina	129	42
Perloe and Curet[56], 1975–1976	Madison General Hospital, Madison, Wisconsin	179	35
Minkoff and Schwartz[47], 1961–1977	Downstate-Kings County Hospital Brooklyn, New York	9,727	27–48
Rehu and Nilsson[63], 1977–1978	State Maternity Hospital Helsinki, Finland	774	21
Farrell et al.[26], 1976–1977	Women's Hospital Ann Arbor, Michigan	457	30
Amirikia et al.[4], 1965–1979	Hutzel Hospital Detroit, Michigan	9,718	18
Richards and Richards[65], 1977–1979	Fourteen Colorado hospitals	1,177	40
Nielsen et al.[51], 1978–1980	Central Hospital Borås, Sweden	1,319	26

Postoperative Morbidity

Postoperative morbidity was significantly more common than intraoperative complications, ranging from 14.5% to 41.9%.[4,22,26,30,38,47,51,56,63,65,77] Infection-related morbidity was 11.3% to 35.5%, with fever secondary to endometritis and urinary tract infection being the most common complications. Other less frequent complications included pneumonia, pelvic abscess, thrombophlebitis, pulmonary embolism, gastrointestinal ileus, and hemorrhage requiring blood transfusion. Long-term morbidity was quite low. In a series of approximately 2,500 cesarean sections there was one vesicovaginal fistula and one ureterovaginal fistula.[38]

Placenta Previa and Placenta Accreta

In 1954, Bender suggested that patients who had a uterine scar were at risk for development of a placenta previa in a subsequent pregnancy.[7] The combination of a transverse uterine incision and placenta previa has been shown to increase the risk for a placenta accreta. In a large study from Los Angeles County–University of Southern California Women's Hospital involving 92,917 women, of whom 4,882 underwent a cesarean section, a clear association was found between a uterine scar and subsequent placenta previa-accreta.[12] In Table 13-8 it can be seen that with no history of a prior cesarean section the incidence of placenta previa was 0.3%. However, this figure rose to 10% with four or more cesarean sections. In patients who had a placenta previa with no history of a cesarean section, there was a placenta accreta in 5% of the cases. How-

Table 13-8 Risk of Placenta Previa/Accreta and Prior Cesarean Section

No. previous cesarean sections	Placenta previa (%)	Placenta previa and accreta (%)
0	0.3	5
1	0.7	24
2	1.8	47
3	3.0	40
≥4	10.0	67

Source: Adapted with permission from *Surgery, Gynecology & Obstetrics* (1954;98:625–628), Copyright © 1954, Franklin H Martin Memorial Foundation.

ever, in those with just one prior cesarean section and a placenta previa, the incidence of placenta accreta was 24%. As almost one in four women today are delivered by cesarean section, one would expect a rise in the incidence of placenta previa and placenta accreta. Furthermore, clinicians should be alerted to the possibility of a placenta accreta if a patient has had a prior cesarean section and has a placenta previa. Such a patient should be counseled about the risk of a cesarean hysterectomy and the appropriate preoperative measures taken.

HAS THE RISE IN THE CESAREAN SECTION RATE IMPROVED PERINATAL MORTALITY?

As described above, over the last 10 years there has been a dramatic rise in the number of cesarean sections performed in the United States. Over the same time period there has also been a decline in perinatal mortality.[9,79] Some investigators have concluded there may be a cause-and-effect relationship between these events. However, the National Maternity Hospital in Dublin has reported a similar decline in perinatal mortality despite a stable cesarean section rate between 4% and 5%. A recent article comparing the perinatal outcome in patients delivered at the Parkland Memorial Hospital in Texas to deliveries in the National Maternity Hospital in Dublin reported that there was an increased perinatal morbidity in Dublin, presumed to be due to the lower cesarean section rate.[39] However, if the comparison between the two institutions covers more years, there is no longer any difference seen in either perinatal morbidity or mortality despite a six times higher cesarean delivery rate at Parkland Memorial Hospital.[76] Furthermore, it is important to note that in this Dublin hospital almost 20% of the patients delivered infants who weighed more than 4,000 g.[76] Thus, a lower incidence of macrosomia is clearly not the reason for their lower cesarean section rate. O'Driscoll et al. attribute their low frequency of cesarean section to active management of labor.[54] This includes early recourse to the use of oxytocin in patients who are already diagnosed as being in the active phase of labor. The contrary point of view has been put forth by Williams and Chen[80] who reported that in California there was a reduction of perinatal mortality in newborns weighing less than 2,000 g due to the advent of neonatal intensive care units and an increase in the cesarean delivery rate. In a study in Georgia done between 1974 and 1978,[71] the effect of cesarean section on the neonatal mortality rate for breech and low birth weight vertex infants was examined. It was shown that in 229,241 singleton deliveries a cesarean section improved neonatal outcome for breech infants and high-risk low birth weight infants presenting by the vertex.

REPEAT CESAREAN SECTION VERSUS TRIAL OF LABOR

The dictum, "Once a cesarean section, always a cesarean" was originally propounded by E.B. Cragin, who was the Chairman of the Department of Obstetrics and Gynecology at Columbia University College of Physicians and Surgeons at the beginning of the 20th century.[15] At that time the frequency of uterine rupture was higher than today because patients were more frequently delivered by classical cesarean section. In contrast, most patients now have a transverse incision made into the lower uterine segment. After this type of cesarean section it has been shown by many investigators to be safe for a patient to have a subsequent trial of labor.[44,55,67] In a review of more than 3,000 vaginal deliveries following a previous cesarean section, the incidence of uterine rupture was 0.7% and that of perinatal loss was 0.93 per 1,000 births.[55] Two of the three perinatal losses occurred in a patient who had had a prior classical uterine incision. This review included 4,729 patients cared for at eleven institutions. Two-thirds of these patients had a successful trial of labor.

The ACOG[1] established guidelines for managing patients who have had a previous cesarean section. The recommendations are that a trial of labor is indicated for all patients except those who have repeating contraindications to a vaginal delivery. There should be a singleton infant presenting by the vertex and not weighing more than 4,000 g. Patients should have had only one prior low transverse incision with no extension and the type of incision confirmed by a written operative report. A trial of labor is indicated even for those patients who have had the first cesarean section for failure to progress in labor. The ACOG guidelines recommend that technical support be available in hospital including skilled nurses and an in-house obstetrician, pediatrician, and an anesthesiologist. Furthermore, an adequate blood bank with compatible blood should be available and staffed 24 hr a day. Electronic fetal monitoring is advisable during labor. Finally, there must be immediate access to an appropriately staffed operating room.

The question is, therefore, given the preponderance of evidence showing that a trial of labor is safe, why do so few patients undergo it? One can only speculate that the reasons might include convenience, exaggerated concern over risks, financial incentive for cesarean, inability of many hospitals to meet ACOG guidelines relating to technical support, and in some cases the patient's request. One of the issues that may have to be addressed in the future is whether it is ethical not to allow a patient a repeat cesarean section even if she prefers it because of the excess costs that would be incurred in comparison to vaginal delivery.

Rupture of the uterus either antepartum or intrapartum is the major concern when allowing the patient who has had a prior cesarean section to labor. In a 53-year review of the incidence of uterine rupture at Duke University Medical Center, the incidence was reported to be one uterine rupture per 1,424 deliveries.[23] During this half-century of clinical experience, the incidence of uterine rupture had not changed. Examining the etiology of the uterine rupture, the investigators found in approximately 21% a history of prior cesarean section; in 13% this was a classical cesarean, and in 8% there was a low transverse incision. Other associations were 17% midforceps delivery, 17% version and extraction, 17% precipitate vaginal delivery, 13% injudicious use of oxytocics, and 13% prolonged labor.

Timing of Repeat Cesarean Section

There are distinct advantages to planning a repeat cesarean section. Among them are that the patient has an empty stomach and, therefore, a lower anesthetic risk, and that there is virtually no risk of uterine rupture. In addition, some patients find some psychosocial advantage in the opportunity to plan the delivery date in advance, and in avoiding the pain of labor. The disadvantages of repeat cesarean section relate to the risk of iatrogenic prematurity, higher cost, longer hospitalization and recuperation, and excess maternal morbidity.

The Department of Obstetrics and Gynecology of Harvard Medical School has recently recommended guidelines for planning a repeat cesarean section. They include: (1) clinical dating of the pregnancy by known last menstrual period in a patient with regular menses and no recent use of oral contraception, (2) early uterine sizing by bimanual examination, (3) antenatal care beginning in the first trimester, and (4) detection of the fetal heart by fetoscope at 20 weeks' gestation or by Doppler examination at 12 weeks' gestation. In addition to these clinical criteria it is strongly recommended that the patient have ultrasonography in the first or early second trimester of pregnancy. If these criteria are not met it is recommended that either the clinician should wait for the patient to go into labor or that an amniocentesis be carried out for evaluation of pulmonary maturity. With respect to dating of a pregnancy by ultrasound, the crown-rump length is utilized between 7 and 10 weeks' gestation. Between 10 and approximately 14 weeks' gestation the measurement of the crown-rump length is less accurate and the biparietal diameter is so small that it is subject to large error. The use of a biparietal diameter is more accurate between 14 and 20 weeks' gestation. However, with respect to predicting the length of gestation, there is an error of at least ±1 week even when the scan was performed at an optimal time.

Vaginal Delivery After Two or More Prior Cesarean Sections

The ACOG has clearly recommended that women with one previous cesarean section be allowed a trial of labor. As there are few data concerning patients who have had more than one cesarean section, it is difficult to know what to recommend for them. There was a recent report of 57 women who had two or more cesarean sections; among them 77% had successful vaginal deliveries.[25] None of these patients had significant complications. Given the paucity of data, individual selection of patients for attempted vaginal delivery may be appropriate with careful counseling.

Trial of Labor: Use of Oxytocin and Epidural Anesthesia

Does oxytocin increase the risk of rupture of the uterus? Without the utilization of oxytocin many patients would not have an adequate trial of labor. The few studies in which this issue has been examined have not found an increased risk.[28,36] Clearly these patients should be carefully monitored and all precautions taken to prevent hyperstimulation of the uterus. One approach is to use 10U of oxytocin in a liter of fluid and to start the use of oxytocin at two mIU/min and to increase the infusion by no more than one mIU/min every 20 min. It was originally thought that the use of an epidural anesthetic would mask the symptoms of impending uterine rupture, and would therefore be contraindicated in patients in labor with a uterine scar. There has been some clinical experience showing that this does not appear to be the case.[28,36] Intrapartum uterine rupture is usually associated with vaginal bleeding and changes in fetal heart rate pattern. Most lower segment scars rupture without severe pain or other catastrophic clinical manifestations.

COST OF CESAREAN SECTION

In an era of cost consciousness in clinical medicine it is clear that the currently very high cesarean section rate adds considerably to the cost of health care. Patients who undergo cesarean section have a longer hospital stay, which is on average 3.1 additional days. They have higher complication rates, require more anesthesia and other medication, and in most instances command a higher doctor's fee than those delivered vaginally. If the patient has a repeat cesarean section, this clearly perpetuates the problem. The difference in direct costs between an uncomplicated cesarean section and an uncomplicated vaginal delivery at Boston's Beth Israel Hospital in 1986 was approximately $3,500. This figure assumes a global fee for obstetric care and thus, the differential will be higher in instances in which physicians bill more for a cesarean than for a vaginal delivery. Moreover, when the excess indirect costs of cesarean delivery (time lost from work, home care and prolonged disability, and so on) are considered, the societal costs of a high cesarean section rate seem daunting. However, a cost-benefit analysis of the problem must balance the costs of cesarean delivery against the costs of the alternative. If even a small proportion of cesarean sections prevent serious disability in mother or offspring, the direct and indirect costs saved by having averted illness may offset the savings that would have accrued had vaginal delivery been done.[13] Obviously, these issues are highly complex and of considerable importance from the standpoint of public health. They have yet to receive thorough and meaningful consideration.

REFERENCES

1. ACOG Newsletter: Committee reports guidelines for vaginal delivery. American College of Obstetrics and Gynecologists, Washington, DC, 1982;26:1.

2. American College of Obstetricians and Gynecologists: *Standards for Obstetrics and Gynecologic Services*. Chicago, American College of Obstetricians and Gynecologists, 1974.

3. American Medical Association: *Action Guide for Maternal and Child Care Committee*. Chicago, American Medical Association, 1974.

4. Amirikia H, Zarewych B, Evans TN: Cesarean section: A 15-year review of changing incidence, indications and risks. *Am J Obstet Gynecol* 1981;140:81–90.

5. Banta HD, Thacker SB: Assessing the costs and benefits of electronic fetal monitoring. *Obstet Gynecol Surv* 1979;348:627–642.

6. Beard RW, Filshie GM, Knight CA, Roberts GM: The significance of the changes in the continuous fetal heart rate in the first stage of labor. *J Obstet Gynaecol Br Commonw* 1971;78:865–881.

7. Bender S: Placenta previa and previous lower segment cesarean section. *Surg Gynecol Obstet* 1954;98:625–628.

8. Bissonnette JM: Relationship between continuous fetal heart rate patterns and Apgar score in the newborn. *Br J Obstet Gynaecol* 1975;82:24–28.

9. Bottoms SF, Rosen MG, Sokol RJ: The increase in the cesarean birth rate. *N Engl J Med* 1980;302:559–563.

10. Bowe ET, Beard RW, Finster M, Poppers PJ, Adamsons K, James LS: Relationship of fetal blood sampling and maternal fetal relationship. *Am J Obstet Gynecol* 1970;107:279–287.

11. Brickell DW: A successful case of caesarean section. *New Orleans J Med* 1868;21:454–466.

12. Clark S, Koonings P, Phelan J: Placenta previa/accreta and prior cesarean section. *Obstet Gynecol* 1985;66:88–92.

13. Cohen WR: The financial cost-effectiveness of cesarean section. *Contemp Ob/Gyn* 1983;19:161–173.

14. Cohen WR, Newman L, Friedman EA: Frequency of labor disorders with advancing maternal age. *Obstet Gynecol* 1980;55:414–416.

15. Cragin EB: Conservatism in obstetrics. *NY Med J* 1916;104:1–3.

16. Crawford J, Lewis M, Davies P: Maternal and neonatal responses related to the volatile inhalation anesthetic agent at cesarean section. *Br J Anaesth* 1985;57:482–487.

17. Crawford JS, Burton M, Davies P: Anesthesia for cesarean section: Further refinements of a technique. *Br J Anaesth* 1973;45:726–732.

18. Dars LK, Rosen SL, Hannon MT: *Cesarean Birth in Massachusetts.* Boston, Boston Department of Public Health, 1984.

19. Datta S, Ostheimer GW, Weiss JB, Brown WV, Alper MH: Neonatal effect of prolonged anesthetic induction. *Obstet Gynecol* 1981;58:331–335.

20. DeLee JB: An illustrated history of the lower cervical cesarean section. *Trans Am Gynecol Soc* 1925;50:90–107.

21. Dewar DM, Floyd HM, Thistlewood JM, Bogard TD, Speilman FJ: Sodium citrate pretreatment in elective cesarean section patients. *Anesth Analg* 1985;64:34–37.

22. Duff P: Pathophysiology and management of post cesarean endomyometritis. *Obstet Gynecol* 1986;67:269–276.

23. Eden RD, Parker RT, Gau SA: Rupture of the pregnant uterus: A 53-year review. *Obstet Gynecol* 1986;68:671–674.

24. Evrard JR, Gold EM: Cesarean section and maternal mortality in Rhode Island. Incidence and risk factors, 1965–1975. *Obstet Gynecol* 1977;50:594–597.

25. Farmakides G, Duvivier R, Schulman H, Schneider E, Biordi J: Vaginal birth after two or more previous cesarean section. *Am J Obstet Gynecol* 1987;156:565–566.

26. Farrell SJ, Andersen HF, Wirj BA: Cesarean section: Indication and post-operative morbidity. *Obstet Gynecol* 1980;56:696–700.

27. Feldman GB, Freeman JA: Prophylactic cesarean section at term? *N Engl J Med* 1985;312:1264–1267.

28. Flamm B, Dunnett C, Fischermann E, Quilligan EJ: Vaginal delivery following cesarean section: Use of oxytocin augmentation and epidural anesthesia with internal tocodynamic and internal fetal monitoring. *Am J Obstet Gynecol* 1984;148:759–763.

29. Frigoletto FD, Ryan KJ, Phillippe M: Maternal mortality rate associated with cesarean section: An appraisal. *Am J Obstet Gynecol* 1980;136:969–970.

30. Green SL, Sarubbi FA: Risk factors associated with post-cesarean section febrile morbidity. *Obstet Gynecol* 1977;49:686–690.

31. Harris RP: Cattle-horn lacerations of the abdomen and uterus in pregnant women. *Am J Obstet* 1887;20:673–685.

32. Harris RP: The operation of gastro-hysterotomy (True Caesarean Section), viewed in the light of American experience and success; with the history and results of sewing up the

uterine wound; and a full tabular record of the caesarean operations performed in the United States, many of them not hitherto reported. *Am J Med Sci* 1878;75:313–342.

33. Harris RP: A study and analysis of one hundred caesarean operations performed in the United States, during the present century, and prior to the year 1878. *Am J Med Sci* 1879;77:43–65.

34. Haynes DE, Regt R, Minkoff H, Feldman J, Schwarz R: Relation of private or clinic care to the cesarean birth rate. *N Engl J Med* 1986;315:619–624.

35. Hooker RS: *Maternal Mortality in New York City. A Study of all Puerperal Deaths, 1930–1932. (By the New York Academy of Medicine Committee on Public Health Relations.)* New York, Commonwealth Fund, 1933.

36. Horenstein JM, Phelan JP: Previous cesarean section: The risks and benefits of oxytocin usage in a trial of labor. *Am J Obstet Gynecol* 1985;151:564–569.

37. Janowsky B, Rodrigues W, Covington DL, Arrunda JM, Morris L: Cesarean delivery in northeastern region of Brazil, 1978–1980. *Am J Pub Health* 1985;75:560–562.

38. Jones OH: Cesarean section in present-day obstetrics. *Am J Obstet Gynecol* 1976;126:521–530.

39. Kenepp NB, Shelley WC, Gabbe SG, Kumar S, Stanley CA, Gutsche BB: Fetal and neonatal hazards of maternal hydration with 5% dextrose before cesarean section. *Lancet* 1982;1150–1152.

40. Leveno K, Cunningham G, Pritchard J: Cesarean section: An answer to the House of Horne. *Am J Obstet Gynecol* 1985;153:838–844.

41. Lowe JA, Klassen DF, Loup RJ: Cesarean sections in United States PAS hospitals. *PAS Rep* 1976;14:1–55.

42. MacDonald D, Grant A, Sheridan-Pereira M, Boyland P, Chalmers I: The Dublin randomized controlled trial of intrapartum fetal heart rate monitoring. *Am J Obstet Gynecol* 1985;152:524–538.

43. Marieskind HI: *An Evaluation of Cesarean Section in the United States.* Department of Health and Human Services, Office of the Assistant Secretary for Planning and Evaluation/Health, 1980.

44. McGarry JA: The management of patients previously delivered by caesarean section. *J Obstet Gynaecol Br Commonw* 1969;76:137–143.

45. McLane JW: The Sloane Maternity Hospital. Report on the first series of one thousand successive confinements from January 1st, 1889, to October 1st, 1890. *Am J Obstet* 1891;24:385–418.

46. Miller JL: Dr. Jessee Bennett (1769–1842), Pioneer Surgeon. Dr. Aquilla Leighton Knight (1823–1897), Humanist. *Va Med Month* 1929;55:711–714.

47. Minkoff HL, Schwarz RH: The rising cesarean section rate: Can it safely be reversed? *Obstet Gynecol* 1980;56:135–143.

48. Moldin P, Hokegard KH, Nielsen TF: Cesarean section and maternal mortality in Sweden 1973–1979. *Acta Obstet Gynecol Scand* 1984;63:7–11.

49. National Center for Health Statistics: *Health in the United States, 1983.* Washington, DC, Public Health Service (DHHS publication no. PAJ 84–1232), 1983.

50. Neutra RR, Greenland S, Friedman EA: Effect of fetal monitoring on the cesarean section rate. *Obstet Gynecol* 1980;55:175–180.

51. Nielsen TF, Hokegard KH: Post-operative cesarean section morbidity: A prospective study. *Am J Obstet Gynecol* 1983;146:911–915.

52. National Institutes of Health (NIH) Consensus Development. Task Force Statement on Cesarean Childbirth. *Am J Obstet Gynecol* 1981;139:902–909.

53. Oakley NW, Beard RW, Turner RC: Effect of sustained maternal hyperglycemia in normal and diabetic pregnancies. *Br Med J* 1972;1:466–469.

54. O'Driscoll K, Foley M, MacDonald D: Active management of labor as an alternative to cesarean section for dystocia. *Obstet Gynecol* 1984;63:485–490.

55. O'Sullivan MJ, Fumia F, Holsinger K, McLeod AGW: Vaginal delivery after cesarean section. *Clin Perinatol* 1981;8:131–143.

56. Perloe M, Curet LB: The effect of internal fetal monitoring on cesarean section morbidity. *Obstet Gynecol* 1979;53:354–357.

57. Petitti D, Olson RO, Williams RL: Cesarean section in California—1960 through 1975. *Am J Obstet Gynecol* 1979;133:391–397.

58. Petitti DB, Cefalo RC, Shapiro SC, Whalley P: Inhospital maternal mortality in the United States: Time trends and relation to method of delivery. *Obstet Gynecol* 1982;59:6–12.

59. Placek PJ: Type of delivery associated with social, demographic, maternal health, infant health and health insurance factors. *Findings from the 1972 US National Natality Survey, Proceedings of the Social Statistics Section, 1977, Part II*. Washington, DC, American Statistical Association, 1978.

60. Placek PJ, Taffel S, Moien M: Cesarean section delivery rates: United States, 1981. *Am J Pub Health* 1983;73:861–862.

61. Placek PJ, Taffel SM: Trends in cesarean section rates for the United States, 1970–1978. *Public Health Rep* 1980;95:540–548.

62. Plass ED: Forceps and cesarean section, in White House Conference on Child Health and Protection. Fetal Newborn and Maternal Mortality and Morbidity. New York, Appleton-Century-Crofts, 1933, pp 215–247.

63. Rehu M, Nilsson CG: Risk factors for febrile morbidity associated with cesarean section. *Obstet Gynecol* 1980;56:269–273.

64. Report on confidential enquiries into maternal deaths in England and Wales 1973–1975. Department of Health and Social Security. Report on Health and Social Security. Her Majesty's Stationery Office, London, 1979.

65. Richards TA, Richards JL: A comparison of cesarean section morbidity in urban and rural hospitals. *Am J Obstet Gynecol* 1982;144:270–275.

66. Richmond JL: History of a successful case of cesarean operation. *West J Med Phys Sci* 1830;3:485–89.

67. Riva HL, Teich JC: Vaginal delivery after cesarean section. *Am J Obstet Gynecol* 1961;81:501.

68. Robillard JE, Sessions C, Kennedy RK: Metabolic effects of constant hypertonic glucose infusion in well oxygenated fetuses. *Am J Obstet Gynecol* 1978;130:199–203.

69. Rubin GL, Peterson HB, Rochat RW, McCarthy BJ, Terry JS: Maternal death after cesarean section in Georgia. *Am J Obstet Gynecol* 1981;139:681–685.

70. Sachs BP, Brown DAJ, Driscoll SG, Schulman E, Acker D, Ransil BJ, Jewett JF: Maternal mortality in Massachusetts: Trends and prevention. *N Engl J Med* 1987; 316:667–672.

71. Sachs BP, McCarthy BJ, Rubin G, Burton A, Terry J, Tyler CW: Cesarean section: Risk and benefits for mother and fetus. *JAMA* 1983;250:2157–2159.

72. Sanger M: Der kaiserschnitt bei uterusfibromen nebst vergleichender methodik der sectio caesarea und der Porro-operation. Leipzig, Engelmann, 1882.

73. Schifrin BS, Dame L: Fetal heart rate patterns. Prediction of Apgar score. *JAMA* 1972;219:1322–1325.

74. Shiono PH, Gielden JG, McNellis D, Rhoads GG, Pearse WH: Recent trends in cesarean birth and trial of labor rates in the United States. *JAMA* 1987;257:494–497.

75. Speert H: Obstetrics and Gynecology in America: A history. The American College of Obstetricians and Gynecologists. Waverly Press, Inc., Baltimore, Maryland, 1980.

76. Stronge JM: National Maternity Hospital Dublin clinical report for the year 1985. *Cahill Printers Ltd*. East Wall Rd, Dublin, Ireland.

77. Taffel SM, Placek PJ, Moien M: One-fifth of United States births by cesarean section. *Am J Public Health* 1985;75:190–196.

78. Watson FC, Placek PJ, Taffel SM: Comparisons of national cesarean section rates. *N Engl J Med* 1987;316:386–387.

79. Williams RL, Chen P: Identifying the sources of the recent decline in perinatal mortality rates in California. *N Engl J Med* 1982;306:207.

80. Williams RL, Chen PM: Controlling the rise in cesarean section rates by the dissemination of information from vital records. *Am J Pub Health* 1983;73:863–867.

81. Williams RL, Hawes WE: Cesarean section, fetal monitoring and perinatal mortality in California. *Am J Pub Health* 1979;69:864–870.

82. World Health Organization: Manual of the International Statistical Classification of Diseases, Injuries and Causes of Death. *Geneva, World Health Organization*, 1977;763–766.

14

Twin Gestation and Labor

David B. Acker and Benjamin P. Sachs

Twin pregnancy is a relatively infrequent obstetric occurrence (approximately 1% of all deliveries) associated disproportionately with high rates of maternal, fetal, and neonatal morbidity and mortality.[6] Ideal management of twin pregnancy requires early detection and appropriate antepartum and intrapartum decisions. This chapter reviews the recent obstetric literature pertaining to the management of twin pregnancy with the goal of providing the clinician with information that may aid in making those decisions.

PERINATAL OUTCOME

Considerable evidence suggests that twin pregnancy is associated with increased risk of adverse perinatal outcome, primarily but not only, related to complications of prematurity.[6,31,34,44,46,71,72,74] Ho and Wu[38] evaluated data obtained from 177 twin pairs who represented a frequency of 8.9 per 1,000 live births in a predominantly indigent population. The incidence of low birth weight (below 2,500 g) was 55% as contrasted with 8% in the singleton population. One-third of the twins were delivered prior to 37 weeks' gestation. Of all neonatal deaths among twins, 91% occurred in preterm infants and 83% in infants whose birth weight was less than 1,500 g. Hyaline membrane disease, necrotizing enterocolitis, and other manifestations of immaturity accounted for 78% of all deaths. Medearis et al.[62] reviewed 3,594 twin births. They represented 1.0% of all deliveries, but accounted for 7% of all stillborns and 13% of all neonatal deaths. Abruptio placentae, placenta previa, other hemorrhagic complications, and premature rupture of membranes were factors associated frequently with the birth of very low birth weight (<1,500 g) infants.

McCarthy et al.[61] evaluated perinatal outcome in 7,000 twins born in Georgia during 1974–1978. The neonatal death rate was almost seven times that for singleton babies. Interestingly, the weight-specific mortality rate was similar to that of singletons; the excess mortality was due to the high rate of prematurity among twins. Many other studies have confirmed the adverse impact of premature delivery on perinatal outcome in twin gestations. Another important contributor to outcome is congenital malformations. Data from the population-based Metropolitan Atlanta Congenital Defects Program disclosed that the overall rate of malformed infants as well as the incidence of several specific defects was higher for twins than for singletons.[50] The elevated risk appears limited to same-sex twins, and is thus presumably related to monozygosity.[86]

Among 1,195 twins evaluated in the Collaborative Perinatal Project, 219 (18.3%) had malformations: 179 (15.0%) were single defects, and 40 (3.4%) were multiple defects.[66] The frequency of malformations was significantly higher in twins than in singletons from the same population; the increased rate was confirmed to be attributable to monozygotic twins. Among them, monoamniotic twins had significantly higher rates of congenital malformations than diamniotic twins. Black twins were malformed more frequently than white, and males more frequently than females. Twins had a significant (more than twofold) increase in cardiovascular and alimentary tract malformations and smaller increases in central nervous system, musculoskeletal, auditory, and respiratory malformations compared to singletons. Significantly increased among specific malformations were macrocephaly, encephalocele, cleft lip and palate, anomalies of the diaphragm, cardiac septal defects, tracheoesophageal fistula, malformations of the alimentary tract, inguinal and umbilical hernias, and cystic kidney. Concordance rates were significantly higher among monozygotic than among dizygotic twins for any malformation as well as for the categories of major, minor, single and multiple malformations. In the majority of cases, the twins were concordant for the same defects.

ANTEPARTUM MANAGEMENT

Early Detection

Early diagnosis of twin pregnancy is an important aspect of antenatal care and an obvious prerequisite for the application of any form of management designed to improve perinatal outcome. A disappointing number of twins are diagnosed late in the third trimester or at the time of delivery.[25] Even a high index of suspicion and a thorough abdominal examination are insufficient screening techniques for detecting twins.[30,73] A discrepancy between uterine size and gestational age or the detection of two fetal heart rates will alert the astute attendant to some, but not all, multiple pregnancies. Indeed, those remaining undetected by such clinical measures may be at highest risk when unexpected delivery occurs without the requisite personnel or equipment available. This is because twins that deliver very prematurely or in whom intrauterine growth retardation exists are least likely to exhibit excessive uterine size.

Measurements of human placental lactogen,[20,34,58,85] human chorionic gonadotropin,[43] and alpha-fetoprotein[9,64] as well as routine ultrasonography [34,53,73] have been proposed as screening tests to identify twin pregnancies. The former two hormonal tests, although of theoretical value, have proved to be of minimal practical use. Maternal serum alpha-fetoprotein is currently measured in many centers as a screening test for open neural tube defects. Approximately 6% of abnormally elevated values detected during prospective screening will, upon further evaluation, be found to be associated with a twin pregnancy.[64] At institutions that use this screening, it is the most common source for the early second trimester detection of multiple gestation.

Ultrasonography has become the most frequently used and reliable method to diagnose multiple gestations in second and third trimesters. Ultrasound screening should detect almost all twin pregnancies, and provide no false-positive results.[73] Levine and Filly[53] evaluated 595 consecutive pregnant patients, referred for a variety of clinical indications, for the presence of multiple gestation. Among 96 in whom multiple gestation was suspected clinically, 20% were indeed found to have twins. At delivery, all diagnosed twin pregnancies were validated and no unsuspected twins were encountered. A prospective evaluation of a larger population was reported initially by Grennert et al.[33] and updated by Persson and Kullander.[73] An intensive ultrasound screening program was carried out during the interval 1971–1977 with 95% of pregnant women in the community participating. The screening, which required 15 min each and was performed by a group of obstetricians and specially trained midwives, detected 97 (88.2%) of 110 twin pregnancies; no singleton pregnancy was diagnosed falsely as a twin pregnancy. The mean gestational age at diagnosis of twins decreased from 35 weeks prior to the study to 30 weeks in 1973 and declined further to 20 weeks in 1977. The percentage of twin pregnancies undiagnosed until delivery decreased from 57% to 2%.

Modern high-resolution ultrasonography can also often distinguish among the varieties of twin placentation.[4,59] Details of the specific status of the intervening chorioamniotic membranes should be sought in all ultrasound evaluations of twin gestations. Accurate information could affect the techniques used for genetic amniocentesis. It may help elucidate the etiology of intrauterine growth retardation. It could also influence the management of a case with fetal death or with twin-twin transfusion syndrome.

Prevention of Premature Labor

Having diagnosed a twin pregnancy, the obstetrician may choose to alter antepartum management to reduce the likelihood of preterm delivery. Were this easily accomplished, the excess risk associated with twin gestation could be reduced considerably. Regrettably, no option has thus far been proved clearly effective.

Bed Rest

Bed rest (either in hospital or at home) has been advocated as a simple and relatively risk-free method to reduce the incidence of premature labor. However, the retrospective analysis of 177 twin pregnancies by Hawrylyshyn et al.[37] emphasized that 70% of the perinatal deaths occurred before the 30th gestational week. They concluded that although bed rest starting after 30 weeks could potentially prolong some pregnancies, its impact was probably too small and it would be applied too late to reduce overall twin perinatal mortality significantly. Jeffrey et al.[42] reviewed 114 twin pregnancies to evaluate the effect of bed rest on perinatal outcome. Three patient groups were identified. The first consisted of 42 patients in whom the diagnosis of twins was made intrapartum. Another 31 patients were diagnosed in the antepartum period but not offered bed rest. The remaining 41 cases were treated with bed rest initiated at 25 to 40 weeks (mean 32.2 weeks) and varying in duration from 2 days to 9 weeks (mean 3.5 weeks). Five of the treated patients had additional interventions (progesterone, intravenous alcohol, or cervical cerclage). Comparison of these three groups revealed only 5 days difference in mean length of gestation; however, the perinatal mortality and incidence of growth retardation was significantly less in the treatment group. The authors noted that 58% of all the twin perinatal mortality occurred in infants born before 30 weeks and concluded that 30 weeks is too late to initiate treatment.

Weekes et al.[90] evaluated 133 consecutive uncomplicated multiple pregnancies. Bed rest was advised for 60 patients, cerclage for 37 patients, and no active form of management for 36 patients. No significant differences in gestational length, frequency of preterm delivery, low birth weight, or perinatal mortality were noted. Hartikainen-Sorri[36] compared perinatal mortality rates for twins whose mothers had been admitted for hospital bed rest to those who attended a special antenatal care unit and could discern no difference. In the only randomized clinical trial relating to this issue, Saunders et al.[82] compared 105 gravidas with twins allocated to bed rest soon after 32 gestational weeks to 107 control patients. Preterm delivery was more common among the bed rest group. The authors speculated that anxiety associated with prolonged separation from family might be contributory.

Clearly, although prophylactic bed rest for prevention of preterm delivery is practiced commonly, proof of its efficacy is wanting. These discouraging observations notwithstanding, Grennert et al.[33] and Persson and Kullander[73] suggested that a communitywide early pregnancy ultrasonographic screening program provided an opportunity to evaluate the effect of early twin pregnancy detection and in-hospital bed rest management on perinatal outcome. Upon detection of a twin gestation, 86 of 97 women accepted immediate cessation of employment and, at 29 weeks, in-hospital weekday rest (alternating with weekends at home). No drug therapy was given for premature contractions and no twin pregnancy that lasted less than 28 gestational weeks was included in the management protocol. For comparison, control groups were composed of 24 women who did not accept hospitalization or whose twin pregnancy was not detected, and 93 twin pairs born at the same hospital before the study period. The bed rest–treated gravidas delivered the fewest growth-retarded and premature twins and delivered no twin weighing less than 1,500 g. Those treated with bed rest also had the lowest perinatal mortality (equivalent to singleton pregnancy) and reduced incidence and diminished severity of preeclampsia. The results supported bed rest treatment, but the strength of that interpretation must be tempered by the limitations imposed by the study design.

Cervical Cerclage

Zakut et al.[93] evaluated the effect of elective cervical suture on perinatal outcome in 133 patients whose pregnancies resulted from gonadotropin administration. If the obstetric history suggested an incompetent cervix or if uterine size (in the first trimester) was at least 2 weeks greater than expected, cervical cerclage was performed in early second trimester. Twenty women with multiple gestation (including three with triplets and two with quadruplets) were thus treated. The control group was a similar number of patients with multiple pregnancies managed at the same center without cerclage. Statistically significant differences included longer duration of pregnancy, lower perinatal loss and shorter hospital stay in the cerclage group. Dor et al.[21] studied 50 twin pregnancies that occurred after ovulation induction. From this group, 25 women underwent elective cervical MacDonald cerclage at the 13th gestational week. The remaining patients served as control subjects. No significant difference in the incidence of premature labor (36.4% in the sutured group and 34.8% in the control subjects), premature rupture of the membranes (9.1% vs. 13.1%) or neonatal death rates (18.2% vs. 15.2%) was noted. Although Zakut et al. recommend prophylactic cerclage, the small number of patients studied, the choice of unmatched control subjects, and the method of data collection by retrospective chart review weaken the conclusions. It seems more reasonable to reserve this procedure only for those gravidas suspected to have an incompetent cervix on standard diagnostic grounds.

Tocolytic Agents

It seems logical to propose that tocolytic drug treatment might benefit women carrying twin gestations. In addition to reducing the risk of premature labor, such drugs might also have fetal growth-promoting effects by increasing uterine blood flow or metabolic substrate. However, available data (admittedly incomplete) do not consistently support the hypothesis that antepartum administration of beta-agonist drugs will reduce complications in twin pregnancy.

O'Leary[68] noted that prophylactic use of oral terbutaline administered to healthy, low-risk women with twin gestations was associated with an increase in mean birth weight compared to a similar group of control patients.[49] However, Cetrulo and Freeman[13] found no difference with respect to gestational age or birth weight in 98 patients treated with ritodrine or placebo. Marivate et al.[60] administered 5 mg oral fenoterol or placebo to 46 women. The two groups were matched for gestational age at entry (mean 32 weeks) and for duration of treatment (mean 5 weeks). No demonstrable benefit accrued to patients who were treated. The authors concluded that prophylactic administration of fenoterol neither enhanced fetal growth nor reduced the frequency of preterm labor. Lipshitz and Schneider[54] criticized this conclusion by summarizing the study's weaknesses: the dose of medication was inadequate to maintain a therapeutic level throughout the day, the number of patients entered in the study was insufficient to allow appropriate statistical analysis, and continuous use of self-administered medications is a difficult goal to achieve or validate. Most other studies that have attempted to evaluate the effectiveness of a specific medicinal treatment to prolong twin pregnancy share these weaknesses.

Fetal Assessment

Once the diagnosis of twin pregnancy has been established, the obstetrician is faced with the need to provide adequate prenatal surveillance. Clinical evaluation by physical examination has considerable limitations in evaluation of twin fetuses. Fetal weight or well-being, cord entanglement, early signs of twin-twin transfusion, and fetal presentations can seldom be determined without modern diagnostic technology.

Fetal Weight

Friedman et al.[27] reviewed 182 sets of twins in which the birth order had been documented. The first twin was heavier in 42.9% of deliveries; however, the mean weight of first-born twins was 21 g larger than that of second-born twins. The apparent paradox was explained by observing that when the first twin was heavier, the difference in birth weights was great (3.2% were heavier by 750 g and 1.6% by 1,000 g), but when the second twin was heavier, the two neonates differed by only a small amount (0.5% of second twins were heavier by 750 g, and none was heavier than the first by 1,000 g). Birth weights were virtually identical for infants weighing less than 2,999 g; but in 31 sets in which at least one twin weighed more than 3,000 g, the difference in weight was significant. Moreover, the differences in weight increased with increasing birth weight.

Sonographic assessment of fetal growth and weight is an integral part of the detection of intrauterine growth retardation in singleton pregnancies. Similarly, estimation of intertwin weight differences is of value. O'Brien et al.[67] noted that weight differences greater than 20% resulted in the birth of at least one small-for-gestational-age infant more than 50% of the time. If the actual birth weight differences were greater than 30%, approximately two-thirds of the smaller infants were small for gestational age. In these weight-discordant groups the incidence of fetal death and distress was also increased. The inherent errors in estimation of fetal weight notwithstanding,[91] ultrasonographic evaluation of fetal weight should be performed routinely at 28 and 34 gestational weeks to best assess fetal size and to identify discordancy. Forewarned by the above associations and alerted by ultrasonographic weight estimates, the clinician may intensify surveillance of potentially affected fetuses. Scheer[83] considered an ultrasonographically detected difference in biparietal diameter of greater than 6 mm to be indicative of significant twin discordancy and noted the incidence of fetal death increased significantly when differences in biparietal diameters were greater than 7 mm. Unfortunately, such biparietal diameter difference is an unreliable indicator of bad outcome.[51,52]

Fetal Well-Being

The routine use of sonographic and serial fetal heart rate testing has been proposed as a method to reduce the risk of third trimester demise, intrapartum complications, and other aspects of neonatal morbidity and mortality in twin gestation. Blake et al.[8] performed serial nonstress fetal heart rate testing upon 94 patients with multiple gestations (193 fetuses). Reactive testing was associated with an uncomplicated perinatal outcome in 89% of the cases. Fetuses with a nonreactive pattern had a significantly higher incidence of perinatal morbidity, including fetal distress in labor (79%), asphyxia (48%), and intrauterine growth retardation (28%). Overall perinatal mortality of 21/1,000) was comparable to that observed in singleton pregnancies. Fetuses with nonreactive tests had a perinatal death rate that was more than six times that of the reactive ones (80 of 1,000 vs. 12 of 1,000). Lenstrup[50] evaluated 122 nonstress tests performed upon 27 sets of twins in the third trimester. Fifty fetuses, including 13 that were small for gestational age, had reactive tests; only 1 (2%) required admission to a neonatal intensive care unit. Four fetuses had nonreactive tests; all required intensive neonatal care. Abnormal cardiotocographic findings included reduced variability, late decelerations, and absence of spontaneous accelerations. Although there was no perinatal mortality, abnormal tests were associated with a statistically significant increased rate of neonatal morbidity, including intrauterine growth retardation and low 1-min Apgar scores. The predictive value of a normal nonstress test to exclude growth retardation was 95.7% and the positive predictive value of an abnormal test to diagnose growth retardation was 75.0%. Knuppel et al.[47] noted no fetal demises among 90 twin pairs in association with weekly nonstress tests that were initiated at 30 gestational weeks and were followed by a contraction stress test if indicated.

Lodeiro et al.[55] found the high sensitivity and specificity of the complete fetal biophysical profile (a nonstress test, fetal breathing movements, fetal tone and movement, amniotic fluid volume, and placental grading) contributed to its accuracy as a method to evaluate fetal well-being in twins. However, because a reactive nonstress test was always followed by a normal biophysical profile, they concluded there is little value in performing a formal biophysical profile if the nonstress test is reactive. In the presence of a nonreactive test, by contrast, the biophysical profile can differentiate between normal transient lack of activity, most likely related to fetal state, and nonreactivity that could result from fetal asphyxia.

Continuous-wave Doppler ultrasonography is a recently introduced noninvasive method to estimate umbilical blood flow. In twins, each umbilical cord pattern can be imaged individually. The method has been reported[24,30] to be useful to detect twin transfusion syndrome and intra-uterine growth retardation. Further evaluation will be necessary to confirm its value.

In summary, antepartum nonstress testing is a highly reliable and predictive tool in the assessment of multiple gestations. For asymptomatic gravidas, serial nonstress testing should begin between the 28th and 32nd gestational week. Ultrasonography should be reserved for evaluation of other suspected complications (congenital defects, growth retardation, twin-twin transfusion) or for follow-up of suspicious or abnormal bioelectric tests.

Management of Fetal Demise

The death of one fetus in the second or third trimester may place both the other twin and the mother in jeopardy. The living fetus remains at risk for complications due to the same factors that contributed to the co-twin's death, or to the transplacental passage of thromboplastin or placental fragments into its circulation.[17,35] The gravida is at risk for complications associated with disseminated intravascular coagulopathy. The degree of risk cannot be ascertained from the small number of cases reported but appears to be partially dependent upon the zygosity of the twins and gestational week at the time of the demise.

Banchi[2] reported the fetal demise of one of three triplets in the 16th gestational week. The other two fetuses were delivered 131 days later without apparent complications. Planned selected abortion at 20 gestational weeks by intracardiac air embolization of one of two dizygotic twins discordant for Tay-Sachs disease was also followed by the uncomplicated progression of the pregnancy and delivery of a normal surviving co-twin.[79] These studies suggest that a fetus may die during the first half of pregnancy without affecting its co-twin adversely. Of note, following early second trimester losses, alpha-fetoprotein (both serum and amniotic fluid) and amniotic fluid acetylcholinesterase determination have been noted to remain elevated for up to 11 weeks.[5]

One hypothetical sequence of events that may be initiated by the death in utero of one monozygotic twin is that of clot formation, followed by occlusion of blood vessels and consequent distal tissue necrosis in the surviving co-twin. Hughes and Miskin[39] provided support for this in their description of a surviving twin whose brain had appeared normal on ultrasonography before the death of the co-twin at 21 gestational weeks. The survivor had the onset of multicystic encephalomalacia that was documented on sequential antenatal sonograms. Choulot et al.[15] reported the stillbirth of one monozygotic twin associated with the birth of the liveborn co-twin, who demonstrated diffuse hypotonia and seizures. Microcephaly and severe encephalopathy were also noted. Szymonowicz et al.[88] described six cases of intrauterine fetal demise that occurred 1 to 11 weeks prior to the delivery of the surviving monozygotic co-twin. All six survivors had central nervous system infarcts and three had pulmonary and hepatic infarcts. Four of the six survivors died and the remaining two had considerable handicaps. D'Alton et al.[18] reviewed 15 cases of fetal demise that occurred in multiple gestations; nine monozygotic twins were represented in the series. Delivery was accomplished if the gestational age was at least 37 weeks, if there was evidence of preeclampsia, or if amniocentesis revealed pulmonary maturity. Steroids were given if the amniotic fluid phospholipid tests revealed immaturity (gestational age ranged from 27 to 39 weeks) or an amniocentesis could not be achieved. All co-twins (and co-triplets) survived; however, one survivor of the monozygotic twin pair had multicystic encephalomalacia.

Hanna and Hill[35] reported three dizygotic twins born at least 3 weeks after the demise of their co-twins. The pregnancies continued without apparent associated complications. However, one surviving co-twin born at 32 gestational weeks demonstrated neurologic deficits; computed tomography revealed dysmorphic changes in the cerebral hemispheres. Although monozygotic multiple gestations appear to be at greater risk for maternal and co-twin coagulopathies than dizygotic pregnancies, insufficient cases have been reported to allow complete confidence in this regard.

Romero et al.[80] described the successful prolongation of such a preterm gestation using intermittent intravenous heparin. Delivery of a more mature fetus was accomplished 10 weeks after the demise of its co-twin and at least 6 weeks after the first documentation of coagulopathy. The placenta was monochorionic-diamniotic. Although this approach cannot yet be considered standard care in these cases, it does lend credence to the notion that fetal thrombosis may play an important role in the outcome for the co-twin.

Of great importance in cases of death of one twin is that the birth of the surviving neonate should not cause the physician to forget to aid and support the parents as they grieve for their lost child. In one reported study 14 such mothers were questioned as to their feelings and all continued to think of their surviving child as a twin; 6 had feelings of resentment toward the survivor, and all felt their loss had been underestimated by the health care providers.[10] The parents' joy and grief must be acknowledged and they must be encouraged to voice their often conflicting but intense feelings.

The infrequency of this complication precludes offering firm recommendations for its management; however, prudent management would include (regardless of the apparent zygosity of the twins) prompt delivery of the remaining co-twin if at or near term or earlier if pulmonary maturity is assured. If remote from term, conservative management may benefit a dizygotic survivor. If monozygosity has been determined, however, delivery should be considered as soon as feasible because there are no currently available tests to permit early detection of co-twin morbidity. All gravidas should be followed by obtaining frequent coagulation profiles and all neonates should be evaluated for multiple infarcts.

Twin-Twin Transfusion Syndrome

The transfusion syndrome has been diagnosed in 5.5% to 14.6% of monochorionic twins. Although vascular anastomoses are present in 85% to 100% of monochorionic placentas, not all are associated with this syndrome. It is characterized classically by a small anemic fetus (the donor), a large plethoric co-twin (the recipient), and varying degrees of fetal stress. A common presenting sign (although a late manifestation of the pathophysiologic sequence) of this syndrome is the acute onset of polyhydramnios in the second trimester. Ten such cases were reported by Schneider et al.[84] Their mean gestational age at diagnosis was 23.5 weeks. All women were hospitalized, except one who underwent termination of pregnancy. Treatment consisted of bed rest, periodic removal of amniotic fluid, and tocolytic therapy. Mean age at delivery was 30.4 weeks. Eight of the 18 newborns survived; none had congenital malformations.

Galea et al.[28] reported 42 liveborn twin pairs with monochorionic placentas. Thirty-two (76.2%) of the placentas had vascular anastomoses and 21 (65.6%) of these had uneventful pregnancies. Twin-twin transfusion of varying severity occurred in 11 affected twin pairs. Twenty-four pairs of stillborn twin fetuses were also studied; 8 (33.3%) had evidence of vascular communications.

Occasionally, cardiac failure in the recipient twin may be noted remote from term. DeLia et al.[19] described the use of maternal digoxin therapy, instituted at 27 gestational weeks, to reverse fetal edema, ascites, and hydramnios. Signs of failure resolved; living twins were delivered at 34 weeks by cesarean section.

Monoamniotic Twins

This variety of twinning (representing less than 3% of all twin gestations) is at highest risk for complications and poor perinatal outcome. In a comparison of the course and outcome of 23 such pregnancies to 1,056 diamniotic twin pregnancies, Lumme and Saarikoski[56] noted the following major complications: polyhydramnios (26% vs. 6% in diamniotic), preterm labor (70% vs. 18%), cesarean section (39% vs. 20%), cord entanglement (17%), and cord prolapse (13%). The perinatal mortality rate was 28% (vs. 5% for diamniotic twins). The most common causes of death were respiratory distress syndrome, congenital abnormalities, and twin-twin transfusion syndrome. Fortunately, the prenatal diagnosis of monoamniotic twins can be made with reasonable confidence using modern sonographic techniques.[87] Forewarned, the obstetrician can plan an elective cesarean birth near term, thereby diminishing late pregnancy complications. In one such case, cord entanglement was diagnosed by ultrasonography; prompt action was associated with survival of both twins.[7]

Conjoined Twins

Conjoined twins occur in approximately 1% of monozygotic twins.[87] The condition has been diagnosed as early as the 13th gestational week.[57] Sakala[81] suggested the following obstetric management: rule out con-

joined twins whenever twins are diagnosed; establish the extent of con-
joining; determine postnatal viability; determine the route of delivery
(and the institution in which delivery will take place); meet parental
psychosocial needs; and provide postpartum counseling and follow-up
of affected families.

Sonographic criteria that will facilitate the diagnosis of conjoined twins
include fetal heads and body parts that are at the same level and imaged
in the same body plane; fetal spines that exhibit unusual extension or
proximity; no change in the relative positions of the fetuses noted after
movement, manipulation, or the passage of time; the presence of a
continuous nonseparated external skin contour; absence of a separating
placental membrane; and the presence of specific fetal anomalies usually
seen with conjoined twins, especially the presence of more than three
vessels within a single umbilical cord.[23,32,48]

INTRAPARTUM MANAGEMENT

Anesthesia

Crawford[16] reviewed 112 patients with multiple pregnancies delivered
under epidural block and concluded that this form of anesthesia could be
beneficial to the infant. Patients were subdivided according to gestational
age (greater or less than 36 weeks) and the presence or absence of
obstetric abnormality. There was no significant difference in 5-min Apgar
scores in any of the groups when babies delivered with epidural anesthesia were compared with those delivered without anesthesia. The epidural
group had, as expected, a longer mean time from full dilatation to
delivery of the first twin; however, the interval between delivery of the
first and second twins was minimally shorter in the epidural group.
Forceps or vacuum-assisted delivery of an infant presenting as a vertex
was more frequent when epidural block was in progress as was the
incidence of breech extraction. In an evaluation of the effect of peridural
bupivacaine on 14 twin and 10 singleton deliveries, James et al.[40] came to
similar conclusions. Acid-base and blood gas values were similar for both
groups of mothers, as they were for first-born twins and for singleton
infants; however, second twins had a significantly lower umbilical artery
pH (7.23 vs. 7.29), higher umbilical vein partial carbon dioxide pressure
(Pco_2), and lower oxygen saturation than singleton control subjects.
Five-minute Apgar scores were seven or greater for all twins. The authors
concluded that epidural was a safe form of anesthesia for twin labor and

delivery because it obviated the need for anesthesia and analgesia which have more potential for central nervous system depression.

Based on experience involving more than 200 singleton breech deliveries managed with epidural block, Gellestad et al.[29] conjectured that epidural anesthesia averts the need for general anesthesia for the operative procedures often required for twin deliveries. They gave epidural blocks to 28 women with twin gestations (9 nulliparas, 19 multiparas). Control patients (4 nulliparas, 20 multiparas) with twins received meperidine, diazepam, and nitrous oxide. The mean duration of labor was increased by 2 hr, and the second stage of labor was often prolonged in the epidural group. This prolongation was the reason for 25% of the operative vaginal deliveries. All infants were liveborn and the distribution of Apgar scores and acid-base values in the two groups was similar. Jaschevatzky et al. confirmed these findings.[41]

The consensus of the most recent reports is that the advantages of epidural anesthesia outweigh its disadvantages for the management of twin labor and delivery. Abnormalities of labor requiring stimulation or operative manipulation are neither increased excessively by the use of epidural anesthesia nor do they appear to pose an insurmountable clinical problem for a well-trained obstetrician. Inhalation anesthesia with its acknowledged greater risks of aspiration and maternal mortality[3,31] is being used with decreasing frequency. Although the issue of anesthetic management for cesarean twin births has not been addressed in clinical trials, it would be prudent, except for emergency situations, to choose conduction anesthesia in these clinical settings. This may need to be supplemented in those unusual circumstances in which inhalational agents are needed for complete myometrial relaxation to facilitate intrauterine manipulation of the second twin.

Choice of Delivery Route

In 1973, Farooqui et al.[25] published an extensive and influential evaluation of 333 consecutive patients who delivered twins. Assisted breech delivery was associated with a small but significant increase in neonatal mortality, as was total breech extraction of the first twin when compared with results of spontaneous and/or low forceps vertex delivery. The author concluded that breech extraction was "relatively safe when indicated . . . in skilled hands." Nonetheless, Taylor[89] commented that Farooqui et al. had actually documented a three- to fivefold increase in perinatal mortality associated with extraction of breeches and advised that cesarean section would be more prudent if one or both twins presented other than as a vertex. Cetrulo et al.[14] also noted that the frequency of abnormal presentation was directly related to the perinatal mortality rate and implied that mortality might be decreased with more liberal use of cesarean section in these situations. Authors of current textbooks[63,75] accept a noncephalic presentation of either twin as a valid indication for cesarean section. Nevertheless, the data base on which such management plans are promulgated is less than ideal in many respects.[45]

Farooqui et al.[25] evaluated clinical events that occurred in the interval 1959–1970. No attempt was made to divide the data into separate time periods to assess whether changes in obstetric or pediatric care over the study interval could have led to improvements in outcome. Virtually no electronic fetal monitoring was carried out in that decade and, as almost one-third of second twins were unsuspected and therefore only diagnosed at delivery, absolutely no monitoring of or pediatric preparation for the delivery of those vaginally delivered second twins was possible. Specific details related to the delivery, the type of anesthesia, the level of experience of the obstetrician, and the neonatal care of the infants who died is lacking. Although Farooqui et al. did document an increase in neonatal deaths in infants delivered by breech extraction, Taylor's[89] conclusion that cesarean section is always the best method of delivery cannot be drawn with certainty from these data. Even Cetrulo and associates'[14] recommendation for more frequent cesarean deliveries is based on observations preceding the current monitoring era and in multiple pregnancies with more than two fetuses.

A retrospective review of 3 years' experience with twin pregnancies diagnosed prior to delivery at the Boston City Hospital and the Brigham and Women's Hospital, Boston, was undertaken to evaluate the relationship of delivery route and perinatal outcome in two tertiary care centers.[1] During the period of study, 45% of twins were delivered by cesarean section. The 111 cesarean births were performed for the following reasons: one or both twins not in a vertex presentation (37.7%), either twin showing evidence of stress (25.2%), uterine scar (21.6%), and maternal complication (9.9%); no indication was recorded in the remaining 5.4%, half of which involved cesarean section for the second twin after vaginal delivery of the first twin. Deleting twins who weighed less than 1,500 g, had fatal congenital anomalies, twin-twin transfusion syndrome, or sudden infant death syndrome, the authors found no neonatal mortality. When similar corrections were applied to 137 vaginally delivered twin pairs, there were also no deaths except for the neonatal death of a second born twin associated with a fatal intracranial hemorrhage from midforceps delivery. There were no neonatal deaths of any infants delivered vaginally from a nonvertex presentation.

Morbidity was evaluated by comparing 5-min Apgar scores for all nonvertex twins delivered by cesarean section from women who had uneventful pregnancies to all second-born twins who were delivered by breech extraction from similarly asymptomatic women with uncomplicated labors. Only three (3.9%) of the 76 infants born by breech extraction had a 5-min Apgar score less than 7, and all did well in the nursery. A similar percentage of the 74 infants born from a nonvertex presentation by cesarean section were also depressed.

Chervenak et al. analyzed 362 twin pairs delivered at Yale-New Haven Medical Center.[11,12] Of 139 (38.4%) twin pairs in the vertex-nonvertex presentation, 35 were delivered by elective cesarean section. Of the remaining 104 twin pairs, 4 (three oblique presentations and one breech presentation) were noted to have spontaneously turned to vertex presentation subsequent to the delivery of the first twin; these were delivered vaginally. External version was attempted upon 24 of the remaining 100 fetuses. It was successful in 19 (79.2%) cases. Cesarean section was performed upon the other five gravidas. The remaining 76 breech-presenting fetuses were delivered vaginally. One difficult total breech extraction resulted in significant birth trauma (unspecified) but the immediate neonatal course of this infant was uncomplicated.

Chervenak et al. concluded that there is general agreement that vaginal delivery is appropriate for vertex-vertex presenting twins and that cesarean section is indicated if the first twin is in a nonvertex presentation. For those vertex-nonvertex twin presentations in which the estimated individual fetal weight is less than 2,000 g (less than 34 gestational weeks) a prudent decision would also be to deliver by cesarean section. But individualization (described below) of the delivery route may be appropriate for the remaining approximately one-third of term or near-term twin pregnancies in which the presentation is vertex-nonvertex.[69,70]

Labor and Delivery

The course of labor in pregnancy complicated by twins has been evaluated by Friedman.[26] Both nulliparas and multiparas exhibit a significant shortening of latent phase that is inversely related to the initial or prelabor cervical dilatation. The length of active phase was related directly to the combined fetal weight. With increasing birth weight, a prolongation of active and deceleration phase and a progressive diminution of the maximum slope of dilatation and descent was observed.

Electronic fetal heart rate monitoring allows surveillance of the state of oxygenation of both fetuses simultaneously. Satisfactory monitoring can sometimes be achieved with two external monitors, although two ultrasound transducers placed close to one another may interfere with each other's signal. A combination of internal (for the first twin) and external (for the second) devices tends to be more useful. Read and Miller[78] presented a method for recording internal uterine pressure on two monitors simultaneously. An internal uterine pressure catheter and a scalp electrode are applied after rupture of the first twin's membranes, as in a singleton pregnancy. The second twin's heart rate is evaluated by any external technique using a second monitor. The outlet of the exhaust valve of one pressure transducer is connected to the dual input connection of the second with intravenous tubing. The exact duplication of the contraction pattern allows evaluation of the relationship of either fetal heart rate pattern to the contraction.

As the second stage of labor nears termination, the obstetrician should confirm that the delivery room, nurses, anesthesiologist, and pediatrician are prepared for the delivery of two babies. Although vaginal delivery may be planned, delivery of one or both babies by cesarean section is an emergency that must be anticipated. It is therefore prudent to conduct the delivery in a room in which surgery can be performed.

Delivery of the vertex-presenting first twin is accomplished as for a singleton. If an epidural block has been placed previously, no additional anesthesia will usually be necessary; however, a local or pudendal block may be used to complement the pain relief provided by the epidural block if necessary. If no epidural anesthetic has been employed, delivery is conducted without anesthesia or under local or pudendal block. A skilled anesthesiologist should be in attendance to administer inhalation anesthesia if necessary. Guiding the vertex of the second twin into the pelvis by Kristeller abdominal pressure (guided by ultrasonography), rupturing membranes, using oxytocin to augment labor and, if indicated, performing operative forceps delivery may be appropriate techniques for use in individual circumstances.

Occasionally after the vaginal delivery of the first twin, the second twin will need to be delivered by cesarean section. Indications include fetal distress, a prolapsed cord, or vaginal bleeding. Rattan et al.[76] reviewed such cases and noted no increase in maternal or perinatal morbidity or mortality when the second twin was thus delivered.

If the second twin remains in a breech presentation or transverse lie, a difficult decision is required as to the route of delivery. Vaginal delivery may be anticipated if the fetal heart rate pattern is normal, the pelvis is adequate, and the fetal head is not hyperextended (as determined by intrapartum radiography or sonography). External version may be attempted by an obstetrician skilled in performing this manipulation. If successful, vaginal delivery of the non-vertex-presenting fetus is conducted as above. If unsuccessful, the clinician may await spontaneous descent of the breech or perform a cesarean section. The only safe option for a persistent transverse lie is cesarean section. If cesarean section is chosen, it can be performed under the previously placed epidural block or, based on the individual circumstance, inhalation anesthesia or newly placed conduction block can be given. Although each case must be judged on an individual basis, it should be borne in mind that total breech extraction may be accompanied by considerable birth trauma, even in a second twin. Good judgment often requires safer alternatives.

Birth Order and Delivery Interval

Young et al.[92] examined differences between 80 firstborn and secondborn twins with respect to Apgar score, umbilical venous and arterial blood gases, and acid-base data. Statistically significant differences favoring the firstborn were found only in 1-min Apgar score, umbilical venous pH, partial pressure of oxygen (Po_2) and Pco_2, and umbilical artery Po_2. When these measurements were examined with respect to route of delivery, zygosity, interval between twins, and presentation, the results still favored the firstborn twin. Comparable findings were obtained by Eskes et al.[22] who examined data on 76 twin pregnancies. Lower Apgar scores and acidemia in the umbilical artery of the second twin were noted, unrelated to the time interval between twins. These differences (despite similar perinatal mortality) suggest that the secondborn twin has potentially greater susceptibility to hypoxia. In the study described above, Farooqui et al.[25] noted that although 95.8% of second twins were delivered within 20 min of their sibling there were no neonatal deaths among those delivered 20 min or more after their older twin. Muller-Holve et al.[65] evaluated umbilical artery pH in 35 vaginally delivered twin pairs in which both were vertex and weighed more than 2,000 g, and noted that although clinical status (not specifically defined) did not correlate well with delivery interval, cord pH less than 7.15 occurred more frequently when the delivery interval was greater than 7 to 10 min. The lack of correlation between the pH and the clinical status was postulated to represent a lag time between the presence of biochemical acidosis and clinical manifestations of hypoxia. The smaller the twins, the authors cautioned, the briefer this lag phase might be; however, they concluded that undue haste should not accompany the delivery of the second twin.

Rayburn et al.[77] evaluated the time interval between delivery of 115 first and second twin pairs. Ultrasonography and continuous electronic monitoring of the fetal heart rate were undertaken while watching for vaginal bleeding. Oxytocin was used if contractions subsided within 10 min of delivery of the first twin. The mean interval was 21 min (range 1 to 134 min) and was not influenced by the type of presentation or the method of delivery. The elapsed delivery interval was within 15 min in 61% of cases, 16 to 30 min in 24%, and more than 30 min in 15%. Apgar scores of the second infant were generally high regardless of the interval (including the longest) and neonatal complications were uncommon.

Early studies evaluating delivery interval were performed prior to the advent of electronic fetal heart rate monitoring. The outcome for the second twin does not seem clearly related to the interval between deliveries as long as the fetal heart rate pattern has remained normal. Based on recent literature and experience, it seems reasonable to monitor the second twin's heart rate pattern and to time delivery based on the state of fetal oxygenation, the evaluation of descent of the presenting part, and the presence of maternal complications. This approach appears to minimize the need for potentially traumatic delivery.

REFERENCES

1. Acker D, Leiberman M, Holbrook RH, James O, Phillippe M, Edelin K: Delivery of the second twin. *Obstet Gynecol* 1982;59:710–711.

2. Banchi MT: Triplet pregnancy with second trimester abortion and delivery of twins at 35 weeks' gestation. *Obstet Gynecol* 1984;64:728–730.

3. Barry AP: I.M.A. maternal mortality report-972. *J Irish Med Assoc* 1973;66:637–644.

4. Barss VA, Benacerraf BR, Frigoletto FD: Ultrasonographic determination of chorion type in twin gestations. *Obstet Gynecol* 1985;66:779–784.

5. Bass HN, Oliver JB, Srinivasan M, Petrucha R, Ng W, Lee JE: Persistently elevated alpha fetoprotein and acetylcholinesterase in amniotic fluid from a normal fetus following demise of its twin. *Prenat Diagn* 1986;6:33–35.

6. Benirschke K, Chung KK: Multiple pregnancy. *N Engl J Med* 1973;288:1276–1283.

7. Bhakthavathsalan A, Heinz L, Wafalosky J, Armstrong CL, Kirkhope TG: Ultrasound diagnosis of monoamniotic twins with cord entanglement: Case report with double survival. *J Clin Ultrasound* 1985;13:137–140.

8. Blake GD, Knuppel RA, Ingardia CJ, Lake M, Aumann G, Hanson M: Evaluation of nonstress fetal heart rate testing in multiple gestations. *Obstet Gynecol* 1984;63:528–532.

9. Brock DJH, Barron L, Duncan P, Scrimgeour JB, Watt M: Significance of elevated midtrimester plasma alpha-fetoprotein values. *Lancet* 1979;1:1281–1282.

10. Bryan EM: The death of a newborn twin: How can support for parents be improved? *Acta Genet Med Gemellol (Roma)* 1986;35:115–118.

11. Chervenak FA: The controversy of mode of delivery in twins: The intrapartum management of twin gestation (Part II). *Semin Perinatol* 1986;10:44–49.

12. Chervenak FA, Johnson RE, Youcha S, Hobbins JC, Berkowitz RL: Intrapartum management of the twin gestation. *Obstet Gynecol* 1985;65:119–123.

13. Cetrulo CL, Freeman RK: Ritodrine HCl for the prevention of premature labor in twin pregnancies. *Acta Genet Med Gemellol (Roma)* 1976;25:321–324.

14. Cetrulo CL, Ingardia CJ, Sbarra AJ: Management of multiple gestation. *Clin Obstet Gynecol* 1980;23:533–547.

15. Choulot JJ, Lecleru MA, Saint Martin J: Cerebral lesion in surviving twins. *Arch Fr Pediatr* 1982;39:105–107.

16. Crawford JS: An appraisal of lumbar epidural blockade in labor in patients with multiple pregnancy. *Br J Obstet Gynaecol* 1975;82:929–935.

17. Dallay D, Soumireu-Mourat J: Problems posed by the death of one fetus in a twin pregnancy. *Rev Fr Gynecol Obstet* 1985;80:877–879.

18. D'Alton MA, Newton ER, Cetrulo CL: Intrauterine fetal demise in multiple gestation. *Acta Genet Med Gemellol (Roma)* 1984;33:43–49.

19. DeLia J, Emery MG, Sheafor SA, Jennison TA: Twin transfusion syndrome: Successful in utero treatment with digoxin. *Int J Gynaecol Obstet* 1985;23:197–201.

20. Dhont M, Thiery M, Vandekerckhove D: Hormonal screening for detection of twin pregnancies. *Lancet* 1976;2:861 (letter).

21. Dor J, Shalev J, Mashiach S, Jongsma HW: Elective cervical suture of twin pregnancies diagnosed ultrasonically in the first trimester following induced ovulation. *Gynecol Obstet Invest* 1982;13:55–59.

22. Eskes TK, Timmer H, Kollee LA: The second twin. *Eur J Obstet Gynecol Reprod Biol* 1985;19:159–166.

23. Fagan CJ: Antepartum diagnosis of conjoined twins by ultrasonography. *Am J Roentgenol* 1977;129:921–925.

24. Farmakides G, Schulman H, Saldana LR, Bracero LA, Fleischer A, Rochelson B: Surveillance of twin pregnancy with umbilical arterial velocimetry. *Am J Obstet Gynecol* 1985;153:789–792.

25. Farooqui MO, Grossman JH, Shannon RR: A review of twin pregnancy and perinatal mortality. *Obstet Gynecol Surv* 1973;28:144–153.

26. Friedman EA: Uterine factors, in Friedman EA (ed): *Labor: Clinical Evaluation and Management*, ed 2. New York, Appleton-Century-Crofts, 1978, pp 216–221.

27. Friedman EA, Sachtleben MR, Friedman LM: Relative birthweight of twins. *Obstet Gynecol* 1976;49:717–721.

28. Galea P, Scott JM, Goel KM: Feto-fetal transfusion syndrome. *Arch Dis Child* 1982;57:781–785.

29. Gellestad S, Sagen N: Epidural block in twin labor and delivery. *Acta Anesth Scand* 1977;21:504–512.

30. Giles WB, Trudiner BJ, Cook CM: Umbilical waveforms in twin pregnancy. *Acta Genet Med Gemellol (Roma)* 1985;34:233–237.

31. Grall JY, Arvis P, Boog G, Bouchet L, Cardi S, Cloup B, Collasson F, Herlicoviez M, Lefevre J, Nolet B, Rouffeteau D: Perinatal mortality in twin pregnancy. 576 case histories. *Gynecol Obstet Biol Reprod (Paris)* 1980;9:471–477.

32. Gray CM, Nix NG, Wallace AJ: Thoracopagus twins: Prenatal diagnosis. *Radiology* 1950;54:398–402.

33. Grennert L, Gennser G, Persson PH, Kallander S, Thorell J: Ultrasound and human placental lactogen screening for early detection of twin pregnancies. *Lancet* 1976;1:4–7.

34. Guaschino S, Spinillo A, Carnevale P, La Penna O, Pesando PC, Rondini G: Assessment of peri-neonatal mortality and morbidity risk in twin pregnancy. *Clin Exp Obstet Gynecol* 1986;13:18–25.

35. Hanna JH, Hill JM: Single intrauterine fetal demise in multiple gestation. *Obstet Gynecol* 1984;63:126–130.

36. Hartikainen-Sorri AL: Is routine hospitalization in twin pregnancy necessary? A follow-up study. *Acta Genet Med Gemellol (Roma)* 1985;34:189–192.

37. Hawrylyshyn PA, Barkin M, Bernstein A, Papsin FR: Twin pregnancies—a continuing perinatal challenge. *Obstet Gynecol* 1982;59:463–466.

38. Ho SK, Wu PYK: Perinatal factors and neonatal morbidity in twin pregnancy. *Am J Obstet Gynecol* 1975;122:979–985.

39. Hughes HE, Miskin M: Congenital microcephaly due to vascular disruption: In utero documentation. *Pediatrics* 1986;78:85–87.

40. James FM, Crawford JS, Davies P, Crawley M: Lumbar epidural analgesia for labor and delivery of twins. *Am J Obstet Gynecol* 1976;127:176–180.

41. Jaschevatzky OE, Shalit A, Levy Y, Grünstein S: Epidural analgesia during labor in twin pregnancy. *Br J Obstet Gynaecol* 1977;84:327–331.

42. Jeffrey RL, Bowers WQ, Delandy JJ: Role of bed rest in twin gestation. *Obstet Gynecol* 1977;43:821–822.

43. Jovanovic L, Landesman R, Saxena B: Screening for twin pregnancy. *Science* 1977;198:738–741.

44. Keith L, Ellis R, Berger GS, Depp R: The Northwestern University multihospital twin study. *Am J Obstet Gynecol* 1980;138:781–791.

45. Kelsick F, Minkoff N: Management of the breech second twin. *Am J Obstet Gynecol* 1982;144:783–787.

46. Khrouf N, Barkallah N, Ben Miled S, Ben Bechr S, Gastli H: Twin pregnancies: Incidence, fetal development and perinatal mortality. *J Gynecol Obstet Biol Reprod (Paris)* 1983;12:619–623.

47. Knuppel RA, Rattan PK, Scerbo JC, O'Brien WF: Intrauterine fetal death in twins after 32 weeks of gestation. *Obstet Gynecol* 1985;65:172–175.

48. Koontz WL, Herbert WNP, Seeds JW, Cefalo RC: Ultrasonography in the antepartum diagnosis of conjoined twins. *J Reprod Med* 1983;28:627–631.

49. Layde PM, Erickson JD, Falek A, McCarthy BJ: Congenital malformation in twins. *Am J Hum Genet* 1980;32:69–78.

50. Lenstrup C: Predictive value of antepartum nonstress test in multiple pregnancies. *Acta Obstet Gynecol Scand* 1984;63:597–601.

51. Leveno KJ, Santos-Ramos R, Duenholter J, Reish JS, Whalley PJ: A table of biparietal diameters for normal twin fetuses and a comparison with singletons. *Am J Obstet Gynecol* 1979;135:727–731.

52. Leveno KJ, Santos-Ramos R, Duenholter J, Reish JS, Whalley PJ: Sonar cephalometry in twin pregnancy: Discordancy of the biparietal diameter after 28 weeks gestation. *Am J Obstet Gynecol* 1980;138:615–619.

53. Levine SC, Filly RA: Rapid B-scan (real time) ultrasonography in the identification of twin pregnancies. *Obstet Gynecol* 1978;51:170–172.

54. Lipshitz J, Schneider JM: Use of fenoterol to delay preterm labor and to promote fetal growth in twin pregnancies. *Am J Obstet Gynecol* 1978;131:230–234.

55. Lodeiro JG, Vintzileos AM, Feinstein SJ, Campbell WA, Nochimson DJ: Fetal biophysical profile in twin gestations. *Obstet Gynecol* 1986;67:824–828.

56. Lumme RH, Saarikoski SV: Monoamniotic twin pregnancy. *Acta Genet Med Gemellol (Roma)* 1986;35:99–105.

57. Maggio M, Callan NA, Hamod KA: The first trimester ultrasonographic diagnosis of conjoined twins. *Am J Obstet Gynecol* 1985;152:833–837.

58. Magiste M, VonSchenk HV, Sjoberg NO, Thorell JI, Aberg H: Screening for detecting twin pregnancy. *Am J Obstet Gynecol* 1976;126:697–698.

59. Mahony BS, Filly RA, Callen PW: Amnionicity and chorionicity in twin pregnancies: Prediction using ultrasound. *Radiology* 1985;155:205–209.

60. Marivate M, DeVilliers KQ, Fairbrothe P: Effect of prophylactic outpatient administration of fenoterol at time of onset of spontaneous labor and fetal growth rate in twin pregnancy. *Am J Obstet Gynecol* 1977;128:707–708.

61. McCarthy B, Sachs BP, Layde P: Epidemiology of neonatal mortality in twins. *Am J Obstet Gynecol* 1981;141:252–256.

62. Medearis AL, Jonas HJ, Stockbauer JW: Perinatal deaths in twin pregnancy. *Am J Obstet Gynecol* 1979;134:413–418.

63. Merkatz IR, Fanaroff AA: Antenatal and intrapartum care of the high risk infant, in Klaus MH, Fanaroff AA (eds): *Care of the High Risk Neonate,* ed 2. Philadelphia, WB Saunders, 1979, pp 1–22.

64. Milunsky A, Alpert E: Results and benefits of a maternal serum alpha fetoprotein program. *JAMA* 1984;252:1438–1442.

65. Muller-Holve W, Saling E, Schwartz M: The significance of the time interval in twin pregnancy. *J Perinat Med* 1976;4:100–105.

66. Myrianthopoulos NC: Congenital malformations in twins: Epidemiologic survey. *Birth Defects* 1975;11:1:39–44.

67. O'Brien WF, Knuppel RA, Scerbo JA, Rattan PK: Birth weight in twins: An analysis of discordance and growth retardation. *Obstet Gynecol* 1986;67:483–487.

68. O'Leary JA: Prophylactic tocolysis of twins. *Am J Obstet Gynecol* 1986;154:904–905.

69. Olofsson P, Rydhstrom H: Management in second stage of labour in term twin delivery. *Acta Genet Med Gemellol (Roma)* 1985;34:213–216.

70. Olofsson P, Rydhstrom H: Twin delivery: How should the second twin be delivered? *Am J Obstet Gynecol* 1985;153:479–481.

71. Osbourne GK, Patel NB: An assessment of perinatal mortality in twin pregnancies in Dundee. *Acta Genet Med Gemellol (Roma)* 1985;34:193–199.

72. Persson PH, Grennert L, Gennser G, Kullander S: An improved outcome of twin pregnancies. *Acta Obstet Gynecol Scand* 1979;58:3–7.

73. Persson PH, Kullander S: Long term experience of general ultrasound screening in pregnancy. *Am J Obstet Gynecol* 1983;146:942–946.

74. Powers WF: Twin pregnancy complications and treatment. *Obstet Gynecol* 1973;42:795–808.

75. Pritchard JA, MacDonald PC: *Williams Obstetrics,* ed 16. New York, Appleton-Century-Crofts, 1982.

76. Rattan PK, Knuppel RA, O'Brien WF, Scerbo JC: Cesarean delivery of second twin after vaginal delivery of the first twin. *Am J Obstet Gynecol* 1986;154:936–939.

77. Rayburn WF, Lavin JP, Miodovnik M, Varver MN: Multiple gestation: Time interval between delivery of first and second twins. *Obstet Gynecol* 1984;63:502–506.

78. Read JA, Miller FC: Technique of simultaneous direct intrauterine pressure recording for electronic monitoring of twin gestation. *Am J Obstet Gynecol* 1977;129:228–230.

79. Redwine FO, Petres RE: Selective birth in a case of twins discordant for Tay Sachs disease. *Acta Genet Med Gemellol (Roma)* 1984;33:35–38.

80. Romero R, Duffy TP, Berkowitz R, Chang E, Hobbins JC: Prolongation of a preterm pregnancy complicated by death of a single twin in utero and disseminated intravascular coagulation. Effects of treatment with heparin. *N Engl J Med* 1984;310:772–774.

81. Sakala EP: Obstetric management of conjoined twins. *Obstet Gynecol* 1986;62:21S–23S.

82. Saunders MC, Dick JS, Brown IM, McPherson K, Chalmers I: The effects of hospital admission for bedrest on the duration of pregnancy: A randomized trial. *Lancet* 1985; 2:793–796.

83. Scheer K: Ultrasonography in twin gestations. *J Clin Ultrasound* 1975;2:197–199.

84. Schneider KT, Vetter K, Huch R, Huch A: Acute polyhydramnios complicating twin pregnancies. *Acta Genet Med Gemellol (Roma)* 1985;34:179–184.

85. Spellacy WN, Buhi WC, Birk SA: Human placental lactogen in multiple pregnancies. *Obstet Gynecol* 1978;52:210–212.

86. Smith DW: *Recognizable Patterns of Human Malformations.* Philadelphia, WB Saunders, 1976.

87. Sutter J, Arab H, Manning FA: Monoamniotic twins: Antenatal diagnosis and management. *Am J Obstet Gynecol* 1986;155:836–837.

88. Szymonowicz W, Preston H, Yu VY: The surviving monozygotic twin. *Arch Dis Child* 1986;61:454–458.

89. Taylor ES: Editorial comment. *Obstet Gynecol Surv* 1976;31:535–536.

90. Weeks ARL, Menzies DN, deBoer CH: The relative efficacy of bed rest, cervical suture and no treatment in the management of twin pregnancy. *Br J Obstet Gynaecol* 1977; 84:161–164.

91. Weinberger E, Cyr DR, Hirsh JH: Estimating fetal weights less than 2000 gm: An accurate and simple method. *Am J Radiol* 1987;141:973–977.

92. Young BK, Suidan J, Antoine C, Silverman F, Wasserman J, Lustig I: Differences in twins: The importance of birth order. *Am J Obstet Gynecol* 1985;151:915–921.

93. Zakut HJ, Inslet V, Serr DM: Elective cervical suture in preventing premature delivery in multiple pregnancies. *Isr J Med Sci* 1977;13:488–492.

15

Induction of Labor

Cassandra E. Henderson and Eric D. Lichter

Maternal and fetal well-being are sometimes affected adversely when pregnancy continues until onset of spontaneous labor. Although cesarean section is used to produce early delivery in many such circumstances, induction of labor is often a more suitable approach. Various forms of medical intervention to initiate labor have been practiced since prior to the 18th century.[20] When induction of labor is indicated, contemporary obstetricians have an array of pharmacologic and mechanical methods from which to choose. Indications and contraindications are similar for all means of induction. However, the efficacy and risk may vary according to the technique of induction and the situation in which it is employed.

INDICATIONS FOR INDUCTION OF LABOR

Labor should be induced when the benefits to be accrued are judged to outweigh those of cesarean section in situations in which delivery is indicated. Some generally accepted maternal medical indications for induction of labor are cardiac disease, hypertensive disorders of pregnancy, chronic hypertension, diabetes mellitus, malignant diseases in which concern for fetal well-being delays or interdicts appropriate maternal treatment, hepatic disease, and logistic factors, such as a multipara who has a history of rapid labors who lives far from the hospital. Reasons for induction that relate to concerns for fetal welfare also exist, including suspicion of fetal distress, prematurely ruptured chorioamniotic membranes, fetal demise, and conditions requiring prompt uterine evacuation, such as chorioamnionitis.

Other fetal indications for labor induction are isoimmunization, intrauterine growth retardation, post-term gestation, and many of the maternal disorders listed above, such as hypertension, that may affect the fetus indirectly by causing a decrease in uterine blood flow. In these situations, a neonatal intensive care unit sometimes provides a less hostile environment than the gravid uterus, and delivery is indicated when the well-being of the fetus is judged to be more at risk in utero in regard to health and survival than it would be in a nursery bed.

CONTRAINDICATIONS TO INDUCTION OF LABOR

Fetal immaturity usually contraindicates labor induction. Exceptions are made if continuation of pregnancy would be life-threatening for mother or fetus. In addition, any condition for which spontaneous labor or vaginal delivery would be inappropriate precludes induction of labor.

Relative contraindications to labor induction include a clinical diagnosis of cephalopelvic disproportion, abnormal fetal presentation, fetal distress, active genital herpes simplex infection, placenta previa, previous cesarean section with the uterine incision involving the uterine corpus, or previous gynecologic surgery that necessitated transection of the myometrium. Induction of labor in women with uterine scars from lower segment cesarean sections is generally safe as long as the cervix is ripe and oxytocin is used judiciously.

While the presence of meconium does not contraindicate induction, it does complicate it. Meconium-stained amniotic fluid that exists in association with abnormal fetal heart tracings, especially late decelerations, is associated with substantially increased perinatal morbidity and mortality.[34,41] When meconium is present, induction should be performed only if the fetal heart rate tracing is completely normal. We perform a scalp blood sample and measure pH to confirm fetal well-being before starting or continuing an induction in the presence of meconium and an abnormal fetal heart rate baseline, with or without recurrent decelerations. However, we do not feel that the presence of meconium mandates scalp blood sampling if the heart rate pattern is completely normal.

RISKS OF LABOR INDUCTION

To the chagrin of obstetricians and patients, the time of onset of labor is quite unpredictable. In Europe, elective induction of labor is performed commonly in gravidas with singleton vertex presentation between 40 and 41 weeks' gestation. Elective induction is convenient for the obstetrician and patient, and the schedules of nursing, anesthesia, and other staff members can be considered when labor is scheduled. There is great potential benefit to fetus and mother if delivery occurs when staffing is optimal.

In the United States, concern about potential fetal and maternal risks has caused elective inductions to be largely abandoned; however, a large amount of European literature attests that there are no significant risks associated with properly conducted elective induction at term.[13,44] In fact, some authors even suggest there may be some maternal and neonatal benefits.[11,51] In a prospective study, Cole et al.[12] found less meconium in labor and a smaller blood loss after elective induction when compared to deliveries after spontaneous onset of labor. In a randomized study of elective induction compared to spontaneous labor at term, no difference in neonatal umbilical vein pH, hemoglobin, bilirubin, or Apgar scores was found between the two groups.[28] Tylleskar et al. observed no increase in obstetric intervention in a randomized prospective study of induced labor compared to spontaneous labor.[44]

Unfortunately, the optimistic findings of these investigators are at odds with data from other studies that have found elective induction to be potentially hazardous. Iatrogenic premature birth and increases in operative intervention—particularly forceps delivery and cesarean section—are complications of elective induction of labor reported recurrently in the obstetric literature.[3,40,43] Hyperbilirubinemia may occur.[6] Amniotomy and the use of internal uterine and fetal monitoring—both generally considered mandatory in these labors—may increase the complications of elective induction. Martell et al. found early amniotomy was associated with a lower cord pH in neonates in comparison with amniotomy performed late in labor.[31] While not usually listed among the complications of labor induction, use of intrauterine pressure catheters is associated, albeit rarely, with intrauterine infection, laceration of placental vessels, and separation of the placenta.[9] Less frequently, perforation of the lower uterine segment and broad ligament[23] have occurred after insertion of an intrauterine pressure catheter.

Perhaps European and American experiences with labor induction are dissimilar because significant differences exist in patient populations, prenatal care delivery systems, or management of labor. The U.S. population is more diverse in ethnic background and socioeconomic status, making it very difficult to identify matched groups to compare the outcomes of spontaneous and induced labor. In particular, limited access to quality prenatal care can affect accurate pregnancy dating and proper evaluation of obstetric and medical diseases. These limitations of care can increase potential complications of elective labor induction, especially iatrogenic preterm birth. Because benefits of elective inductions do not clearly outweigh the risks of the intervention, the procedure is not currently acceptable in the United States, and the Food and Drug Administration (FDA) does not approve use of synthetic oxytocin to induce labor without a medical or obstetric indication to do so.

METHODS OF LABOR INDUCTION

Drugs

Oxytocin

Pharmacologic agents used to induce labor affect cervical dilatation by stimulating uterine contractions. While research continues to search for safer and more effective agents, most clinicians continue to use oxytocin as the drug of choice for induction of labor.[1] Oxytocin probably has no direct influence on the cervix, but rather causes cervical dilatation through its effect on myometrial smooth muscle.[19]

Endogenous oxytocin is synthesized in the supraoptic and paraventricular nuclei of the hypothalamus. Secretion of oxytocin from the posterior pituitary can be initiated through sensory stimulation of the breast, cervix, and vagina, or by increases in plasma osmolality.[13,19,32] Contractile activity in uterine smooth muscle is more forceful and frequent in the presence of this hormone. Although the precise mechanisms of oxytocin action on the uterus are not understood completely, it is likely that oxytocin stimulates prostaglandin release from endometrial tissue, leading to enhancement of calcium transport through plasma membranes, and activation of the actomyosin phosphorylation system. These effects are modulated by the existing hormonal milieu of pregnancy. Specifically, estrogen maintains myometrial cellular structure and excitability, and progesterone has a negative influence on uterine activity.[32]

Even though oxytocin remains the preferred agent for labor induction its usefulness is limited to late in the third trimester. While oxytocin can initiate uterine contractions at any time, very high doses are needed early in pregnancy[7] and the likelihood of success is diminished considerably when the drug is used remote from term.

Direct intravenous injection of concentrated oxytocin, which relaxes vascular smooth muscle, may lead to decreased systolic and diastolic blood pressure, flushing, and reflex tachycardia. Therefore, variable speed electronic infusion pumps are used to administer oxytocin safely diluted in a 5% dextrose solution. Careful titration of oxytocin to provide the smallest dose necessary to produce adequate uterine contractility minimizes the complications of its use. A 10 mU/mL concentration (usually 5 U of oxytocin in 500 mL 5% dextrose) can be used for most inductions. The use of buccal or intramuscular oxytocin, or intravenous administration not regulated by an electronic infusion pump is unwarranted and is potentially dangerous.

The infusion is usually started at 1 to 2 mU/min and increased by 1 or 2 mU/min every 15 to 30 min until approximately three contractions in each 10-min period are achieved. Because the equilibration of oxytocin takes 12 to 17 min on average, increasing the dose more frequently than every 15 min may result in myometrial hyperstimulation. In fact, the major risks of oxytocin relate not to the drug itself, but to its effects on uterine contractility. The rate of oxytocin infusion is often increased more rapidly than necessary. Seitchik[2,38] emphasized that a steady state of plasma concentration and maximal contractile effect for any infusion rate is not generally attained until 30 to 40 min. It is probably unnecessary to increase dose rates at more frequent intervals for most patients. Nevertheless, some women may, by virtue of individual differences in myometrial sensitivity to the drug or in drug plasma clearance rates, require higher than usual doses, or more rapid incremental change in the infusion rate. Although individualization of dose schedules is sensible, it must be emphasized that to ensure optimal safety, careful continuous monitoring of fetal heart rate and uterine contractions is mandatory.

An excess of uterine activity in the form of tetanic contractions, polysystole, or increased basal tonus can cause fetal asphyxia or, if sufficiently prolonged, fetal death. Uteroplacental blood flow, normally 500 mL/min at term, is effectively stopped during the course of normal uterine contractions in a term labor.[22,36]

The placenta is perfused by maternal blood from branches of uterine arteries that traverse the myometrium and terminate at the intervillous space. Flow through these arteries (and therefore delivery of oxygen to the fetus) occurs only when the mean arterial pressure exceeds the intramyometrial pressure. During the peak of a normal uterine contraction, intramyometrial pressure approaches or exceeds that of the uterine artery, and intervillous flow diminishes or ceases. Under normal circumstances, these brief intermittent episodes of decreased intervillous flow are tolerated with equanimity by the fetus. They will result in potentially serious decrements in fetal oxygenation if fetal oxygen reserves are already diminished. The practical importance of this fact is that many of the conditions for which labor induction is required (e.g., hypertension, postmaturity) are associated with depleted fetal reserve. If the contraction is unusually intense or prolonged, the effects on the fetus can be devastating. For these reasons, carefully monitored slow infusion of oxytocin is mandatory. Its use should be proscribed in the presence of fetal asphyxia or conditions that have seriously compromised uterine blood flow.

In addition to fetal risks, excess uterine activity probably increases the likelihood of uterine rupture. This is an uncommon event, but one with potentially catastrophic consequences. Niswander[35] reviewed 19,000 cases of elective induction without any reported uterine rupture, but rupture does occur, albeit rarely, with oxytocin and/or prostaglandin use to augment labor.[10] Oxytocin infusion should be discontinued at the first sign of excessive uterine contractions or evidence of fetal distress, for example, bradycardia, decelerations, or change in fetal baseline rate. The short half-life of oxytocin usually allows rapid uterine relaxation and fetal recovery. If the fetal heart rate pattern returns to normal, the infusion can be often restarted at 1 to 2 mU/min and then increased very cautiously.

All commercially available preparations of oxytocin are synthetic; however, like the natural hormone they have antidiuretic properties when used in large doses. Infusion rates higher than 20 mU/min are associated with a decrease in free water clearance by the kidneys. When higher doses of oxytocin are required, care must be taken to avoid water intoxication and subsequent convulsions. High doses are administered more safely in diluted saline solution than in dextrose. Also, close monitoring of the gravida's intake and output and, when appropriate, serum sodium concentration will help to avoid serious water intoxication during induction of labor.

Prostaglandins

Prostaglandins comprise another class of pharmacologic agents used to induce labor.[27] Since 1978, prostaglandin E_2 has been available in the United States for induction of labor in cases of fetal demise. Although now employed widely in Europe for labor induction under many circumstances, the use of prostaglandins in labor with a living fetus remains investigational in the United States.

Prostaglandins are 20-carbon fatty acids that exert important physiologic effects on smooth muscle. Series E and F, abundant in menstrual flow and amniotic fluid, may be used pharmacologically to stimulate labor. They can be administered by a variety of routes including oral, intravenous, vaginal, intracervical, and extraamniotic. In addition to initiation of uterine contractions, prostaglandins have been given orally or locally to soften the cervix prior to oxytocin induction.

Any route of prostaglandin administration can be accompanied by severe side effects. Prostaglandins in the E series are potent vasodilators and have a direct inotropic effect on cardiac muscle. Prostaglandin E_1 inhibits platelet aggregation, as does prostaglandin E_2 at high levels. However, at low concentrations prostaglandin E_2 potentiates platelet aggregation. Although prostaglandin F and E usually relax bronchial and tracheal smooth muscle, severe bronchospasm may occur in asthmatics. While prostaglandin E_2 relaxes circular smooth muscle in the gastrointestinal tract, prostaglandin E and F frequently cause contraction of longitudinal smooth muscle resulting in profuse diarrhea. The thermoregulatory sensors in the hypothalmus are also affected by prostaglandin E and F, resulting in transient pyrexia that may be quite extreme.

Prostaglandins E_2 and $F_2\alpha$ are clinically useful for labor induction. Unfortunately, the potentially severe maternal side effects of large doses of prostaglandin—myometrial hyperstimulation, pyrexia, vomiting and diarrhea—have limited the enthusiasm for their use in women with viable pregnancies who might require long labors. For uncertain reasons, these drugs work with extraordinary speed and efficiency when labor is stimulated in the presence of a dead fetus.

Several promising reports of the use of low-dose prostaglandins to soften the cervix prior to induction with oxytocin have appeared in the literature. While several studies have employed oral prostaglandins, local application to the cervix to simulate physiologic production of the hormone has become the technique of choice. In contrast to the large doses used for induction of labor, low doses of prostaglandin E_2 suppositories or prostaglandin E_2 gel[5,21,25,39,46,47,49,50] are used to prime or soften an unripe cervix before induction. When applied to the cervix, prostaglandin E_2 has been shown to separate collagen fibers and increase the amount of ground substance,[45] while intracervical prostaglandin E application increases collagenase activity.[14] These changes in cervical connective tissue composition and morphology may be the mechanism by which prostaglandins induce cervical change in the absence of myometrial stimulation.

The success of labor induction is proportional to the ripeness of the cervix at the time induction is begun.[18] In 1964, Bishop[4] described a scoring system to facilitate uniform assessment of the cervical readiness for labor (Table 15-1). The attainable score ranges from 0 (unripe) to 12 (ripe cervix). A prelabor score of 9 or more is associated with a good prognosis for successful labor induction. Unfortunately, inductions must frequently be attempted when the cervix is unripe. To reduce the incidence of failed induction and the concomitant high cesarean section and instrumental delivery rate, and frequent chorioamnionitis, serial induction using intravenous oxytocin for limited periods on successive days or

Table 15-1 Assessment of Bishop Score

Characteristic	Bishop score			
	0	1	2	3
Dilatation (cm)	0	1–2	3–4	5–6
Effacement (%)	0–30	40–50	60–70	80
Station	−3	−2	−1, 0	+1, +2
Consistency	Firm	Medium	Soft	—
Position	Post	Mid	Anterior	—

locally applied low-dose prostaglandin gels have been employed to make the cervix more favorable.

Protocols for serial induction generally employ 10 to 12 hr of intravenous oxytocin infusion daily for 2 to 3 days. Clearly, there are some inherent problems associated with serial induction. Several days of hospitalization and intravenous therapy are expensive, anxiety provoking, and uncomfortable for the patient. In addition, intensive staff time is required for maternal management and continuous fetal monitoring. Obviously, serial induction is contraindicated when 2 to 3 days of uterine contractions would affect existing maternal or fetal well-being adversely. In spite of these problems, serial induction may be useful for some parturients with, for example, mild preeclampsia or postdate gestation, in whom the benefits of these persistent attempts to induce labor are judged to be safe and preferable to prompt delivery.

Even though prostaglandin E_2 gel is felt to work locally without myometrial effect, continuous uterine and fetal monitoring is indicated because even low doses can stimulate uterine contractions in some individuals.[49] In addition to fetal concerns, recent reports of uterine hyperstimulation and uterine rupture using prostaglandin gel and suppositories[8,10] have appeared in the literature.

Relaxin

Because the use of prostaglandins and oxytocin is not without risks, the search for better methods of labor induction continues. Relaxin appears to hold the most promise as an effective means of cervical ripening,[24,29] although its use is still experimental. Intracervical or vaginal use of relaxin improved Bishop scores by an average of 3.3 points and resulted in spontaneous labor in 30% of the patients studied by MacLennon et al.[30] Furthermore, Evans et al.[16] reported a shorter induction duration when intravaginal relaxin suppositories were used before the start of an oxytocin induction. These reports of favorable outcome and cervical ripening with no apparent stimulation of uterine contractions should encourage more investigation of the therapeutic role of relaxin in induction of labor.

Mechanical Methods

Oxytocin, prostaglandins, and relaxin are all endogenous hormones administered pharmacologically to effect onset of labor prior to its spontaneous initiation. Breast stimulation and artificial rupture of membranes probably stimulate labor by causing the release of endogenous hormones and these mechanical approaches for induction or stimulation of labor are often advocated.

Breast Stimulation

Nipple stimulation causes release of oxytocin from the posterior pituitary.[32] Physiologic effects of this endogenous release may be painfully obvious to the breastfeeding mother. Oxytocin produces contractions of the myoepithelial cells in the alveoli and small milk ducts, resulting in expression of breast milk. Often strong uterine contractions accompany the oxytocin response to suckling.

Recently, investigators have used nipple massage or breast pumps to stimulate uterine contractions. Obvious potential advantages of breast stimulation to induce labor—no intravenous infusions or need for administration of pharmacologic agents—have aroused enthusiasm about this modality. However, one disadvantage, namely, the inability to control oxytocin release closely, has caused concern about the potential for uterine hyperstimulation. In fact, Curtis et al. observed hyperstimulation in 55% of the patients undergoing a modified oxytocin challenge test using nipple stimulation.[13] Another potential problem is the gravida anxious to deliver who, once having been instructed in nipple stimulation, continues the practice unsupervised at home.

Nevertheless, investigations of nipple stimulation to induce labor continue and some suggest potential benefits. Salmon et al.[37] reported improved Bishop scores in women using breast stimulation. The study group consisted of women instructed to stimulate their breasts for 90 min/day. During the initial 3 days, continuous fetal heart rate monitoring was used. After documenting fetal well-being during the first

3 days, the duration of nipple stimulation was increased to 3 hr/day and was performed at home for 3 days without fetal monitoring. Of considerable interest is the lack of uterine hypertonus reported in this group. The risks and benefits of this procedure will become better delineated as more experience is gathered. Until then, breast stimulation for labor induction remains investigational.

Amniotomy

Success with other mechanical means of labor induction have been varied. Manipulating amniotic membranes is the most frequent such intervention. Stripping or separating the chorioamniotic membranes from the lower uterine segment with the examining finger has long been considered a safe and effective means to induce labor. Unfortunately there are no objective data to support the benefit of this widespread practice. Swan studied a group of 221 patients, 147 of whom had their membranes stripped on 3 consecutive days near term.[42] Unexpectedly, membrane stripping increased maternal and fetal morbidity without any significant increase in the frequency of spontaneous labor. More recently, Weissberg and Spellacy confirmed the high failure rate of membrane stripping.[48]

Amniotomy is performed commonly prior to initiating oxytocin therapy for labor induction. This approach probably shortens the duration of induction and permits documentation of the presence of meconium in amniotic fluid and application of a fetal scalp electrode. Despite these benefits of amniotomy certain liabilities may accrue from its use.

Risks of amniotomy include maternal and fetal infections and umbilical cord prolapse. Early work by Bishop[4] indicates clearly that if the cervix is dilated sufficiently to permit amniotomy, it is likely to respond favorably to any attempt at labor induction. The mechanism by which amniotomy hastens the onset of labor has not been fully elucidated. It is likely that membrane rupture results in release of prostaglandins, and that these compounds mediate all the enhancing effects of amniotomy on the initiation of labor. Although there is little doubt that amniotomy results in onset of labor in many individuals, an accelerating effect of rupturing membranes on already established labor has not been documented. It is sometimes appropriate to begin labor induction and to withhold amniotomy until it is clear that the patient is in labor. This approach may serve to reduce the risk of infection associated with long-ruptured membranes, and it retains the option to terminate the induction without the need for delivery if successful stimulation of uterine contractions should fail.

Laminaria and Balloon Catheters

Laminaria and Foley catheters have been proposed as mechanical cervical dilators to improve cervical ripeness and to initiate labor. Laminaria, a hygroscopic dried seaweed, is thought to enhance cervical dilatation by drawing water from the collagen complexes, thereby facilitating cervical softening and slow dilatation. In a recent prospective study evaluating cervical ripening using a synthetic laminaria tent, less uterine activity, fetal distress, and more normal deliveries were observed when compared to the use of intravaginal prostaglandin gel for cervical ripening.[25] Earlier retrospective studies of the use of laminaria report a 60% postpartum endometritis and a 20% neonatal sepsis rate. Obviously, more investigation is required before laminaria may be recommended for use in labor induction.

Ezimokhai and Nwabineli reported that the use of a Foley catheter placed in the extraamniotic space and inflated with 35 to 40 mL of saline improved Bishop scores in primigravidas as well as did vaginal prostaglandin E_2 gel.[17] They reported no infection or accidental rupture of amniotic membranes. In another investigation, Embrey and Mollison[15] used 50 cc of sterile saline to inflate the Foley balloon. Although they reported success in ripening the cervix, vaginal bleeding occurred in one patient from an undiagnosed partial placenta previa. The mechanism by which Foley catheters can make the cervix more favorable for induction, like many other mechanical means of labor induction, is probably mediated through prostaglandins.

MANAGEMENT

While complete understanding of the physiologic events surrounding the onset of human labor remains elusive, it is probable that under most circumstances spontaneous labor is less hazardous than induced labor irrespective of what method is used to produce uterine contractions. Nevertheless, in the presence of adverse maternal or fetal conditions, awaiting the onset of spontaneous labor can increase perinatal and maternal morbidity and mortality. If immediate delivery is required, cesarean section is obviously indicated. When induction of labor is judged to be appropriate, the obstetrician must include in the patient's chart thorough documentation that the benefits outweigh expected risks of the procedure. It is equally important to document the patient's awareness and understanding of these risks and benefits.

Obviously, determination of fetal lung maturity would reduce an uncommon but extremely serious complication of induction of labor, namely, iatrogenic preterm birth. The authors perform amniocentesis prior to induction whenever delivery is not urgent, and the gestational age is not known with certainty. Even with well-documented fetal age, determination of fetal lung maturity may be appropriate in fetuses of

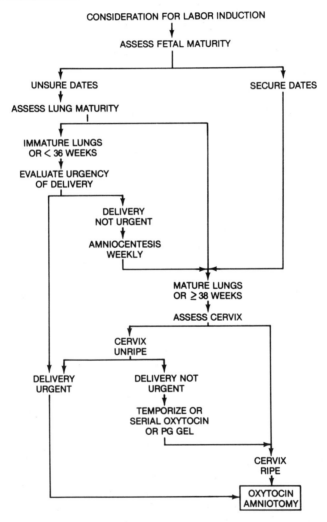

Figure 15-1 Paradigm for approach to induction of labor. If indication to deliver is compelling, risk of awaiting lung maturation or cervical ripening may justify attempts to induce labor, despite the high probability of failure.

diabetic mothers. In these cases, lung maturation may develop later in gestation than usual, particularly if glycemic control has not been optimal. Once induction of labor is deemed indicated, we follow an obstetric management plan as outlined in Figure 15-1. The Bishop score should be used to choose the method of induction. If the cervix is unfavorable, cervical ripening with prostaglandin gel or relaxin might prove useful followed by oxytocin induction. However, because neither agent has received FDA approval for cervical ripening, serial induction with oxytocin is generally chosen. We perform amniotomy as soon as it is technically possible once uterine contractions have been established with oxytocin.

Failed Induction

Several factors influence the probability that induction of labor will be successful. Paramount among these is the Bishop prelabor score. If the induction is begun with an unripe cervix, one may anticipate that the

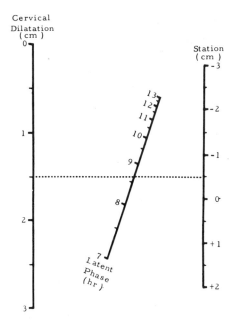

Figure 15-2 Nomogram to predict duration of latent phase from cervical dilatation and fetal station at onset of labor in nulliparas. A straight line connecting dilatation (left scale) with station (right scale) will intersect the center scale at the expected average duration of the latent phase. The horizontal dashed line connects average values for all three parameters. *Source:* Reprinted with permission from *American Journal of Obstetrics and Gynecology* (1965; 93:541), Copyright © 1965, The CV Mosby Company.

latent phase will be quite long, particularly in nulliparas. Although the anticipated length of an induced labor cannot be predicted with precision, inferences may be drawn from information gleaned from study of spontaneous labors. The nomogram in Figure 15-2 indicates the mean duration of latent phase in relation to cervical dilatation and fetal station at the onset of labor. Based on this information it is clear that considering an induction to have failed in a woman with an unripe cervix after only 6 to 8 hr have elapsed in the latent phase is not reasonable. Sometimes attempts at induction may be abandoned after only a few hours based on concerns about maternal or fetal condition, and the ability of either to tolerate a long period of labor. When there is a compelling reason to terminate the pregnancy promptly, lengthy attempts at induction should not be condoned if the initial Bishop score was low. However, lengthy induction is to be expected when the cervix is unripe. Sometimes allowing the mother to sleep after 8 to 12 hr of oxytocin infusion and beginning anew the next day will result in success. Obviously, all such decisions must be based on a continuing assessment of the relative risks of available alternatives.

Once the labor has entered the active phase, factors unrelated to uterine contractility (e.g., fetal status, presence of cephalopelvic disproportion, or chorioamnionitis) influence the probability that vaginal delivery will occur. An induction should therefore probably be considered successful once the labor is in active phase, rather than using vaginal delivery as an endpoint.

REFERENCES

1. ACOG Technical Bulletin: *Induction and Augmentation of Labor*. No. 110. Washington, DC, American College of Obstetricians and Gynecologists, 1987.

2. Amico JA, Seitchik J, Robinson AG: Studies of oxytocin in plasma of women during hypocontractile labor. *J Clin Endocrinol* 1984;58:274–279.

3. Bergsjo P, Bakketeig LS, Eikhorn SN: Case-control analysis of post-term induction of labor. *Acta Obstet Gynecol Scand* 1982;61:317–324.

4. Bishop EH: Pelvic scoring for elective induction. *Obstet Gynecol* 1964;24:266–268.

5. Buchanan D, Macer J, Yonekura ML: Cervical ripening with prostaglandin E$_2$ vaginal suppositories. *Obstet Gynecol* 1984;63:659–663.

6. Calder AA, Orensted MK, Morr VA, Turnbull BA: Increased bilirubin levels in neonates after induction of labor by intravenous prostaglandin E$_2$ or oxytocin. *Lancet* 1974;25:1339–1342.

7. Caldeyro-Garcia R, Posiero JJ: Oxytocin and contractility of the pregnant human uterus. *Ann NY Acad Sci* 1959;75:813–825.

8. Chamberlin RO, Cohen GR, Knuppel RA: Uterine hyperstimulation resulting from intravaginal prostaglandin E$_2$. *J Reprod Med* 1987;32:233–235.

9. Chan WH, Paul RH, Toews J: Intrapartum fetal monitoring. *Obstet Gynecol* 1973;41:7–13.

10. Claman P, Carpenter RJ, Reiter A: Uterine rupture with the use of vaginal prostaglandin E_2 for induction of labor. *Am J Obstet Gynecol* 1984;150:889–890.

11. Clinch J: Induction of labour—a six year review. *Br J Obstet Gynaecol* 1979;86:340–342.

12. Cole RA, Howie PA, MacNaughton MC: Elective induction of labour. *Lancet* 1975;31:767–770.

13. Curtis P, Evans S, Resnick J, Ramon R, Lynch K, Carlson J: Uterine responses to three techniques of breast stimulation. *Obstet Gynecol* 1986;67:25–28.

14. Ekma G, Malmstrom A, Uldbjerg N, Ulmstern U: Cervical collagen: An important regulation of cervical function in term labor. *Obstet Gynecol* 1986;67:633–636.

15. Embrey MP, Mollison BG: The unfavorable cervix and induction of labour using a cervical balloon. *J Obstet Gynaecol Br Commonw* 1967;74:44–48.

16. Evans MI, Dougan M, Moawad AH, Evans WJ, Bryant-Greenwood GD, Greenwood FC: Ripening of the human cervix with porcine ovarian relaxin. *Am J Obstet Gynecol* 1983;147:410–414.

17. Ezimokhai M, Nwabineli JN: The use of Foley's catheter in ripening the unfavorable cervix prior to induction of labour. *Br J Obstet Gynaecol* 1980;87:281–286.

18. Friedman EA, Niswander KR, Bayonet-Rivera NP, Sachtleben MR: Relation of prelabor evaluation to inducibility and the course of labor. *Obstet Gynecol* 1966;28:495–501.

19. Gilman AG, Goodman LS, Rall TW, Murod F: *The Pharmacological Basis of Therapeutics.* New York, Macmillan, 1985.

20. Graham H: *Eternal Eve: The History of Gynaecology and Obstetrics.* Garden City, NY, Doubleday, 1951.

21. Granes GR, Baskett MB, Gray JH, Luther ER: The effect of vaginal administration of various doses of prostaglandin E_2 gel on cervical ripening and induction of labor. *Am J Obstet Gynecol* 1985;151:178–181.

22. Henderson CE, Cohen WR: Uteroplacental circulation: Obstetrician's view, in Datta S, Ostheimer GW (eds): *Common Problems in Obstetric Anesthesia.* Chicago, Year Book Medical Publishers, 1987, pp 53–57.

23. Haverkamp AD, Bowes WA: Uterine perforation: A complication of continuous fetal monitoring in high risk pregnancy. *Am J Obstet Gynecol* 1972;110:667–669.

24. Hisaw FL: Experimental relaxation of the pubic ligament of the guinea pig. *Proc Soc Exp Biol* 1926;23:661.

25. Johnson IR, MacPherson MBA, Welch RC, Filshshie GM: A comparison of Lamicel and prostaglandin E_2 vaginal gel for cervical ripening before induction of labor. *Am J Obstet Gynecol* 1985;151:604–607.

26. Kazzi GM, Bottoms SF, Rosen MG: Efficacy and safety of laminaria digitata for preinduction ripening of the cervix. *Obstet Gynecol* 1982;60:440–443.

27. Lange I, Collister C, Johnson J, Cote D, Torchi M, Freund G, Mannis F: The effect of vaginal prostaglandin E_2 pessaries in induction of labor. *Am J Obstet Gynecol* 1984;148:621–625.

28. Leiyon I, Finnstrom O, Hedenskog S, Ryden G, Tylleskar J: Spontaneous labour and elective induction. A prospective randomized study. Behavioral assessment and neurological examination in the newborn period. *Acta Paediatr Scand* 1979;68:553–560.

29. MacLennon AH: The role of relaxin in human reproduction. *Clin Reprod Fertil* 1983;27:77–81.

30. MacLennon AH, Green RC, Bryant-Greenwood GD, Greenwood FC, Seamark C: Ripening of the human cervix and induction of labor with purified porcine relaxin. *Lancet* 1980;24:220–227.

31. Martell M, Belizan JM, Nieto F, Schwarcz R: Blood acid-base balance at birth in neonates from labor with early and late rupture of membranes. *J Pediatr* 1976;89:963–967.

32. McNeilly AS, Robinson ICA, Houston MJ, Howie PW: Release of oxytocin and prolactin in response to sucking. *Br Med J* 1983;286:257–259.

33. Miller FC: Uterine motility in spontaneous labor. *Clin Obstet Gynecol* 1983;26:78–85.

34. Miller FC, Sacks DA, Yeh S-Y, Paul RH, Schifrin BS, Martin CB, Hon EH: Significance of meconium during labor. *Am J Obstet Gynecol* 1975;122:573–580.

35. Niswander KR: Elective induction of labor, in Reid D, Barton T (eds): *Controversy in Obstetrics and Gynecology*. Philadelphia, WB Saunders, 1969, pp 121–132.

36. Ramsey EM, Martin CB Jr, McGaughey HS, Kaiser IH, Donner MW: Venous drainage of the placenta in rhesus monkeys: Radiographic studies. *Am J Obstet Gynecol* 1966; 95:948–955.

37. Salmon YM, Kee WH, Tan SL, Jen SW: Cervical ripening by breast stimulation. *Obstet Gynecol* 1986;67:21–24.

38. Seitchik J: The management of functional dystocia in the first stage of labor. *Clin Obstet Gynecol* 1987;30:42–49.

39. Sheperd J, Pearce JMF, Sims CD: Induction of labor using prostaglandin E_2 pessaries. *Br Med J* 1979;14:108–110.

40. Smith LP, Nagourney FH, Usher RH: Hazards and benefits of elective induction of labor. *Am J Obstet Gynecol* 1984;148:579–585.

41. Starks GC: Correlation of meconium-stained amniotic fluid, early intrapartum fetal pH and Apgar scores as predictors of perinatal outcome. *Obstet Gynecol* 1980;56:604–609.

42. Swan RO: Induction of labor by stripping membranes. *Obstet Gynecol* 1958;11:74–78.

43. Tew M: Do obstetric extranatal interventions make birth safer? *Br J Obstet Gynaecol* 1986;93:659–674.

44. Tylleskär J, Finnström O, Leijon I, Hedenskog S, Ryden G: Spontaneous labor and elective induction. A prospective randomized study—effects on mother and fetus. *Acta Obstet Gynecol Scand* 1979;58:513–518.

45. Uldbjerg N, Ekman G, Malmstrom A: Biochemical and morphological changes of human cervix after local application of prostaglandin E_2 in pregnancy. *Lancet* 1981;27:267–268.

46. Valentine BH: Intravenous oxytocin and oral prostaglandin E_2 for ripening of the unfavorable cervix. *Br J Obstet Gynaecol* 1977;84:846–850.

47. Weiss RR, Tejani N, Israeli I, Evans MI, Bhakthavathsalan A, Mann LI: Priming of the uterine cervix with oral prostaglandin E_2 in the term multigravida. *Obstet Gynecol* 1975;46:181–184.

48. Weissberg SM, Spellacy WN: Membrane stripping to induce labor. *J Reprod Med* 1977;19:125–127.

49. Williams JK, Wilkerson WG, O'Brien WF, Knuppel RA: Use of prostaglandin E_2 topical cervical gel in high risk patients. A critical analysis. *Obstet Gynecol* 1985;66:769–773.

50. Wilson PD: A comparison of four methods of ripening the unfavorable cervix. *Br J Obstet Gynaecol* 1978;85:941–946.

51. Yudkin P, Frumar AM, Anderson ABM, Turnbull AC: A retrospective study of induction of labor. *Br J Obstet Gynecol* 1979;86:257–265.

16

Effects of Labor and Delivery Procedures on the Fetus

Emanuel A. Friedman

It is generally accepted that much of the toll in neurologic and developmental handicaps among children is unrelated to labor and delivery events. This is based on the high relative frequency of cases with unknown cause or with causes documented to have had their deleterious effect well before labor begins.[48,56,57,60] The reassurance this offers to parents and obstetricians alike cannot be misinterpreted to indicate that the birth process is entirely risk-free. Even those who absolve birth attendants of essentially all responsibility in regard to adverse outcome do acknowledge that damage can and does occur at times from peripartum asphyxia and trauma.[20,36,49,50,52,70] There is a very clear association between intrapartum hypoxia and neonatal encephalopathy (especially seizures).[43,44,62] Encephalopathy is in turn a well-recognized predictor of permanent brain damage.[47,64] In fact, from one-quarter to one-half of term infants surviving hypoxic ischemic encephalopathy related to an intrapartum hypoxic insult are likely to have demonstrable neurologic deficits in later life.[1,19,37,65]

In recent decades, increasingly sophisticated measures have been introduced for detecting such hypoxia during labor. Moreover, changing practice trends have favored less traumatic delivery procedures. At the same time (and perhaps as a result of these influences), both the neonatal mortality rate and the frequency of cerebral palsy among term-size infants (over 2,500 g) have fallen in parallel.[32,33,40,66] However, because prematurity contributes so strongly to neurologic damage and more very small premature infants (who are at especially high risk) are surviving, the overall incidence of neurologic problems among infants does not seem as yet to be appreciably affected.

Despite the fact that perinatal events probably have only a relatively small overall impact on outcome, it is nevertheless logical to focus on the labor and delivery to ascertain which conditions or procedures can be considered risk factors by virtue of their association with poor results among exposed infants. This will serve to help alert obstetric personnel to such potentially serious risk factors. Given the current extreme sensitivity to liability issues among healthcare professionals, it should be clearly stated at the outset that the available data deal only with associations between labor-delivery events and outcome. While causation can some-times be inferred, especially if a mechanism is identifiable by means of which damage is likely to occur, one must be cautious in applying the general observation to the specific case. Knowledge about the rela-tionship between a risk factor and its associated adverse result is impor-tant because it forewarns the practitioner that the prevailing condition or event warrants attention in the form of astute evaluation and close surveillance (if not aggressive intervention) or that the proposed pro-cedure carries a potential hazard which must be counterbalanced by a clearly defined benefit.

All studies from which we can draw information for assessing the potential fetal and infant impact of labor and delivery have design defi-ciencies that limit the validity of interpretation. Since it is no longer feasible to undertake a critically controlled laboratory-type study to resolve such matters today, we are forced to rely on experiential reports in which the results are derived from anecdotal material without controls or from comparative study utilizing controls of questionable value. The principal problem with such studies is their failure to take concurrent confounding factors into account. This means the findings are always somewhat suspect because one cannot be sure some factor other than the one being examined may be responsible for the effect encountered. Such skepticism is healthy, of course, but there is obvious need to resolve doubts, if possible, to ensure optimal outcome for both mother and fetus by modifying clinical practices in their interests.

A recent attempt to supply such resolution utilized the extensive resources of the National Collaborative Perinatal Project (NCPP), consist-ing of data collected prospectively from nearly 60,000 pregnant women and their infants between 1958 and 1974. The data source and collection methodology have been detailed previously.[51] A total of 2,441 factors were examined as related to a spectrum of potentially relevant influences on the fetus and infant, such as labor progression, drugs and anesthesias, and delivery procedures, conditions, and complications, while control-ling for a wide range of concurrent intrinsic maternal, fetal, and pelvic variables. Outcome assessment of risk was based on perinatal death, severe neonatal depression, 8-month mental and motor evaluations, 1-year neurologic tests, 3-year battery of speech, language and hearing evaluations, and 4- and 7-year intelligence surveys. Specific attention was limited to cases yielding term-sized infants free of anomalies and compatible with normal development. In all there were 17,935 infants with sufficiently detailed labor data to study. The analytic sequence and results have been presented in monographic form.[23]

The investigation identified the fetal and infant risk factors associated with labor and delivery while fully addressing the confounding and interactional effects of as many other factors as possible within the constraints of current computer technology. Although the data were collected in the era before wide availability of electronic fetal heart rate monitoring, they can nonetheless be considered reasonably applicable to current obstetric practice because close fetal auscultatory surveillance was maintained in most cases. This form of monitoring has been determined to be quite satisfactory for practical purposes with results essentially indistinguishable from those obtained by continuous electronic means.[34,35] This applies especially in low-risk populations in which the predictive value of fetal monitoring is recognized to be poor as a screening test.[3,61] While practice patterns have changed over the years, the analytic methodology readily took this factor into account, making the results quite applicable to today's clinical practice. Moreover, the elapsed time permitted critical long-term follow-up of surviving infants to be accomplished, thus providing data that could not otherwise be obtainable; they may actually constitute a unique resource which is unlikely to be duplicated ever again.

PROLONGED LATENT PHASE

The several types of labor abnormalities identifiable by objective clinical means (see Chapter 1) may have very disparate effects on the gravida and her fetus. Earlier studies showed evidence, for example, that the common disorder of prolonged latent phase was innocuous. Delivery outcome seemed to depend entirely on the pattern that evolved later in the patient's active phase and second stage with no discernible adverse additive influence from the antecedent latent phase abnormality.[27] Furthermore, patients with prolonged latent phase did not appear to be at any increased risk of developing a major labor abnormality later in the course of their labor. The infant also fared well both in the immediate perinatal period[25] and during early childhood.[30,31] The perinatal mortality rate encountered among term-sized infants delivered of nulliparas with prolonged latent phase only (i.e., without a subsequent protraction or arrest disorder in the same labor) was 4.0 per 1,000 (as compared to 4.9

per 1,000 after a normal labor pattern). Neonatal depression as defined by a 5-min Apgar score below 5 occurred in 4.6% (vs. 3.2%, not a significant difference). Abnormal speech, language, and hearing results at age 3 years were disclosed in 8.1% (7.7% with a normal labor). Mean intelligence quotient at 4 years was entirely unaffected. When controlled for the impact of other labor progress variables in the aforementioned NCPP study, prolonged latent phase was shown to be significantly associated with poor perinatal outcome in multiparas (relative risk 2.00, $p = 0.002$), but not in nulliparas, and was without any detectable effect on long-term results.[23] The perinatal influence of prolonged latent phase among offspring of multiparas persisted at a statistically significant level (relative risk 1.77, $p = 0.024$) even when all concurrent intrinsic, drug, and delivery factors were assessed simultaneously.

FALSE LABOR

Spurious or false labor is recognized to be present in a proportion (about 10%) of patients with prolonged latent phase, diagnosable only by hindsight. This segment of the population was not specifically investigated in the NCPP study, but the possibility that false labor is an adverse factor was raised by Arulkumaran et al.[2] They examined 168 gravidas who had had a recent prior episode of false labor and found a significantly higher incidence of fetal distress (16.7% vs. 3.8%) and more operative intervention (20.2% vs. 8.0% cesarean section and 20.8% vs. 10.8% operative vaginal delivery) than in a normal control group. While cases were preselected to ensure comparability in regard to intact membranes and absence of high-risk antenatal factors, the degree of comparability between index cases and controls was unclear. Premature labor, for example, a factor known to be associated with episodic false labor, was not addressed at all. Moreover, there was overt dissimilarity in regard to the excessively frequent rate of oxytocin induction and augmentation of labor in the false labor group (15.5% and 35.7% vs. 0 and 19.7%). When stratified for oxytocin use, the analysis showed depressed babies needing neonatal intensive care to occur exclusively among those exposed to oxytocin within the study group (5.5% vs. 0, an insignificant difference). Thus, the observed effects could have been related to this or other factors, although the incidence of fetal distress was significantly higher in the false labor group even among those who received no oxytocin (7.3% vs. 2.6%). A contrary finding was reported by Quinn et al. who failed to detect any adverse effect from preceding false labor in a similarly flawed study.[58] The issue, therefore, remains unresolved, but it seems worthy of attention. It is reasonable to consider false labor a possible risk factor so as to be duly alerted.

PROTRACTION DISORDERS

The major labor aberrations of protracted active phase dilatation and protracted descent have been found to place the fetus and surviving infant at serious risk. They were initially determined to yield a perinatal mortality more than threefold greater than after normal labor patterns (15.2 per 1,000 vs. 4.9 per 1,000) in an essentially uncontrolled study.[26] Abnormal speech, language, and hearing results occurred more than twice as often at age 3 years than expected (16.2% vs. 7.7%) and significant lowering of the mean 4-year intelligence quotient by an average of 4.6 points was also verified.[30] At age 7 years, the intelligence quotient was reduced on average by a remarkable 8.4 points as shown in an analysis that dealt with a limited number of possible confounders by means of a matching technique.[31] Much more extensive weighting for confounding factors, made possible by the NCPP investigation described earlier, verified that abnormally slow active phase progress was deleterious to the fetus and infant, affecting both perinatal outcome and, to a lesser extent, long-term development.[23] The perinatal relative risk was 1.57 for children of nulliparas and 2.40 for those of multiparas when all other relevant factors were taken into account. The hazard is apparently enhanced by operative intervention utilized for purposes of effecting delivery in these cases.[21,22,25,26,30,31]

These observations confirm long-held impressions that prolonged labors are potentially perilous, especially if followed by forceps delivery. Tucker and Benaron, as far back as 1953, found neonatal apnea much more common after prolonged labor with forceps than after normal labor (23.9% vs. 4.1%).[69] Similarly, there were nearly five times the perinatal deaths encountered (5.2% vs. 1.1%). Remote effects were less clear-cut among survivors, except for some increase in emotional disturbance (21.3% vs. 16.3%), infantile behavior (14.9% vs. 9.3%), and low intelligence quotient scores (7.5% vs. 2.5% below 71).[4] More recently, Duignan et al. showed an inverse correlation between second stage duration and Apgar score.[17] The relationship was examined in more detail by Cohen, who verified the trend for 1-min Apgar scores, entirely corrected by fetal monitoring, but not for 5-min scores.[10] Ott demonstrated abnormal fetal heart rate patterns in 25.6% of patients with abnormally slow active phase labor (as contrasted with 15.4% in normal labors); even corrections for oxytocin use and high-risk status failed to diminish this effect (24.4% vs. 11.0%).[55] The intrinsic risk from this condition thus seems clearly established.

PRECIPITATE LABOR

Excessively rapid labors impact adversely on the fetus on the basis of a combination of physical trauma and hypoxia, usually from the excessive uterine contractility that is so commonly associated with precipitate labor patterns and the rapid compression-decompression of the fetal head (so-called "blast" injury) that occurs in the course of rapid descent. Although the frequency of neonatal apnea was only slightly increased in the cases reviewed by Tucker and Benaron (5.5% vs. 4.1%), there was a substantive increase in perinatal mortality (15.5 per 1,000 vs. 10.7 per 1,000, a statistically significant difference) with impressive numbers of traumatic intracranial hemorrhage disclosed at autopsy among infants who died (18.8%).[69] Late developmental deficiencies were encountered more often than expected in these cases as well, including mental retardation (20.0% vs. 7.0%) and intelligence quotients of 70 or less (20.0% vs. 2.5%).[4]

Analysis of the NCPP data with all confounders weighted showed adverse perinatal and long-term effects following labors with very short active phase in nulliparas only (perinatal relative risk 1.68, $p = 0.031$, and composite relative risk 1.29, including outcomes to 7 years, $p = 0.042$).[23] Paradoxically, there was a protective effect with labors characterized by a precipitate descent pattern (relative risk 0.71, $p = 0.015$ for composite outcome). The discrepancy could not be completely explained away, but it was felt related somehow to the common association of this condition with oxytocin use and tumultuous uterine contractions, the risk effects of which were accounted for by the analytic method. The failure to demonstrate poor results from precipitate labor in multiparas may have been due to these factors coupled with the frequent occurrence of this phenomenon in otherwise normal cases, diluting any potentially adverse effect it might have.

ARREST DISORDERS

A number of published comparative studies have demonstrated that arrest disorders of labor can be very serious. There is no doubt that as markers for cephalopelvic disproportion, with which they are so often associated, they are important indicators of potentially obstructed labor.

As such, cesarean delivery is commonly needed and operative vaginal delivery can be expected to be hazardous. These delivery trends have been verified, up to 56% of cases being subjected to operative delivery by cesarean section or midforceps.[24,28] The immediate results to the infant included high rates of mortality and neonatal depression.[26] In one study, the perinatal death rate was more than six times that for infants delivered after a normal labor pattern (36.6 per 1,000 vs. 4.9 per 1,000); even when corrected for the type of delivery procedure done in these cases, there were many more deaths than expected (16.1 per 1,000 vs. 1.5 per 1,000 after spontaneous delivery).[21]

Nelson and Broman applied discriminant function analysis to determine perinatal risk factors leading to serious motor and mental handicaps, examining 133 such factors simultaneously.[46] They found none of 60 antenatal factors was useful as a discriminator of later neurologic problems, but 3 of 26 intrapartum factors were, namely, low fetal heart rate, arrest of labor progress, and use of midforceps. There was nearly three times the frequency of arrested labor among handicapped infants than expected (18.0% vs.6.6%). Bottoms et al. studied cases with brief periods of arrested dilatation—between 1 and 2 hr—and reported more operative deliveries, maternal trauma, fetal acidosis, shoulder dystocia, meconium staining, and depressed infants than for normal labors.[6] Using the more generally accepted criteria for arrest disorders, as defined in Chapter 1, they were able to verify adverse effects, especially as regards low Apgar scores (relative risk 1.6), need for neonatal intensive care (relative risk 1.4, a significant finding), and neurologic damage (relative risk 1.7).[5] It was clear that patients with arrest disorders differed in other aspects from those with normal labor in important ways. For example, the frequencies of midforceps and cesarean section were increased fivefold among them. Stratifying by delivery route showed the poor infant outcome impact of arrest disorders to be relatively more common among cases delivered vaginally; indeed, the relationship was no longer evident after cesarean section.

Preliminary examination of the extensive NCPP data illustrated comparable adverse perinatal effects from arrest of dilatation and arrest of descent in both nulliparas (relative risk 1.54 and 1.53) and multiparas (relative risk 1.68 and 4.02), but no demonstrable residual effect later in life.[23] The perinatal effects diminished, moreover, to a statistically insignificant level when the impact of other concurrent labor disorders was weighed simultaneously, and they essentially vanished when the aggregate effect of other intrinsic drug and delivery factors was assessed at the same time. Thus, it is logical to ascribe the influence of arrest disorders to other risk variables acting on the gravida and her fetus concomitantly.

This should not be interpreted to absolve the labor aberration from all responsibility, however, because these other factors, such as uterotonic stimulation or forceps delivery, may have had their inherent peril magnified by the labor disorder; that is, we can postulate that the labor disorder somehow sensitizes the fetus so that the effect of an otherwise relatively innocuous risk factor becomes overtly manifest. This would emphasize the need to recognize the abnormality and manage it in a manner that can be relied upon to minimize risk (see Chapter 1).

INDUCTION AND AUGMENTATION OF LABOR

The hazards of oxytocin have long been known because complications are well recognized to occur occasionally from hypercontractility, including tetanic contractions, uterine rupture, abruptio placentae, amniotic fluid embolism, and fetal distress. Careful titration of dilute solutions with delicately controlled pump delivery systems, coupled with intensive surveillance of mother and fetus, have reduced the risk, but the potential peril is always present. This consideration motivated the Food and Drug Administration to interdict elective use altogether. Whether the fetal risk from oxytocin administration can be justified on balance when it is invoked for an indicated use remains to be assessed.

Short-term controlled and limited usage for purposes of undertaking contraction stress testing of fetoplacental status by Scanlon et al. showed no demonstrable neonatal neurobehavioral impact of any kind.[63] In their series of 54 cases, the results of all the oxytocin challenge tests were negative so the possible adverse synergistic effect of oxytocin on marginally compromised fetuses could not be determined. By contrast, Crowell et al. found significant alteration in neurophysiologic function in regard to resting brain activity defined in terms of autoregressive spectral estimates or coefficients among newborn infants delivered after labors induced with oxytocin or prostaglandin $F_2\alpha$.[12] They encountered no such difference in electroencephalographic responses to auditory, visual, tactile, or olfactory stimuli. Ott also showed adverse effects in the form of fetal heart rate abnormalities, although the impact of the fetal risk status and labor aberration was greater.[55] This confirmed earlier studies illustrating that oxytocin-stimulated term labors were more likely to show variable and late fetal heart rate decelerations than unstimulated labors, principally correlated with uterine hypercontractility.[29] A well-designed, randomized clinical study of elective oxytocin induction at term in Sweden by Leijon et al. demonstrated no discernible differences in neonatal behavior or neurologic status.[41] A large-scale epidemiologic study of elective labor induction and stimulation was conducted by Rindfuss et al., using multiple regression analysis and taking a limited number of demographic and obstetrical factors into account.[59] It clearly showed significantly increased frequencies of neonatal depression. In contrast, it has been reported by Studd et al. that augmentation of labor with oxytocin to accelerate progress in patients whose labor was not advancing in a satisfactory manner reduced the incidence of low Apgar scores.[67] Furthermore, two long-term follow-up studies of infants born after elective induction of labor disclosed no identifiable neurologic or developmental problems.[45,53]

The results of the extensive NCPP study designed to give a more definitive answer to the question of oxytocin effect left the issue somewhat unresolved.[23] Labor augmentation with oxytocin, considered collectively without distinction as to the preparation used, showed significantly deleterious perinatal effects in offspring of both nulliparas (relative risk 1.93, $p = 0.0009$) and multiparas (relative risk 1.65, $p = 0.022$) when all drug effects were weighed together. Parallel impact was encountered for oxytocin induction, but only in infants delivered of multiparas (relative risk 4.15, $p = 0.0005$). When the effects of all other relevant labor, delivery, and intrinsic variables were also accounted for, oxytocin augmentation (but not induction) was still shown to have a significant residual perinatal influence, especially in nulliparas (relative risk 1.61, $p = 0.039$). No long-term effects could be documented. Inexplicably, the two prevailing pharmaceutical preparations of oxytocin, namely, Pitocin and Syntocinon, were examined separately and found to have very disparate effects, one strongly adverse and the other somewhat protective. Focusing preliminarily on the preparations themselves, the study showed Pitocin to have markedly adverse perinatal (relative risk 3.27, $p = 0.009$) and composite outcomes (relative risk 2.46, $p = 0.0007$) in nulliparas only. Syntocinon showed no comparable effect and was actually protective in regard to long-term results in multiparas (relative risk 0.68, $p = 0.030$). Correcting for all other concurrent risk factors still left a significantly adverse composite effect from Pitocin on children of nulliparas (relative risk 2.30, $p = 0.029$) plus protective effects from Syntocinon on short- and long-term outcomes in multiparas, although the latter were no longer statistically significant. While these findings are difficult to interpret, it seems likely they were affected by the conditions prevailing in the patients to whom the drugs were given (and for which the agent may have been indicated), even though those factors were supposed to be fully accounted for by the analytic technique. In the overview, however, the weight of the data does suggest an adverse effect from oxytocin. This warrants limiting use to patients in whom the benefit of uterotonic stimulation can be shown to outweigh its possible risk.

FORCEPS

Much controversy still exists in regard to the effect of forceps on the fetus and infant. This may be due to the fact that there is no ethical way to carry out the kind of controlled clinical experiment that would be necessary to determine the real effect objectively and resolve the issue definitively. It may also be related to an understandable reluctance on the part of experienced obstetricians to relinquish a skill acquired only with difficulty and diligence. Nevertheless, there are a number of clinical studies that, when considered in composite, support a contention that some types of forceps procedures are inherently hazardous. This applies specifically to midforceps operations. There is no evidence that low forceps (defined as application with the fetal skull advanced to the maternal perineum, the scalp visible at the introitus without spreading the labia, and the sagittal suture directed anteroposteriorly) carries substantive risk when skillfully done.

Most descriptive studies tend to be anecdotal in nature, lacking controls for meaningful comparison. Retrospective surveys of the type of delivery to which damaged infants had been subjected, while also of limited value, may offer some useful insights. A series of 27 deaths at term from traumatic intracranial hemorrhage, for example, were found by O'Driscoll et al. to be consistently related to forceps delivery in nulliparas.[54] By banning Kielland forceps use altogether, they reduced the frequency sevenfold. Fenichel et al. similarly determined that nine of ten subarachnoid hemorrhages and five of eight intraventricular hemorrhages, all found on computed tomography scanning of term newborn infants, occurred in conjunction with traumatic forceps operations.[18] These impressive observations corroborate reports that show a correlation between birth trauma and midforceps procedures[42] and reduction in perinatal mortality paralleling the decline in midforceps use.[39]

Retrospective comparative studies tend to be somewhat more reliable, but the choice of control groups is always open to question. Nearly all point to the same conclusion, namely, that midforceps procedures are potentially harmful, although the data do not necessarily stand up to rigorous statistical probing. Indicated midforceps were shown to be associated with increased neonatal depression (relative risk 1.8), birth trauma (relative risk 1.9), and morbidity (relative risk 3.7) by Dudley et al.[16] Cooke compared easy and difficult midforceps procedures and confirmed a very marked and statistically significant increase in neonatal trauma (relative risk 16.1).[11] Matching cases delivered by Kielland forceps with those delivered vaginally by other means, Chiswick and James demonstrated significantly elevated mortality principally from tentorial tears (4.7% vs. 0%) as well as increased need for intensive neonatal care (relative risk 2.6), prolonged resuscitation (relative risk 5.0), birth trauma (relative risk 4.3), and neurologic damage (relative risk 10.1).[9]

Controlling for labor pattern among term-sized infants, we found perinatal mortality significantly increased with midforceps compared to spontaneous delivery (relative risk 8.6).[21] In addition, there were nearly three times as many children with disordered communications skills at age 3 years (relative risk 2.9), and this adverse relationship was magnified in conjunction with foregoing protracted or arrested labor patterns.[30] Similar effects were seen in the intelligence quotient scores at 4 years with an average reduction of 4.4 points.[30] Limited matching of cases showed a 5.8-point mean intelligence quotient loss at 7 years.[31] Dierker et al. also showed significantly increased rates of neonatal depression (relative risk 1.8) and cephalohematoma (relative risk 4.9) and statistically insignificant elevations in seizures and neuropathies.[14] Follow-up study of these infants for 2 years, however, showed no detectable residual effect.[15] Hughey et al. verified impressively high rates of perinatal death, neonatal depression, and neurologic damage when they compared results of midforceps delivery with those of cesarean section done in arrested second stage.[38] A similar study by Bowes and Bowes showed significantly increased neonatal morbidity relative to cesarean section (relative risk 3.7), mostly of a traumatic nature.[7] The same kind of investigation by Traub et al. revealed more deaths (15.2 per 1,000 vs. 0), neonatal intensive care (relative risk 1.4), and abnormal neurologic signs (relative risk 1.4), but none was statistically significant.[68]

Examining temporal trends of changing obstetric practice and their effects on outcome, Cyr et al. noted an increase in both cesarean section and midforceps over two decades, accompanied by a proportional reduction in neonatal deaths due to asphyxia and trauma, plus fewer cases of neonatal encephalopathy or permanent central nervous system damage, but with more peripheral neuropathies and fractures, including skull fractures.[13] Many of these latter traumatic injuries occurred in term infants with asphyxia and encephalopathy, and these children in turn had often been delivered by midforceps. The linear discriminant function analysis conducted by Nelson and Broman, mentioned earlier in respect to arrest of labor, showed that midforceps procedures were a statistically significant discriminator of severe neurologic handicap (relative risk 2.9) when their effect was investigated while taking into account the simultaneous impact of 132 other possible risk factors.[46]

The extensive study of the NCPP data, controlling for many more concurrent factors, found a number of forceps related variables to affect the infant in important ways.[23] Forceps application at stations 0 to +2 (referring to the level of the forward leading edge of the fetal presenting part on a centimeter scale with reference to zero station at the plane of the ischial spines) had a particularly strong adverse composite effect (short- and long-term combined) in children delivered of nulliparas (relative risk 8.6). Other factors related to forceps use that were determined to be seriously deleterious included difficult and failed forceps operations. Those procedures in which the traction was deemed difficult, as judged by trained dispassionate observers, more than doubled the composite harm in nulliparas (relative risk 2.2) and if very difficult, there was an eightfold effect on perinatal results in multiparas (relative risk 8.2). Difficult forceps rotation showed comparable hazard, especially in multiparas (perinatal relative risk 8.3, composite 3.4). Failed rotation magnified the latter impact markedly (relative risk 11.7).

Still greater risk was determined in cases in which there was failure to achieve vaginal delivery by any interventive means, including forceps attempts principally (perinatal relative risk in multiparas 21.9). The peril attendant upon failed forceps has been verified in a recent study reported by Boyd et al.[8] Although cesarean section after failed forceps yielded the same frequency of moderate and severe neonatal depression as cesarean section for failure to progress in the second stage (13.2% and 13.4% respectively), the rate was significantly greater than for infants delivered spontaneously (relative risk 5.7) or by low forceps (relative risk 6.6). Signs of neonatal encephalopathy occurred more often after failed forceps than in the control cesarean section group (5.7% vs. 2.4%) and they were rarely encountered after uncomplicated vaginal delivery (0.1%). Fractures and nerve palsies were also more frequent (3.8% vs. 0 and 0.7%, respectively). The need for neonatal intensive care was equally high in both cesarean section groups (24.5% and 23.2%), but significantly increased over spontaneous vaginal delivery (relative risk 3.10).

IMPLICATIONS FOR PRACTICE

It should follow logically from the material presented here that some labor and delivery conditions and practices are either themselves hazardous to the fetus or so closely associated with peril as to serve as important risk markers. While one can argue that the risk for a given factor may not be irrefutably proved in the scientific sense, the preponderant weight and relative consistency of evidence warrants sufficient concern to justify modifying clinical practices. Those relevant labor problems that expose the fetus and infant to danger must be recognized, evaluated expeditiously, and treated appropriately. The programs reviewed in Chapters 1 and 2 offer tested recommendations by which patients with specific labor aberrations can be effectively managed so as to minimize risk to their offspring. In the decade following introduction of these management programs at Boston's Beth Israel Hospital, the midforceps rate fell steadily from 10.7% to 1.2% in inverse relationship to the rising primary cesarean section rate which increased from 5.4% to 14.0%. At the same time, the neonatal mortality for infants weighing 1,000 g or more fell progressively from 11.3 per 1,000 to 3.8 per 1,000 (8.0 per 1,000 to 2.1 per 1,000 if corrected for fatal anomalies). Similar trends were reported by Iffy et al.[39]

It is clear that a number of other changes in medical practice took place during this time, including more sophisticated use of electronic fetal heart rate monitoring and other biophysical means for assessing fetal well-being, diminished use of narcotic analgesics and uterotonic agents in labor, and improved neonatal intensive care. The gratifying mortality trend, therefore, cannot be attributed entirely to the labor management programs and resulting changes in delivery mode. Experienced pediatricians specializing in neonatal care are uniformly impressed about how much less often they are called upon to care for the severely depressed and traumatized babies so commonly seen in the past. There can be little doubt that both survival and quality of life have benefitted. This goal should be readily attainable in all institutions at which obstetric services are offered. It is unlikely that further major improvements in outcome can be made unless those risk factors still remaining are uncovered and dealt with in an appropriate manner. Some of the areas needing attention have been addressed here. In our collective quest to optimize results for the mother and fetus whose welfare we are entrusted with, we cannot become complacent with the good that has been achieved to date. We must avoid assuming a self-satisfied attitude that we have accomplished the best we can, but rather continue to probe and improve the care we offer.

REFERENCES

1. Adsett DB, Fitz CR, Hill A: Hypoxic-ischemic cerebral injury in the term newborn: Correlation of CT findings with neurological outcome. *Dev Med Child Neurol* 1985; 27:155–160.

2. Arulkumaran S, Michelson J, Ingemarsson I, Ratnam SS: Obstetric outcome of patients with a previous episode of spurious labor. *Am J Obstet Gynecol* 1987;157:17–20.

3. Banta HD, Thacker SB: Assessing the costs and benefits of electronic fetal monitoring. *Obstet Gynecol Surv* 1979;34:627–642.

4. Benaron HBW, Brown M, Tucker BE, Wentz V, Yacorzynski GK: The remote effects of prolonged labor with forceps delivery, precipitate labor with spontaneous delivery, and natural labor with spontaneous delivery on the child. *Am J Obstet Gynecol* 1953;66:551–568.

5. Bottoms SF, Hirsch VJ, Sokol RJ: Medical management of arrest disorders of labor: A current overview. *Am J Obstet Gynecol* 1987;156:935–939.

6. Bottoms SF, Sokol RJ, Rosen MG: Short arrest of cervical dilatation: A risk for maternal/fetal/infant morbidity. *Am J Obstet Gynecol* 1981;140:108–116.

7. Bowes WA Jr, Bowes C: Current role of the midforceps operation. *Clin Obstet Gynecol* 1980;23:549–557.

8. Boyd ME, Usher RH, McLean FH, Norman BE: Failed forceps. *Obstet Gynecol* 1986;68:779–783.

9. Chiswick ML, James DK: Kielland's forceps: Association with neonatal morbidity. *Br Med J* 1979;1:7–9.

10. Cohen W: Influence of the duration of second stage labor on perinatal outcome and puerperal morbidity. *Obstet Gynecol* 1977;49:266–269.

11. Cooke WAR: Evaluation of the midforceps operation. *Am J Obstet Gynecol* 1967;99:327–332.

12. Crowell DH, Sharma SD, Philip AGS, Kapuniai MB, Waxman SH, Hale RW: Effects of induction of labor on the neurophysiologic functioning of newborn infants. *Am J Obstet Gynecol* 1980;136:48–53.

13. Cyr RM, Usher RH, McLean FH: Changing patterns of birth asphyxia and trauma over 20 years. *Am J Obstet Gynecol* 1984;148:490–498.

14. Dierker LJ Jr, Rosen MG, Thompson K, Debanne S, Linn P: The midforceps: Maternal and neonatal outcomes. *Am J Obstet Gynecol* 1985;152:176–183.

15. Dierker LJ Jr, Rosen MG, Thompson K, Linn P: Midforceps deliveries: Long-term outcome of infants. *Am J Obstet Gynecol* 1986;154:764–768.

16. Dudley AG, Markham SM, McNie TM: Elective versus indicated midforceps delivery. *Obstet Gynecol* 1971;37:19–23.

17. Duignan NM, Studd JWW, Hughes AO: Characteristics of normal labour in different racial groups. *Br J Obstet Gynaecol* 1975;82:593–601.

18. Fenichel GM, Webster DL, Wong WKT: Intracranial hemorrhage in the term newborn. *Arch Neurol* 1984;41:30–34.

19. Fitzhardinge PM, Flodmark O, Fitz CR, Ashby S: The prognostic value of computed tomography as an adjunct to assessment of the term infant with postasphyxial encephalopathy. *J Pediatr* 1981;99:777–781.

20. Freeman J (ed): *Prenatal and Perinatal Factors Associated with Brain Disorders.* NIH Publication no. 85-1149. Bethesda, MD, US Department of Health and Human Services, 1985, p 13.

21. Friedman EA: Patterns of labor as indicators of risk. *Clin Obstet Gynecol* 1973; 16:172–183.

22. Friedman EA: *Labor: Clinical Evaluation and Management.* New York, Appleton-Century-Crofts, 1978.

23. Friedman EA, Neff RK: *Labor and Delivery: Impact on Offspring*. Littleton, MA, PSG Publishing, 1987.

24. Friedman EA, Niswander KR, Sachtleben MR, Ashworth M: Dysfunctional labor: IX. Delivery outcome. *Am J Obstet Gynecol* 1970;106:219–226.

25. Friedman EA, Niswander KR, Sachtleben MR: Dysfunctional labor: XI. Neurological and developmental effects on surviving infants. *Obstet Gynecol* 1969;33:785–791.

26. Friedman EA, Niswander KR, Sachtleben MR, Naftaly N: Dysfunctional labor: X. Immediate result to infant. *Obstet Gynecol* 1969;33:776–783.

27. Friedman EA, Sachtleben MR: Dysfunctional labor: I. Prolonged latent phase in the nullipara. *Obstet Gynecol* 1961;17:135–148.

28. Friedman EA, Sachtleben MR: Dysfunctional labor: III. Secondary arrest of dilatation in the nullipara. *Obstet Gynecol* 1962;19:576–591.

29. Friedman EA, Sachtleben MR: Effect of oxytocin and oral prostaglandin E_2 on uterine contractility and fetal heart rate patterns. *Am J Obstet Gynecol* 1978;130:403–407.

30. Friedman EA, Sachtleben MR, Bresky PA: Dysfunctional labor: XII. Long-term effects on infant. *Am J Obstet Gynecol* 1977;127:779–783.

31. Friedman EA, Sachtleben-Murray MR, Dahrouge D, Neff RK: Long-term effects of labor and delivery on offspring: A matched-pair analysis. *Am J Obstet Gynecol* 1984; 150:941–945.

32. Hagberg B, Hagberg G, Olow I: Gains and hazards of intensive neonatal care: An analysis from Swedish cerebral palsy epidemiology. *Dev Med Child Neurol* 1982;24:13–19.

33. Hagberg B, Hagberg G, Olow I: The changing panorama of cerebral palsy in Sweden: IV. Epidemiological trends 1959–1978. *Acta Paediatr Scand* 1984;73:433–440.

34. Haverkamp AD, Orleans M, Langendoerfer S, McFee J, Murphy J, Thompson HE: A controlled trial of the differential effects of intrapartum fetal monitoring. *Am J Obstet Gynecol* 1979;134:399–408.

35. Haverkamp AD, Thompson HE, McFee JG, Cetrulo C: The evaluation of continuous fetal heart rate monitoring in high-risk pregnancy. *Am J Obstet Gynecol* 1976;125:310–317.

36. Hensleigh PA, Feinstat T, Spencer R: Perinatal events and cerebral palsy. *Am J Obstet Gynecol* 1986;154:978–981.

37. Hill A, Volpe JJ: Seizures, hypoxic-ischemic brain injury and intraventricular hemorrhage in the newborn. *Ann Neurol* 1981;10:109–121.

38. Hughey MJ, McElin TW, Lussky R: Forceps operations in perspective: I. Midforceps rotation operations. *J Reprod Med* 1978;20:253–259.

39. Iffy L, Bilenki I, Apuzzio JJ, Ganesh V, Sun SC, Thomas H, Erian M, Kaminetzky HA: The role of obstetric factors in perinatal mortality trends. *Int J Gynaecol Obstet* 1986;24:85–95.

40. Kudrjacev T, Schoenberg BS, Kurland LT, Groover RV: Cerebral palsy: Trends in incidence and changes in concurrent neonatal mortality, Rochester, MN, 1950–1976. *Neurology* 1983;33:1433–1438.

41. Leijon I, Finnström O, Hedenskog S, Ryden G, Tylleskär J: Spontaneous labour and elective induction: A prospective randomized study. *Acta Pediatr Scand* 1979;68:553–560.

42. Levine MG, Holroyde J, Woods JR Jr, Siddiqi TA, Scott M, Miodovnik M: Birth trauma: Incidence and predisposing factors. *Obstet Gynecol* 1984;63:792–795.

43. Low JA, Galbraith RS, Muir DW, Killen HL, Pater EA, Karchmer EJ: The predictive significance of biological risk factors for deficits in children of a high-risk population. *Am J Obstet Gynecol* 1983;145:1059–1066.

44. Low JA, Galbraith RS, Muir DW, Killen HL, Pater EA, Karchmer EJ: The relationship between perinatal hypoxia and newborn encephalopathy. *Am J Obstet Gynecol* 1985; 152:256–260.

45. McBride WG, Lyle JG, Black B, Brown C, Thomas D: A study of five year old children born after elective induction of labour. *Med J Aust* 1977;2:456–462.

46. Nelson KB, Broman SH: Perinatal risk factors in children with serious motor and mental handicaps. *Ann Neurol* 1977;2:371–377.

47. Nelson KB, Ellenberg JH: Neonatal signs as predictors of cerebral palsy. *Pediatrics* 1979;64:225–232.

48. Nelson KB, Ellenberg JH: Antecedents of cerebral palsy: Multivariate analysis of risk. *N Engl J Med* 1986;315:81–86.

49. Niswander KR: The obstetrician, fetal asphyxia, and cerebral palsy. *Am J Obstet Gynecol* 1979;133:358–361.

50. Niswander KR: Does substandard obstetric care cause cerebral palsy? *Contemp Ob Gyn* 1987;30:42–60.

51. Niswander KR, Gordon M (eds): *The Collaborative Perinatal Study of the National Institute of Neurological Disease and Stroke: The Women and Their Pregnancies.* Philadelphia: WB Saunders, 1972.

52. Niswander KR, Henson G, Elbourne D, Chalmers I, Redman C, Macfarlane A, Tizard P: Adverse outcome of pregnancy and the quality of obstetric care. *Lancet* 1984;2:827–830.

53. Niswander KR, Turoff BB, Romans J: Developmental status of children delivered through elective induction of labor: Results of a 4-year follow-up study. *Obstet Gynecol* 1966;27:15–20.

54. O'Driscoll K, Meagher D, MacDonald D, Geoghegan F: Traumatic intracranial haemorrhage in firstborn infants and delivery with obstetric forceps. *Br J Obstet Gynaecol* 1981;88:577–581.

55. Ott WJ: Relationship of normal and abnormal late labor patterns to perinatal morbidity. *Clin Obstet Gynecol* 1982;25:105–110.

56. Paneth N: Birth and the origins of cerebral palsy (editorial). *N Engl J Med* 1986;315:124–125.

57. Paneth N, Stark RI: Cerebral palsy and mental retardation in relation to indicators of perinatal asphyxia: An epidemiologic overview. *Am J Obstet Gynecol* 1983;147:960–966.

58. Quinn MA, Murphy AJ, Gallagher J: "Spurious" labour: Does it matter? *Aust NZ J Obstet Gynaecol* 1984;21:167–172.

59. Rindfuss RR, Gortmaker SL, Ladinsky JL: Elective induction and stimulation of labor and the health of the infant. *Am J Pub Health* 1978;68:872–878.

60. Rosen MG, Debanne S, Thompson K, Bilenker RM: Long-term neurological morbidity in breech and vertex births. *Am J Obstet Gynecol* 1985;151:718–720.

61. Sachs BP, Friedman EA: Antepartum and intrapartum assessment of the fetus: Current status and does it influence outcome? *Clin Anesthesiol* 1986;4:53–65.

62. Sarnat HB, Sarnat MS: Neonatal encephalopathy following fetal distress. *Arch Neurol* 1976;33:696–705.

63. Scanlon JW, Suzuki K, Shea E, Tronick E: Clinical and neurobehavioral effects of repeated intrauterine exposure to oxytocin: A prospective study. *Am J Obstet Gynecol* 1978;132:294–296.

64. Scott H: Outcome of very severe birth asphyxia. *Arch Dis Child* 1976;51:712–716.

65. Shaywitz BA: The sequelae of hypoxic-ischemic encephalopathy. *Semin Perinatol* 1987;11:180–190.

66. Stanley FJ: Spastic cerebral palsy: Changes in birthweight and gestational age. *Early Hum Dev* 1981;5:167–178.

67. Studd J, Clegg DR, Sanders RR, Hughes AO: Identification of high risk labours by labour nomogram. *Br Med J* 1975;2:545–547.

68. Traub AI, Morrow RJ, Ritchie JWK, Dornan KJ: A continuing use for Kielland's forceps. *Br J Obstet Gynaecol* 1984;91:894–898.

69. Tucker BE, Benaron HBW: The immediate effects of prolonged labor with forceps delivery, precipitate labor with spontaneous delivery, and natural labor with spontaneous delivery on the child. *Am J Obstet Gynecol* 1953;66:540–550.

70. Visscher HC: Physical birth trauma is not a major source of brain damage. *ACOG Newslett* 1985;29(6):1–5.

17

Critical Care of the Parturient

Ellen Harrison and Wayne R. Cohen

The specialty of critical care has evolved rapidly over the past two decades. This progress has been fueled primarily by technologic developments that have made sophisticated monitoring and intervention at the bedside possible, and by the availability of devices to support failing cardiopulmonary function. Modern critical care approaches have been applied in disparate patient populations, from neonates to combat soldiers and geriatric cardiac patients, and in settings that range from intensive care units to transport helicopters. The practice of critical care must be reevaluated and adapted for each unique application; this is especially true when intensive care medicine is extended to parturient women. Although few labors are more taxing for the physician to manage than those in critically ill women, fewer still provide as much gratification.

This chapter focuses on the unique aspects of applying critical care to the grave conditions that may complicate or be complicated by parturition. Ways to prevent critical illness during labor and delivery are considered. Modalities of monitoring and therapeutic intervention, ranging from the commonplace, but crucial, to the more dazzling technologically advanced choices are discussed, with emphasis on their use during labor.

While obstetricians with an interest and proficiency in critical care are making great contributions to this field, the diseases encountered are so varied and the techniques and therapies used so infrequently in obstetrics that in most settings, care is provided through the collaboration of obstetricians and colleagues from other specialties. This chapter is intended as an obstetrician's resource for that collaboration. It reviews basic aspects of intensive care and highlights the pitfalls of applying them to this unique population.

SCOPE OF CRITICAL CARE DURING PARTURITION

A broad spectrum of conditions may warrant intensive care in the peripartum period. Hemorrhagic shock, pulmonary edema, disseminated intravascular coagulation, adult respiratory distress syndrome (ARDS), septic shock, thyroid storm, intracerebral hemorrhage, renal cortical necrosis, and hepatic rupture are a few examples that demonstrate the breadth of the problems encountered. Women at risk to become critically ill form a continuum from the completely well to the chronically ill. Conditions seen may be unavoidable or, sometimes, iatrogenic. Life-threatening diseases may be an unpredictable complication of labor in a healthy woman, as in amniotic fluid embolism, or an anticipated outcome of birth in a patient known to face extreme risks in parturition. An example of the latter is Eisenmenger's syndrome, in which the anticipated maternal mortality is 30% to 70%.[42] Intensive care techniques may be employed in a relatively stable patient in anticipation of difficulties, or used in the atmosphere of unexpected acute and profound clinical deterioration. The degree to which the pregnancy must be considered in shaping the treatment plan can vary greatly, depending in large part on the age of gestation.

The wide array of conditions that comprise critical illness in labor and delivery can be categorized in a variety of ways. Classification by their causal relationship to parturition is useful because it helps bring into focus the possibilities for prevention, to be discussed below.

Childbirth may provoke critical illness in an otherwise healthy woman. Although the great majority of parturients are healthy, complications in this category (e.g., postpartum hemorrhage, placental abruption with disseminated intravascular coagulation, sepsis) represent a commonly encountered class of serious disorders. Their unexpected nature may find the obstetrician unprepared to deal with them promptly.

Labor and delivery may produce critical illness in patients by exacerbating a coexisting disease. Grave illness is far more likely to occur in an individual with a serious underlying disease than in a well woman. The disease process can be transformed adversely by labor and delivery, as when hyperthyroidism accelerates into thyroid storm or a cerebral arteriovenous malformation ruptures. Labor and delivery may impose an intolerable burden on a system with inadequate reserves. For example, the enormously increased cardiovascular demands of pregnancy may outstrip the reserve of a compromised heart and precipitate pulmonary edema. A bleeding diathesis, so mild as to cause no significant problems with everyday minor traumas can, in the face of delivery, be responsible for severe hemorrhage.

An acute illness may initiate parturition. Many kinds of acute severe illness may trigger labor. Multiple trauma and hemorrhage, pyelonephritis, or other forms of acute febrile illness, diabetic ketoacidosis, or acute cardiac or pulmonary decompensation are sometimes complicated by the appearance of labor. Similarly, a drug abuser may be catapulted into labor by use of cocaine and may need to be delivered while dangerously intoxicated. Serious illness may result indirectly in delivery when the disease is judged to be an indication to terminate pregnancy; the induction of labor or cesarean section in an eclamptic gravida would be such a case.

During labor and delivery, patients may go without drugs they usually take. The cessation of needed medications can have disastrous consequences in several ways. If the underlying condition requires continuous suppression and if the medication's effects are not sustained long after discontinuation, as is true of many antiarrhythmic drugs, a problem that had been well controlled may recur during labor and delivery. A previously controlled disorder can reemerge in a more virulent form than ever if the medication that was controlling it is stopped; such rebound phenomena can occur after the cessation of certain antihypertensive, anticonvulsant, and antianginal agents. Hypertensive crisis, status epilepticus, and unstable angina may be provoked in this manner. Wittingly or unwittingly an abused substance, such as alcohol, barbiturates, narcotics, or diazepam may be withheld, putting the patient (and the fetus) at risk for intrapartum or postpartum withdrawal.

Medications and procedures during labor and delivery can precipitate critical illness. Certain medications used during parturition may have adverse effects because of the underlying illness, a drug interaction, or an allergy. For example, aminoglycoside antibiotics, magnesium sulfate, and many drugs used during anesthesia can precipitate weakness and respiratory depression in a patient with myasthenia gravis. Women with no known contraindication to an agent may also be at risk, as when an unknown penicillin allergy declares itself with anaphylaxis after appropriate intrapartum treatment for a streptococcal infection. An error in administering medication can be disastrous as well. Procedures performed during labor and delivery such as endotracheal intubation, central venous line placement, and administration of anesthesia also have the potential to cause grave complications.

Rarely, *critical illness may coincide with labor and delivery by chance alone* and bear no causal relationship to it. The parturient is susceptible to the same risks of acute serious illness as young women in general.

PREVENTION OF CRITICAL ILLNESS

Among the factors that distinguish critical illness from its milder counterparts is the possibility of death or permanent impairment. The goal of intensive care is to reduce these risks insofar as possible; but no matter how scrupulous the care, the chance of adversity can never be eliminated. It is evident from the preceding categorization of critical illness complicating labor and delivery that many conditions are predictable, and some are preventable. To eliminate those that are preventable and to prepare for what can be foreseen are important aspects of reducing the frequency and risks of critical illness.

Prevention strategies are uniquely applicable to the obstetric patient population. For patients with a disease or condition that may worsen during labor the obstetrician often has the enviable advantage of knowing months in advance that a crisis is approaching, approximately when it will occur, and what the nature of it will be. Labor and delivery can usually be made to occur at a prearranged time, if that would be beneficial. These conditions afford the obstetrician an opportunity for prevention and preparation that is unparalleled in critical care.

The preventive approach is most applicable to women with known conditions that put them at risk, but it should be recognized that preventive measures are built into the accepted regimens of prenatal and peripartum care for all women. For example, the use of antacids to reduce gastric acidity prior to cesarean section is a prophylactic measure against aspiration pneumonia and adult respiratory distress syndrome.

Prenatal Care

Prevention begins during prenatal care. A scrupulous history, physical examination, and medical record review are the first steps to prevent perinatal catastrophe, because risk reduction is inconceivable without risk recognition. A thorough grasp of the patient's past problems and current health status is the cornerstone of all further planning for testing, monitoring, and treatment. Armed with such understanding, the physician can, in some instances, avert intrapartum disaster by prenatal treatment. The threat of thyroid storm to mother and fetus can, for example, be minimized by appropriate prenatal control of hyperthyroidism.

Prenatal treatment may not necessarily be targeted specifically to prevent intrapartum events, but may do so as part of a broader strategy. For instance, prescribing digoxin for a patient with mitral stenosis and a previous paroxysm of atrial fibrillation will prevent rapid tachycardia if this arrhythmia recurs. While digoxin exerts its protective effect throughout pregnancy, it is of more vital importance when the detrimental hemodynamic effects of tachycardia would be superimposed upon the heavy cardiovascular burden of parturition.

A preventive prenatal approach remains an option even when prenatal treatment cannot prevent catastrophic intrapartum events. Testing can be performed to clarify the risks, and diagnostic surveillance strategies can be altered to identify and address pathologic events early so that patients do not enter labor and delivery in a severely compromised state.

Plans for Labor and Delivery

An essential component of prenatal care for women at risk is the development of a comprehensive delivery plan. The aim of the plan is to prevent or to minimize the impact of hazardous events. Table 17-1 outlines the basic components of the labor and delivery plan.

With appropriate foresight, some threats to well-being can be avoided. For some conditions, the plan may specify treatment regimens such as corticosteroid administration to prevent addisonian crisis in susceptible women, or cryoprecipitate to prevent bleeding in a patient with von Willebrand's disease.[9] Prevention may entail optimization of the patient's condition as she enters labor. If a woman with heart disease put at risk for pulmonary edema by the cardiac demands of parturition is treated so she begins labor with a volume state at the lower end of her acceptable range, she will have a wider margin to tolerate abrupt volume shifts without pulmonary congestion.

Recrudescence of a chronic previously stable condition can be forestalled by a plan for administration of chronic medications, such as bronchodilators in a severe asthmatic or anticonvulsants in an epileptic. The plan should call attention to contraindicated drugs that might otherwise be used. For example, in patients with paroxysmal tachyarrhythmias due to abnormal conduction pathways, treatment of their arrhythmias with commonly used drugs like verapamil or digoxin can precipitate far more rapid and dangerous disturbances, including ventricular fibrillation. The plan should identify common medications that, if needed, would be used in a nonroutine way. For example, magnesium sulfate or certain antibiotic doses must be modified in the presence of renal disease.

Preventive measures also involve obstetric decisions relating to the conduct of labor and mode of delivery. The decision may sometimes be to circumvent labor in women with certain diseases to prevent dreaded intrapartum complications; but in other situations, cesarean delivery might accrue maternal risks deemed best avoided.

Disorders capable of precipitating life-threatening illness do not necessarily do so, and the ability to respond expeditiously can keep an ominous

Table 17-1 Prenatal Planning for Labor and Delivery

---

1. Who will be involved in caring for the patient during labor and delivery? Have all necessary consultations been performed?
2. Will labor occur spontaneously or be induced? Will the pregnancy be allowed to continue post-term?
3. What is the preferred mode of delivery? What intrapartum events would change this choice?
4. What type of anesthesia will be employed for vaginal delivery? For cesarean section?
5. Where should the patient labor and deliver? Labor room, delivery room recovery, or operating room? Sometimes proximity to the operating room or facility for aortic counter-pulsation will dictate choice. Is referral to another institution appropriate?
6. What complications might occur in the peripartum period? What treatments will be employed for them?
7. What nonroutine tests, if any, should be ordered on presentation?
8. What medications, if any, are contraindicated?
9. Are any prophylactic drug regimens indicated?
10. Is treatment or further evaluation of any existing disorder needed prior to delivery?
11. Should the patient have an intravenous line placed? What kind? What types of fluids should be administered and at what rate?
12. Should blood be cross-matched? Is excessive bleeding anticipated? Is difficulty with cross-matching anticipated?
13. If the patient is on chronic medications how will they be handled in the peripartum period? Is there any danger connected with missing one or more doses? Should a parenteral substitute for oral medications be given?
14. What type of monitoring will be performed? Electrocardiogram (ECG)? Arterial line? Swan-Ganz catheter? Foley catheter? Pulse oximeter?
15. Is it anticipated that any medications or equipment not commonly kept or used on a labor floor will be needed? If so, how can they be obtained, how should they be used and who will be familiar with their use?
16. Should a pediatrician attend the delivery? Is any special equipment or medication needed in the delivery room? Does fetal condition warrant transfer for delivery?
17. What will ensure that the patient's record and this plan will be available at delivery?
18. What health professionals will comprise the team during labor and delivery? Have their individual responsibilities been defined? Who will have overall responsibility for clinical decision making?

---

event from achieving its full potential for disaster. A carefully designed plan for management of labor and delivery may promote readiness in several ways. Rapid recognition of a developing problem is a prerequisite for prompt response; plans must be made for evaluation, observation, and monitoring to achieve this end. The ability to intervene speedily must also be assured; this involves having made available in advance the personnel, facilities, equipment, and drugs that could be needed. One must see that equipment and medicines required rarely on an obstetric service are made available and that the appropriate caregivers are familiar with their use.

Deciding controversial management issues in advance can save precious time. Attention to detail is required to handle powerful but unfamiliar drugs and devices safely. Doctors and nurses may need to familiarize themselves with drug use protocols.

Planning ideally serves to promote rapid response to grave situations by having dispensed with conflict, controversy, and reluctance in advance; no time need be wasted establishing the available options if a careful program has already been developed by the physicians most familiar with the patient. The plan should be discussed with the patient during prenatal care. In fact, discussing what she can expect and what may be asked of her will help to alleviate anxiety and to promote cooperation; moreover, obtaining informed consent for a needed intervention can be streamlined if the patient already understands the procedure.

While this chapter addresses critical illness in the mother only, it is important to point out that women with potential for critical illness in labor and delivery often have offspring at risk; no labor and delivery plan is complete unless concerns centering on the fetus have been met. Some diseases may affect both directly. Mother and infant may both be at risk of thyroid storm in untreated Graves' disease, or of hemorrhage in isoimmune thrombocytopenic purpura. The fetus and newborn may be at peril in a more indirect way from maternal cardiovascular or pulmonary compromise. Assembling the appropriate team of professionals with the facilities and expertise to handle serious complications in the fetus and newborn is of obvious importance.

PROVISION OF INTENSIVE CARE

Bedside Care

In view of the array of sophisticated equipment found in critical care units, it is no surprise that intensive care has been equated with bioelectronic wizardry. Advanced technology is surely a crucial part of the provision of critical care; but it cannot be overemphasized that the most important and sophisticated intensive care monitoring system is a clinician at the bedside. No electronic data can replace what is learned from talking with and examining the patient, whose perceptions of her symptoms provide unique insights into the disease process. There is, for example, no better way to obtain information about pain, blurred vision, orthopnea, or a change in fetal movement. Nothing can improve on the ability of a severe preeclamptic patient's complaint of marked right upper quadrant pain to warn of a possible supcapsular hepatic hematoma. The evaluation of mental status is a function that can be done only by a person at the bedside. Sometimes simply touching a patient and finding her skin cold or hot or clammy can alert the clinician to a serious problem. The physical examination is invaluable in other self-evident ways too numerous to mention.

Careful bedside assessment can at times obviate the need for more invasive methods of evaluation, but physical examination is especially important in patients receiving complex monitoring and intervention. It can identify complications or technical problems, and provide a safeguard against acting solely on the basis of bioelectronic information that may sometimes be misleading.

The history and physical examination must be evaluated by someone who understands the expected physiologic changes of pregnancy. Findings that are normal in an obstetric population may be viewed by a consultant unfamiliar with pregnant patients as pathologic, or important abnormalities may be overlooked. For example, heart failure might be diagnosed erroneously in a healthy pregnant woman with a physiologic heart murmur, ankle edema, and shortness of breath when supine if the examining physician were unaware these could be normal findings in pregnancy. The development of a common understanding of the patient based on a shared interpretation of the findings is an important part of a successful collaboration between obstetrician and medical or surgical colleagues.

Electrocardiographic Monitoring and Electrical Cardioversion

Continuous electrocardiographic (ECG) monitoring allows assessment of heart rate, rhythm, and conduction patterns. It is of value during labor in women with serious rhythm or conduction disturbances, a history of cardiac ischemia, and patients, such as those with mitral stenosis, in whom even moderate tachycardia could precipitate decompensation. Electrocardiographic monitoring should be used routinely in women on mechanical ventilators, those with pulmonary artery catheters, and those receiving arrhythmogenic drugs. Occasionally, patients without primary cardiovascular disease may require monitoring, such as when cocaine intoxication accompanies labor, thus obliging one to conduct the labor and delivery of a patient at risk for cardiac arrhythmias and myocardial ischemia. The only direct risk of monitoring is skin irritation due to the electrode gel.[25]

Laboring women may move about considerably. To interfere minimally with their activities while maintaining a technically acceptable ECG tracing, place the electrodes over the sternum and clavicles; these bony prominences will be less affected by respiratory motion and muscular activity than other portions of the chest wall. It is better to adjust the equipment to give the patient freedom when possible rather than to restrict her unnecessarily. Special exercise electrodes are available that will be less likely to fall off if the patient is sweating.

Electrical cardioversion to convert supraventricular and ventricular tachyarrhythmias immediately to sinus rhythm has been used in a small number of pregnant women without apparent adverse sequelae. The number of cases reported is too small to be certain about the risks entailed,[56] but the technique should not be withheld if standard pharmacologic measures prove fruitless, or if immediate cardioversion is necessary to prevent or treat cardiac decompensation or life-threatening arrhythmias. In the latter circumstances the hemodynamic benefits of returning to sinus rhythm outweigh any potential risk.

Arterial Blood Gases

Blood gas analysis consists of measurement of partial pressures of oxygen and carbon dioxide and the pH of arterial blood samples. It yields information about oxygenation, ventilation, and acid-base balance. Oxygen saturation or content can be measured directly only with an oximeter. Arterial blood gas analysis is used in adults primarily to assess aspects of pulmonary function. It provides useful data relating to acid-base balance and the relative contribution of metabolic and respiratory processes that influence blood pH. Sampling of arterial blood may be accomplished by arterial puncture or from an indwelling catheter. Catheters are preferred when multiple samples are required or when continuous blood pressure monitoring is desirable. Attention to detail in blood sampling, storage, and analysis is important if results are to be accurate.

Usually the radial artery is used, after ensuring that collateral ulnar circulation exists. The risks of arterial puncture are arterial occlusion with ischemia, distal embolization, hemorrhage, infections and injury to adjacent structures. These are encountered quite rarely as a consequence of simple arterial puncture, but are more common when arterial catheters are used. There are no documented additional complications of arterial sampling in pregnancy. Arterial puncture carries a heightened risk in patients with bleeding and clotting disorders. This is especially important to the obstetrician because hemostatic defects characterize many of the syndromes responsible for critical illness in parturients. Carpal tunnel syndrome is a known complication of radial artery puncture when bleeding into the wrist occurs. It is prudent to be especially vigilant for signs of median nerve compression because pregnant patients are predisposed to the problem by upper extremity edema, particularly in preeclampsia.

Physicians unfamiliar with pregnant women need to take special care in evaluating arterial blood gases; their correct interpretation requires an appreciation of the physiologic changes of pregnancy. The physiologic metabolic acidosis may be misinterpreted as a sign of possible grave illness and treated accordingly, to the patient's detriment. Conversely, important pathologic conditions may be overlooked if nonpregnancy standards are applied to the blood gases of pregnant women. For example, the degree of respiratory depression in a gravida may be vastly underestimated if the baseline level of partial pressure of carbon dioxide (Pco_2) is assumed to be the higher normal level found in nonpregnant women.

Progesterone, produced in vast quantities during pregnancy, increases the sensitivity of the respiratory center to carbon dioxide, producing central hyperventilation, hypocarbia, and a chronic respiratory alkalosis. Metabolic compensation is achieved by a decrease in serum bicarbonate that counteracts the alkalosis and restores the pH to normal. The partial pressure of oxygen (Po_2) rises as a result of hyperventilation. Because of these physiologic changes, blood gas values in late pregnancy are pH 7.40 to 7.45, Pco_2 27 to 32 torr, Po_2 100 to 104 torr, and serum bicarbonate 18 to 21 mEq/L.[58]

Noninvasive Assessments of Arterial Oxygenation

Pulse oximetry is a method for the spectrophotometric determination of arterial oxygen saturation using a device that fits on the earlobe or fingertip. Light of specific wavelengths is directed across a pulsating arterial bed. Changes in light transmission during each pulse are detected and analyzed, and arterial oxygen saturation is displayed.[61] Compared to the in vitro analysis of sampled blood, its advantages are that it (1) provides continuous rather than intermittent monitoring; (2) does not necessitate phlebotomy; (3) is painless; and (4) carries no direct risk.

Pulse oximetry can obviate the need for some, but not all, arterial sampling. Oximetry has two important limitations. It is not useful in shock states when a pulse cannot be detected by the device. Also, because it measures saturation and not Po_2, and because the oxygen-hemoglobin dissociation curve is nearly flat when the Po_2 exceeds 70 torr, considerable changes in partial pressure above 70 torr cause only small changes in saturation.[15] Movement artifact is the only special consideration in applying this method to sick laboring women. It is the best available method for noninvasive arterial oxygen monitoring.

Transcutaneous Po_2 measurement is another continuous noninvasive monitoring technique. It detects oxygen tension produced at the skin surface by oxygen that diffuses through the skin from dermal and subcutaneous capillaries, and is an index of oxygen delivery to the peripheral tissues, rather than a direct reflection of arterial Po_2.[3] It will therefore decrease not only when arterial oxygenation falls, but also when perfusion is poor, as when cardiac output is low or local vasoconstriction limits flow. Thus, this parameter cannot be used as a reliable substitute for direct measurement of arterial Po_2, particularly in hemodynamically unstable patients.[3] It is noninvasive and provides continuous data, but it is somewhat cumbersome to use and may cause local harm to the skin.[61]

Arterial Pressure Monitoring

Blood pressure can be monitored by sphygmomanometry, automated noninvasive monitors, or direct intra-arterial measurement. Sphygmomanometry is simple, familiar, reasonably reliable,[8] noninvasive, and free of risk; it is adequate for most purposes. An often overlooked secondary benefit is that it brings a clinician to the patient's bedside. It has important drawbacks in the care of critically ill patients. Relying on measurement of the auscultated blood pressure results in underestimation of intra-arterial pressure in hypovolemic patients, those in shock, and those with vasoconstriction of any etiology, including vasopressor therapy.[24,25] Also, it provides only intermittent data and thus is an inefficient early warning system. For this reason it is of limited value for assessment of patients receiving drugs with the potential to raise or lower blood pressure rapidly.

Several types of automated noninvasive blood pressure monitors are available. They use an automatically inflating cuff and during deflation measure either pressure changes (oscillotonometry), sound (electronic auscultation), or both.[30] These devices permit very frequent monitoring of blood pressure with comparatively little effort. They are likely to be inaccurate when the blood pressure is low, and some models lose accuracy at the high end of the spectrum as well.[30] Some arrhythmias render measurements inaccurate and thus preclude the use of these devices.

In addition to providing easy and painless access for arterial blood withdrawal when frequent sampling is necessary, intra-arterial lines are used for continuous measurement of arterial pressure. They are particularly valuable when extreme hypotension renders noninvasive methods inaccurate and when infusion of powerful intravenous vasoactive drugs, which may alter blood pressure precipitately, necessitates constant monitoring. Accurate pressure recordings will be obtained only with scrupulous attention to all relevant technical requirements.[24]

Arterial cannulation may be performed in many sites, but the radial artery is chosen most commonly because it is readily accessible and because the hand generally has a dual blood supply, a protection in the event of radial arterial thrombosis. Prominent complications include thrombosis, embolization, ischemia or infarction of the distal extremity, infection, vasospasm, and hemorrhage. Disconnection of the tubing can lead to exsanguination within minutes.[44] Continuous monitoring with an automatic alarm system and maintenance of the entire line and entry site within full view, when possible, are important safeguards. While intra-arterial pressure recording is the gold standard in blood pressure monitoring, remember that the pressure in only the cannulated artery is being measured. In shock states or when vasoconstricting drugs are used, peripheral blood pressure may differ significantly from central blood pressure.

During labor when the patient may move vigorously, special care must be taken to avoid disconnection and arterial trauma, a factor that predisposes to thrombotic complications. Because the factors that are correlated with increased risk of complications of arterial lines (advanced age, low cardiac output, underlying arterial disease, and prolonged cannulation) are generally absent in parturients, these patients may be expected to have fewer complications than would be anticipated from the literature.

Body position can alter blood pressure readings in all patients; the effects of vasodilation and of aortocaval compression on blood pressure make postural effects an even more important concern in women in late pregnancy. No matter what system of measuring blood pressure is used, uniformity of position during measurements, and preferably measurement in the left lateral recumbent position, will increase the reliability and precision of the readings.

Endotracheal Intubation and Mechanical Ventilation

Endotracheal intubation is performed for much the same reasons in a parturient as in a nonpregnant patient: to maintain a patent airway, prevent aspiration, permit suctioning, allow assisted ventilation, and give inhalational anesthesia.

One special caution that applies to obstetric patients relates to the edema of preeclampsia and eclampsia that can involve the upper airway and on occasion cause stridorous breathing. While this edema per se is almost never an indication for endotracheal intubation, it can make required intubation difficult. Moreover, the edema can be exacerbated by the presence of the tube and present problems after extubation. Although it will rarely prove to be necessary, it is prudent in planning extubation to be prepared to reintubate these patients immediately.

Mechanical ventilation is indicated when neurologic or muscular disorders cause hypoventilation or when medications that may produce hypoventilation must be given, as in status epilepticus. Ventilators are also necessary in the presence of hypoxemia refractory to oxygen supplementation, as in adult respiratory distress syndrome, or when airway obstruction leads to acute respiratory failure in status asthmaticus. Sometimes assisted ventilation is necessary to reduce the work of breathing, and thus improve the balance between cardiac work and cardiac demands. This may be beneficial for patients in septic or cardiogenic shock.

The special challenge of caring for a woman on a ventilator during labor and delivery is the problem of matching ventilation to needs that may be changing rapidly. If the patient can trigger the ventilator, and ventilatory drive is unimpaired, she can determine her own respiratory rate to respond optimally to changing metabolic demands. One concern is the development of hypocapnia and alkalosis between contractions if each breath is a full cycled ventilatory volume. In some patients, use of the intermittent mandatory ventilation mode may obviate this problem, but this is not an option for all intubated parturients and may be a deleterious choice in some. This decision must be made on an individual basis. End-tidal carbon dioxide monitoring is useful to ascertain the adequacy of ventilation and may reduce the need to perform frequent arterial blood gas analysis.

The most difficult problems arise in the management of a patient whose ventilatory failure prohibits her, even while on the ventilator, from being able to meet the increased demand. This may occur in a patient in status asthmaticus. Here attention must be focused on correcting the underlying abnormality.

In general, provision of adequate oxygenation is less problematic than adjusting ventilation. Administration of supplemental oxygen can usually maintain an acceptable Po_2; if not, positive end-expiratory pressure (PEEP) can be added. PEEP may affect uterine blood flow adversely by decreasing cardiac output and blood pressure, or by increasing venous pressure. This can be minimized by manipulation of central blood volume and/or adjustment of the level of PEEP applied. One must balance the benefits of relieving hypoxemia with PEEP against the adverse hemodynamic consequences of it in individual patients. Adjustments in the PEEP settings should be followed by a close assessment of maternal blood pressure, pulse, blood gases and, if a Swan-Ganz catheter is in place, cardiac output, as well as continued vigilance for evidence of fetal compromise.

Unstable patients sometimes require monitoring with a variety of systems that may include pulse oximetry, arterial blood gases, end-tidal Co_2, and mixed venous oxygen saturation (SvO_2) measurements. What system is appropriate must be determined by the nature of the respiratory disease that prompted mechanical ventilation.

When the disorder that necessitated mechanical ventilatory support is acute and reversible, discontinuing mechanical ventilation presents little difficulty. Most of the common problems encountered in the setting of labor and delivery, such as asthma, drug overdose, pulmonary edema, pneumonia, and aspiration, are of this type. In these instances, when the acute process is resolved, and criteria for discontinuing ventilatory support are met, mechanical ventilation can usually be withdrawn without elaborate regimens.[27] Long-standing respiratory failure presents more formidable problems in weaning.

CENTRAL VENOUS PRESSURE MONITORING

Measurement of central venous pressure (CVP), long used as an index of central blood volume, has undergone a reappraisal since introduction of the Swan-Ganz catheter has allowed simplified comparison of the filling pressures of the right heart (CVP) and the left heart (pulmonary capillary wedge pressure). In people without cardiopulmonary dysfunction, CVP generally reflects left atrial pressure indirectly. This relationship is disrupted in critically ill patients.[50] In many common conditions the CVP may be elevated for reasons independent of volume status and may be discordant with simultaneous left heart filling pressures. Some of these conditions may be seen in obstetric patients, for example, pulmonary embolism, amniotic fluid embolism, long-standing mitral stenosis, adult respiratory distress syndrome, or any cause of pulmonary hypertension.[36,46,50] In contrast, the CVP may not be elevated despite high left heart pressures. This has been demonstrated amply in a variety of critical illnesses in parturient women, including amniotic fluid embolism,[12] mitral stenosis,[13] and pregnancy-induced hypertension.[10,17,18]

Cotton et al.[17] compared 207 determinations of CVP and wedge pressure in 18 women with severe pregnancy-induced hypertension. While a significant linear relationship was found between the two variables, the wide variation in wedge pressure for a given CVP reading made substitution of one for the other on an individual clinical basis unacceptable. In patients whose CVP was 8 torr, wedge pressures ranged from low to high (3–21 torr).

The technique of CVP assessment consists of measuring pressure via fluid-filled tubing placed in the superior vena cava or right atrium and linked to a fluid column manometer or an electronic transducer. There are no special considerations in using CVP readings in parturient women, apart from possible difficulty in identifying the zero reference point, the right mid-atrium. This is important because without a reliable zero point, the absolute pressure readings can be erroneous.[22]

Central venous catheters may be inserted in any of several access sites. The most common are the internal jugular and subclavian veins. When a hemostatic defect complicates the condition, access from an antecubital vein is preferred because any bleeding is evident immediately and tamponade can be accomplished easily. Complications of central line placement vary with the access site and include pneumothorax, arterial puncture or cannulation, hemothorax, hydrothorax, thoracic duct injury, thrombosis, embolism, sepsis, shearing off and embolization of the catheter, local infection, and cardiac arrhythmia. Special care must be taken during the introduction and removal of these catheters, and they should remain in place no longer than necessary.

SWAN-GANZ CATHETER

The Swan-Ganz catheter is a pulmonary artery catheter with a circumferential balloon just proximal to the tip. The prototype has two lumens: one is fluid-filled for measuring pressure and extends to the catheter tip; the other is used to inflate the balloon with air.[53] Two subsequent modifications have become standard: a third lumen opening into the right atrium and a thermistor for cardiac output determination. Other available additions include a fiberoptic channel for continuous mixed venous oxygen saturation monitoring and cardiac pacing wires.

To understand this kind of monitoring, one must begin with an understanding of the catheter. Insertion begins much like central venous catheter placement. Once the catheter is in a central vein, the balloon is inflated, allowing blood flow to guide it through the right heart until the balloon floats into a branch of the pulmonary artery with a lumen too small to permit the catheter to advance any further. There, with the balloon deflated, the catheter tip lies in a pulmonary artery and measures pulmonary artery pressure; but when the balloon is inflated, it temporarily occludes the artery in which it lies, isolating the tip of the catheter from pulmonary artery pressure. Blood flow in the arteries, capillaries, and veins distal to the balloon ceases. The catheter tip then lies at the head of a column of nonflowing blood that extends to the point where the veins of the balloon-occluded circuit converge with pulmonary veins in which blood continues to flow. Because pressure equilibrates in a static fluid column, the pressure recorded at the tip of the catheter is identical to the pressure in the pulmonary veins that lie at the other end of the occluded vascular bed. When the balloon is inflated, it is the pulmonary venous pressure that is being read. This pressure is called the pulmonary artery occlusion pressure, the pulmonary capillary wedge pressure, or, in intensive care unit vernacular, simply the wedge pressure.

What makes the wedge pressure valuable is that, although imperfect, it is the best available bedside indicator of two other crucially important hemodynamic variables: (1) the left ventricular preload, which is a primary determinant of the force of left ventricular contraction; and (2) the pulmonary capillary hydrostatic pressure, which controls in large part the development of pulmonary congestion and edema.

Wedge Pressure and Left Ventricular Preload

The force of left ventricular contraction is determined by, among other variables, the volume in the heart prior to contraction, which is the left ventricular end-diastolic volume or preload. It derives its clinical value by assessing left ventricular function, determining the etiology of hypotension and shock, and guiding therapy. The wedge pressure is used to reflect the preload, because no more direct means is readily available or practical for repeated bedside measurement.

Before basing a clinical decision on this measurement, one must appreciate the series of assumptions that permit use of the pulmonary artery wedge pressure to elucidate left ventricular volume and the circumstances that may make these assumptions invalid. Conditions likely to be encountered in an obstetric population that may make the wedge pressure an unreliable indicator of preload include mitral stenosis, mitral regurgitation, aortic insufficiency, dilated cardiomyopathy, and all causes of left ventricular hypertrophy, most notably hypertension, aortic stenosis, and hypertrophic cardiomyopathy.

Wedge Pressure and Pulmonary Capillary Hydrostatic Pressure

The hydrostatic pressure in the pulmonary capillaries is a major determinant of fluid flux into the lungs, and is approximated by the wedge pressure, which is used to assess the causes of, or the propensity for, pulmonary congestion. Normally, the pulmonary capillary hydrostatic pressure is only a few torr higher than the pulmonary capillary wedge pressure, and parallels it closely; but in ARDS, pulmonary hypertension, and other conditions characterized by increased pulmonary vascular resistance, the gap between wedge and capillary hydrostatic pressure may widen and the wedge pressure may underestimate the tendency for fluid flux into the pulmonary interstitium.[16,34,60]

The wedge pressure is crucial in differentiating cardiogenic from noncardiogenic pulmonary edema, but it is less helpful in predicting the onset of pulmonary edema, for three reasons. First, it is only one of several variables that determine net fluid flux, and factors such as capillary permeability, alveolar injury, oncotic pressure, and central nervous system events can influence fluid movement independent of the wedge pressure. Second, pulmonary edema is the net result of fluid moving into and being cleared from the lung. The wedge pressure correlates with the tendency for fluid to enter the pulmonary interstitium, but lymphatic clearance determines how much fluid is carried out. Enhanced clearance of transudated fluid occurs when pulmonary venous pressure is elevated chronically, as it often is in mitral stenosis.[40,47] These patients may therefore tolerate higher hydrostatic pressures without developing pulmonary edema. Third, some skepticism and judgment are required in using wedge pressures. Reliance on the absolute pressure alone is unwise; relative changes and trends are more useful clinically.

Given the critical nature of the decisions made on the basis of wedge pressure readings, it is essential to know how reliable the data are and how to guarantee that the best possible information is available. Erroneous wedge pressure data are not infrequent. Morris et al.[37,38] showed that 23% to 49% of readings in various intensive care unit (ICU) settings were based on specious waveforms; this resulted in errors in wedge pressure of 4 torr or more, with occasional flagrantly spurious readings. In addition to these problems, errors can occur because the catheter tip is not sensing a true wedge pressure, the waveform being transmitted is distorted for technical reasons, monitoring equipment misreads the waveform, or the human interpreter misreads the data displayed. If wedge pressures are to reflect physiologic conditions accurately, several conditions must be met. While a detailed discussion of all the technical considerations that make Swan-Ganz catheter pressure data reliable is beyond the scope of this chapter, those with special implications for obstetrics will be discussed.

Aortocaval Compression

The standard position in which to obtain pressure readings in nonpregnant patients is supine. This position may be unfavorable for women in late pregnancy because the inferior vena cava and aorta may be compressed by the gravid uterus. This results in impaired venous return, a drop in central filling pressures and volumes, and diminished cardiac output. These adverse hemodynamic effects are an issue for any woman in late pregnancy, but assume a far greater clinical significance in patients with pathology severe enough to warrant invasive hemodynamic monitoring. These compromised women and their threatened offspring are far less likely to tolerate the hemodynamic adversity that may occur in the supine position than their healthy counterparts with greater reserves.

Ill women, with few exceptions, should be maintained in the lateral decubitus position to relieve aortocaval compression. The degree of rotation needed to displace the uterus ranges from 0 to 45 degrees[32] and varies among individuals depending on, among other things, uterine size, fetal position, and maternal anatomy. The problems with returning the patient to the supine position for every reading are that it may compromise placental perfusion and that the change in position will itself alter all the central pressures so that readings will not reflect the conditions that prevail when the patient is returned to a lateral posture. Leaving the patient in a lateral decubitus position may itself create problems; body position has bearing on two aspects of pressure monitoring, zero reference points and Zone III position.

Zero Reference Point

When reading pulmonary artery pressures the manometry system must be set to equate atmospheric pressure at the level of the left atrium with a reading of zero. All subsequent readings are performed relative to this zero reference point and any error in locating it will distort all pressure readings commensurately. Unlike systemic arterial blood pressure, the wedge pressure operates in a very narrow range (Figure 17-1) and wedge pressure differences that would be trivial between systemic arterial pressure readings are given significant weight in clinical decision making. One important way to avoid erroneous readings is to zero the manometry system correctly, but this may present special problems in parturition when the patient may need to be monitored in a lateral

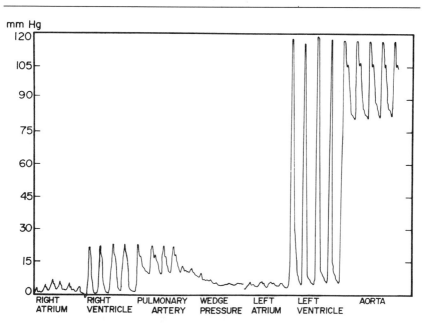

Figure 17-1 Pressure at various segments of the vascular system. The narrow range in which pulmonary capillary wedge pressure fluctuates in comparison to systemic arterial pressure is demonstrated. *Source:* Reprinted from *Textbook of Critical Care* (p 118) by WC Shoemaker, WL Thompson, and PR Holbrook (Eds) with permission of WB Saunders Company, © 1984.

position. While guidelines are available to locate the position of the atria in supine nonpregnant patients,[21] there are no standard references to guide the clinician in locating the atria in patients who are pregnant and/or on their side.

In the supine position the atria lie side by side in the same horizontal plane and the landmark for both is the midaxillary line. In the parturient lying on her side, locating the vertical level of the left atrium can be challenging. One solution that will work sometimes is to use the Swan-Ganz data to define just how far a patient needs to be turned before aortocaval compression is relieved. A small pillow under the hip which barely affects rotation of the upper trunk will suffice in some women. If this is not satisfactory, it is important to do the measurements with the patient in the same position every time. One might try turning the patient for readings into the full left lateral decubitus position—it is more reproducible than interim positions—and using the left sternal border as the atrial level marker. If both the right atrial pressure and the wedge pressure need to be read, as they always are during catheter insertion, pressure readings from each atrium will require a different zero reference point.

Zone III Position

It is possible to obtain a true wedge pressure reading only when the catheter tip lies in an area of the lung in which pulmonary arterial and venous pressure exceed alveolar pressure. Only in this region, called Zone III by West et al.,[59] is one of the necessary conditions for a wedge pressure reading met—a continuous column of blood extends from the balloon-occluded artery across the capillary bed to the pulmonary veins. In non-Zone III positions in which the vascular pressures are exceeded by the alveolar pressure, small vessels collapse and the continuity between the pulmonary artery and the pulmonary veins is lost. These pulmonary zones are functional, not anatomic; conditions that increase alveolar pressures (e.g., PEEP) or decrease pulmonary venous pressure (e.g., hypovolemia) may change the zone boundaries and result in spurious wedge pressure readings.[49,54]

One reason lung zone positioning is not usually of much concern is because when placed and employed with the patient supine, most Swan-Ganz catheters float into a position dorsal to the heart, where pulmonary venous pressure is highest. Most catheters (75%–85%) lie in the right lung.[4,33] When a patient whose catheter is in the right lung is turned toward the left, the catheter and the artery it is in will rotate into a position superior to the heart. When this happens, local pulmonary venous pressure falls. If it falls below alveolar pressure, the catheter tip will no longer be exposed to the true pulmonary capillary wedge pressure, and readings will be spurious. It is prudent to confirm that a true wedge pressure tracing is still present after repositioning the patient, and to be aware that even small changes in alveolar or vascular pressures may shift the boundaries of Zone III under some circumstances. If such problems occur and the catheter tip is in the right lung, it might be advantageous to turn the parturient into the right (rather than left) lateral position, provided this does not cause aortic or vena caval compression.

The last technical consideration in using Swan-Ganz catheters in laboring women relates to the skill and experience of the staff. Scrupulous care must be taken in inserting, maintaining, monitoring, and reading the information from these lines. Otherwise the data may be at best meaningless and potentially harmful if relied upon.

Thermodilution Cardiac Output Determination

Cardiac output can be determined by the thermodilution method using a Swan-Ganz catheter. An exact quantity of cold fluid of known temperature is injected into the proximal (right atrial) port of the catheter. A thermistor is located in a portion of the catheter in the pulmonary artery. The cardiac output is related to the rate at which the cold injectate reaches the thermistor. The curve relating the change in temperature over time is analyzed by a bedside computer that calculates cardiac output. This form of measurement has become a mainstay of monitoring because of its simplicity and comparability to standard methods.

The limitations of the method must be understood so that correct inferences can be made from the data. It is unwarranted to rely on a single value; in clinical practice, the mean of three or more values with technically adequate temperature curves is used. Under these circumstances, a 15% change is sufficient to assume clinical significance.[52] Careful attention to technical requirements of performing the measurement is important to obtain the most precise data.

When cardiac output is determined in the context of various pressure measurements, comprehensive assessment of the patient's cardiovascular status may be obtained. When a Swan-Ganz and peripheral arterial catheter are used, a variety of hemodynamic variables can be derived that give a fuller view of the patient's physiologic state: systemic vascular resistance (SVR), pulmonary vascular resistance, stroke volume, stroke work, oxygen delivery, and oxygen consumption.

Mixed Venous Oxygen Saturation

A modification of the pulmonary artery catheter makes possible continuous monitoring of mixed venous oxygen saturation (SvO_2). A fiberoptic channel in the catheter allows light of known wavelengths to be directed toward pulmonary arterial blood; the relative amounts of oxygenated and deoxygenated hemoglobin present are ascertained by spectrophotometric analysis of the reflected light.[23] Mixed venous oxygen saturation is best thought of as a measure of the balance between oxygen delivery and oxygen uptake by the body as a whole. The SvO_2 is basically a measure of how much oxygen is left in the blood after it has completed a pass through the body.

Interpretation of SvO_2 requires an understanding of the many variables that can influence it. A fall in SvO_2 may occur in the presence of acute blood loss, other causes of decreased cardiac output, pulmonary edema, or seizures, among others. Some authors use SvO_2 monitoring as an all-purpose warning system;[39] others emphasize its ability to provide a continuous, real-time reflection of cardiac output in patients in whom oxygen demand, hemoglobin, and pulmonary function are relatively stable.[7]

Many of the variables that determine SvO_2 often change during labor and delivery. Breathing patterns fluctuate during labor, and variation in arterial Po_2 is especially common during panting and pushing. Cardiac output, already increased at term approximately 40% over nonpregnancy levels, rises 15% or more with each contraction, and overall may rise during the course of labor by an additional 40%. In the immediate postpartum period, a 60% to 80% rise over prelabor levels is achieved.[29] Hemoglobin concentration may change due to bleeding, hydration, transfusion, hemorrhage, or vasoconstriction. Oxygen demands may rise and fall throughout labor and delivery as a result of dramatic changes in muscular activity.

With so many variables that affect it changing at once, interpretation of variations in SvO_2 may be difficult. For instance, during a second stage contraction a patient's breathing pattern and increased muscle activity may tend to lower the SvO_2 while the surge in cardiac output may tend to increase it. After delivery blood loss would tend to decrease the SvO_2 while the increased cardiac output would augment it.

SvO_2 has the potential to become an extraordinarily useful tool in critically ill patients. Oxygen utilization by tissues is the ultimate index of circulatory function, and SvO_2 is the best index of tissue perfusion that can be monitored continuously with available technology. It is premature to recommend it for clinical use in obstetric patients during parturition, but research is underway to delineate its role.

Risks of Swan-Ganz Catheterization

Pulmonary artery catheterization is an invasive procedure that entails both the general risks of obtaining central circulatory access (discussed under Central Venous Pressure Monitoring, above) and the risks unique to the Swan-Ganz catheter placement and maintenance (Table 17-2).

Risks during insertion are related to the experience of the physician, the duration of the procedure, and the patient's condition. Once inserted, the safety of an indwelling line requires the continuous presence of medical professionals who fully understand and are familiar with its use. After the catheter is in place, it is often carried more distally into a small arterial radicle. There inflation of the balloon may rupture the pulmonary artery, or the tip may lodge in a vessel and lead to segmental pulmonary infarction. The catheter may also fall back into the right ventricle and cause arrhythmias. Protocols for using the balloon safely to obtain wedge pressure readings must deal with speed of inflation, volume of air used, monitoring the tracing during inflation, how to deflate, when attempting

---

Table 17-2 Risks of Swan-Ganz Catheterization

Arrhythmias
  Atrial fibrillation, supraventricular tachycardia, premature ventricular contractions,
    ventricular tachycardia, ventricular fibrillation
Right bundle branch block
Damage to valve cusps, chordae tendinae, papillary muscles
Knotting of catheter
Pulmonary artery rupture
Pulmonary infarction
Pulmonary embolism
Balloon rupture
Venous thrombosis
Sepsis
Endocarditis
Incorrect readings with resultant inappropriate treatment
All complications of securing central venous access

Source: Critical Care Medicine (1986;14:195–197), Copyright © 1986, Williams & Wilkins Company; *Anesthesiology* (1984;61:271–275), Copyright © 1984, JB Lippincott Company.

---

inflation can be dangerous, and how to tell if the balloon has ruptured. It is not the purpose of this chapter to be a primer on Swan-Ganz catheter use, but it is important to emphasize that these catheters require continuous monitoring and scrupulous attention to multiple details to maintain safety and to obtain meaningful data.

Pulmonary Artery Catheterization in Obstetrics

In recent years many descriptions have been published of Swan-Ganz catheter use in the peripartum period. Clark et al. report[11] of 1 year's experience in the Los Angeles County Hospital obstetric service gives an overview of the potential range of indications for the device. Seventy-two catheterizations were performed for the following conditions: severe preeclampsia/eclampsia with oliguria or pulmonary edema, Class III/IV (New York Heart Association) cardiac disease in labor, Class II/III cardiac disease and severe preeclampsia in labor, septic shock, adult respiratory distress syndrome, amniotic fluid embolism, and hypovolemic shock unresponsive to fluids. Coronary artery disease manifested by angina or prior myocardial infarction has also been used as an indication for pulmonary artery catheterization.[14,28] This field of investigation is still very new, and many fundamental questions remain unanswered. Carefully designed studies and broader experience will determine in which situations the same information could be obtained by less invasive means. More knowledge about the risk/benefit ratio and the appropriate therapeutic goals in various conditions require clarification. Before the role of pulmonary artery catheterization in obstetrics is elucidated fully, several major issues need to be addressed. The first among these is the lack of normative data.

There are no studies of normal pregnant women during labor and delivery in whom Swan-Ganz catheters were used to measure vascular pressures, cardiac output, and mixed venous oxygen saturation. Much of the existing hemodynamic data come from studies done in the 1950s and 1960s. These were done often with women in the supine position and thus may not represent true basal data.[31,32] In a careful study of 20 women during labor and delivery, Ueland and Hansen found cardiac output, determined by dye dilution technique, to range from 3.3 to 13.0 L/min during parturition in the lateral position.[55]

Given the paucity of intrapartum measurements, data obtained in women late in pregnancy have been used to determine norms. In a small but valuable study, Groenendijk et al. used the Swan-Ganz catheter to study four normal women at 28 to 34 weeks' gestation.[26] The pulmonary capillary wedge pressure ranged from 6 to 12 (mean 9) torr; the cardiac index was 3.96 to 4.97 (mean 4.53) L/min/m^2; and the SVR was 805 to 1,021 (mean 886) dyne•sec•cm^{-5}. These are the only available normative data determined by using a Swan-Ganz catheter. Kerr[31] studied five third trimester women and found a mean cardiac output of 6.26 L/min and a mean SVR of 1,119 dyne•sec•cm^{-5}. Cotton et al.[19] have proposed a set of pregnancy norms based on a review of seven prior studies using disparate techniques performed between 1949 and 1984. They suggest using these values: cardiac index 3 to 5 L/min/m^2, pulmonary capillary wedge pressure 6 to 12 torr, and CVP 4 to 8 torr.

It is important to remember that norms established for late pregnancy cannot be assumed to represent intrapartum values adequately. Moreover, vast and fluctuating changes in cardiac output, stroke volume, central blood volume, and oxygen consumption may occur during labor. If the cardiac output does not increase as expected during labor, it may be considered abnormal even if the absolute value is not unusually low. Not enough is known to make subtle judgments in this regard with certainty.

A further problem with assessing hemodynamic variables in pregnancy occurs with the use of data expressed as an index. Index calculations divide measurements data such as cardiac output, stroke work, or SVR by body surface area. This adjusts these values for body size and makes comparison between individuals or between an individual and population norms more meaningful. The striking change in body shape that characterizes late pregnancy no doubt changes the surface area and the relationship between height and weight, from which body surface area is calculated. The use of indexed values may be useful to correct for extremes of height and weight in the pregnant population, but it should be recognized that the formula has never been adjusted for index measurements in pregnant women.

Another major issue to be confronted is the need to identify optimal values of monitored hemodynamic variables. In addition to our ignorance of values in normal pregnant women, we know little about what might be optimal for those with specific illnesses. A striking example of the importance of this principle was demonstrated in the study of Shoemaker et al. in high-risk surgical patients.[51] They compared the hemodynamic profiles of high-risk patients who ultimately survived with those of similar patients who died, and identified features that characterized the survivors. They designed a protocol that used the survivor's profile as the therapeutic endpoint despite the fact that several of these values were well outside of the normal range. They achieved a dramatic diminution in mortality by using these clinically meaningful values rather than normal values as their goal.

In obstetrics, we have just begun to define disease-specific hemo-dynamic standards. For pregnant mitral stenosis patients with Class III or IV disease, Clark et al. recommend that a Swan-Ganz catheter be placed and that the wedge pressure, if elevated, be cautiously lowered to about 14 torr, as long as this level does not compromise cardiac output or blood pressure.[13] An even lower wedge pressure might be considered optimal in an intubated parturient with aspiration pneumonia; a higher pressure might well be suitable in a patient with myocardial ischemia.

The determination of what hemodynamic manipulations are optimal and appropriate must ultimately be based on demonstrated improve-ment in relevant outcome parameters. There is considerable controversy over the value of Swan-Ganz catheterization in medicine in general, largely because its effect on outcome has rarely been assessed in carefully controlled studies. Neither has this been done in obstetrics, although the exploration of the role of this technology is still in an early stage in this specialty.

There is no uniformity of opinion about what the best hemodynamic profile ought to be or about how best to achieve it in particular obstetric situations. Judgments about the value of a Swan-Ganz catheter are pre-mature until the protocols for altering hemodynamic variables have been established. The catheter is, of course, only a diagnostic tool with no intrinsic ability to safeguard or improve the patient's condition. If the information about pressure, blood flow, cardiac work, and oxygen econ-omy can be put to use, then the catheter will prove efficacious. If its inherent risks are not countervailed by benefits, use of the catheter may on balance prove detrimental. This is emphasized by the work of Shoe-maker et al. mentioned previously.[51] They studied a group of surgical patients with an expected mortality of 30%. Patients randomized to be monitored with a Swan-Ganz catheter and treated according to a protocol aimed at reproducing survivor's hemodynamic profiles had a mortality rate of 5%; those monitored with a Swan-Ganz catheter with the data used in the conventional manner of the service had a 29% mortality; they were indistinguishable from the historical control subjects and from patients randomized to be monitored without a pulmonary artery catheter.

NONINVASIVE CARDIAC OUTPUT DETERMINATION

Electrical impedance cardiography is a noninvasive method of deter-mining cardiac output. Changes in thoracic electrical impedance caused by variations in aortic blood flow are measured. From this information, cardiac output is derived.[5] Recent refinements of the technique have made it more acceptable as a clinical tool, but experience with it remains limited. Appel et al. have demonstrated that it is reliable even in unstable critically ill patients.[2] Its chief advantages over the commonly used thermodilution technique are that it is noninvasive, carries no known risk beyond skin irritation from electrodes, provides continuous data, and consumes minimal staff time. It correlates as well with dye dilution and thermodilution methods as they do with one another.[2,5,35] One serious limitation of impedance cardiography is that it overestimates low cardiac outputs.[5] Other conditions in which it cannot be relied upon are aortic insufficiency, ventricular septal defect, rapid tachycardia, irregular cardiac rhythms, chaotic ventilatory patterns, sepsis in the hyperdynamic phase, and abnormal body proportions.[2,5,6]

Several features of pregnancy might interfere with the accuracy of this method: the changes in thoracic shape and fluid volume, position of the heart, blood composition, contour, and the vasodilation and marked increase in fluid volume in the thoracic skin and muscles. Milsom et al.[35] studied women in the third trimester of pregnancy and compared cardiac outputs derived by dye dilution and electrical impedance. They found good correlation between the two methods, although the impedance cardiac outputs consistently underestimated its dye dilution counterpart. This is the reverse of what is described in the nonpregnant state. Thus, this method might not be useful for following women over the course of gestation, because over the time span that their cardiac output is rising dramatically, the impedance method might underestimate the true cardiac output by a widening margin. This does not in any way impugn its ability to monitor changes in cardiac output over short periods. A reliable, noninvasive method to obtain cardiac output could have a significant impact on the care of the critically ill parturient woman. Whether or not impedance cardiography will prove to be reliable and accurate during the tumultuous hemodynamic events of labor and delivery is as yet unknown.

PHARMACOTHERAPY

When drugs are administered during labor and delivery, special considerations arise. These relate to possible effects on uterine perfusion and contractility, fetal oxygenation, or fetal heart rate patterns. Problems may arise with extrapolating data about the known efficacy and safety of an oral preparation in pregnancy to the effects of the same drug given intravenously in a different quantity during an intrapartum emergency. The possibility of neonatal effects of intrapartum medications is also a concern. For example, diazoxide, a very rapidly acting antihypertensive agent, commonly provokes hyperglycemia, and babies born during maternal treatment may become hypoglycemic. Other medications may compromise the neonate directly. The treatment of maternal pulmonary edema with morphine or antihypertensives may lead to respiratory depression and/or hypotension in the neonate.

Considering the panoply of disease states that can cause critical illness in parturients, it is evident that any of hundreds of medications might be needed during labor. Vasopressor drugs, antiarrhythmics, and potent antihypertensives are three groups of agents that may be unfamiliar to obstetricians, and are likely to be used in critically ill parturients. It is not within the scope of this chapter to review each medication, but some general points will be made.

Most drugs commonly used in critical care have not been evaluated sufficiently in pregnant women to allow a confident opinion regarding safety. The drug may not have been fully evaluated for the specific indications for which its use is being contemplated. For example, Cotton et al.[20] described a clinical trial of intravenous nitroglycerin, a potent vasodilator whose predominant effect is on the venous bed. When nitroglycerine was used in severe preeclamptic women prior to volume expansion cardiac output and oxygen delivery fell substantially, and some fetuses developed evidence of hypoxemia. These data remind us that venodilating an already volume-depleted patient will shift the heart down the Starling curve and be deleterious to cardiac function. It is an example of the importance of finding appropriate goals of therapy. Nitroglycerin did lower blood pressure effectively in these severe preeclamptic gravidas, but achieving an effect on blood pressure was not synonymous with improving the clinical condition of the woman or her fetus. This study does not tell us that nitroglycerine is a dangerous drug. In another setting in which the initial hemodynamic state was characterized by volume overload (e.g., pulmonary edema due to peripartum cardiomyopathy), the drug would be expected to have more favorable hemodynamic consequences.

The potential adverse or beneficial effects of potent vasoconstrictors and vasodilators comes more from their hemodynamic effects than from intrinsic qualities of the drug. The setting in which the agents are used assumes paramount importance in judging their worth. Pharmacologic intervention should always be designed with the underlying pathophysiology in mind. Intrapartum pulmonary edema provides an excellent example of this principle.

When pulmonary edema exists in a patient with isolated mitral stenosis, the essential problem is obstruction to flow across the mitral valve with consequent increase in intravascular pressure in the left atrium, pulmonary veins, and capillaries antegrade to the obstruction. This increased hydrostatic pressure causes transudation of fluid into the pulmonary interstitium. The anatomic obstruction cannot be structurally relieved intrapartum, but functional obstruction can be minimized. Slowing the heart rate by beta-blockade with propranolol increases time spent in diastole, the portion of the cardiac cycle when the mitral valve is open, thus facilitating blood flow across the valve. In the intrapartum setting, in which large volume shifts occur, particularly following delivery, sequestering or removing that volume by venodilators or diuretics is valuable. Because the left ventricle functions normally in this disease, efforts to help resolve the pulmonary edema with inotropic agents like dobutamine and digoxin or with afterload reduction will be to little avail.

When pulmonary edema occurs in peripartum cardiomyopathy, it is a weakened myocardium that is at the root of the problem. In this instance, drugs such as nitroglycerine and morphine that venodilate and thus sequester central volume peripherally, treatment with diuretics that lead to volume loss, and medications that improve left ventricular function are warranted. Myocardial function can be enhanced by inotropic agents; the best agent in the acute setting is dobutamine, a synthetic catecholamine that increases myocardial contractility without provoking tachycardia or increased afterload. Myocardial function can also be enhanced by decreasing the afterload against which the left ventricle must pump. In the acute setting, nitroprusside, a potent dilator of both arterioles and venules, is optimal because it is rapid acting and can be reversed in minutes. In congestive heart failure from cardiomyopathy, propranolol, mentioned above in connection with treating mitral stenosis, would be absolutely contraindicated, because it would further weaken myocardial contraction.

When pulmonary edema develops in association with preeclampsia, a third set of pathophysiologic factors is operative. In this disease, marked increase in the systemic vascular resistance, low oncotic pressure, decreased ventricular compliance, and myocardial depression may all play a role to varying degrees.[10,19,43,57] Since a markedly increased systemic vascular resistance is a near-universal finding and is probably responsible in most instances both for poor ventricular compliance and depressed cardiac output, efforts to decrease afterload should be the primary thrust of treatment.

Thus, for therapy of intrapartum pulmonary edema to be effective, its source must be understood and therapy tailored to that etiology as well as to the individual details that characterize the patient's illness. This principle can be applied to the pharmacotherapy of most critical disorders.

STAFFING AND DATA

The management of labor and delivery in women who require critical care techniques is complex and challenging. Few generalists and only a small proportion of maternal-fetal medicine specialists are sufficiently conversant with intensive care techniques to manage such cases independently. In fact, to do so is rarely sensible because judging maternal and fetal condition during the dynamic, rapidly changing, and sometimes unpredictable events of labor requires interaction and close collaboration among several specialties. Often the team must consist of an obstetrician (usually a specialist in maternal-fetal medicine), internist (critical care specialist, cardiologist, or others as appropriate), obstetric anesthesiologist, and nurses. Nurses play a vital role in obtaining and recording data from the patient and various monitoring devices. The presence of the husband or any individual of the patient's choice can be very important to provide emotional support. All involved personnel must bear in mind that they are dealing with a woman who is not only experiencing a serious illness, but is at the same time experiencing a momentous event in her life. Childbirth is a physically and emotionally demanding time under the best of circumstances; to undergo it in the presence of grave illness and bewildering technology requires great courage and conviction on the part of the parturient and unusual sensitivity to her needs and feelings on the part of her caretakers.

The necessity for meetings among medical personnel prior to the labor has been emphasized. Meetings with the patient and her family are of equal importance. They should be aware of all planned (and possible) interventions in some detail. This education usually serves to minimize anxiety during the labor. Sometimes difficult ethical issues must be confronted with the patient relating to her desires for therapy in the event of cardiac arrest or other catastrophic complications (see Chapter 21). Above all, these preliminary conferences serve to develop a bond of trust between the patient and her medical providers. This bond will serve everyone well if unanticipated situations arise. It is therefore highly advantageous to have the patient meet the members of the team prior to labor, to be educated thoroughly about what to expect, and to be encouraged to express her own concerns and fears.

The medical staff should also meet prior to the planned event. In general it is wise to assign one individual as the team leader through whom all decisions regarding therapy should filter. Usually the perinatologist would serve this role, but anyone with a broad general under-

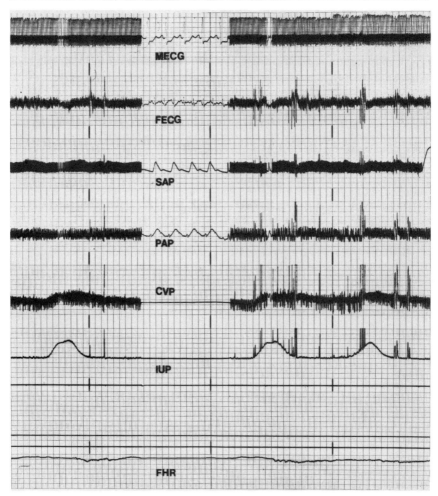

Figure 17-2 Sample of recording from a laboring patient with aortic and mitral valve prostheses and heart failure. Simultaneous observations of maternal and fetal data facilitate interpretation of physiologic events. CVP, central venous pressure; FECG, fetal electrocardiogram; FHR, fetal heart rate; IUP, intrauterine pressure; MECG, maternal electrocardiogram; PAP, pulmonary artery pressure; SAP, systemic arterial pressure.

standing of the relevant obstetric, medical, nursing, and anesthetic issues and with the ability to unify a diverse group is appropriate.

The daunting task of managing complex patients is made easier by an organized and systematic method of data collection. Flow sheets appropriate for the particular problem at hand are extremely helpful and facilitate the assessment of trends quite readily. It is also advantageous to maintain a continuous hard copy record of cardiovascular data. We have been successful with a standard eight-channel physiologic recorder used to print maternal and fetal data simultaneously (Figure 17-2). This kind of record serves to identify cardiovascular changes promptly and to monitor effects of interventions. In addition, it provides a marvelous teaching tool because it allows for subsequent review.

REFERENCES

1. Alderman EL, Glantz SA: Acute hemodynamic interventions shift the diastolic pressure-volume curve in man. *Circulation* 1976;54:662–671.

2. Appel PL, Kram HB, Mackabee J, Fleming AW, Shoemaker WC: Comparison of measurements of cardiac output by bioimpedance and thermodilution in severely ill surgical patients. *Crit Care Med* 1986;14:933–935.

3. Barker SJ, Tremper KK, Gamel GM: A clinical comparison of transcutaneous PO_2 and pulse oximetry in the operating room. *Anesth Analg* 1986;65:805–808.

4. Benumof JL, Saidman LJ, Arkin DB, Diamont M: Where pulmonary artery catheters go: Intrathoracic distribution. *Anesthesiology* 1977;336–338.

5. Bernstein DP: Continuous noninvasive real-time monitoring of stroke volume and cardiac output by thoracic electrical bioimpedance. *Crit Care Med* 1986;14:898–901.

6. Bernstein DP: A new stroke volume equation for thoracic electrical bioimpedance: Theory and rationale. *Crit Care Med* 1986;904–909.

7. Birman H, Haq A, Hew E, Aberman A: Continuous monitoring of mixed venous oxygen saturation in hemodynamically unstable patients. *Chest* 1984;86:753–756.

8. Brest AN: *Cardiovascular Disorders.* Philadelphia, FA Davis, 1968.

9. Chediak JR, Alban GM, Maxey B: Von Willebrand's disease and pregnancy: Management during delivery and outcome of offspring. *Am J Obstet Gynecol* 1986;155:618–624.

10. Clark SL, Greenspoon JS, Aldahl D, Phelan JP: Severe preeclampsia with persistent oliguria: Management of hemodynamic subsets. *Am J Obstet Gynecol* 1986;154:490–494.

11. Clark SL, Horenstein JM, Phelan JP, Montag TW, Paul RH: Experience with the pulmonary artery catheter in obstetrics and gynecology. *Am J Obstet Gynecol* 1985;152: 374–378.

12. Clark SL, Montz FJ, Phelan JP: Hemodynamic alterations associated with amniotic fluid embolism: A reappraisal. *Am J Obstet Gynecol* 1985;151:617–621.

13. Clark SL, Phelan JP, Greenspoon J, Aldahl D, Horenstein J: Labor and delivery in the presence of mitral stenosis: Central hemodynamic observations. *Am J Obstet Gynecol* 1985; 152:984–988.

14. Cohen WR, Steinman T, Patsner B, Snyder D, Satwicz P, Monroy P: Acute myocardial infarction in a pregnant woman at term. *JAMA* 1983;250:2179–2181.

15. Comroe JH: *Physiology of Respiration*. Chicago, Year Book Medical Publishers, 1983.

16. Cope DK, Allison RC, Partmentier JL, Miller JN, Taylor AE: Measurement of effective pulmonary capillary pressure using the pressure profile after pulmonary artery occlusion. *Crit Care Med* 1986;14:16–22.

17. Cotton DB, Gonik B, Dorman K, Harrist R: Cardiovascular alterations in severe pregnancy-induced hypertension: Relationship of central venous pressure to pulmonary capillary wedge pressure. *Am J Obstet Gynecol* 1985;151:762–764.

18. Cotton DB, Jones MM, Longmire S, Dorman KF, Tessem J, Joyce TH: Role of intravenous nitroglycerin in the treatment of severe pregnancy-induced hypertension complicated by pulmonary edema. *Am J Obstet Gynecol* 1986;154:91–93.

19. Cotton DB, Lee W, Huhta JC, Dorman KF: Presenting hemodynamic profile of severe pregnancy-induced hypertension. *Am J Obstet Gynecol* (in press).

20. Cotton DB, Longmire S, Jones MM, Dorman KF, Tessem J, Joyce TH: Cardiovascular alterations in severe pregnancy-induced hypertension: Effects of intravenous nitroglycerin coupled with blood volume expansion. *Am J Obstet Gynecol* 1986;154:1053–1059.

21. Cross CJ, Cain HD, Deaton WJ, Summerhill S, Stevens PM: Vertical relationships of the pulmonary artery catheter tip and transducer reference point in estimation of the left atrial pressure (abstr). *Am Rev Respir Dis* 1978;117(Suppl):105.

22. Debrunner F, Buhler F: "Normal central venous pressure," significance of reference point and normal range. *Br Med J* 1969;3:148–150.

23. Divertie MB, McMihan JC: Continuous monitoring of mixed venous oxygen saturation. *Chest* 1984;85:423–428.

24. Gardner RM, Hollingsworth KW: Optimizing the electrocardiogram and pressure monitoring. *Crit Care Med* 1986;14:651–658.

25. Goldenheim PD, Kazemi H: Cardiopulmonary monitoring of critically ill patients. *N Engl J Med* 1984;311:717–720, 776–780.

26. Groenendijk R, Trimbos JBMJ, Wallenburg HCS: Hemodynamic measurements in preeclampsia: Preliminary observations. *Am J Obstet Gynecol* 1984;150:232–236.

27. Hall JB, Wood LDH: Liberation of the patient from mechanical ventilation. *JAMA* 1987;257:1621–1628.

28. Hankins GDV, Wendel GD Jr, Leveno KJ, Stoneham J: Myocardial infarction during pregnancy: A review. *Obstet Gynecol* 1985;65:139–146.

29. Hansen JM, Ueland K: The influence of caudal analgesia on cardiovascular dynamics during normal labor and delivery. *Acta Anaesth Scand* 1966;(Suppl 23):449–452.

30. Johnson CJH, Kerr JH: Automatic blood pressure monitors: A clinical evaluation of five models in adults. *Anaesthesia* 1985;40:471–478.

31. Kerr MG: Cardiovascular dynamics in pregnancy and labour. *Br Med Bull* 1968;24: 19–24.

32. Kerr MG: Maternal cardiovascular adjustments in pregnancy and labor, in Goodwin JW, Godden JO, Chance GW (eds): *Perinatal Medicine: The Basic Science Underlying Clinical Practice*. Baltimore, Williams & Wilkins, 1976, pp 395–408.

33. Kronberg GM, Quan SF, Schlobohm RM, Lindauer JM, Goodman PC: Anatomic locations of the tips of pulmonary-artery catheters in supine patients. *Anesthesiology* 1979; 51:467–469.

34. Laine GA: Pulmonary capillary pressure? *Crit Care Med* 1986;14:76–77.

35. Milsom I, Forssman L, Sivertsson R, Dottori O: Measurement of cardiac stroke volume by impedance cardiography in the last trimester of pregnancy. *Acta Obstet Gynecol Scand* 1983;62:473–479.

36. Moore PG, James OF, Saltos N: Severe amniotic fluid embolism. *Anaesth Intensive Care* 1982;10:40.

37. Morris AH, Chapman RH, Gardner RM: Frequency of technical problems encountered in the measurement of pulmonary artery wedge pressure. *Crit Care Med* 1984; 12:164–170.

38. Morris AH, Chapman RH, Gardner RM: Frequency of wedge pressure errors in the ICU. *Crit Care Med* 1985;13:705–708.

39. Nelson LD: Continuous venous oximetry in surgical patients. *Ann Surg* 1986; 203:329–333.

40. O'Quin R, Marini JJ: Pulmonary artery occlusion pressure: Clinical physiology, measurement, and interpretation. *Am Rev Respir Dis* 1983;128:319–326.

41. Patel C, Laboy V, Venus B, Mathru M, Wier D: Acute complications of pulmonary artery catheter insertion in critically ill patients. *Crit Care Med* 1986;14:195–197.

42. Perloff JK: Pregnancy and cardiovascular disease, in Braunwald E (ed): *Heart Disease: A Textbook of Cardiovascular Medicine.* Philadelphia, WB Saunders, 1980.

43. Phelan JP, Yurth DA: Severe preeclampsia: I. Peripartum hemodynamic observations. *Am J Obstet Gynecol* 1982;144:17.

44. Pierson DJ, Hudson LD: Monitoring hemodynamics in the critically ill. *Med Clin North A* 1983;67:1343–1360.

45. Raper R, Sibbald WJ: Misled by the wedge? The Swan-Ganz catheter and left ventricular preload. *Chest* 1986;89:427–434.

46. Schlant RC: Altered cardiovascular function of rheumatic heart disease and other acquired valvular disease, in Hurst JW, Logue RB, Schlant RC, Wenger NK (eds): *The Heart: Arteries and Veins.* New York, McGraw-Hill, 1982.

47. Schlant RC: Altered physiology of the cardiovascular system in heart failure, in Hurst JW, Logue RB, Schlant RC, Wenger NK (eds): *The Heart: Arteries and Veins.* New York, McGraw-Hill, 1982.

48. Shah KB, Rao TLK, Laughlin S, El-Etr AA: A review of pulmonary artery catheterization in 6,245 patients. *Anesthesiology* 1984;61:271–275.

49. Shasby DM, Dauber IM, Pfister S, Anderson JT, Carson SB, Manart F, Hyers TM: Swan-Ganz catheter location and left atrial pressure determine the accuracy of the wedge pressure when positive end-expiratory pressure is used. *Chest* 1981;80:666–670.

50. Shoemaker WC: Monitoring of the critically ill patient, in Shoemaker WC, Thompson WL, Holbrook PR (eds): *Textbook of Critical Care.* Philadelphia, WB Saunders, 1984, pp 105–121.

51. Shoemaker WC, Bland RD, Appel PL: Therapy of critically ill postoperative patients based on outcome prediction and prospective clinical trials. *Surg Clin North Am* 1985; 65:811–833.

52. Stetz CW, Miller RG, Kelly GE, Raffin TA: Reliability of the thermodilution method in the determination of cardiac output in clinical practice. *Am Rev Respir Dis* 1982; 126:1001–1004.

53. Swan HJC, Ganz W, Forrester J, Marcus H, Diamond G, Chonette D: Catheterization of the heart in man with use of a flow-directed balloon-tipped catheter. *N Engl J Med* 1970;283:447.

54. Todd TRJ, Baile EM, Hogg JC: Pulmonary arterial wedge pressure in hemorrhagic shock. *Am Rev Respir Dis* 1978;118:613–616.

55. Ueland K, Hansen JM: Maternal cardiovascular dynamics. II. Posture and uterine contractions. *Am J Obstet Gynecol* 1969;103:1–7.

56. Ueland K, McAnulty JH, Ueland FR, Metcalfe J: Special considerations in the use of cardiovascular drugs. *Clin Obstet Gynecol* 1981;24:809–823.

57. Wasserstrum N, Cotton DB: Hemodynamic monitoring in severe pregnancy-induced hypertension. *Clin Perinatol* 1986;13:781–799.

58. Weinberger SE, Weiss ST, Cohen WR, Weiss JW, Johnson TS: Pregnancy and the lung. *Am Rev Respir Dis* 1980;121:559–581.

59. West JB, Dollery CT, Naimark A: Distribution of blood flow in isolated lung: Relation to vascular and alveolar pressures. *J Appl Physiol* 1964;19:713–724.

60. Wiedemann HP, Matthay MA, Matthay RA: Cardiovascular-pulmonary monitoring in the intensive care unit. *Chest* 1984;85:537–549, 656–668.

61. Yelderman M, New W: Evaluation of pulse oximetry. *Anesthesiology* 1983;59:349–352.

18

Cardiopulmonary Resuscitation in Labor and Delivery

Steven S. Schwalbe and Gertie F. Marx

Pregnancy is most often thought of as a benign process that occurs in young, healthy women. While this may be true for the vast majority of pregnancies, it is, unfortunately, not always the case. For example, Ginz[19] estimated the rate of myocardial infarction to be about 1 in 10,000 deliveries, with an overall mortality rate of 28%. Sullivan and Ramanathan[57] reported that the prevalence of heart disease in pregnancy ranged from 0.4% to 4.1%, and that among gravid women in Class III or IV of the New York Heart Association's functional classification, the maternal mortality was as high as 6.8%.

Causes of cardiac arrest during pregnancy are numerous and include hemorrhage,[48] pulmonary embolism,[22] amniotic fluid embolism,[34,43] myocardial infarction,[55] pheochromocytoma,[5] laryngeal edema secondary to preeclampsia,[21] local anesthetic toxicity,[2] hypoxia from anesthetic mishap,[39] electrocution from operating room equipment,[8] motor vehicle accidents,[6] and lightning injuries.[46] Such occurrences are far from routine in the delivery suite; nevertheless, the labor team must be conversant with basic resuscitative techniques, and have a clear understanding of how resuscitative efforts must be adapted for the pregnant woman.

PHYSIOLOGY OF PREGNANCY

Several pertinent aspects of the physiology of pregnancy will be reviewed prior to a discussion of resuscitative measures.

Hemodynamics

The position of the heart is changed during normal pregnancy, being displaced anteriorly and to the left due to the upward movement of the

515

abdominal contents and diaphragm by the enlarging uterus. Chamber dilatation and hypertrophy also occur. As a result, the electrocardiogram of a parturient may display left axis deviation, Q-waves, ST segment changes, and T-wave changes, without necessarily indicating the presence of heart disease.[45]

Total blood volume increases markedly during the course of pregnancy, with the rise in plasma volume (30%–40%) exceeding that of the cell mass (20%–30%).[47] Both reach their maximum values early in the third trimester, when they level off and become constant throughout the remainder of gestation.[33] Most of this increase in blood volume is accommodated by enhanced perfusion of the gravid uterus; but there is also added flow to the enlarged breasts as well as to the kidneys, skeletal muscle, and skin. As a result of this flow redistribution, the normal gravida does not exhibit signs of fluid overload. Her central venous pressure remains unchanged and responds normally to fluid infusion.[61] One significant exception to this is the woman with preeclampsia, who tends to have a contracted plasma volume due to a shift of intravascular fluid to the extravascular compartment.

Cardiac output rises with the increase in blood volume, reaching a maximum of 30% to 40% above normal before the 34th week of gestation. The rise is due to increases in both heart rate and stroke volume.[4] Blood pressure in the normal gravida remains constant or decreases slightly. In view of the high cardiac output, this suggests a decrease in peripheral vascular resistance. Pregnancy can thus be viewed as a state of high output and low resistance. This hyperdynamic state may result in the development of functional murmurs, but it does not impair cardiac reserve in the healthy gravida.

Cardiac output is further increased during labor, with each strong uterine contraction raising stroke volume an average of 33%.[59] Following delivery and elimination of the transplacental arteriovenous shunt, the heart rate slows while stroke volume increases to at least 50% above predelivery values. The left ventricular work at this point is approximately 40% greater than in the beginning of labor.[1] Thus, the early postpartum period may be one of significant myocardial stress.

Position of a pregnant woman near term can markedly affect both the venous and arterial sides of her circulation. Radiographic evidence demonstrates that when a gravida lies supine, the enlarged uterus almost completely occludes the inferior vena cava.[26] Despite some collateral flow via the paravertebral veins and azygos system, venous return and preload are reduced significantly, resulting in a decreased cardiac stroke volume. Although most women are able to compensate for this reduction by increasing peripheral resistance and/or heart rate, up to 15% of patients develop signs of shock, in what Howard et al.[23] named the "supine hypotension syndrome." High sympathetic blockade, such as occurs with regional block analgesia or deep general anesthesia, increases this figure to 60% to 80% of women.

The lower aorta and its branches may be involved as well. Bieniarz et al.[7] showed the subrenal part of the aorta to be displaced and partially occluded when the third trimester gravida was lying in the supine position. Uterine contractions virtually divided the maternal circulation into two zones. Distal to the obstruction, blood flow and arterial pressures were reduced. Proximal to the obstruction, aortic pressure was increased. Such aortic compression may lead to inadequate renal and uteroplacental perfusion, with the latter resulting in fetal asphyxia. These effects may be enhanced if cardiac output has already been decreased as a consequence of caval compression or other factors.

Respiration

Respiratory changes during pregnancy are both mechanically and hormonally induced. Minute ventilation at term is about 50% higher than prior to conception, primarily as a result of a hormonally induced increase in tidal volume. This maternal hyperventilation lowers the arterial carbon dioxide tension ($PaCO_2$) to about 32 torr; pH, however, is maintained in the normal range by compensatory renal mechanisms, which lower the serum bicarbonate level from the usual 26 mEq/L to about 22 mEq/L.[38]

Oxygen consumption increases throughout gestation and, at term, is 50 to 60 mL/min above nonpregnant levels, a rise of approximately 20%. During labor, oxygen consumption increases further in proportion to the frequency and intensity of the myometrial contractions, and may reach 300% above normal values at rest in nonpregnant women. After delivery, oxygen consumption does not decline immediately, suggesting that an oxygen debt is incurred during delivery.

From the fifth month of gestation onward, there is a progressive decline in the functional residual capacity, primarily a result of elevation of the diaphragm. This reduction, about 20% at term, is accentuated further in the recumbent position. One-third to one-half of parturients develop airway closure during normal tidal ventilation when in the supine position. These changes result in a markedly diminished oxygen reserve which, when combined with the higher oxygen consumption, make the pregnant woman very susceptible to hypoxia. Even a short period of apnea may cause a dangerous fall in arterial oxygen tension (PaO_2). Archer and Marx[3] found a mean reduction of 139 torr in the PaO_2 of pregnant women during the first minute of apnea, as opposed to a decrease of only 58 torr in nonpregnant control subjects.

Chest wall and total respiratory compliance are decreased during pregnancy.[40] These compliance changes increase the work of breathing in the spontaneously breathing woman, and make positive pressure ventilation more difficult when that modality is employed. The decrease in respiratory compliance is even greater if the pregnant woman is in the lithotomy position compared to being supine. This effect is primarily a result of the enlarged uterus elevating the diaphragm.[61] Therefore, both chest wall and total respiratory compliance increase dramatically following delivery.

A progressive reduction in alkali reserve makes the gravida prone to the development of metabolic acidosis. This is exaggerated during labor due to a variety of factors, such as renal loss of bicarbonate as compensation for respiratory alkalosis, increased oxygen consumption and skeletal muscle activity as a response to pain, and reduced carbohydrate intake.[38]

CARDIOPULMONARY RESUSCITATION (CPR)

The first step in resuscitation for a suspected cardiac arrest should always be a check for consciousness. Loss of consciousness ensues 5 to 11 sec following the loss of cerebral blood flow.[52] Therefore, a patient who is even slightly arousable cannot have suffered a cardiac arrest. Once unconsciousness has been confirmed, the next steps are the classic ABCs of resuscitation: Airway, Breathing, and Circulation.[31]

Airway

A patent airway must be achieved immediately. The goal is to relieve the obstruction that occurs when there is loss of muscle tone. Most often such obstruction in the unconscious patient is due to the tongue. Three methods of opening the airway have been recommended: the head tilt-neck lift maneuver, the head tilt-jaw thrust maneuver, and the head tilt-chin lift maneuver. Although all three methods can, if properly performed, result in a patent airway, there is evidence that the chin lift and jaw thrust maneuvers may be superior to the neck lift.[20]

Head tilt-chin lift can be performed by using the palm of one hand to apply backward pressure on the patient's forehead. The fingers of the other hand are placed under the mandible to lift the chin upward (Fig-

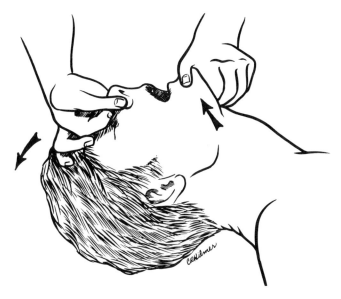

Figure 18-1 The head tilt-chin lift method of opening the airway. *Source*: Reprinted from *Anesthesia*, ed 2, by RD Miller (Ed) with permission of Churchill Livingstone Inc, © 1986.

ure 18-1).[18] Care must be taken not to press on the soft tissues underneath the mandible, as this may occlude the airway.

The head tilt-jaw thrust maneuver involves placing the fingers of both hands under the angles of the mandible to displace the jaw forward and tilt the head back at the same time (Figure 18-2).[18] Once again, care should be taken not to obstruct the airway by compressing the soft tissues of the neck.

Breathing

After opening the airway, any vomitus or foreign material visible in the oropharynx should be wiped away, and a check made for the presence of spontaneous breathing. Sometimes, in cases of respiratory arrest, merely relieving the obstruction and opening the airway by one of the maneuvers described above may be all that is necessary to restore spontaneous respiration. There should, however, be no unnecessary delay at this point. As mentioned earlier, a pregnant woman, particularly one in labor, has little oxygen reserve.[3] Even brief periods of apnea will not be tolerated well by either mother or fetus. In the presence of apnea, artificial respiration should begin immediately. Due to the possibility of commu-

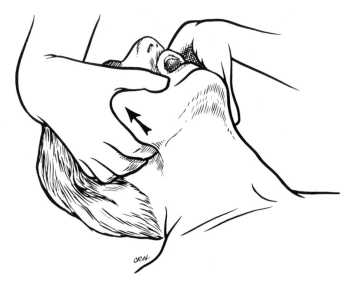

Figure 18-2 The head tilt-jaw thrust method of opening the airway. *Source*: Reprinted from *Anesthesia*, ed 2, by RD Miller (Ed) with permission of Churchill Livingstone Inc, © 1986.

nication of infectious diseases, mouth-to-mouth ventilation has become increasingly controversial. In the hospital setting, equipment such as a bag-valve-mask device or a pocket mask should be readily available and is the preferred mode of therapy to deliver supplemental oxygen. The jaw thrust maneuver can be used to maintain the patient's airway while using these devices. If mouth-to-mouth ventilation is chosen outside the hospital, it should begin with two full breaths of 1 to 1.5 sec each. This differs from the old technique of four quick initial breaths, which is more likely to force air into the esophagus, leading to regurgitation and pulmonary aspiration.[54]

Aspiration is an ever-present danger in the unconscious parturient. A combination of mechanical and hormonal factors retards gastric emptying in the parturient to the point at which food may be retained for more than 24 hours.[13] Therefore, even if ventilation is thought to be adequate by either the mouth-to-mouth or the bag-valve-mask technique, these should be considered only temporary measures. Control of the airway by endotracheal intubation must be secured as soon as possible.

Circulation

Once the airway has been opened and artificial ventilation has begun, the next step is to palpate the carotid artery. If pulsations are absent, the diagnosis of cardiac arrest is confirmed, and external chest compression (closed-chest cardiac compression) should begin. Clearly, if pulses are absent there should be no hesitation to begin cardiac compressions. However, the importance of first checking for pulselessness must be emphasized, since chest compression does entail a notable risk of injury, such as fractured ribs, pneumothorax, and laceration of the liver or spleen.

With the hands over the lower sternum, and not overlying the xiphoid, the sternum should be compressed 1.5 to 2 inches with each effort, at a rate of 80 to 100 compressions per min. The ratio of compressions to ventilation should be 5 to 1, with a 1- to 1.5-sec pause for ventilation.[54]

It had long been thought that these cardiac compressions generate blood flow by a direct compression of the heart between the sternum and spine, the "cardiac pump" mechanism proposed by Kouwenhoven et al. in 1960.[29] There is now growing evidence to suggest that a second mechanism may be of equal or greater importance for maintaining blood flow during CPR.[44,53,60] This "thoracic pump" mechanism is based on the observation that external chest compression increases the intrathoracic pressure, which is transmitted equally to all thoracic structures. Since arteries tend to resist collapse, such a pressure increase should be almost fully transmitted to the extrathoracic arteries. Venous collapse and the presence of valves in the venous system prevent full transmission of this pressure increase to extrathoracic veins. A pressure gradient is created between the extrathoracic arteries and veins, causing antegrade flow during compression. During the relaxation phase between compressions, the intrathoracic pressure falls below the extrathoracic venous pressure, resulting in venous return to the right side of the heart.

With this mechanism in mind, it is clear that even minor degrees of aortocaval compression imposed by the gravid uterus may have a profound effect on the success or failure of the resuscitative efforts. Any compression of the inferior vena cava will seriously impede the venous return to the heart. In addition, obstruction of the lower aorta would represent a significant obstacle to flow, hindering the development of an appropriate arteriovenous pressure gradient during chest compressions.

It is therefore imperative that uterine displacement be maintained during CPR. A wedge or sandbag should be placed under the right hip to provide a left lateral tilt to the pelvis of approximately 30 degrees. The position of the torso will not be greatly affected and chest compressions should still be possible without difficulty. If circumstances make this approach cumbersome or impractical, the uterus can be deviated manually by having the patient's abdomen displaced to the left and slightly cephalad.

If hemodynamic stability still cannot be achieved despite attempts at uterine displacement, then abdominal delivery of the baby must be performed with dispatch. It would be a serious mistake to defer cesarean section until the mother has been "stabilized," since such stabilization may never occur without delivery and relief of the aortocaval compression.[31] Several cases have occurred in which prompt delivery led to adequate maternal resuscitation and recovery.[16,35]

A recent review of agonal and postmortem cesarean sections also demonstrates the importance of this procedure to the infant.[25] Most of the children who survived such emergency cesarean section were delivered within 5 min of the onset of maternal cardiac arrest. As the time to delivery extends beyond 5 min, the chances for survival of the fetus diminish markedly, and the probability of severe neurologic damage increases. This is demonstrated clearly in Table 18-1.

In the first and second trimesters the degree of aortocaval compression exerted by the uterus may be minimal, and an emergency abdominal delivery may offer little in terms of effective resuscitation at this time in pregnancy.

If CPR fails to maintain peripheral circulation, emergency thoracotomy with open chest cardiac massage should be considered as a last resort.[31]

Table 18-1 Survival Rate of Infants According to Interval between Cardiac Arrest and Delivery

Cases	No. Patients	Percent
0–5 min	42 (normal infants)	70
6–10 min	7 (normal infants)	13
	1 (mild neurologic sequelae)	
Subtotal	8	
11–15 min	6 (normal infants)	12
	1 (severe neurologic sequelae)	
Subtotal	7	
16–20 min	1 (severe neurologic sequelae)	1.7
21 + min	2 (severe neurologic sequelae)	
	1 (normal infant)	3.3
Subtotal	3	
Total	61	100

Source: Reprinted with permission from the American College of Obstetricians and Gynecologists from "Perimortem Cesarean Delivery" by VL Katz, DJ Dotters, and W Droegmueller in *Obstetrics and Gynecology* (1986;68:571–576).

In selected clinical situations (e.g., chest trauma, severe emphysema, cardiac tamponade), open chest massage may be necessary to produce adequate perfusion of brain and heart.[54]

Acid-Base Balance

The primary mode of therapy for acid-base imbalances during a cardiac arrest is the establishment of adequate alveolar ventilation.[17] To this end, frequent determination of arterial blood gas values can be used to assess the adequacy of ventilation and guide further therapy. In late pregnancy, the $PaCO_2$ should be kept between 30 and 34 torr. If the patient remains severely acidotic at this level of normocapnia, sodium bicarbonate should be administered in an initial dose of 1 mEq/kg. Hyperventilation to the point at which the $PaCO_2$ falls below 28 torr is to be avoided, as is overuse of bicarbonate, since both of these events will have a deleterious effect on placental transfer of oxygen.

Vasopressors

Since the uterine vascular bed probably lacks autoregulation, uterine blood flow is dependent directly on mean perfusion pressure. Therefore, hypotension has severe consequences for the fetus. Although the uterine vascular bed is almost maximally dilated under normal conditions, it can respond with marked vasoconstriction to any exogenous or endogenous alpha-adrenergic stimulation. Ralston et al.[49] demonstrated that uterine blood flow was well maintained by administration of ephedrine, but that agents with alpha-adrenergic activity reduced uterine blood flow as they raised maternal blood pressure. Ephedrine, through its predominant beta-adrenergic effects, increases cardiac output, blood pressure, and uterine blood flow without deleterious effects on the fetus, making it the agent of choice for maternal hypotension.

During cardiac arrest, ephedrine may not be a sufficient myocardial stimulant. Epinephrine has been used in these situations primarily for its alpha-adrenergic properties[50,62] and the value of its beta-adrenergic effects in this situation is controversial.[54] The recommended intravenous dose of epinephrine (0.5–1.0 mg every 5 min during resuscitation) is more than enough to reduce uterine blood flow and adversely affect an already compromised fetus.[51] As mentioned above, early delivery of the infant gives the child the best chance of survival.

Direct Current Cardioversion

Some concern has been raised as to the risk of fetal morbidity during the treatment of maternal arrhythmias with direct current (DC) shock. Few cases of DC cardioversion for supraventricular arrhythmias have been reported during pregnancy, and the experience with ventricular defibrillation is even more limited. However, a recent review of these cases, which employed energies as high as 300 joules, showed no adverse infant outcomes related to the use of this therapy.[15] At present, there appears to be no contraindication to the use of direct current shock.

Specific Therapies

The 1985 National Conference on Standards and Guidelines for Cardiopulmonary Resuscitation has established suggested algorithms for the treatment of specific dysrhythmias.[54] The treatment algorithms for ventricular fibrillation, asystole, electromechanical dissociation, and bradycardia are presented in Figures 18-3 through 18-6.

SPECIAL SITUATIONS

The resuscitative regimens for two special syndromes are detailed below. Prompt appropriate management may save the lives of mother and fetus in these unusual, but extremely morbid, situations.

Amniotic Fluid Embolism

Amniotic fluid embolism (AFE), an uncommon complication of pregnancy, is nevertheless one of the most dangerous, having a reported maternal mortality rate of 86%.[41] Clinically, the awake patient often presents with anxiety, shivering, coughing, and sudden respiratory distress, almost always without chest pain. Besides the mechanical blockage of the pulmonary vessels by amniotic fluid and other fetal debris, an anaphylactoid reaction may also develop, causing bronchospasm and enhancing pulmonary artery constriction. The result is severe hypoxia and an acute pulmonary hypertension which may lead to acute pulmonary edema. Twenty-five to 50% of AFE patients die in the first hour from this initial insult.

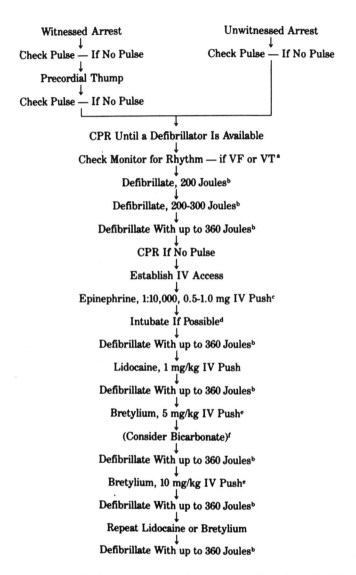

Witnessed Arrest → Check Pulse — If No Pulse → Precordial Thump → Check Pulse — If No Pulse

Unwitnessed Arrest → Check Pulse — If No Pulse

CPR Until a Defibrillator Is Available
↓
Check Monitor for Rhythm — if VF or VT[a]
↓
Defibrillate, 200 Joules[b]
↓
Defibrillate, 200-300 Joules[b]
↓
Defibrillate With up to 360 Joules[b]
↓
CPR If No Pulse
↓
Establish IV Access
↓
Epinephrine, 1:10,000, 0.5-1.0 mg IV Push[c]
↓
Intubate If Possible[d]
↓
Defibrillate With up to 360 Joules[b]
↓
Lidocaine, 1 mg/kg IV Push
↓
Defibrillate With up to 360 Joules[b]
↓
Bretylium, 5 mg/kg IV Push[e]
↓
(Consider Bicarbonate)[f]
↓
Defibrillate With up to 360 Joules[b]
↓
Bretylium, 10 mg/kg IV Push[e]
↓
Defibrillate With up to 360 Joules[b]
↓
Repeat Lidocaine or Bretylium
↓
Defibrillate With up to 360 Joules[b]

Figure 18-3 Ventricular fibrillation (VF) and pulseless ventricular tachycardia (VT). Flow of algorithm presumes that VF is continuing. [a]Pulseless VT should be treated identically to VF. [b]Pulse and rhythm should be checked after each shock. If VF recurs after transiently converting, whatever energy level has previously been successful for defibrillation should be used. [c]Epinephrine should be repeated every 5 min. [d]Intubation is preferable but ventilation without it may be necessary. [e]Repeated boluses of lidocaine may be preferred, given in 0.5 mg/kg boluses every 8 min to a total dose of 3 mg/kg. [f]Value of bicarbonate is uncertain. *Source*: Reprinted with permission from *Journal of the American Medical Association* (1986;255:2905–2984), Copyright © 1986, American Medical Association.

**If Rhythm Is Unclear and Possibly Ventricular
Fibrillation, Defibrillate as for VF. If Asystole is Present[a]**

↓

Continue CPR·

↓

Establish IV Access

↓

Epinephrine, 1:10,000, 0.5 - 1.0 mg IV Push[b]

↓

Intubate When Possible[c]

↓

Atropine, 1.0 mg IV Push (Repeated in 5 min)

↓

(Consider Bicarbonate)[d]

↓

Consider Pacing

Figure 18-4 Asystole. [a]VF, ventricular fibrillation; IV, intravenous. Flow of algorithm presumes that asystole is continuing. [a]Confirm asystole in two leads. [b]Epinephrine should be repeated every 5 min. [c]Intubation is preferable, when possible. [d]Value of bicarbonate is uncertain. *Source:* Reprinted with permission from *Journal of the American Medical Association* (1986;255:2905–2984), Copyright © 1986, American Medical Association.

Of the patients who do survive this period, most develop a diffuse intravascular coagulopathy. This clotting defect is usually thought of as a late development, but it can be an early event. In Morgan's review of 272 cases,[41] the presenting signs and symptoms were respiratory in 51%, cardiovascular in 27%, and hematologic in 12% of cases. Convulsions were the first signs in 10% of patients.

Diagnosis is often difficult and rests upon a high index of suspicion combined with recovery of fetal squames and other amniotic debris from a central venous catheter inserted into the mother's right atrium.[27] Recent investigations, however, have shown that squames and trophoblastic cells can be recovered from the maternal circulation even in pregnancies where there is no overt clinical evidence of amniotic fluid embolism.[11,30,32] The question of how much amniotic fluid is necessary to precipitate the clinical picture of embolism has yet to be answered.

Treatment of AFE must be geared toward (1) improvement of oxygenation, (2) support of the cardiovascular system, and (3) treatment of the coagulopathy. Severe ventilation-perfusion inequalities usually develop following entry of amniotic fluid into the pulmonary vasculature, leading

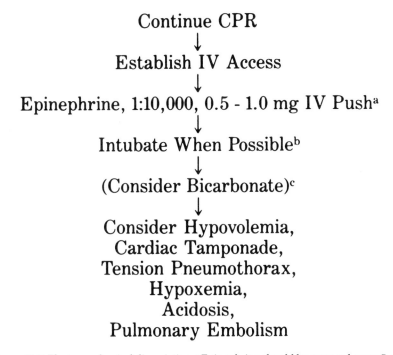

Continue CPR
↓
Establish IV Access
↓
Epinephrine, 1:10,000, 0.5 - 1.0 mg IV Push[a]
↓
Intubate When Possible[b]
↓
(Consider Bicarbonate)[c]
↓
Consider Hypovolemia,
Cardiac Tamponade,
Tension Pneumothorax,
Hypoxemia,
Acidosis,
Pulmonary Embolism

Figure 18-5 Electromechanical dissociation. [a]Epinephrine should be repeated every 5 min. [b]Intubation is preferred. [c]Value of bicarbonate is uncertain. *Source*: Reprinted with permission from *Journal of the American Medical Association* (1986;255:2905–2984), Copyright © 1986, American Medical Association.

to profound hypoxia. Intubation and positive pressure ventilation with 100% oxygen should be instituted promptly in an effort to enhance oxygenation. Positive end-expiratory pressure (PEEP) is often beneficial.[14] A bronchodilating agent, such as terbutaline, isoproterenol, or aminophylline, may aid in relieving bronchospasm. Hydrocortisone, 2 to 4 g IV, may help reduce pulmonary edema.

As mentioned above, a central venous catheter should be inserted to aspirate blood for examination for fetal squames and amniotic debris. Blood should also be obtained for coagulation studies and for cross-match of blood. A pulmonary artery catheter should be placed as soon as is practicable, in order to monitor the patient's hemodynamic status properly. Although historically the teaching has been to watch for acute failure of the right heart secondary to pulmonary hypertension, there may be as much to fear from left-sided heart failure. A review by Clark et al.[10] of reported data from AFE patients with pulmonary artery catheters in place

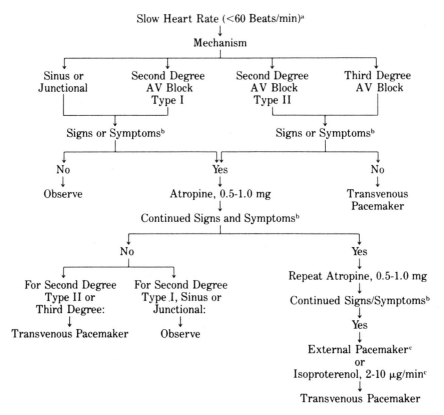

Figure 18-6 Bradycardia. AV, atrioventricular. [a]A solitary chest thump or cough may stimulate cardiac electrical activity, resulting in improved cardiac output, and may be used at this point. [b]Hypotension, premature ventricular contractions, altered mental status or symptoms (e.g., chest pain or dyspnea), ischemia, or infarction. [c]Temporizing therapy. *Source*: Reprinted with permission from *Journal of the American Medical Association* (1986;255:2905–2984), Copyright © 1986, American Medical Association.

revealed a general pattern of left heart failure, even in patients with only mildly elevated pulmonary artery pressure. This suggests that inotropic support may often be necessary, and may be guided by data obtained with the pulmonary artery catheter. Rapid digitalization, dopamine, or dobutamine may be utilized for this purpose. Cardiac dysrhythmias should be treated in the appropriate fashion, as described above.

There is some evidence that early use of intravenous heparin, 2,500 to 5,000 U, may help to prevent amniotic fluid-induced coagulopathy.[56] This is controversial, but there are anecdotal reports of its efficacy.[9]

Intravascular volume must be maintained and replacement of clotting factors with fresh frozen plasma and platelets should continue as necessary.

In addition to the cardiopulmonary and hematologic complications, uterine atony is often a problem in these cases, and should be treated in the standard fashion. The potential adverse consequences of severe hypovolemia in these patients is considerable, and efforts to control uterine bleeding promptly are vital.

Bupivacaine Cardiotoxicity

Bupivacaine, a relatively new potent local anesthetic, has become popular in obstetrics owing to its excellent analgesic properties combined with long duration of action. Unfortunately, these advantages are offset by the potential for cardiotoxicity when the drug is unintentionally injected intravascularly.[2]

Although high plasma levels of all local anesthetics possess the propensity to cause ventricular arrhythmias, the cardiotoxic effects of bupivacaine are significantly greater than those of other local agents. In awake, unmedicated sheep, convulsant doses of bupivacaine, but not of lidocaine, produced severe ventricular arrhythmias in the absence of hypoxia or acidemia.[28] In addition, pregnant sheep required smaller doses of bupivacaine than nongravid animals to initiate symptoms of cardiovascular depression.[42] This may explain why more parturients than surgical patients have suffered fatal cardiac arrest from the access into the general circulation of clinical doses of this drug. In most of these cases, the concentration of bupivacaine was 0.75%, leading to a letter (1983) from the drug's manufacturers advising that this concentration should no longer be used in obstetrics. However, several healthy parturients died after receiving 0.5% bupivacaine for lumbar epidural block and a few succumbed after single-dose injections of 0.25% bupivacaine into the caudal canal. This indicates that the patient's peak plasma level of bupivacaine depends not on the concentration employed but on the actual dose injected.[36,37] Therefore, strict adherence to the recommended safeguards for epidural blockade, that is, appropriate test dosing, fractionation of the therapeutic dose, and ready availability of drugs and equipment for treatment of adverse effects is imperative for all concentrations of this anesthetic.

Cardiac depression due to bupivacaine has been particularly difficult to reverse, due in part to a prolonged blockade of cardiac sodium channels. Lidocaine blocks these channels in a fast-in–fast-out manner, resulting in a rapid recovery from the blockade, while bupivacaine blocks these channels in a fast-in–slow-out fashion, resulting in delayed recovery during diastole.[12] If tachyarrhythmias should develop during bupivacaine administration, they are probably best treated with bretylium and DC cardioversion, rather than with lidocaine.

Since the cardiac toxicity of bupivacaine is further aggravated by hypoxia and acidemia,[58] resuscitative efforts must begin at the first sign of dysrhythmia. Control of the airway, ventilation with 100% oxygen, and correction of acid-base imbalances are of key importance here, as they are with other causes of cardiac arrest. Diazepam or barbiturates may be given parenterally for control of any seizure activity.

The importance of relieving aortocaval compression with dispatch cannot be overemphasized. Marx[35] reported the fate of five healthy gravidas who received 0.75% bupivacaine during attempted epidural anesthesia for cesarean section. All five had a short grand mal seizure followed by disappearance of pulse and blood pressure. All required external cardiac compression for more than 10 min. In three the infant was delivered with no delay and the mother survived intact. In the other two, delivery was postponed for several minutes, and both suffered irreversible brain damage. Kasten and Martin,[24] using a dog model, also demonstrated that relief of aortic and caval compression was a necessity for effective resuscitation from a bupivacaine-induced cardiac arrest.

CONCLUSION

The goal of cardiopulmonary resuscitation—the establishment of an adequate flow of oxygenated blood to vital organs—is identical for pregnant and nongravid subjects. The basic tenets of resuscitative measures are also the same. However, consequent to the physiologic changes induced by pregnancy, there are special considerations in the gravid woman. First, her oxygen consumption is increased while her oxygen reserve is decreased. This makes immediate controlled ventilation with 100% oxygen imperative. Second, the increased susceptibility to the development of metabolic acidosis in response to uterine contractions and seizure activity (e.g., bupivacaine-induced convulsions) emphasizes the importance of early blood gas determinations to detect the need for intravenous sodium bicarbonate. Third, and most importantly, although in nonpregnant patients external cardiac compression is most effective when performed with the patient lying in the supine position on an unyielding surface, this is the very position that in pregnancy produces aortocaval compression with its progressive decrease in venous return to the heart. This impediment to cardiac filling hinders effective restoration of the circulation and must be avoided by manual displacement of the uterus or rapid delivery of the neonate.

REFERENCES

1. Adams JQ, Alexander AM: Alterations in cardiovascular physiology. *Obstet Gynecol* 1958;12:542–548.

2. Albright GA: Cardiac arrest following regional anesthesia with etidocaine or bupivacaine. *Anesthesiology* 1979;51:285–287.

3. Archer GW, Marx GF: Arterial oxygen tension during apnoea in parturient women. *Br J Anaesth* 1974;46:358–360.

4. Assali NS, Brinkman CR III: Disorders of maternal circulation and respiratory adjustments, in Assali NS, Brinkman CR III (eds): *Pathophysiology of Gestation. Maternal Disorders.* New York, Academic Press, 1972, vol 1, pp 278–285.

5. Batts JA, Tchilinguirian NGO, Passmore J: Pheochromocytoma in pregnancy: A case report and review of the pathophysiology. *Am J Obstet Gynecol* 1974;118:576–577.

6. Beco J, Thoumsin H, Lambotte R: Pregnancy and traffic accidents. *Rev Med Liege* 1986; 41:75–83.

7. Bieniarz J, Crottogini JJ, Curuchet E, Romero-Salinas G, Yoshida T, Poseiro JJ, Caldeyro-Barcia R: Aortocaval compression by the uterus in late pregnancy. *Am J Obstet Gynecol* 1968;100:203–217.

8. Chambers JJ, Saha AK: Electrocution during anaesthesia. *Anaesthesia* 1979;34:173–175.

9. Chung AF, Merkatz IR: Survival following amniotic fluid embolism with early heparinization. *Obstet Gynecol* 1973;42:809–814.

10. Clark SL, Montz FJ, Phelan JP: Hemodynamic alterations associated with amniotic fluid embolism: A reappraisal. *Am J Obstet Gynecol* 1985;151:617–621.

11. Clark SL, Pavlova Z, Greenspoon J, Horenstein J, Phelan JP: Squamous cells in the maternal pulmonary circulation. *Am J Obstet Gynecol* 1986;154:104–106.

12. Clarkson CW, Hondeghem LM: Mechanism for bupivacaine depression of cardiac conduction: Fast block of sodium channels during the action potential with slow recovery from block during diastole. *Anesthesiology* 1985;62:396–405.

13. Crawford JS: Some aspects of obstetric anesthesia. *Br J Anaesth* 1956;28:201–208.

14. Cruikshank DP: Amniotic fluid embolism, in Berkowitz RL (ed): *Critical Care of the Obstetric Patient.* New York, Churchill Livingstone, 1983, pp 431–442.

15. Cullhed I: Cardioversion during pregnancy. *Acta Med Scand* 1983;214:169–172.

16. Depace NL, Betesh JS, Kotler MN: "Postmortem" cesarean section with recovery of both mother and offspring. *JAMA* 1982;248:971–975.

17. Donegan JH: New concepts in cardiopulmonary resuscitation. *Anesth Analg* 1981; 60:100–108.

18. Donegan JH: Cardiopulmonary resuscitation, in Miller RD (ed): *Anesthesia,* ed 2. New York, Churchill Livingstone, 1986, pp 2111–2147.

19. Ginz B: Myocardial infarction in pregnancy. *J Obstet Gynaecol Br Commonw* 1970; 77:610–615.

20. Guildner CW: Resuscitation—opening the airway: A comparative study of techniques for opening an airway obstructed by the tongue. *J Am Coll Emergency Phys* 1976;5:588–590.

21. Hein HAT: Cardiorespiratory arrest with laryngeal oedema in pregnancy-induced hypertension. *Can Anaesth Soc J* 1984;31:210–212.

22. Hibbard LT: Maternal mortality due to cardiac disease. *Clin Obstet Gynecol* 1975; 18:27–36.

23. Howard BK, Goodson JH, Mengert WF: Supine hypotension syndrome in late pregnancy. *Obstet Gynecol* 1953;1:371–377.

24. Kasten GW, Martin ST: Resuscitation from bupivacaine-induced cardiovascular toxicity during partial inferior vena cava occlusion. *Anesth Analg* 1986;65:341–344.

25. Katz VL, Dotters DJ, Droegmueller W: Perimortem cesarean delivery. *Obstet Gynecol* 1986;68:571–576.

26. Kerr MG, Scott DB, Samuel E: Studies of the inferior vena cava in late pregnancy. *Br Med J* 1964;1:532–533.

27. Killam A: Amniotic fluid embolism. *Clin Obstet Gynecol* 1985;28:32–36.

28. Kotelko DM, Shnider SM, Dailey PA, Brizgys RV, Levinson G, Shapiro WA, Koike M, Rosen MA: Bupivacaine-induced cardiac arrhythmias in sheep. *Anesthesiology* 1984;60:10–18.

29. Kouwenhoven WB, Jude JR, Knickerbocker GG: Closed chest cardiac massage. *JAMA* 1960;173:1064–1067.

30. Kuhlman K, Hidvegi D, Tamura RK, Depp R: Is amniotic fluid material in the central circulation of peripartum patients pathologic? *Am J Perinatol* 1985;2:295–299.

31. Lee RV, Rodgers BD, White LM, Harvey RC: Cardiopulmonary resuscitation of pregnant women., *Am J Med* 1986;81:311–318.

32. Lee W, Ginsburg KA, Cotton DB, Kaufman RH: Squamous and trophoblastic cells in the maternal pulmonary circulation identified by invasive hemodynamic monitoring during the peripartum period. *Am J Obstet Gynecol* 1986;155:999–1001.

33. Lund CJ, Donovan JC: Blood volume during pregnancy. *Am J Obstet Gynecol* 1967; 98:393–403.

34. Mainprize TC, Maltby JR: Amniotic fluid embolism: A report of four probable cases. *Can Anaesth Soc J* 1986;33:382–387.

35. Marx GF: Cardiopulmonary resuscitation of late-pregnant women. *Anesthesiology* 1982;56:156.

36. Marx GF: Cardiotoxicity of local anesthetics—the plot thickens. *Anesthesiology* 1984; 60:3–5.

37. Marx GF: Bupivacaine cardiotoxicity—concentration or dose? *Anesthesiology* 1986; 65:116.

38. Marx GF, Bassell GM: Physiologic considerations of the mother, in Marx GF, Bassell GM (eds): *Obstetric Analgesia and Anaesthesia*. New York, Elsevier, 1980, pp 21–51.

39. Marx GF, Finster M: Difficulty in endotracheal intubation associated with obstetric anesthesia. *Anesthesiology* 1979;51:364–365.

40. Marx GF, Murthy PK, Orkin LR: Static compliance before and after vaginal delivery. *Br J Anaesth* 1970;42:1100–1103.

41. Morgan M: Amniotic fluid embolism. *Anaesthesia* 1979;34:20–32.

42. Morishima HO, Pedersen H, Finster M, Tsjui A, Hiraoka H, Feldman HS, Arthur GR, Covino BG: Is bupivacaine more cardiotoxic than lidocaine? (abstr). *Anesthesiology* 1983;59(Suppl):A409.

43. Mulder JI: Amniotic fluid embolism: An overview and case report. *Am J Obstet Gynecol* 1985;152:430–435.

44. Niemann JT, Rosborough J, Hausknecht M, Brown D, Criley JM: Cough-induced cardiac compression: Self-administered form of cardiopulmonary resuscitation. *JAMA* 1976;236:1246–1250.

45. Perloff JK: Pregnancy and cardiovascular disease, in Braunwald E (ed): *Heart Disease*. Philadelphia, WB Saunders, 1980, pp 1871–1892.

46. Pierce MR, Henderson RA, Mitchell JM: Cardiopulmonary arrest secondary to lightning injury in a pregnant woman. *Ann Emerg Med* 1986;15:597–599.

47. Pritchard JA: Changes in the blood volume during pregnancy and delivery. *Anesthesiology* 1965;26:393–399.

48. Pritchard JA: Haematological problems associated with delivery, placental abruption, retained dead fetus, and amniotic fluid embolism. *Clin Haematol* 1973;2:563–586.

49. Ralston DH, Shnider SM, deLorimier AA: Effects of equipotent ephedrine, metaraminol, mephentermine, and methoxamine on uterine blood flow in the pregnant ewe. *Anesthesiology* 1974;40:354–370.

50. Redding JS, Pearson JW: Evaluation of drugs for cardiac resuscitation. *Anesthesiology* 1963;24:203–207.

51. Rosenfeld CR, Barton MD, Meschia G: Effects of epinephrine on distribution of blood flow in the pregnant ewe. *Am J Obstet Gynecol* 1976;124:156–163.

52. Rossen R, Kabat H, Anderson JP: Acute arrest of cerebral circulation in man. *Arch Neurol Psychiatry* 1943;50:510–528.

53. Rud MT, Maughan WL, Effron M, Freund P, Weisfeldt ML: Mechanism of blood flow during cardiopulmonary resuscitation. *Circulation* 1980;61:345–352.

54. Standards and Guidelines for Cardiopulmonary Resuscitation (CPR) and Emergency Cardiac Care (ECC). *JAMA* 1986;255:2905–2984.

55. Stokes IM: Myocardial infarction and cardiac arrest in the second trimester followed by assisted vaginal delivery under epidural analgesia at 38 weeks gestation. Case report. *Br J Obstet Gynaecol* 1984;91:197–198.

56. Strickland MA, Bates GW, Whitworth NS, Martin JN: Amniotic fluid embolism: Prophylaxis with heparin and aspirin. *South Med J* 1985;78:377–379.

57. Sullivan JM, Ramanathan KB: Management of medical problems in pregnancy—severe cardiac disease. *N Engl J Med* 1985;313:304–309.

58. Thigpen JW, Kotelko DM, Shnider SM, Foutz SE, Levinson G, Koike M, Rosen MA: Bupivacaine cardiotoxicity in hypoxic-acidotic sheep (abstr). *Anesthesiology* 1983; 59(Suppl):A204.

59. Ueland K, Hansen JM: Maternal cardiovascular dynamics II. Posture and uterine contractions. *Am J Obstet Gynecol* 1969;103:1–7.

60. Werner JA, Greene HL, Janko CL, Cobb LA: Visualization of cardiac valve motion in man during external chest compression using two-dimensional echocardiography. Implications regarding the mechanism of blood flow. *Circulation* 1981;63:1417–1421.

61. Wollman SB, Marx GF: Acute hydration for prevention of hypotension of spinal anesthesia in parturients. *Anesthesiology* 1968;29:374–380.

62. Yakaitis RW, Otto CW, Blitt CD: Relative importance of alpha and beta adrenergic receptors during resuscitation. *Crit Care Med* 1979;7:293–296.

19

Contemporary Issues in Childbirth

Maureen Guarino McRae and Frances V. Mervyn

Dramatic and pervasive changes in obstetric care occurred in the United States during the 1960s and 1970s. The conflict between burgeoning technologic abilities and renewed interest in psychoprophylactic techniques for labor and other trappings of the "natural childbirth" movement produced a climate of unrest. Relations between consumers and health professionals were often strained and mutually mistrustful. Gratifyingly, the strength of the women's movement and related social and medical forces have produced a population of women far more knowledgeable and better able to assess and understand obstetric options and choices than their predecessors. In addition, the medical community has, at least in many areas, responded to pressure from consumers (and from some health care professionals) and initiated important changes in obstetric care. Two decades of struggle for control and power by the childbearing woman have resulted in a new environment for the practicing obstetric physician, nurse, and nurse midwife. Thus, the 1980s have become a time of reduced conflict and defensiveness for childbearing women and their health caretakers.

HISTORICAL PERSPECTIVE

Women in search of the optimal delivery experience consistent with the prevailing social and cultural climate have always considered alternatives that would allow them to fulfill their childbirth aspirations. In late 19th century America, the maternal role was dictated culturally as one of childbearing and childrearing exclusively. It was culturally acceptable that the father (then considered the undisputed family provider) be absent completely from the birth events. Women sought relief from pain

535

and suffering as they accomplished their biologic obligation, and chloroform anesthesia became accepted for relieving childbirth pain.

The early 20th century brought the founding of the Twilight Sleep Association, a group of women committed to liberation from childbirth suffering, and the medical profession was accused of being indifferent to women's pain. In this climate, the use of heavy sedation or anesthesia for labor and delivery became commonplace.

Later in this century, influenced once again by changing social and cultural attitudes (the movement for sexual equality and acknowledgement of the importance of the paternal role in family development), a new generation of childbearing concepts emerged. The belief in childbirth and motherhood as one means of a woman's emotional fulfillment—rather than her biologic obligation—brought social, psychologic, and cultural issues to the forefront with a new focus. Women began to expound on feelings of powerlessness, isolation, and passive dependence, which the traditional hospital birthing environment engendered. They had new aspirations, none of which could be realized under the influence of drug-induced amnesia. Thus, in the 1940s began a challenge to the medical establishment's domination of the birth process and to the entire obstetric climate that had prevailed in the previous four decades. This challenge would accelerate dramatically coincident with the surge of the women's rights movement of the 1970s.

At that time, the new literature stressed that the vast majority of women in labor would not need analgesia if they had appropriate prenatal education, and the new philosophy of psychoprophylaxis was promulgated.[16] This approach was based on active parental participation in childbirth and viewed techniques such as analgesia as unnecessary interventions. Seeds of conflict were thus sown because the natural childbirth philosophy emerged when the prevalent tendency in obstetrics (a response, in part, to previously expressed societal preferences) was to use medication that would provide analgesia or even complete anesthesia and amnesia during labor and delivery. In the context of new value systems regarding childbirth, this latter approach was interpreted in much of the lay literature as representing attempts to dominate childbirth by the largely male medical community. In fact, when viewed in historical context, it was consistent with a growing reliance upon science (and perhaps especially on medical science) to provide pervasive solutions to our problems. The subsequent trend toward unmedicated birth was part of a general societal upheaval and a growing distrust of science and its potential for controlling human endeavors. This distrust and concern appeared to reach a peak in the 1970s; certain aspects have continued into the present.

Today's unrest has a powerful agenda. Patients' expectations often exceed outcomes. They have responded by focusing blame on the physician and nurse. Technologic advances thought initially to be panaceas are, in a sense, worthy of both applause and denigration.[26] The persistence of authoritarian medical systems, the continuing poor communication between women and health professionals, and the emergence of medicolegal agendas have created dissatisfaction. Corea,[9] Arms,[1] and Rich[32] have pointed out continued discontent among women about their health care. Current practices of postponing parenting and enhancing paternal roles convey to health professionals new messages that require continued emphasis on communication and trust.

ALTERNATIVES FOR BIRTHING

The introduction of alternatives for labor, birth attendants, and place of confinement has allowed women freedom of choice and increasingly active participation in the birthing process. Grantly Dick-Read published his initial concepts of "childbirth without fear" in 1942,[13] at which time his theory had limited support. His notions were popularized by Ferdinand Lamaze in France.[24] In 1952, he renewed interest in techniques of psychoprophylaxis, a method of pain control based upon the development of new conditioned responses to discomfort.

In 1975, Frederick Leboyer's book[25] *Birth without Violence* brought a focus on the need for a peaceful transition for the newborn to the extrauterine environment. Sensitivity and gentleness were concepts promulgated in the Leboyer method. Even underwater birth has been suggested as a means to ensure smooth transition to extrauterine life.[29] This alternative has not received much attention and is limited by the lack of information regarding safety. Nevertheless, it is emblematic of the apparent extremes to which alternative birthing has progressed. Although the concepts put forth by Leboyer are generally considered radical, and although the reputed benefits of the technique cannot be proved, his influence on contemporary obstetric practice is not inconsiderable. His emphasis on an ambiance of quiet and calmness in the delivery room and on birth as an emotionally fulfilling experience forms the basis of many of our current attitudes toward childbirth.

Desires for a birth experience that allows early attachment and bonding of mother, father, and newborn have focused increasingly on the potential benefits of parental involvement with the newborn at birth. Bowlby,[4] Kennell et al.,[20] Klaus et al.,[23] and Brazelton[5] have addressed the importance of contact between mother and infant, and considerable research suggests significant benefits from early parental bonding. In 1974, 27% of fathers were present in the delivery room in our hospital; currently participation by the father (or another individual chosen by the patient) is almost universal. Also, we have begun to understand the importance of bonding even with the very premature infant (which was once thought impossible or harmful). The advantages of early initiation of breastfeeding with both the term and the premature infant further support the need for professionals to be aware of continued advances that encourage the growth of the family. Modern changes in prenatal care, especially regarding premature infants, have created new challenges for professional sensitivity to the needs of birthing women and families. Nevertheless, it now appears that initial near-fanatic insistence on early bonding was exaggerated. Although there is no doubt that early establishment of maternal-infant interaction is pleasant and desirable, it is by no means a prerequisite for normal evolution of the parent-child relationship.

POSTPONED PREGNANCY

One of the most prevalent contemporary choices is to postpone pregnancy until the mother's career or personal goals have been achieved.[17,35] Thus, the number of older nulliparas in the obstetric population has increased. Once considered a high-risk situation to be avoided, advanced maternal age has become a deliberately planned event in many families. To term gravidas "elderly" at the age of 35 years or greater was a designation adopted by the Council of the International Federation of Obstetricians and Gynecologists in 1958. In 1985, Kirz et al.[22] argued for a more gentle and less pejorative designation of this population and have coined the term "mature gravida."

The projected 37% increase in the next decade in the number of women bearing their first child in their 30s and 40s is a result of many factors. Kirz et al.[22] cite the maturation of the postwar baby boom cohort, women's career priorities, advanced education, infertility, control over fertility, late, and second marriages, and financial concerns as factors contributing to advanced maternal age.

Some research has suggested increased risk to these women and their infants, including high cesarean section rates, and frequent labor abnormalities.[20,27,30,38] Nevertheless, some data support the idea that healthy older women (without diabetes mellitus, hypertension, or other diseases known to complicate pregnancy) are at no greater obstetric risk than their younger counterparts. In a critical review of the literature linking maternal age to adverse pregnancy outcomes, Kernoff and Mansfield[21] found little support for the view that late childbearing is necessarily more hazardous than that which occurs in younger women. The ability to detect fetal chromosomal abnormalities, which increase in frequency with maternal age, has allowed women the option to postpone pregnancy with a more confident outlook. Midlife childbirth is an issue that will require increased availability of sophisticated prenatal care services, such as genetic counseling, antenatal diagnosis, ultrasonography, and electronic fetal heart rate testing.[12]

From a nursing perspective, advanced maternal age is an issue that requires sensitivity to many psychosocial needs. Issues of maternal adaptation, self-esteem, control, role transition, and prenatal and intrapartum support are just beginning to be understood.[2,14,28,33] The lay literature abounds with advice and reassurance for the older mother. The mature gravida will undoubtedly have issues unique to career, postponed birthing, and transition to parenting. The need for communication, assessment of needs, and responsiveness to new issues cannot be overstated. If these women are in hospital for birth, this locus must continue to accommodate individual needs. The mature gravida, if considered high risk, will require professional surveillance; but such care must also encourage autonomy. This population may be more educated, more prepared, and committed to higher expectations and outcomes than their younger counterparts.

Eichholz and Offerman-Zukerrberg[14] found that pregnancy in women over age 35 required negotiation of the psychosocial tasks of pregnancy in the context of the physical and psychosocial impact of aging. They recognized many differences in the needs of women based on age. To deliver good obstetric care requires that these new and unique issues be addressed. Individual assessment is essential. Winslow[38] interviewed 12 primigravidas aged 35 to 44 and found important psychosocial differences in their deferred childbearing. She suggested caregivers should anticipate goal-directed behavior, a sophisticated consumption of a wide range of resources, and a need to evaluate whether they have done the task well. These women saw pregnancy as a project; this conceptual framework was important to them and to those who cared for them. We must take care to avoid unnecessary intervention but rather emphasize more appropriate responsiveness. Future research is necessary for us to understand the special needs of this population fully.

LITIGATION

The concept of alternative choices in childbirth must be addressed in the context of the current litigious climate.[29] Analysis of the concept of informed consent includes the need to discuss with the patient the controversy surrounding proffered medical recommendations. Whether or not to have genetic amniocentesis is an example cited of a choice between reasonable alternatives, not between good and bad medicine.[26] The current legal climate demands communication and decision making that must include the expectant parent. It may be argued that optimal care includes an awareness of the need to include the couple in decision making and to advocate for women so that they remain "active" participants in their birth experience. Health professionals must continue to be attentive to the social and psychologic aspects of childbirth in addition to the mandate to be educated and skilled in obstetric technology.

Suggestions and support for alternatives such as the squatting position for second stage labor, early breastfeeding, and the importance of the paternal role are all inherent in the role of the nurse. Professional nurses must be ever-cognizant of their susceptibility to litigation. Nurses are no longer considered physicians' handmaidens who play a passive role. Highly educated professionals in their own right, nurses in the 1980s are responsible for assessment, intervention, decision making, and documentation as expected standards of care. Malpractice litigation attacks the professional nurse as frequently as it does the physician.

Good obstetric nursing demands knowledge and sensitivity, and an acute sense of a commitment to adherence to standards of care; these should interface with attending to the physical and psychosocial needs of the patient. Nursing care extends well beyond physiology and therefore responsibility extends beyond clinical skills. The ability to communicate and collaborate with both the patient and the medical staff is one of the most challenging aspects of obstetric nursing.

COMMUNICATION AND DECISION MAKING

The quality of communication and decision making is essential to building good rapport between the individual physician and expectant parent(s). Joint communication and decision making is needed to address the foremost underlying issue, namely, the degree of control and responsibility each woman or family can have over the birth of the child. The outcomes of these discussions may well prove critical to that larger concern about the relationship between obstetrics as a profession and its now increasingly vocal and litigious public.

The importance of establishing a strong rapport is not new; however, the prevailing methods are. Previously, one primary approach was to encourage the gravida to develop dependency on the authoritative obstetrician to provide a secure milieu in which any subject could be discussed.[18] Even now this is acceptable in some relationships or at certain times in these relationships. Although many women currently have a very sophisticated understanding of perinatal events, not all are equally informed. There are women who have not had the opportunity to learn any relaxation or breathing techniques even though such information is widely available. Those who are uninformed may be unprepared to take responsibility in the birth experience and may need to continue to rely on an authoritative physician. However, the increasingly well informed and sometimes angry public sector, focusing on a psychologically and physically optimal birth and demanding more control over the process, views the traditional stance as unnecessary authoritarianism that may create overdependency in the pregnant woman. The feminist literature abounds with descriptions of the ways in which sex role stereotypes interfere with health care services.[3,6,32]

It would be useful if consumers and physicians alike could view each other's conduct and objectives rationally and in proper context. Just as the current consumer perspective has drawn from many sources of experience and study, so has the physician's. These sources include the previous reality of an uninformed public interfacing with a well-informed medical profession. Also, the psychoanalytic view of pregnancy as a state involving maturation but also normal regression lent credence to an approach responsive to the dependent, suggestible components of female psychologic functioning. A simplistic view of the active male/passive female dynamic in relationships has helped to mold physicians' attitudes, as has our society's pervasive reliance on technologic solutions to problems.

The challenge for both physician and consumer is how to respond to the positive aspects of each other's view and get beyond the anger and frustration that may be generated by differing perspectives on optimal outcomes and responsibility for decision making during birth. Anger is an emotion experienced commonly when one moves from a dependent to a more self-reliant role or when one is challenged angrily. Understanding that is of some intellectual help, but hardly suffices when irate physician and patient confront each other regarding differing opinions on the birth process. The heat of this debate in obstetrics may have constructively engaged those who would otherwise remain uninvolved; but it may also have served to sharpen already existing dichotomies and to entrench otherwise potentially flexible caregivers and consumers. It has some characteristics of a crisis: the opportunity to develop new ways to communicate about choices in labor and birth side by side with the danger of retrenchment to the old authoritarian physician/passive patient role. Unfortunately, fear of litigation may hasten this retrenchment. Indeed, Summey and Hurst[37] view current obstetrics as having shifted away from managing childbirth and toward surveillance and monitoring of the unborn child. They question whether the technologic advances of the period will result in the mother being a teammate in this endeavor or a passive receptacle.

Even though there have been important changes in hospital practice in response to current family need, the strain of decision making persists. It has been 11 years since the Interprofessional Task Force on Health Care of Women and Children[19] offered its guidelines for family-centered, hospital-based maternity and newborn care. This group recognized the difficulties entailed in changing attitudes so that family-centered care would become the norm. Sugarman[36] suggested modifications to that plan 2 years later that included greater understanding of humanistic needs, prevention strategies, and the utilization of less expensive, more cost effective, less technologically sophisticated alternatives where appropriate. But with the rise of litagation it seems as if physicians find themselves relying more on "objective" technologic devices, and less on simple communication and patient-generated data.

Obstetrician: Specialist, Primary Care Physician, Team Player, or Litigant

In 1976, Burkons and Willson evaluated medical interventions of 1,008 women in five Michigan hospitals.[7] They found that 86% saw only their obstetrician-gynecologist and that 41% reported their obstetrician-gynecologist treated them for nongynecologic conditions. They concluded that both obstetric training and practice needed revision to encompass the reality of a primary physician role. They also recommended utilization of a team approach for the provision of general and specialized health care services to women. Recognizing that working as a team leader was not necessarily a role for which obstetric education had adequately prepared one, Burkons and Willson stressed that the obstetrician-gynecologist stood to gain: the roles and responsibilities would expand, not contract, as a result. In his 1981 presidential address to the American College of Obstetricians and Gynecologists, Rhu supported this position of expanded responsibilities in a primary physician role to women.[31] He emphasized the extraordinary degree of understanding and compassion required to do so in today's society in which women want to participate actively in decisions concerning their care.

This encompassing of new roles—primary physician, team leader, educator, or coparticipant in decision making—requires education. Only recently has there been recognition that the medical curriculum needs to teach effective communication skills. One problem had been that the classic intensive methods utilized to enhance self-understanding (and, presumably, communication) would take too much time from an already sated curriculum. Casey and Wuerscher worked on this problem by experimenting with physicians' role playing and videotaped mock interviews between obstetrician and patient.[8] They suggested these techniques be considered as both economic of time and effective for enhancing the physician's capacity for open interpersonal relationships. These same techniques are found effective in training psychotherapists. For the practicing obstetrician, incorporation of such opportunity for role playing in continuing education courses may prove to be an important method of coping with the increased expectations for communication inherent in the expanding obstetrician role (and in averting the potential adverse outcome of poor communication, namely, litigation).

INTERPERSONAL INTERACTIONS IN OBSTETRICS

There are two research studies relating to interpersonal interactions in obstetrics that offer a sensitive view of some relevant problems and a schema for understanding some of the variables encountered in this time of transition.

In 1976, Danziger, a sociologist, studied the use of expertise in physician-patient interactions in two clinic and three hospital settings over an 8-month period.[10] A continuum of interactional postures was conceptualized. Physicians took a technical expert role when there was little interest in discussing the plan for care; a counselor role when more general wisdom, not merely technical information, was shared and authoritative guiding through a therapeutic process was the mode; or a co-participant role in which the clients' need for valid information was recognized and participation in decision making encouraged. Patients took roles as a mere passive recipient who did not seek information nor respond to it; as an active dependent recipient who sought information primarily about the physician's reliability and competence; or as a potentially knowledgeable participant, whose interest in the physician's expertise exceeded this minimum, and who was willing to share in the responsibility of decision making. The outcome of each encounter was viewed by Danziger in terms of the manner in which participants conveyed their respective notions of how expert knowledge is to be shared.

Danziger presented a schema for understanding those interactions that are compatible and those that are conflictual:

1. When the physician acted as technical expert and the patient as passive recipient there was no conflict, but the provision of service was perfunctory, resulting in no transmission of expertise and no patient involvement in the decision or assessment process.
2. When the physician acted as counselor and the patient as active-dependent recipient, there was also no apparent conflict. Some information was shared and the style was characteristic of a benefactor-beneficiary relationship.
3. The other compatible interaction occurred when both acted as co-participants, resulting in cooperative decision making and a relatively open feedback situation.
4. Two conflictual types of interactions occurred when the physician and patient acted most dissimilarly regarding information sharing. First, when the physician acted as co-participant and the patient as passive recipient, the result was an antagonistic type of hostility on the part of the physician. Second, when the physician acted as technical expert and the patient acted as a potentially knowledgeable participant, the result was an arrogant type of hostility on the part of the physician. In both cases, the patient's expressed attitude toward information was defined by the physician as inappropriate.

These were clearly compatible and incompatible interchanges. In the middle range on the continuum—for example, physician as co-participant or expert and patient as active dependent—subtle nuances determined the outcomes, which were quite variable. Danziger postulated what is experienced today: changing frequencies in types of exchanges reflect changes in society and technology. For example, if the feminist movement is having an impact on medicine, one would expect feminist women to intensify their assertiveness. This would result in an increase in the number of hostile and/or co-participant educative relationships, depending upon the physician's reaction to the heightened interest of patients in medical knowledge and decision making. The changing technology of obstetric care should encourage physicians to act more like technical experts, while the growing advocacy of patients' rights in birthing should motivate them to act more like counselors and co-participants. Thus, there will be many different types of relationships emerging in obstetric practice of the future.

In a second study, Danziger analyzed themes in interactions during pregnancy and labor over a 4-month period in two Midwestern hospitals.[11] She found three major themes: that professionals attempted to assert control over the social process of labor; that patients were not usually presented with treatment choices; and that although there was enormous variation in analgesic aids and techniques used to stimulate labor, there was little variation in either the style or the content of the interactions with the patients. Caregivers acted as though giving more information would be stressful in labor, where calming activities were the focus. (Information giving was not considered calming, an assumption that one might question.) General assumptions about the needs of birthing women were made by staff to fit their conception of their own work, while individual patients proceeded to birth in their own way and attempted to avoid staff disruption. Neither group seemed aware of the extent to which their perspectives diverged. Danziger's study emphasized the importance of understanding the potential impact of interactions around birthing. During that time of normal crisis, when a woman is even more susceptible to the influence of those about her, staff communication may serve as a mediating influence not only on preconceptions about birthing but also on subsequent parenting.[11]

APPLICATION TO OBSTETRICIAN-PATIENT INTERACTIONS

It will take time for the practicing obstetrician responding to current trends regarding expanded decision-making power of the patient and expanded roles of obstetricians to come to a personal position of comfort regarding these changes. This becomes especially important as litigation is frightening some physicians away from the field. But this integration is essential because only then can that position be communicated to the prospective parent(s) early enough in the provider-patient relationship to allow negotiation. Moreover, should physician and patient find their views too divergent, it gives the opportunity for terminating the relationship in a timely way. It will present a challenge to see such early decision making as one element of optimal care, and not as simply rejection should the patient choose to go elsewhere.

In this pluralistic society with its current variety of beneficial medical practices and societal rituals for childbirth, it would be a mistake to designate any one practice best for all. Seiden[34] cautioned against entrapment in the familiar myths: of the one best solution; the one best family constellation for birthing (nuclear); and the idea of the "feminine" personality with its passive, dependent, inept, emotionally labile, and sexually inhibited components.

Coming to a personal position on birthing options that may be communicated to the patient is good practice for other reasons. Principles of primary prevention in health care emphasize the likelihood of better coping when one is well prepared. An obstetrician (or midwife) and a patient (or couple) who have had the time to discuss expectations and negotiate differences will be in a much better position to weather the unexpected occurrences of labor and birth than they would if unprepared. For example, should an emergency surgical intervention be necessary despite expectations to the contrary, the patient who has had the opportunity to discuss options, gain trust, and develop rapport will be better able to interpret the decision within that context as a legitimate response to an unexpected emergency. Therefore, the previous context of the relationship carries even more weight. By context is meant the accumulation of satisfying or unsatisfying exchanges, not the comprehensive discussion of all possible eventualities. Such discussion is often impractical, or weights the pregnancy too heavily in the direction of abnormality. It is worthy to note, however, that for some individuals such thorough review alleviates rather than generates anxiety. More often an approach that focuses on the discussion of the patient's areas of particular concern regarding labor or birth is most useful.

Inevitably, in each prenatal visit the stage is being set for that final performance: labor and birth. If the stage setting requires repeated questioning and even revision, it must be remembered that in the successful mastery of the normal crisis of birth, a woman is greatly strengthened, and the obstetrician can be justifiably proud to assist in that achievement. In contrast, a woman who experiences an emergency procedure in the context of a nonsharing noneducative relationship may even feel it has been foisted upon her, especially if her unshared expectations of birth without medical or analgesic interventions were strong. It is in these kinds of situations that the idea of litigation may arise. Birth is one crucible of a woman's life: the residues of birth disappointments remain to affect all important relationships. Therapists working with patients who have postpartum depressions attest to the impact of loss associated with unrealized and unrecognized birth expectations.

Another advantage for the obstetrician who comes to a considered personal position in response to today's trends is that it prevents a superficial response to societal demands. Seiden[34] gives the example of allowing fathers to be present but then intimidating them into inactivity by hospital rules. When there is unexamined ambivalence about who should be in control of the birth, there is the potential for a new kind of infantilization; whereas, when the physician is confident in his or her own position, it becomes easier to listen and to respect the reasons patients give for their birth preferences and to make appropriate decisions. Seiden[34] emphasized how important such active listening is, citing evidence which suggests that the best outcomes in health care in pregnancy are obtained when women's own preferences are a major determinant of care.

Active listening is a skill in and of itself. Sometimes physicians feel they are not providing medical care when merely listening. Consider that pregnancy represents a unique experience of altered physiologic and psychologic states. Even if the patient has had previous children the unique constellation of forces surrounding the pregnancy may create unpredictable emotional and physical responses, and listening to the patient's concerns can be viewed as one way to alleviate both present and future anxiety through the steady building of a strong rapport that occurs when a patient feels she is being heard. For example, an experience of terror in labor may arise suddenly and be inexplicable in the light of the current situation. Only later might it be recognized as the upsurge of a painful past association to a present procedure. It is expecting too much for either obstetrician, patient, mate, or other attendants to unravel the reasons for such a response at the time of its occurrence. Instead, an appropriate expectation would be that the patient be supported during that occurrence, that her concerns be heard, and that she be given whatever reassurance is realistic given the present situation. Such listening to the need to be assisted, supported, told that something is supposed to happen that way, or told that though the terror exists, there is no reason in the present for the alarm, will offset the weight of the negative unconscious associations that are dominating the response, and will be experienced as extremely helpful.

Several writers address legitimate concerns about the physician's time constraints. Seiden[34] and Gray and McGinnis[15] offered this experience: more time given initially, because it increases trust and rapport, saves time later. It may also save litigation. Burchell[6] made a concrete suggestion: instruct the person making the appointments to ask patients if they would like discussion time. Scheduling for a long appointment in such instances eases the sense of time constraint, and allows the participants to prepare for discussion.

There are some specific questions the obstetrician could choose to discuss with patients during the course of prenatal care. The purpose is not to have immediate answers, but to address the questions posed as one more way to assess and to enhance coping skills.

1. Are there particular concerns you have for the pregnancy or for the birth?

2. Do you know how you cope with the unexpected?
3. What do you know now about what helps you cope best?
4. Do you know what is the best learning situation for you: one-to-one discussion, group discussion, film, written materials, tour of facilities?
5. Do you know how you feel about the use of technology?
6. Are you aware of the educational and support child care resources available to you during pregnancy and after giving birth? What are your own plans for support?

SUMMARY

We have examined the current trends affecting the nature of the obstetrician-patient interaction. The practicing obstetrician who reflects on the variety of forces operant and clarifies his or her own position regarding the roles and rights of patients and physicians will be able to communicate that information to patients and negotiate a relationshp based upon that explicit sharing. Such a change in interaction would constitute a great leap forward toward optimal communication. Obstetric caregivers need the support of each other that such clear communication can provide.

Obstetricians have long occupied a powerful position in relation to women's health and lives. We have attempted to convey ways in which this significant relationship may be updated for the challenges of this era and thereby enhanced for the benefit of both obstetricians and the families whose lives they touch so deeply.

REFERENCES

1. Arms S: *Immaculate Deception*. Boston: Houghton Mifflin, 1975.

2. Bing E, Coleman L: *Having a Baby After 30*. New York: Bantam Books, 1980.

3. Boston Women's Health Collective: *Our Bodies Ourselves*, ed 2. New York: Simon & Schuster, 1976.

4. Bowlby J: *Attachment and Loss*, Vol 1. New York: Basic Books, 1969.

5. Brazelton TB: *The Neonatal Behavioral Assessment Scale*. William Heineman, London, 1973.

6. Burchell RC: Counseling in gynecologic practice: An overview. *Clin Obstet Gynecol* 1978;21:165–172.

7. Burkons D, Willson JR: Is the obstetrician-gynecologist a specialist or primary physician to women? *Am J Obstet Gynecol* 1976;121:808–816.

8. Casey MJ, Wuerscher A: Identification of skills involved in effective interactions between physicians and patients. *J Med Educ* 1977;52:602–603.

9. Corea G: *The Hidden Malpractice*. New York: Harper and Row, 1985.

10. Danziger S: The uses of expertise in doctor-patient encounters during pregnancy. *Soc Sci Med (Med Psychol/Med Sociol)* 1978;12:359–367.

11. Danziger S: Treatment of women in childbirth: Implications for family beginnings. *Am J Pub Health* 1979;69:895–901.

12. Davidson EC Jr, Fukishima T: The age extremes for reproduction: Current implications for policy change. *Am J Obstet Gynecol* 1985;152:467–473.

13. Dick-Read G: *Childbirth without Fear. The Principles and Practices of Natural Childbirth*, ed 4. London, Pan Books, 1960.

14. Eichholz A, Offerman-Zukerrberg J: Later pregnancy, in Blum BL (ed): *Psychological Aspects of Pregnancy, Birthing, and Bonding*. Human Sciences Press, New York, 1980, pp 94–103.

15. Gray MJ, McGinnis S: Role of the gynecologist and the emerging woman. *Clin Obstet Gynecol* 1978;21:173–180.

16. Greenhill MP, Friedman EA: *Biological Principles and Modern Practice of Obstetrics*. Philadelphia: WB Saunders, 1974, pp 149–154.

17. Griffith JW: Women's stressors according to age groups. *Issues Health Care Women* 1983;6:311–326.

18. Hansen JP: Older maternal age and pregnancy outcome: A review of the literature. *Obstet Gynecol Surv* 1986;41:726–742.

19. Interprofessional Task Force on Health Care of Women and Children. *The Development of Family Centered Maternity/Newborn Care in Hospitals*. Chicago: American College of Obstetricians and Gynecologists, 1978.

20. Kennell J, Jerauld R, Wolfe H: Maternal behavior one year after early and extended post partum contact. *Dev Med Child Neurol* 1974;16:172–179.

21. Kernoff R, Mansfield P: Re-evaluating the medical risks of late childbearing. *Women and Health* 1986;11:37–60.

22. Kirz DS, Dorchester W, Freeman RK: Advanced maternal age: The mature gravida. *Am J Obstet Gynecol* 1985;152:7–12.

23. Klaus M, Jerard R, Kreger NC: Maternal attachment: Importance of the first post partum days. *N Engl J Med* 1972;286:460–463.

24. Lamaze F: *Painless Childbirth, Psychoprophylactic Method*. Chicago, H. Regnery Co, 1970.

25. Leboyer F: *Birth without Violence*. Knopf, New York, 1975.

26. Lenke RR, Nemes JM: Wrongful birth, wrongful life: The doctor between a rock and a hard place. *Obstet Gynecol* 1985;5:719–722.

27. Martel M, Wachholder S, Lippman A, Brohan J, Hamilton E: Maternal age and primary cesarean section rates: A multivariate analysis. *Am J Obstet Gynecol* 1987;156: 305–308.

28. Mercer R: *First-time Motherhood: Experience from Teens to Forties*. New York: Springer, 1986.

29. Odent M: Birth Under Water. *Lancet* 1983;2:1476–1477.

30. Queenan HT, Freeman RK, Niebyl JR, Resnick R, Simpson HL: Managing pregnancy in patients over 35. *Contemp Ob/Gyn* 1987;29:180–198.

31. Rhu HS: The American College of Obstetricians and Gynecologists—Past, Present and Future (Presidential Address). *Obstet Gynecol* 1981;57:513–515.

32. Rich A: *Of Woman Born: Motherhood as Experience and Institution*. Bantam Books, New York, 1977, pp 117–182.

33. Robinson GE, Garner DM, Gore DJ, Crawford B: Psychological adaptation to pregnancy in childless women more than 35 years of age. *Am J Obstet Gynecol* 1987;156:328–333.

34. Seiden A: The maternal sense of mastery in primary care obstetrics. *Primary Care* 1976;3:717–724.

35. Stein A: Pregnancy in gravida over age 35 years. *Nurse Midwife* 1983;28:17–20.

36. Sugarman M: Regionalization of maternity and newborn care: How can we make a good thing better? *Perinate/Neonate* 1978;39–44.

37. Sumney P, Hurst M: Obstetrics and gynecology on the rise: The evolution of professional ideology in the twentieth century Part II. *Women and Health* 1986;11:102–114.

38. Winslow W: First pregnancy after 35: What is the experience? *Am J Mat Child Nurs* 1987;12:92–96.

20

Ethical Dilemmas in Labor Management

Alan R. Fleischman and Nancy K. Rhoden

Women and their caregivers have always realized that there are ethical dilemmas inherent in the process of pregnancy and birth. Before surgical delivery was possible, a choice often had to be made between saving the woman or the baby. Historically, physicians and midwives, sometimes in consultation with the pregnant woman, made medical decisions concerning pregnancy, weighing the benefits of proposed medical and surgical interventions against the potential risks to both mother and fetus. These decisions have often been viewed as purely medical decisions made in the corridors of the labor and delivery floor, with little recognition of their ethical components. But modern technology to assess fetal status has made it increasingly difficult to deny the complex value judgments inherent in the treatment of two patients, one nestled within the other.

This chapter will analyze the ethical dilemmas in labor management. The most obvious and well known of these arise when a woman acts in a manner that is contrary to her physician's recommendations and that is detrimental to the health or well being of mother or fetus. However, there are many less obvious but far more common dilemmas in labor and delivery. Hence we will begin by reviewing issues a physician may face in making recommendations to women who are completely willing to abide by medical advice. Such issues may arise in normal labors, or in ones in which the fetus is premature or has some diagnosed abnormality. After considering these seldom-discussed dilemmas that do not involve conflict, we will analyze the case of forthright conflict between woman and physician.

Several ethical principles will be utilized in this analysis. The first principle is known as "respect for persons." This principle incorporates two ethical convictions: that individuals should be treated as autonomous agents, and that persons with diminished autonomy are entitled to protection.[14] This principle supports the right of any person capable of participating in decision making to determine what happens to his or her own body. Furthermore, persons with diminished autonomy and incapable of participating in decision making for themselves are entitled to protection from harm.

The second applicable principle of bioethics is the principle of "beneficence." This principle states that persons are treated in an ethical manner not only by respecting their decisions and protecting them from harm, but also by making efforts to secure their best interests or well-being. Beneficent actions attempt to maximize possible benefits and to minimize possible harms. Specifically in the case of labor management, the health care provider has a duty to protect and to promote the best interests of both mother and fetus. This requires an objective assessment of the various options and the implementation of those that promote the best interests of both parties. The outcome thus would secure the most favorable balance of benefits over harms.[6]

The principle of beneficence should apply as well to the decisions and actions of the pregnant woman. She might be said to have a moral obligation to act in the best interests of her fetus, at least insofar as she has allowed the fetus to come to term as a wanted offspring and as her actions will not place her at undue risk. Of course, decisions by women concerning their fetuses involve more than a consideration of the best interests of the fetus. Such decisions must also take into account the woman's interest in her own bodily integrity and physical well-being. Thus, a woman making a decision for her fetus is at the same time an autonomous decision maker for herself and a proxy decision maker for her fetus. It is important to point out that treatments that may benefit the fetus directly have the potential to place the mother at significantly increased risk.[5] The central dilemma in weighing the appropriate decision is the potential for maternal-fetal conflict.

In addition, the principle of beneficence may place the physician and the pregnant woman's other health care providers in significant conflict. While desiring to protect and promote the best interests of both the woman and her fetus when a potential intervention may benefit one while placing the other at potential risk, the physician may be faced with a conflict. This poses the dilemma of divided loyalties and the need to determine where the physician's ultimate responsibility lies. How will the physician weigh the conflicting obligations to protect and promote the best interests of both patients? Does the duty to promote the best interests of the woman obligate the physician to place the fetus at significant risk, or does the obligation to be concerned for the ultimate outcome of the fetus obligate the physician in that direction?

This chapter will attempt to deal with some of these ethical dilemmas and value conflicts and set a framework for analysis of those complex ethical issues that arise on a daily basis in the management of normal and abnormal labor.

ISSUES IN NORMAL TERM LABOR

Needless to say, obstetricians would be delighted if all patients went into natural labor at term, with no unusual risk factors or detected or suspected fetal problems; but even such desirable situations are not without potential ethical dilemmas. There is, for example, controversy about the validity of and necessity for electronic fetal monitoring (EFM) in the low-risk labor. The obstetrician who prefers to forgo monitoring may wonder about the ethics or the potential legal liability of doing so. The obstetrician who prefers to monitor all parturients may be faced with patient requests or demands for a less technologically intensive birth experience. Furthermore, in a variety of situations, physicians have to decide how to respond to ambiguous or abnormal data and how (or whether) to disclose uncertainties or ambiguities to the laboring woman.

Significant conflict among physicians about the optimal form of treatment or the value of a particular treatment modality frequently gives rise to ethical dilemmas and value conflicts. For example, physicians who disagreed as to what surgical procedure was best for breast cancer were likely to disagree about precisely how information about this conflict should be presented to the woman or, if indeed it should be presented at all. The physician who believed that survival after "lumpectomy" had not been fully substantiated as being equivalent to that after more extensive surgery, and that choosing this course was inappropriate, would be unlikely to feel his or her obligation to preserve life was discharged by a completely neutral presentation of the data. The debate over EFM yields similar value conflicts for practitioners.

In brief, the disagreement about EFM concerns whether women who have no unusual risk factors should be monitored routinely during labor. The logic of the justification for monitoring—that physicians should try to detect problems in the fetus before they can cause any permanent damage—seems incontrovertible. The value of monitoring in high-risk pregnancies is largely undisputed. The major debate is over whether routine monitoring in low-risk women succeeds in enhancing neonatal outcome. Proponents claim that prompt detection of abnormal heart rate patterns permits early intervention. Opponents claim that many of the abnormal patterns detected result in unnecessary interventions, and that controlled studies do not show a difference in neonatal outcome between low-risk women monitored electronically and those monitored by auscultation.

This longstanding scientific debate cannot be resolved here. Rather, we wish to examine how this medical uncertainty may lead to moral uncertainty concerning how to advise the low-risk woman about the use of EFM during her labor. Because medical uncertainty is difficult to convey to patients—and may undermine their confidence—there is a strong temptation to avoid discussing it. This is so even if the physician's personal views favor neither approach. If the physician strongly prefers one alternative, it may be even harder to present the data neutrally and to let the patient decide. As Jay Katz pointed out, the problem of shared decision making posed by medical uncertainty is not that physicians are unaware of it; rather, it is that this awareness vanishes when the physician moves from theoretical discussion to practical decision making.[10]

What are the obligations of the physician who believes that EFM is not necessary for low-risk women? Obviously, the patient should be informed about the goals of EFM, the controversy over its effectiveness, the claim that it leads to an increase in cesarean sections for the false-positive diagnosis of fetal distress, and any other relevant data. Some would argue strongly that this is all the woman should be told, and that the physician should give no recommendation either way. While such purely nondirective counseling—simply presenting the medical and statistical data—is probably the most neutral way to proceed, it is unsatisfactory to many physicians and patients. Often the patient will ask, "But you're the doctor; what do you recommend?" Are there ethical or legal difficulties in recommending that the patient forgo EFM unless unexpected problems in labor arise?

An ethical problem would be raised if the physician who did this thereby neglected his or her obligation to protect the interests of the fetus and optimize the chances of fetal health. However, the controversy over the effectiveness of EFM has led some physicians to conclude that not using EFM in low-risk pregnancies does not compromise outcome. The uncertain benefit of the intervention makes allowing the thoroughly informed woman to choose whether or not to have continuous EFM in a low-risk labor an ethical course of action.

The tendency among physicians to rely upon controversial technology is reinforced significantly by fear of legal liability. With good reason, physicians fear that if an unmonitored birth results in an impaired child, the physician will be criticized or sued on the grounds that monitoring could have prevented the tragedy. We feel strongly that physicians should not base their treatment decisions on fear of legal liability, though we realize that this is easier to recommend than to implement. But as long as the woman is informed adequately, understands the information, and chooses for herself, the physician has acted in a manner that is ethically appropriate and defensible in the event of litigation. Such is the case whether or not the physician has made a recommendation.

The same analysis should apply when a physician who favors EFM recommends it to a low-risk woman and she refuses. This situation is uncomfortable for the physician, because the patient's decision was contrary to the physician's recommendation, and was made after full discussion of the reasons for the recommendation. Despite the physician's discomfort, however, this is not a situation in which the woman is clearly compromising the fetal interests, since responsible medical opinion differs as to the value of EFM in low-risk labors. Hence, although gentle attempts at persuasion are perhaps appropriate, and suggestions for compromise (e.g., a baseline monitoring and occasional or intermittent monitoring thereafter) are likewise legitimate, these situations should not be classified as full-fledged conflicts in which the woman's actions are indisputably deemed to place the fetus at potential risk.

In summary, decisions about EFM in low-risk women can be dealt with by a combination of careful and comprehensive informed consent, acknowledgment of medical uncertainty, respect for patient choice, and an attempt to forge compromises acceptable to both patient and physician. The high-risk woman who refuses EFM presents a different sort of problem, however, because her action is contrary to accepted medical opinion and does have a potentially adverse impact on the fetus. We will discuss such outright conflicts subsequently in this chapter.

An additional ethical quandary may arise in the care of a normal labor at term. Frequently, a physician may be faced with a woman in normal labor whose fetal monitor tracing becomes abnormal. Once the physician has tried unsuccessfully to correct the abnormality a complex series of decisions must evolve. Experts sometimes disagree on the interpretation of various abnormal fetal heart rate patterns. How does a physician deal with the threshold decision of when to inform the woman there might be a problem, knowing that such information could scare her needlessly and that inducing anxiety in the laboring woman might have other deleterious effects?

The ethical issue here is more complex than merely the question of truth telling because the physician may be uncertain as to what the truth is. Each situation will differ, and we can, of course, offer no absolute guidelines on when to disclose, what to disclose, or how to proceed. However, a physician should keep in mind that threshold decisions of monitor interpretation, while seemingly medical in nature, may also implicate the physician's approach to uncertainty. They may raise ethical issues concerning the amount of information the patient ought to be told and the possibility that there will be a difference in the approach to uncertainty between the patient and physician. For example, a physician who recognized a pattern as abnormal but also knew that this pattern was not generally believed to be ominous, and who thus decided to continue to observe it, might, in doing so, withhold information from a patient who would wish to be far more cautious in response to an abnormal pattern. Likewise, a physician who took a very cautious approach and recommended an emergency cesarean section in the face of a somewhat nonreassuring pattern might be acting very differently from the way his or her patient would act if she knew all the data. This dilemma is not new to medicine. It illustrates the danger of paternalistically "protecting" the patient by withholding information she needs to make an autonomous choice.

When time constraints are superimposed on the medical uncertainty, such dilemmas cannot be eliminated entirely. Moreover, women in the throes of labor often are not in the best state of mind to decipher the intricacies, ambiguities, and potential inaccuracies of EFM data and to render an informed opinion as to how to proceed. Indeed, if a woman is in severe discomfort, or has had analgesics for pain, one could raise questions about her capacity either to refuse or to consent to any course of treatment. The ethical and legal presumption, however, is that persons are competent to consent to treatment unless deemed otherwise. The physician should presume competence and err in the direction of providing more information rather than less. Additionally, if a physician has adequately explained prior to the onset of labor, or early in labor, the various problems that can arise during labor and the limitations of EFM, then the woman's decision is much more likely to reflect her general values and not simply the pressure of the moment. Such prior discussion best allows the treatment decision to be collaborative in nature rather than merely prescriptive.

ISSUES IN PREMATURE LABOR

Preterm labor raises additional, and often far more complex, ethical issues. Preterm deliveries account for only about 8% of all births, but contribute the vast majority of perinatal deaths. Whatever the reason for the preterm labor, ethical as well as medical dilemmas may arise, particularly if the labor is extremely premature, and the fetus is at the threshold of viability. The obstetrician must decide whether to treat the situation as a miscarriage, a premature birth, or something in between.

The Threshold of Viability

The threshold of viability is approximately 24 weeks' gestation. Neonates born at a gestational age of less than 24 weeks and a weight less than 500 g have almost no chance of surviving. Survival of the 500- to 600-g neonate born at approximately 24 weeks of gestation is 10%, increasing to approximately 15% to 20% for the 600- to 700-g, 25-week-gestation newborn.[11,17]

It is clear that there is a biological threshold below which present day technology will not allow extrauterine survival. The most crucial organ in this regard is the lung. Gas exchange cannot occur until the air sac-capillary interfaces are developed sufficiently to permit the diffusion of oxygen. Precisely when the fetal lungs become mature enough for diffusion differs widely among fetuses, but anatomic studies suggest that it almost never occurs before 23 weeks of gestation and it has usually taken place by 26 weeks.

Many perinatal specialists have argued that more aggressive obstetric intervention in premature labor would enhance newborn survival and outcome.[16] This has certainly been the case for infants of approximately 1,000 g or 26 to 28 weeks' gestational age. It is not as clear that more aggressive management of premature labor in infants of less than 26 weeks' gestation will result in a similar enhancement of outcome.

Recommendations about treatment for the fetus in premature labor should take these data into account. A woman in premature labor should be given a realistic assessment of her fetus' chance of survival. In addition to the regional or national data, such an assessment should include the capacity of one's own institution to maintain extremely premature babies successfully. A danger here is creating a self-fulfilling prophecy: writing off a 25-week fetus because its chances are so poor, and thereby ensuring its death or causing it to survive in a far more impaired condition than necessary. Awareness of this danger should not lead physicians to succumb to the opposing pitfall of optimistically downplaying biologic, technologic, and institutional limitations.

Physicians should also carefully include in their counseling the uncertainties inherent in estimating gestational age. Ultrasonography is the most accurate available means of assessing gestational age; but even in the best of hands, ultrasonography in the third trimester may be inaccurate by ± 14 days.[2] Deciding not to monitor a labor or not to act to relieve fetal distress because the fetus is believed to be too immature can be disastrous if it turns out the fetus was more advanced than physicians believed it to be.

The Cesarean Section Controversy

It is generally agreed that the fragile premature fetus is benefited by a delivery that is atraumatic. There are conflicting data concerning the efficacy of cesarean section in the very low birth weight infant, and controversy reigns as to whether vaginal or cesarean delivery will result in better survival rates, less intraventricular hemorrhage, and lower morbidity in the newborn. There appears, however, to be a consensus on the benefit of fetal monitoring in premature labor.[3] Inherent in the use of EFM for the premature gestation is the commitment to immediate cesarean section when fetal distress is detected.[4] This intensive perinatal management of very low birth weight infants appears to result in good outcome without the routine use of cesarean section for all prematures.

In assessing the benefits to the fetus of cesarean section in premature labor, one must consider the risks to the woman of the surgical procedure, which is often a classic cesarean section. A classic uterine incision places the woman at risk not only during this surgical procedure but also increases her jeopardy in subsequent pregnancies and affects the route of delivery for future fetuses. The woman's willingness to undergo the surgical procedure for the sake of her fetus often will be based not only on her hope for the baby's survival but also on the belief that the baby's neurologic outcome will be enhanced. Hence, women in these circumstances must be informed carefully of mortality and morbidity data for extremely premature newborns in order for them to make an informed choice.

An Ethical Analysis

Physicians and patients face massive uncertainty in making decisions about treatment of premature labor. Gestational age, weight, and level of development of the fetus are often uncertain. The benefits of the various routes of delivery to the fetus and the risks to the woman may also be unclear. The mortality and morbidity data of newborn outcome add additional ambiguities. It is impossible to predict which very low birth weight fetuses will survive and flourish outside of the uterus. It is crucial that physicians recognize the basic strategy they use to deal with multiple uncertainties is affected by psychologic factors and personal values that will have a profound impact on which course of action is deemed most appropriate.

In the context of choice under certainty, one may pursue a policy that focuses upon the worst potential outcome and avoids it at all cost. This is known as a "maximin" strategy.[18] Inherent in it is the ambiguity as to what is the worst possible outcome that must be avoided. This could be assessed variously as the death of the mother, the birth of a premature newborn who survives devastatingly impaired, or the death of a fetus who would have been a healthy infant. Regardless of the course of action or the treatment that is proposed by the physician or patient, it is important to realize that these strategies for decision making are not value-neutral.

An additional perspective to add to the assessment of the appropriate course of action in premature labor is an analysis of the decision-making approach utilized in the neonatal intensive care unit. It has become standard for virtually all infants with any chance of survival to be treated aggressively by pediatricians in the delivery room and stabilized in the intensive care nursery. Some neonatal units involve parents in decision making for their critically ill newborns and allow withdrawal of treatments from infants if death or a terribly impaired life seems inevitable. In other units, aggressive intervention is maintained for all infants regardless of their future potential, and parental involvement in decision making is minimal or absent. Obstetricians must take into account the propensities of the neonatal unit and share this information honestly so that women opting for aggressive intervention in labor realize all its implications.

There are three possible treatment approaches in premature labor. First, there is an aggressive approach to perform a cesarean section in all labors that cannot be stopped in order to attempt to maximize benefits to the fetus. Second, one can write off the extremely low birth weight yet potentially viable 24- to 26-week-gestation fetus, assuming that the potential risks to the woman of cesarean section outweigh the possible benefits to the fetus of active intervention. Third, it is possible to monitor the potentially viable fetus intensively and to intervene promptly with a cesarean section if the fetus shows signs of deterioration. For the sake of this analysis, we will assume that the woman will go along with whatever course of action is recommended by her physician. This does not mean the physician should consider her completely passive; rather, he or she should explore her approach to uncertainty and take this into account when making recommendations.

Routine delivery by cesarean section for all premature labors that cannot be stopped will result in increased maternal risks for somewhat questionable benefits to the premature infant. The recommendation should only be made when it is clearly consistent with the woman's values and her preferred approach to risk and uncertainty.

The second option, writing off the very premature fetus, or treating it basically as a miscarriage, presupposes that the chances for survival are so slim as not to warrant subjecting the woman to additional risks. There are several problems with this approach. The fetus believed to be 25 weeks may, upon delivery, turn out to be 27 weeks' gestation. If it had not been monitored, it may have suffered from undiagnosed fetal distress and thus may survive with preventable neurologic deficits. Even if survival with severe neurologic handicap is deemed worse than death, this approach cannot ensure that the outcome will be death rather than permanent devastating impairment. Hence, we do not believe that the physician should recommend this approach unless there is virtual certainty that the fetus is less than 25 weeks' gestation.

In general, the appropriate recommendation is the "middle of the road" course of treatment. The explanation to the woman of all of the uncertainties involved is essential, but the recommendation to assess fetal well-being carefully and to intervene promptly in an attempt to optimize fetal outcome appears to be appropriate, particularly in light of the inability to predict with certainty the death of a particular fetus prior to or after birth.

ISSUES IN LABOR WITH AN ABNORMAL FETUS

Another set of ethical dilemmas arises when a woman enters labor carrying a fetus with a known severe congenital anomaly, chromosomal disorder, or infectious disease that is not immediately lethal to the newborn. Such disorders might include complex congenital heart disease, trisomy 13 or 18, and acquired immunodeficiency syndrome (AIDS). The issue may be complicated by how long the diagnosis has been known. If the diagnosis was made early in gestation and the woman declined the opportunity to abort the fetus, she may voice the desire to do everything possible for her fetus during labor. Alternatively, she may be opposed to abortion but not in favor of extraordinary efforts to prolong the life of her fetus or newborn. If the diagnosis of the fetal abnormality was made after the opportunity for an abortion had passed, the woman may have a whole host of feelings about what potential risks she would endure for the sake of her unborn child and what level of intensive fetal and neonatal care she might wish.

The analysis of the appropriate course of treatment is clouded by uncertainty, particularly because prediction of the neonate's duration and quality of life may not be possible. If there is reasonable certainty about the type of congenital abnormality, then the prognostic potential for that infant will be far clearer than in cases in which the anomaly is difficult to diagnose.

The new problem of the pregnant woman who is carrying the virus associated with AIDS is a complex issue. Recent data suggest that the majority of fetuses carried by a seropositive mother will be seropositive and go on to develop AIDS. This development of overt AIDS may take many months or years, however, and with the intense efforts presently being made toward finding a cure or a means to alleviate some of the basic problems in AIDS, it is possible the current grave prognosis for affected individuals may change in the future. Thus, it is difficult to predict whether the newborn will have a long or short life span.

With these infants, as with extremely premature ones, writing off the fetus may result in a liveborn baby in a far worse condition than would have occurred if the labor had been managed aggressively. The problem with the writing off approach is that death of the fetus or newborn is not inevitable, even though that might be the intended outcome. At the same time, surgical delivery inevitably poses greater risks for the woman, and a physician or patient may justifiably believe that these risks are not worth taking when the infant's prospects for survival are extremely grim.

Given the uncertainty about the infant's future quality of life, and the complex and subjective value judgments involved, the woman should be the primary decision maker here and the physician's task should be to help her understand all the relevant factors fully. Many consultants, including pediatricians, geneticists, surgeons, and others, may be needed to assist the obstetrician and the woman in evaluating the future potential of the fetus. Some members of the consulting team may need to communicate directly with the woman to clarify this information. The more specific and certain the information about the infant's abnormality, the more help the caregivers will be in making recommendations about the appropriate course of treatment. The better the fetus' chances of a reasonable quality of life, the greater the obligation of the health care providers to recommend treatment that will help it realize that potential. The poorer the fetus' chances, the more likely it is that the physician's obligations to promote the woman's best interests will lead to a recommendation against fetal monitoring or surgical delivery.

ISSUES OF CONFLICT IN LABOR

A host of physician/patient conflicts may arise during labor. We have already mentioned several. Without ignoring the other potential conflicts we will focus here upon one paradigm of physician/patient conflict—the situation in which the physician recommends a cesarean section and the patient refuses to consent. This may occur either in cases in which the woman's condition makes vaginal delivery hazardous for both woman and fetus (e.g., placenta previa), or in which the medical situation indicates that only the fetus is threatened by vaginal delivery (e.g., an ominous EFM tracing). We will treat both cases alike. We focus on this paradigm both because it is the most common sort of overt conflict that occurs during labor and delivery, and because it is one of the obstetric conflicts that has been litigated in at least a few states and analyzed by a number of commentators.

Although the purpose of this chapter is to analyze the physician's ethical obligations, such obligations are, needless to say, related to how courts deal, or are likely to deal, with these dilemmas. Hence we will discuss some of the judicial decisions on this topic briefly, although we should note at the outset that the law is by no means settled in this area. Also, cases of this sort tend to be unreported trial court decisions, making them of very limited precedential value and also making it difficult, if not impossible, to know how many such cases there are or how most cases were decided. Hence, reference to or reliance on the law in this area is problematic at best, and ultimately an ethical analysis of each case will be essential.

Cases Authorizing Nonconsensual Cesarean Sections

In *Jefferson v. Griffin Spalding County Hospital Authority*,[9] the only case that has been officially reported and the only one to be appealed to the highest state court, Mrs. Jefferson was diagnosed as having placenta previa, but refused a cesarean section based upon religious beliefs precluding surgery. The Georgia Supreme Court upheld the lower court's order authorizing nonconsensual surgery. It found that the severe nature of the potential harm to the fetus warranted imposing the relatively low risk of surgery upon Mrs. Jefferson. It supported its decision by reference to *Roe v. Wade*,[19] the 1973 abortion decision, which held that after the fetus is viable, the state can prohibit abortion unless it is needed for the woman's life or health. It also relied on the well-established principle that parents who refuse needed medical care for their child are committing child neglect, suggesting that just as a court can order care for a neglected child, a court can order surgery needed for the survival of a viable fetus.

A few other courts have issued similar (though unpublished) orders.[12] These include *In re Jeffries*,[7] another case in which the woman had placenta previa, and *North Central Bronx Hospital v. Headley*[15] in which the woman had hypertension and preeclampsia and the physicians thought surgical delivery might be needed, though they were by no means certain of this. *Jeffries* and *Headley*, like the *Jefferson* case, involved women whose religious convictions precluded surgery. In other cases in which the fetal monitor indicated severe fetal distress, it is reported that the women refused surgery based not upon religious convictions, but rather based on their fear of the risks of surgery. Each judicial decision held that although the woman had a general right to refuse treatment, the harm to the viable fetus that might accrue from this refusal outweighed this right.

In at least one case,[8] the judge refused to authorize a nonconsensual cesarean section. The judge simply held that an adult who is competent has a right to refuse treatment, despite the potentially tragic consequences to herself or her fetus. The woman involved held no strong religious convictions, but having had ten previous pregnancies, believed firmly in natural childbirth and also disbelieved the physicians' dire warnings. As it turned out, although the umbilical cord was wrapped around the fetus' neck, vaginal delivery proceeded much more rapidly than expected with good outcome for the baby.

The outcomes in these reported cases are important. In *Jefferson*, the diagnosis of placenta previa proved incorrect, and Mrs. Jefferson delivered vaginally. In *Jeffries*, Mrs. Jeffries went into hiding and delivered vaginally elsewhere. Mrs. Headley never returned to the hospital, and delivered vaginally at home. Although it is unclear precisely what conclusions can be drawn from these data, it should help us keep in mind the limitations and uncertainties of medical predictions in these areas.

Legal and Ethical Issues Raised by Court-Ordered Cesarean Sections

As mentioned previously, courts have invoked *Roe* to support nonconsensual cesarean delivery, reasoning that since states can prohibit the intentional termination of fetal life after viability, they can likewise protect viable fetuses by preventing vaginal delivery when it will result in death of the viable fetus. At first glance, this analysis appears attractive since the state has a compelling interest in protecting the viable fetus. The fact that states have an interest in preventing certain consequences, however, does not mean that any and all action to prevent such consequences is constitutional. That the state can prohibit intentional fetal destruction at a certain time in pregnancy does not mean that it can necessarily go even further and mandate major surgery to protect and preserve fetal life. There is a quantum leap between prohibiting active destruction of the fetus and requiring surgery on a competent adult to prevent potential harm to the fetus.

The analogy to child neglect has equally serious problems. It is quite true that parents cannot legally or ethically refuse needed medical care for their children, even if provision of such care violates their most cherished religious beliefs. However, a problem with the argument that refusing care needed for fetal health is the prenatal equivalent of child neglect is that while parents have historically had a host of legal duties to their children, women have not heretofore been held to have legally enforceable duties to fetuses. Of course, until recently we have lacked the technology for visualizing the fetus, diagnosing problems in it, and hence recommending procedures for its benefit. Some writers have suggested that the development of such techniques is sufficient to create new maternal duties to the fetus. Moreover, even if one argues that the new technology increases the woman's ethical duty to act in the best interests of her fetus, at a minimum this duty is not unmitigated, and it is a far different matter to conclude that she has a legal obligation to sustain personal risks in order to fulfill her obligation.

In analyzing the issue of fetal neglect, one can see the pregnant woman as primary and the fetus as secondary, or the reverse. If one views the fetus as primary, one would discern its needs and then require the woman either to meet those needs or to justify her failure to do so. The opposite point of view would insist that the woman be seen as primary, with the question being when, if ever, the state can invade her body to protect potential life. Whether or not one ultimately concludes that some nonconsensual procedures are justified, there are serious problems with approaching the issue by asking what the fetus needs and forcing the woman to justify failing to meet these needs. Such an approach denies the importance of the fact that the fetus is, no matter how fully developed, still inside the woman. While no fetus can be treated without breaching the maternal barrier, no similar breach is necessary to treat children of parents who refuse necessary medical treatments. Hence, this breach must first be justified. In other words, if one approaches this issue by looking first at what the fetus needs, there is a tendency to forget the woman is there—or to forget that she is more than, as George Annas put it, a "fetal container."[1] Instead, one must approach it by asking if her bodily integrity can be violated—with the justification being the important interest of protecting the potential life within her.

This analysis raises the issue of a competent patient's right to refuse treatment and the reasons that can override this right occasionally. Competent persons can legally refuse medical treatment, even when it means their death. Respect for a person's autonomy ethically mandates respecting a patient's refusal of recommended treatments. Even though the state has an interest in preserving life which can be arrayed against a treatment refusal that will result in death, respect of a person's bodily integrity precludes overriding that refusal. Most other treatment refusals do not have such a direct and devastating effect upon third parties. Courts must weigh the right of an individual to refuse in these cases against the interest in preserving a third party's life—an interest that makes these cases unique.

The most relevant analogy to the current dilemma is the extremely rare situation in which one person's refusal of a medical procedure will result in another's death. Although there is, for obvious reasons, a dearth of legal precedent in this area, there is one case that is relevant. In *McFall v Shimp*,[13] a man dying of aplastic anemia asked the court to mandate that his cousin, who was the only compatible relative, be forced to donate bone marrow to save him. The court called the relative's refusal to donate morally reprehensible, but held that for the law to "sink its teeth into the jugular vein or neck of one of society's members and suck from it sustenance for *another* member, is revolting to our hard-wrought concepts of jurisprudence. Such would raise the spectre of the swastika and the Inquisition, reminiscent of the horrors this portends."

McFall makes plain society's general position on mandating bodily invasions to save third parties: although it may be deemed ethically appropriate, it cannot be mandated legally. This follows directly from the refusal of Anglo-American law to create a general duty to rescue. There may, of course, be an ethical duty to rescue even in the absence of a legal one. However, even within those special relationships in which the law imposes a duty on an individual to rescue another (innkeeper/guest, parent/child), there is no duty to undertake risky rescues. Bone marrow donation, though not nearly so hazardous as surgery such as cesarean section, is by no means risk-free, and could not be imposed upon a relative. However, to many commentators and observers the cesarean section cases *feel* different from these analogous situations involving forced intrusions on one individual to save another. This is because cesarean deliveries are common and relatively safe; the potential harm to the baby is very serious; and the harm will occur here and now, not later and perhaps elsewhere as with a refusal to donate bone marrow. Moreover, pregnancy is simply unique. No matter how dire his or her need, a dying relative, even a child, is a separate, physically independent person.

Furthermore, the unique physical and emotional bond between a woman and her fetus engenders a more intense feeling of duty of one toward the other.

Bioethics is an area in which emotional responses certainly should not be disregarded. But neither should they necessarily rule. These special features of pregnancy make it understandable that physicians become very uncomfortable when a woman appears ready to risk her fetus' life and health for the sake of her religious faith or her personal values. Indeed, trivial reasons for running this risk may let us justifiably cast moral aspersions on the woman's conduct. The problem with all this is that despite the uniqueness of pregnancy, and despite the strength or weakness of the competent woman's reason for refusal, what the state does when it imposes a cesarean section on a woman is to compel risk and bodily invasion, similar to mandatory marrow donation.

A court, or any individual, can contemplate surgery for a pregnant woman only as a third party bystander, albeit a careful and concerned bystander. It can assess the objective risks of surgery to the woman and the corresponding benefits to the fetus. Nonetheless, its ability truly to understand the situation is radically limited. Some limitations simply relate to the impossibility of extrapolating from statistical statements of risks, which apply to groups, to the risks pertaining to a particular individual. The court cannot know the exact risk it will impose on the individual woman, because statistics cannot predict this. Other limitations relate to the particular, and undoubtedly unusual, circumstance: the risks may be increased if the surgery is done on an emergency basis, and likewise may be magnified by its nonconsensual nature. Perhaps the most significant limitations are that a third party cannot possibly know or take into account the woman's subjective response to these risks, or to the proposed violation of her deeply held religious beliefs. In short, these decisions simply cannot be rendered objective.

By ordering surgery, the court is rendering objective a determination that cannot rightfully be anything but subjective. When it subjugates the woman's subjective beliefs to its objective assessment of the action deemed right on the basis of potential consequences, it essentially makes an interpersonal risk/benefit comparision—that is, it holds that she must run a risk to prevent a greater risk from occurring to the baby. Objectively, this may well be the proper assessment. But in our society, decisions about surgery on unconsenting competent adults simply are not delegated to third parties. In our opinion, such judgments inevitably treat the woman as a means—a vehicle for rescuing an imperiled fetus— and not as an end in herself. Thus, despite the potentially tragic consequences to the fetus, we must conclude the appropriate course is to respect the woman's refusal.

How do these conclusions impact on the physician's options and obligations? Some physicians might maintain that in cases of forthright physician/patient conflict, in which the woman's refusal may harm the fetus, the physician's best and most neutral course of action is simply to ask the court to adjudicate the respective claims and interests of woman and fetus. As such, despite the compelling circumstances and emotional turmoil such conflicts cause, the act of seeking a court order has the same ethical problems as the act of issuing one. Given the nature of litigation, seeking a court order is an adversarial undertaking that can never be neutral. Court proceedings, rather than seeking compromise, pit the parties against one another. If physicians seek court orders to force women to comply with recommended treatments, this action will have significant and detrimental effects on the nature of the physician/patient relationships in the specific cases and on obstetric practice in general.

Obviously, a physician faced with a maternal refusal of surgery that is thought necessary for the fetus' health should make sure the woman realizes the import of what she is doing. Ideally, if the woman has had prenatal care, these contingencies should have been discussed with her in advance. Advance discussions, especially with women who have unusual religious or medical beliefs, should be undertaken whenever possible. But sometimes there will be situations in which a woman with whom there have not been previous discussions refuses emergency surgery. These cases are probably the hardest to deal with because they arise unexpectedly. Refusals can be most difficult to handle when they are based not on firm religious convictions, but on a seemingly irrational refusal to understand or accept medical recommendations. Indeed, these refusals can sometimes call into question the woman's decision-making capacity.

Along with ensuring that any woman refusing treatment understands that this can kill her infant or result in a child with profound and lifelong mental retardation and physical disability, physicians should assess the competency of the woman who is refusing, if this appears to be war-ranted. We believe that holding religious beliefs opposed to surgery is not, in and of itself, a reason to question the woman's competency. However, some cases in which the woman's refusal lacks any apparent firm basis raises questions about her competency, and a psychiatric assessment would be wise. While refusals arising out of stubbornness or disbelief are the hardest to deal with (because it is difficult to be sure that the refusal really reflects the woman's values), these women often can be persuaded to change their mind. We believe it is ethically appropriate to attempt to persuade the patient by calling in other health care professionals, social workers, or clergy to talk with her, involving her husband or other close relatives, and giving her a clear understanding of how severely impaired her child might be.

If one assumes the woman has been found competent and is adamant in her refusal, what should be done? Should the physicians and the hospital try to overturn her refusal legally? Despite our critique of judicially mandated surgery, the chances are fairly good that if an order for nonconsensual surgery is sought, it will be granted. For one thing, the woman is unlikely to be in any position to oppose the hospital's petition, and in an emergency situation, the judge is likely to take the route that preserves the fetus' life. Will obtaining an order satisfactorily resolve the individual problem?

In many cases it will. In a Colorado case,[5] for example, after the order the woman became more compliant, surgery was performed, and the infant, though depressed at birth, was resuscitated and appeared to suffer no lasting damage. But some cases will not be resolved so satisfactorily. Mrs. Jeffries, for example, went into hiding after a court order was obtained. Mrs. Headley never returned to the hospital and instead had a home birth with a lay attendant. Home births for high-risk women are much more risky for mother and fetus than hospital births even with surgery precluded as an option. In one sense, if the woman never returns to the hospital, it is not the physician's problem; he or she has been relieved of a problem patient and will have no fears of liability if the infant is impaired. In another sense, however, in taking action likely to turn the woman away from the medical system, the physician who obtains an order has increased the risk for woman and fetus. If she is a member of a religious community, this may likewise cause other members to avoid prenatal care and thereby increase their risk.

Assuming the woman does return to the hospital or is already there, another serious problem may arise: what to do if the court order does not induce compliance. Should the physicians forcibly hold her down and anesthetize her? How much effort should they make to enforce the order once they have obtained it? Merely asking these questions demonstrates the violence lurking in the notion that physicians and judges can force women to have surgery they have refused. Although the violence is being done for the most benevolent of reasons, we think that if physicians focus on this repugnant behavior, they may well become less comfortable with the idea of asking the court to authorize such intervention.

Even if the woman complies with the order and no overt violence is needed, as will most likely be the case if she remains in or returns to the hospital, the act of obtaining the order may solve an individual problem but may create greater physician/patient dilemmas for subsequent cases. A physician who knows that he or she will seek a court order has a duty to inform a patient with unusual religious or medical beliefs of this practice early in her prenatal care. Providing such information is not likely to improve the physician/patient relationship, because a probable result is that the patient will not return. If she is a person of means, she can simply seek another physician. But if she is a public patient, she may have no other choice but to avoid health care entirely. Hence, a policy of seeking court orders could cause members of religious communities that oppose surgery to be unable to obtain prenatal care compatible with their convictions, and could thus increase the risk to these mothers and fetuses.

There is a final risk—albeit a future one—of physicians increasingly seeking to override maternal refusals with which they disagree. As seeking court intervention becomes better established, it may be harder for the physician who wishes to respect a woman's refusal to feel safe in doing so. Physicians have little choice in whether to abide by the refusal of a Jehovah's Witness parent to consent to a blood transfusion for her child in a life-endangering situation. They simply must obtain a court order and perform the transfusion in the best interests of the child. If the law, through the instigation of suits by physicians, comes to equate "fetal neglect" with child neglect, then physicians will increasingly be obligated to seek these orders. Even if the law does not go this far, but seeking court intervention becomes the medical norm, the physician who does not seek it could be at risk if the child is indeed impaired and someone (the father, a guardian of the child, or even the mother, having come to regret her decision) sues, alleging the physician should have sought to override the patient's refusal. Thus, it is not only the individual physician/patient relationship that is jeopardized by court involvement. There is also a threat to the future of patient autonomy in medical decision making and to physician autonomy in making reasonable medical judgments.

CONCLUSION

When the physician and the woman are in conflict concerning the appropriate course of treatment to benefit the fetus, we believe that the woman has a moral obligation to act in the manner that promotes the best interests of her fetus, but that this obligation is not unlimited. In addition, it is the duty of the physician to try to convince the woman to comply with a recommended treatment that is deemed to be in the best interests of the fetus and also imposes minimal risk to her. An individual physician may find it difficult to be sympathetic to a woman's refusal to act in the prescribed manner and may wish to use all available forms of moral persuasion to change the woman's mind. The physician, however, should not be party to overriding the woman's autonomous judgments by forcibly restraining her or by inflicting nonconsensual treatment upon her. This position is based on the "respect for persons" principle, which gives rise to a duty to the woman that may supersede the duty to act beneficently to the fetus.

In addition, a woman's refusal of a recommended cesarean section should be respected. The significantly increased risk of her dying during childbirth is sufficiently high to respect as binding her weighing of risks to herself from the surgery as greater than the potential risks to her fetus from forgoing the cesarean section. Although medical risks and benefits can be determined objectively, a patient's assessment of the degree of risk she is willing to assume for the sake of predictive benefits to another is a subjective matter. Even when the degree of risk can be ascertained with some accuracy based on well-documented statistics, reasonable people disagree on the question of which of life's risks are worth taking to attain desired benefits.

The unique physical, emotional, and moral relationship between the pregnant woman and her fetus results in myriad complex ethical dilemmas. Respect for both parties, the woman and the fetus, requires that caregivers weigh all of the consequences of proposed treatments, make recommendations that appear to maximize benefits to both, and use moral persuasion when necessary to convince women to take reasonable risks to optimize fetal outcome. But caregivers should not let their concern for one party denigrate their respect for the other. Recommendations in ambiguous cases should take into account the woman's values and preferences. Moreover, when conflict does arise, physicians should ultimately let the woman's choice prevail. A woman in labor will almost always make decisions consistent with the best interests of her fetus. Knowing that the professionals in the labor room respect her ability to decide and her concern for her fetus will help a woman to evaluate the recommended treatments carefully, and to reach decisions optimizing benefits to all concerned.

REFERENCES

1. Annas GJ: Women as fetal containers. *Hastings Cent Rep* 1986;16:13–14.

2. Berkowitz RL, Birnholz JC: Ultrasound characterization of fetal growth. *Ultrason Imaging* 1980;2:135–149.

3. Bowes WA, Gabbe SG, Bowes C: Fetal heart rate monitoring in premature infants weighing 1500 grams or less. *Am J Obstet Gynecol* 1980;137:791–799.

4. Bowes WA, Halgrimson M, Simmon MA: Results of intensive perinatal management of very low birth weight infants (501 to 1500 gms). *J Reprod Med* 1979;23:245–252.

5. Bowes WA, Selgestad B: Fetal versus maternal rights: Medical and legal perspectives. *Obstet Gynecol* 1981;58:209–214.

6. Chervenak FA, McCullough LB: Perinatal ethics: A practical method of analysis of obligation to mother and fetus. *Obstet Gynecol* 1985;66:442–446.

7. *In re Jeffries*, No. 14004 Jackson County, Mich. P. Ct. May 24, 1982.

8. Interview, Judge Margaret Taylor, NY Family Court, November 6, 1985.

9. *Jefferson v. Griffin Spalding County Hospital Authority*, 147 GA 86, 274 S.E. 2d 247 (1981).

10. Katz J: *The Silent World of Doctor and Patient*. New York: Free Press, 1984.

11. Kitchen W, Murton LJ: Survival rates of infants with birth weights between 501 and 1000g. *Am J Dis Child* 1985;139:470–471.

12. Kolder VEB, Gallagher J, Parsons MT: Court-ordered obstetrical interventions. *N Engl J Med* 1987;316:1192–1196.

13. *McFall v. Shimp* 10 Pa. D.&C. 3d 90 (1978).

14. National Commission for the Protection of Human Subjects: *The Belmont Report*. Washington, DC: U.S. Government Printing Office, 1979.

15. *North Central Bronx Hospital v. Headley*, No. 1992-85, NY Sup.Ct. January 6, 1986.

16. Paul RH, Koh KS, Monfared AH: Obstetric factors influencing outcome in infants weighing from 1001 to 1500 grams. *Am J Obstet Gynecol* 1974;118:529–536.

17. Raju TNK: An epidemiologic study of very low and very very low birth weight infants. *Clin Perinatol* 1986;13:233–250.

18. Rhoden NK: Treating Baby Doe: The ethics of uncertainty. *Hastings Center Rep* 1986;4:34–42.

19. *Roe v. Wade*, 410 U.S. 113 (1973).

21

Medical-Legal Implications of Labor and Delivery

Jeffrey A. Shane

Medical-legal considerations, and specifically medical malpractice risk management and prevention, have become as much a part of obstetric medicine as are fetal surveillance or surgical techniques. It is probably most appropriate that medical-legal issues be viewed as a routine part of doing business in medicine and not, as some see them, as dark clouds on the horizon of practice. Many consumer groups feel, with some justification, that the attention to detail that good risk management entails is a positive factor in enhancing the quality of patient care. Unfortunately, the recent excessive emphasis on attempting to reform the tort system through legislative remedies actually has made the physician's life more, rather than less, difficult. Without getting further into the debate over the advantages and disadvantages of tort reform and the beneficial and deleterious effects of malpractice lawsuits, it is certainly true that practicing health care providers will continue to live, as they have in the past, with the potential of being sued for their acts. This fact goes far back into the history of American jurisprudence. It is reported that the first medical malpractice case in America was filed in 1794.[3]

Certainly, in terms of high medical risk, the labor floor and delivery room represent one of the most perilous areas in medical practice. The reasons for this are several, and relate to the kind of life-threatening illnesses that can occur in otherwise healthy women, and also to the perception that there is a relationship between obstetric practice and long-term human health. Of importance is the feeling of many that risks can be lessened by modifying behavior of health care providers, perhaps resulting in improved quality of medical care. In this sense, the recent emphasis on risk management issues is a positive step that individuals and health care groups can view as a means of optimizing patient care.[4]

From the patient's viewpoint, the expectation in today's society is that pregnancies will be normal, babies will be healthy, mothers will go home happy and intact, and that all this can be accomplished with less and less intervention by health care providers and more and more participation by the patient and her family. Perhaps as important, however, is the simple fact that the financial and emotional devastation caused by a handicapped child is of remarkable magnitude, and it is not unreasonable that under these circumstances many patients will seek legal counsel to discover whether the tragedy that they face could and should have been prevented. Their motivation may range from a simple desire to unearth the truth about the case to a realistic need for money to help care for a seriously ill child. More than one health care provider has become a plaintiff when his or her child or spouse has been injured, even when the defendant provider is a colleague or friend.

Like the patients who have been injured and are looking for a simple answer to why adverse events occurred, today's health care providers seek a simple solution to the liability problem when, in fact, there is none. No advice or action will prevent lawsuits from being filed or assure that a suit, if filed, will be successfully defended by the health care provider. There are, however, some situations that have resulted repetitively in lawsuits in the past and for which risks can be lessened to some degree. It is quite appropriate that this chapter is placed at the end of a volume such as this. If the reader has gone through this book in an orderly fashion, he or she has taken an important step in risk control, namely, acquisition of knowledge of current practice. However, expertise is of little help to the patient who is in a well-equipped hospital with the most modern equipment unless the person who has the knowledge and is able to interpret the data is available.

DEFINITIONS

"Malpractice" is a somewhat inflammatory and not particularly useful term. It is used as a shorthand for professional negligence. The legally defined elements of a medical negligence action include (a) presence of duty to the patient; (b) breach of duty; (c) causation, direct and proximate; and (d) damages. A breach of duty is usually defined in medical actions as a failure to do that which a reasonable and prudent practitioner would do (omission), or doing that which a reasonable and prudent practitioner would not do (commission). If these negligent actions upon an individual to whom one owes a duty of due care cause an injury, a cause of action in negligency (or some other similar, but differently phrased, action) may follow.

Other legal actions that are somewhat different in their proof may arise out of medical care, including, for example, assault and battery, libel and slander, breach of contract or warranty, and even intentional infliction of emotional distress. Some courts have allowed these actions, although the trend today is for courts to consider many of these problems that occur in the context of medical treatment as merely different aspects of a negligence cause of action.

The physician should be aware of two important facts. Different states have their own bodies of law, developed over the years within their own court systems. To find out how your state laws function, speak to an experienced malpractice attorney there. Also, one of the most important protections you have is your professional liability insurance policy. You should be familiar with its contents, limitations, and the duties that you have under the policy to be sure that you are sufficiently protected. Generally, the insurer will appoint an attorney to represent you, and the attorney's canon of ethics requires that you receive full and proper representation. But the insurance company has an important financial interest in the case, and often exercises some control over the litigation process and its ultimate resolution. If the potential exists for a judgment against you in an amount in excess of your policy, or if you feel inadequately represented by your assigned attorney, you may wish to consider hiring your own personal counsel (at your expense) to represent you in addition to the insurance company's selected attorney.

THE MEDICAL RECORD

In the evaluation of a malpractice case the most telling witness of the actions (or, often of equal importance, inactions) of health care providers is the medical record itself. This is especially true if the events at the time seemed rather routine and complacency allowed the medical records to become abbreviated and incomplete. Remember that for the patient, care for her health and her infant's well-being are virtually never routine events, and her recollections, whether or not entirely correct, will often be substantially more vivid than those of her health care providers.

For the plaintiff's attorney, the medical record is usually the starting place for investigation. He or she looks to the record for a description of the care, and is attuned to pick up inconsistencies, missed clues, and, perhaps most damaging of all, evidence of missing, altered, or otherwise inaccurate information. So important are the records to the documentation of medical care that many states have statutes relating to the necessity for maintaining records. Virtually all hospitals have regulations regarding record keeping, and accrediting bodies routinely evaluate hospital medical record maintenance systems. At least one state's courts have held that failure to maintain customary records that a plaintiff might require to prove her case creates a rebuttable presumption of negligence.[2]

Medical records more often help than hurt the physician. Well documented, honest, and complete records that reflect appropriate and well-reasoned care often do more than just help to win a case; they may, in fact, help prevent a case from being filed. The keynote in this regard is honesty. An attempt to create a record different from the facts—aside from being quite unethical and, in some states, illegal—may be courting courtroom disaster. There are simply too many other sources of entry in the record or other sources of discovery that make it unlikely the truth will not be uncovered. A jury that finds a health care provider both negligent and dishonest will be most unsympathetic.

PRENATAL CARE

Although the focus of this chapter is the labor and delivery area, those who deal in malpractice risk prevention recognize that often by the time the patient reaches the delivery floor, the die may very well be cast for an inevitably bad outcome. This is especially true if prenatal care has failed to identify a high-risk situation in sufficient time to allow planning for appropriate labor and delivery care.

One must remember that it may be difficult to recall every patient and her individual problems, especially when a call is received from the labor floor at 3 o'clock in the morning, or if the patient's primary health care provider is someone other than yourself. It is therefore appropriate that the files of patients with special problems be marked so that potentially serious complications can be readily recognized by anyone who examines the chart.

An important practical footnote relates to this issue of medical records. It is common for obstetricians to send medical records from their office to the hospital labor and delivery unit at some time late in the pregnancy. If this is done, one must ensure that additional necessary records of care are sent on a timely basis to supplement that chart should a problem develop after that initial record has been sent to the hospital. This will keep the labor and delivery personnel current concerning potential risk factors. Even in the absence of a new problem, current records are always useful.

There are many ways in which good prenatal care serves to improve the quality of management of labor. For example, undertaking heroic measures detrimental to maternal health in order to attempt to rescue an infant with an undiagnosed fatal genetic abnormality could lead to litigation if the fetal abnormality should reasonably have been identified prior to labor. Similarly, if a patient delivers a significantly immature fetus, neonatal outcome may be poor even if all the care rendered for that labor and delivery was appropriate. If the prenatal care was proper and well-documented, there would be no reason to expect a lawsuit. However, if the record reveals the patient has a previous history of early third trimester losses, and if additionally she has a history of previous induced abortion or cervical conization and no prenatal evaluation was done for evidence of cervical incompetence, the obstetrician may become involved in a very expensive lawsuit.

Other issues of importance regarding prenatal care include accurate assignment of gestational age, appropriate screening for gestational diabetes, and prompt recognition of preeclampsia. A recent article[1] that reviewed 100 plaintiff allegations revealed that 40 related to hypertension, 22 to diabetes mellitus, 13 to prolonged pregnancy, 10 to fetal antenatal compromise, and 21 to uncertain gestational age or discrepancies between uterine size and menstrual dates. One of the more helpful measures to help prevent these kinds of errors is a well-designed prenatal chart that reminds the obstetrician to seek out and identify problems at the earliest possible time.

Personal injury attorneys who prepare initial client interview sheets often provide themselves with footnotes to identify potential problems directly on the interview sheet. For example, the statute of limitations for filing an action is often recorded in a conspicuous location at the top and sometimes, in an especially efficient firm, docketed on a computer system. A similar procedure for identifying high-risk problems as they occur and placing them outside of the routine progress notes and in a more obvious and visible place serves as a useful reminder of the potential complications ahead.

LABOR AND DELIVERY FLOOR

One way to help prevent obstetric problems and thereby minimize the risk of medical liability suits is to be sure that the labor and delivery unit is designed for the expeditious management of complications. Relevant issues range from the complex to the mundane. Is the physical layout of the labor and delivery area sufficient to meet the needs of the sickest patients? For example, are there physical barriers to access and movement? Can the patient with a prolapsed cord or placenta previa be moved immediately from the examining or labor area to the cesarean section room? Does the delivery room have cesarean section capability? Can the patient with severe postpartum hemorrhage be operated upon on the delivery table; alternatively, how long will it take to move the patient to an area where anesthesia can be administered and surgery undertaken? If the patient must be transported elsewhere in the hospital, as is the case in some institutions in which the operating theater is on a different level than the delivery floor, access to an elevator must be immediately available. Equipment and medication for cardiopulmonary resuscitation of mother and infant should be on hand and in good working order. Documentation of regular inspections of this equipment is mandatory.

In addition to considering the physical facility, ensure that certain personnel who have an important preventive role, such as pediatricians and/or anesthesiologists, can be present in a reasonable time in the event of an emergency. Blood bank personnel and technicians for urgent laboratory procedures should also be readily available in hospitals that have an obstetric service.

GENERAL GUIDELINES

Experience with medical malpractice related to labor and delivery has revealed certain situations and circumstances that occur repeatedly. These suggest several guidelines that deserve special attention.

1. Minimize the use of "routine" printed orders in the delivery suite. When the patient first arrives on the labor unit, several steps should be taken by the staff. The patient's prenatal chart should be examined, vital signs obtained, and the responsible health care provider called. The provider may wish to authorize further examination or evaluation at that time. The provider should know the abilities of the individual(s) designated to act for him or her and, sometimes, must be prepared to assume legal responsibility for the errors they might make.

2. Keep a written record of the date, time, and contents of all conversations (including those made by telephone) with the patient. Record your advice and prescriptions given. Pay particular attention to information regarding the reported status of fetal heart rate patterns, fetal presentation, and labor progress. Note who was spoken to and what instructions were given. If you were contacted about a patient during the night, review the notes in the morning.

3. Keep a record of all consultations in the medical record and try to require all consultants to enter a note in the chart. When you are

consulted, write a note you would be proud to have displayed as an example of a complete evaluation. Unrecorded curbside consultations are, as has been said about oral agreements, not worth the paper they're written on.

4. Set a firm policy that no laboratory report is to be filed away in the back of a chart (or worse, in the record room) without being seen by someone competent to evaluate and act upon it.

5. Be sure that operative reports, discharge summaries, and so forth, are completed in a timely manner. Read them before signing them. Keep track of what you dictate or what someone else is to complete for you.

6. Try to write prescriptions and orders legibly. Check the proper dosage of medications with which you are unfamiliar.

7. Whenever you know you will be otherwise occupied, even for what you think will be a brief time, arrange for competent coverage.

PROBLEM AREAS

The area of obstetric practice that causes the greatest risk of liability is the delivery of a brain-damaged infant. Notwithstanding all of the information that implicates other factors in the causation of cerebral palsy or other neurologic injury, a labor characterized, for example, by evidence of fetal hypoxia and delivery of a depressed infant with cerebral injury, has an extremely high risk of loss in the lawsuit that will often follow. If compounded by other features that could be construed as evidence of negligence (e.g., oxytocin augmentation in a patient unattended by the obstetrician, unnecessarily prolonged arrest of labor, or difficult forceps delivery), the likelihood of loss at suit becomes very high. The plaintiff's attorney often has a very sophisticated knowledge of obstetric management. Oxytocin administered by a manually controlled system rather than by an electronic infusion pump, or oxytocin administered without continuous electronic fetal heart rate monitoring will raise strong suspicions about the quality of care administered. An abnormal fetal heart rate tracing will send the attorney immediately to consultants for evaluation.

DEFENDING A CASE

Several factors may be helpful in the defense of a lawsuit involving permanent neurologic injury. Thorough gross and histologic evaluation of the placenta may reveal evidence of an in utero problem that may have resulted in brain damage long before labor. Similarly, serologic studies on the newborn infant to reveal an unrecognized maternal or fetal infection may be helpful. A thorough neurologic evaluation of the handicapped child may sometimes reveal explanations for the brain damage unrelated to the labor. The defendant physician should work with his or her attorneys to plan a defense strategy, to be sure the lawyers understand the medical nuances of the case, and to evaluate the expert witnesses to be used.

The fetal monitoring tapes should be retained as well as the rest of the medical records. Since brain damage may not become manifest for many years after delivery and statutes of limitation (the time within which a suit must be brought) are often quite long for cases that involve perinatal injury, all of the records should be kept and safely stored for many years. Some states mandate minimum retention times, but these are not long enough to protect from later lawsuit. Discussion with an experienced attorney in each state is probably necessary to determine exactly how long to retain the records.

If a patient presents an unusual or difficult problem, write down what you are doing and why. Record consultations and special considerations. Generally, neither juries nor the law demands a perfect outcome—only reasonable and competent treatment. Juries want to know that the physician was present, was thinking, was doing the proper things, and was getting help when in doubt. If they find all of these to be true, they will more often than not overcome their natural sympathy for the severely injured plaintiff and find for the provider.

Traumatic neurologic injuries are also a common cause for a lawsuit. The two most frequent sources are shoulder dystocia and breech delivery. Complete description of the steps taken to manage the shoulder dystocia or the breech delivery may often provide a defense against later allegations of negligence. Included in the record should be a clear expression of the rationale for the decision to attempt vaginal breech delivery.

Timely notification of the pediatrician in circumstances when an injured or ill newborn is delivered (or, even better, when the delivery of one is anticipated) can both decrease the extent of the injury and reduce the chance of later legal action.

SUMMARY

The following suggestions may help to lessen the stress inherent in obstetric practice, to improve patient care, and to provide some degree of protection against professional negligence lawsuits.

1. Read and carefully study the literature pertaining to the changes and developments in the practice of obstetrics; keep your knowledge up-to-date.
2. Apply current knowledge to every patient, and never assume that her course will be uncomplicated. However, resist meddlesome intervention or treatments done only for your (or the patient's) convenience. Use special tools or procedures only when indicated.
3. Invite the patient's participation in decision making and keep her informed of what you are doing and why.
4. Document in your medical records your thoughts and the treatment you provide regardless of how routine things sometimes seem.
5. Try to anticipate problems insofar as possible.
6. Don't be embarrassed to get help from your colleagues when the problem is beyond your ken.
7. When there is an unexpected outcome, investigate the cause immediately, rather than waiting for the discovery phase of a lawsuit. In doing so you may help the patient, since the problem could be one that will recur. You may even have a duty to investigate the cause, if future recurrence is preventable.
8. Protect your financial security with adequate liability insurance.
9. If a lawsuit is filed, don't become obsessed with it, but don't ignore it either. Cooperate with your attorney maximally in helping him or her to understand the details of the case.

The system of laws under which we live is generally quite efficient. Juries are in most cases more favorably inclined toward, rather than against, health care professionals. Juries are reluctant to believe that a physician or nurse was negligent. If they find the care was reasonable, the provider was competent and attentive, and he or she gave credible testimony, they will usually find in favor of the defendant physician.

REFERENCES

1. Iffy L: Antenatal pitfalls in primary care practice: How to avoid them. *Med Malpractice Prev (Primary Care)* 1987;March–April:40–42.

2. *Public Health Trust of Dade County vs. Valcin*, 507 So. 2d. 596 (FL, 1987).

3. Roberts KD, Shane JA, Roberts ML: *Confronting the Malpractice Crisis.* Kansas City, KS: Eagle Press, 1985.

4. See EG, Fiscina SF: *Medical Law for the Attending Physician.* Carbondale: Southern Illinois University Press, 1982.

Index